REPERTORY

TO THE

MORE CHARACTERISTIC

SYMPTOMS

OF THE

MATERIA MEDICA

ARRANGED BY

CONSTANTINE LIPPE, A.M., M.D.

Copyrighted 1879 by Constantine Lippe.

OF NEW YORK.
STEAM PRESS OF BEDELL & BROTHER.
3RD AVENUE 175TH STREET

TO

Doctor CONSTANTINE HERING,

OF PHILADELPHIA, PA.,

This Book

IS RESPECTFULLY DEDICATED.

PREFACE.

This work is offered to the profession as an index to the more characteristic symptoms of the Materia Medica ; and my endeavor has been to present only such symptoms as the experiments and experience of many have proved to be characteristic. This work is based on the Repertory to the Manual published in Allentown in 1838 by Dr. C. Hering and the faculty of the College at that place. and which, I believe, was the first Repertory and Materia Medica published in the English language ; to this have been added selections from Boenninghausen's works, Ad. Lippe's Materia Medica, Bell on Diarrhœa N. H. Guernsey, Hering, and Jahr. Many of the books referred to are out of print. To the student this repertory may be of value as it will give at a glance the corresponding remedies to symptoms sought for, and further comparison with the Materia Medica will, in the differences of conditions, or locality, or combinations, give the differences between the remedies having a general symptom in common. I have given first the mental symptoms, and then followed in the order as pursued in the Materia Medica Pura. All of the sections are to be compared with *Generalities*. Being well aware that a work of this kind is necessarily imperfect, and that many very characteristic symptoms are omitted which are known to others, I will gratefully receive any suggestions or communications.

C. L,

January 1st, 1880.

CONTENTS.

SECT.		PAGE.
" 1.	Mind and disposition,	1
" 2.	Sensorium, cloudiness, dizziness, Vertigo,	16
" 3.	Head interior, headache, congestion of blood, heaviness, fulness, &c.,	20
" 4.	Scalp,	33
" 5.	Eyes and sight,	37
" 6.	Ears and hearing,	48
" 7.	Nose and smell,	53
" 8.	Face, lips and lower jaw,	58
" 9.	Teeth and gums,	68
" 10.	Cavity of mouth, palate and tongue,	74
" 11.	Fauces, pharynx and oesophagus,	81
" 12.	Appetite and taste, hunger and thirst,	86
" 13.	Ailments during and after meals,	93
" 14.	Eructation, nausea, vomiting, hiccough, heartburn and waterbrash,	100
" 15.	Stomach and pit of stomach,	108
" 16.	Hypochondres, kidneys, diaphragm, liver and spleen,	113
" 17.	Abdomen, groin and flatulency,	116
" 18.	Stool and anus,	126
" 19.	Urine and urinary organs,	140
" 20.	Male sexual organs,	149
" 21.	Female sexual organs,	155
" 22.	Coryza,	165
" 23.	Larynx and trachea,	169
" 24.	Cough,	174
" 25.	Respiration,	184
" 26.	Internal chest and heart,	190
" 27.	External chest and mammœ,	198
" 28.	Neck, back and sacrum,	201
" 29.	Upper extremities,	209
" 30.	Lower extremities,	222
" 31.	Sleep and dreams,	237
" 32.	Fever,	246
" 33.	Skin,	265
" 34.	Generalities, aggravations and ameliorations,	283

REPERTORY.

1. Mind and Disposition.

Abusive, Hydroph. Hyosc.
Activity, (love of being busy), *Bar-c.* Lach. Mosch. *Sep.* Stann. *Verat.*
— with physical debility, Mosch.
Acuteness, *Anac.* Asa-f. *Aur. Coff.* Lach. Op. Verat. Viol-od.
Alone, when, state of mind worse, Elaps. Phosp. Stram.
Alternations of humor, *Acon.* Agn. Alum. Ambr. Anac. Arg. Ars. *Bell.* Bov. Borax. Cannab. Caps. Carb-an. Caust. Chin. Cocc. *Croc.* Cupr. Cycl. Dig. Ferr. Gels. Graph. Hyosc. *Igt.* Iod. Kali-c. Lach. Lachn. Lyc. Meny. Merc. Mez. Ntr-c. Ntr-m. Nitr-ac. Nux-m. Petr. *Plat.* Ran-b. Sabad. Sass. Seneg. Sep. Spig. Spong. Staph. *Stram.* Sulph-ac. Tart. Valer. Verat. Verb. *Zinc.*
— anxiety with indifference, Ntr-m.
— — — jollity, Spig. Spong.
— burst of passion with gaiety, Croc.
— complaining with delirium, Bell.
— dejection with gaiety, Petr.
— disgust of life with laughing, Aur.
— distraction with gaiety and singing, Spong.
— easily startled and frightened, with low spirits, Zinc.
— fearfulness with mania, Bell.
— gaiety with vexation, Caust. Cocc. Croc. Ntr-m. Spong. Tart.
— — — hatred of work, Spong.
— — — seriousness, Plat.
— — — melancholy, Ferr.
— — — ill humor, peevishness, Ntr-m. Tart.
— — want of sympathy, Merc.
— — sorrowfulness, depression, Caust. Ferr. Ntr-c. Sep.
— gaiety with tearfulness, Acon. Arg. Cannab. Carb-an. Igt. Iod. Spong.
— — — mania, Bell. Cannab. Croc.
— — — bursts of indignation, Aur. Caps. Croc. Igt.
— — — groaning with laughter, Stram.
— — — dancing, Bell.
— hatred of work with gaiety, Spong.
— hope with faint heartedness, despair, Acon. Kali-c.
— ill humor with jollity, Chin. Merc. Plat. Spig.
— — — gaiety, Cycl. Ntr-c. Tart.
— — — liveliness, Lyc.
— — — tenderness, Plat.
— indifference with anxiety, Ntr-m.
— — — vexation, Chin.
— — — irritability, Bell. Carb-an.
— irritability with lowness of spirits, Zinc.
— — — cowardice, Ran-b.
— — — care, Ran-b.
— — — wrath, Zinc.
— jollity with vexation, Borax.
— — — melancholy, Zinc.
— — — shouting, Chin.
— — — sorrowfulness, Cannab. Croc. Graph. Nitr-ac. Plat. Sep. Zinc.
— — —tearfulness, Bell. Plat.
— laughter with vexation, Croc. Stram.
— — — seriousness, Nux-m. Plat.
— — — violence, Croc. Stram.
— — — groaning, Stram.
— — — sorrowfulness, Stram.
— — — frenzies, Hyosc.
— — — tearfulness, Acon. Alum. Aur. Caps. Graph. Lyc. Sep. Stram.
— — — whining, Verat.
— mania with anxiousness and dread, Bell.
— — — gaiety and laughing, Acon. Bell. Caust. Croc.
— — — disgust for life, Bell.
— — — tearfulness, Acon. Cannab.
— melancholy with vexation, Zinc.
— — — gaiety, Ferr. Zinc.
— pusillanimity with vexation, Ran-b.
— — — exaltation, Sulph-ac.
— — — irritability, and quarrelsomeness, Ran-b.
— quarrelsomeness, with gaiety and laughter, Croc. Spong.

I. MIND AND DISPOSITION.

Alternations, quarrelsomeness singing, Croc.
— — — care and discontent, Ran-b.
— singing with vexation, Croc.
— — — hatred of work, Spong.
— — — tearfulness, Acon Bell. Stram.
— — — distraction, Spong.
— — — burst of anger, Croc.
— sorrowfulness, with serenity, Cannab. Casc. Graph. Nitr-ac. Petr. Plat. Sep. Zinc.
— — — gaiety and laughter, Canth. Caust. Ferr. Ntr-c. Zinc.
— — — intense excitement, Petr.
— sudden anger with gaiety, Aur.
— tearfulness with vexation, Bell.
— — jollity, Borax. Plat.
— violence with gaiety, Aur. Croc. Stram.
— wrath with gaiety, Aur. Caps. Igt.
— — — quick repentance, Croc. Mez.
— — — tenderness, Croc.
Amorous, *Ant.* Bell. Calc. Canth. Carb-veg. Chin. *Hyosc.* Igt. Lach. Lyc. Ntr-m. Nux. *Op.* Phosp. Plat. Puls. Sep. *Stram.* Ver..t.
— fits, Acon. Op.
Anger, Acon. Aloe. Ars. Bufo. Caust. Cham. Coloc. Igt. Kali-c. Led. Lyc. Meph. Mur-ac. Ntr-c. Ntr-m. Niec. Nux. Petr. Phosp. Plat. Ran-b. Sang. Scill. Sep. Staph. Stront. Sulph. Thuj.
— at trifles, Ars. Meph. Ntr-m. Nitr-ac. Scill.
— after being angry has a red face and is chilly, Bry.
— — — — tip of nose is red, Vinca-m.
— — — — chilliness, thirst, heat and vomiting, Nux.
— from least contradiction, Nicc.
— rage, violence and heat, Cham.
— throwing away what is in the hand, Staph.
— followed by headache, Petr.
Answer, will not, Ambr. Arn. Coloc. Euphr. Phosp-ac. Verat.
Anxiety, *Acon. Aeth.* Aloe. Alum. *Amm-c.* Anac. Arn. *Ars. Aur.* Bar-c. Bar-m. *Bell.* Berb. *Bry. Calc.* Camph. *Carb-veg* Caust. Cham. Chin. Cina. *Cocc. Coff.* Coloc. Con. Cupr. Cycl. Dig. Dros. Evon. Ferr. *Graph. Hell. Hepar.* Hyosc. Igt. Iod. Ip. *Jatr.* Kali-c. Lach. Lact. Lam. *Laur. Lyc.* Mgn-c. Mgn-m. Meny. *Merc.* Mez. Mosch. Mur-ac. *Ntr-c.* Nitr-ac. Nitr. *Nux.* Op. Petr. *Phosp.* Plat. *Plb. Puls.* Ran-sc. Raph. *Rhus.* Ruta. *Sabad. Samb. Sec-c. Seneg.* Sep. Sil. Spig. Spong. Stann. *Stram.* Sulph. *Tabac.* Thuj. *Verat.* Viol-tr.
Anxiousness, *Acon.* Alum. *Ambr.* Amm-c *Anac. Arg. Arn.* Aur. Bar-c. Bell. *Bry.* Calad. *Calc. Canth.* Caust. *Cham.* Cic. *Cocc. Coff.* Con. Cu.pr. *Dros.* Euph. *Ferr. Graph.* Grat. Kal.-c. Kali-nitr. Led.

Lyc: Mgn-m. *Mgn-s. Mosch. Mur-ac. Ntr-c.* Ntr-m. Nicc. *Nitr-ac.* Nitr. Nux. Op. Petr. *Phosp. Puls.* Ruta. *Sabad.* Sass. *Scill. Sep.* Sil. *Spig. Spong.* Staph. Stront. *Sulph.* Tart. Thuj. Valer. *Verat.*
Anxiety timid, *Alum. Amm-m.* Calad. Calc. *Canth. Caust.* Cina. *Mgn-s.* Meny. *Merc.* Nicc. Phell. Sep. *Spig. Stront.* Sulph-ac. *Tabac.* Tart. *Verat.*
— fearful, Amm-c. *Aur. Calc. Caust.* Cocc. *Coff. Dig.* Ferr. *Graph. Hep.* Kali-c. Kali-jod. Lach. *Mgn-s.* Meny. Sulph. *Verat.*
— by thoughts, excitable, Calc.
— compelling rapid walking, Arg.
— by weeping, relieved, Dig. Graph. *Tabac.*
— in chest, Phosp.
— of conscience, Ferr.
— in pregnant women, Con.
Anxiety, in the morning. Alum. Anac. Ars. Carb-veg. Caust. Chin. *Graph.* Igt. Ip. Lyc. Nitr-ac. Nux. Plat. Puls. Rhus. Sep. Sulph. Verat.
— 3 A M., Ars.
— in the forenoon, Ran-b.
— — afternoon, Aeth. *Amm-c.* Bell. Bov. Calc. Carb-an. *Carb-veg.* Mgn-c. Ntr-c. *Nitr. Nux.* Phosp-ac. Puls. *Tabac.*
— — evening, *Ambr. Ars.* Bry. Calad. *Calc.* Carb-an. *Carb-veg.* Cocc. *Dig.* Dros. Graph. *Hepar.* Kali-jod. *Laur.* Lyc. Mgn-c. Merc. Nitr-ac. *Nux.* Phosp. *Rhus.* Sep. Sulph.
— — — relieved, Amm-c.
— — — in bed, *Ambr.* Amm-c. Ars. *Bar-c.* Carb-veg. Caust. *Cocc. Graph.* Hepar. Laur. *Lyc. Mgn-c.* Mgn-m. Nitr. Nux. Phosp. Puls. Sabin. Sep. Sil. Stront. Sulph. Verat.
— — twilight, Ambr. Ars. *Calc.* Carb-veg. Dig. Laur. Nux. Rhus. Sep.
— — night, Acon. Alum. Arn. *Ars. Bell. Calc.* Cannab. Carb-an. *Carb-veg. Caust. Cham.* Chin. Dig. Ferr. *Graph.* Hepar. Hyosc. *Igt.* Kali-c. Lyc. Mgn-c. *Merc.* Ntr-m. Nitr-ac. Nux. Petr. *Phosp.* Plb. Puls. Ran-sc. *Rhus.* Sep. Sil. Sulph. *Verat.* Zinc.
— periodical attacks, Ars. Cham. Cocc. Ntr-c. Ntr-m. Phosp. Plat. Sep. Spong. Sulph.
Anxiety, when alone, *Dros.* Mez. *Phosp.*
— in children, Borax. Calc. Kali-c.
— on awaking, Amm-c. Calc. Carb-veg. Caust. Chin. Con. Graph. Igt. Ip. Lyc. Nitr-ac. Nux. Phosp. Plat. Puls. Rhus. Samb. Sep. Sil. Sulph.
— in company, in a crowd, Bell. Lyc. Petr. Plat.
— on falling asleep, Calc. Lyc.
— from noise, Caust. Sil.

I. MIND AND DISPOSITION.

Anxiety when riding in a carriage, Borax. Lach.
— — sitting, Caust. *Graph.*
— — rising from sitting, Verat.
— — speaking, Alum. Ambr. Plat.
— during a storm, Ntr-c. Ntr-m. Nitr-ac. Phosp.
— — walking, Anac. Arg. Arg-n. Bell. Cina. Hepar. Igt. Nux. Plat. Staph.
— — — rapidly, Staph.
— — the approach of others, Lyc.
— during mental labor, Ntr-c.
— from meditation, Acon. Ars. Calc. Camph. Cham. Nux. Puls. Rhus. Sec-c. Verat.
— in open air, Cina.
— — — relieved, Laur. Mgn-m.
— after vexation Lyc. Verat.
— hypochondriacal, Amm-c. Arn. Ars. Asa-f. Calad. Canth. Cham. Dros. Kali-chl. Mosch. Ntr-m. Nitr-ac. Phosp. Phosp-ac. Valer.
— hysteric, Asa-f. Con.
— tremulous, as if death were near, Ars. Bell. Ntr-c. Plat. Psor. Puls. Sass. Tart.
— with pains in abdomen, Ars. Aur. Cham. Cupr-ac.
— burning in stomach and coldness of body, Jatr.
— congestion, Calc.
— dyspnœa, Ars. Creos. Hydroc-ac. Plat. Seneg.
— headache, Acon. Alum. Bell. Bov. Calc. Carb-veg. Caust. Graph. Laur. Mgn-c. Phosp. Puls. Ruta. Sulph.
— head sweat of, Ars. Carb-veg. Nux. Phosp. Sep.
— with pain at heart, Nux. Spong.
— — pressure at, tearing in loins and restlessness, Rhus.
— — — palpitation, *Acon.* Aur. Calc. Cham. *Dig.* Ferr. Igt. Lyc. Mosch. Ntr-m. Nux. Plat. *Puls.* Ruta. *Spig.* Tart. Verat.
— heat, *Alum.* Arn. *Ars.* Bry. Calc. Carb-an. Chin. Dros. Grat. Hepar. *Mgn-c.* Mgn-m. Ntr-m. Nux. Phosp-ac. Plat. Puls. Ruta. Sep. Spong.
— humming in ears, Puls.
— shuddering, Bell. Calc. Carb-veg. Ntr-c. Plat. Puls. Tabac Verat.
— perspiration, Ars. Graph. Nux.
— pupils dilated, Nux.
— syncope, Ars.
— tremor, Ars. Plat. Puls. Sass. Tart.
— weakness, Amm-c.
— with nausea, Bar-m. Graph. Nux. Puls.
Apathy, mental, *Hyosc.* Phosp-ac. Stram.
Apprehensions, Acon. Amm-c. Bar-c. Bell. Bry. Calc. Caust. Chin. Clem. Cocc. Coff. Dig. Glon. Graph. Hell. Hepar. *Hyosc.* Iol. Kali-c. Kali-jod. Lach. Laur. Mgn-c. Mgn-s. Merc Meny. Nicc. Op. Sulph. Sulph-ac. Tabac. Verat.

Arrogance, Alum. Arn. Chin. Cupr. Ferr. Hyosc. Ip. *Lach.* Lyc. Par. *Plat. Stram.* Verat.
Assumption of importance, Cupr. Ferr. *Hyosc.* Lyc. *Stram.* Verat.
Avarice, envy, Ars. Bry. Calc. Lyc. Ntr-c. *Puls.* Sep.
Aversion to company, (compare Love of solitude,) Ambr. Bar-c. Carb-veg. Ntr-c.
— — everything, Nux. Therid. Thuj.
— — laugh, Alum. Ambr.
— — life, Ambr. Amm-c. Ant. Ars. Aur. Bell. Berb. Carb-veg. Creos. Lach. Merc. Ntr-c. Phosp. Plumb. Sep. Sil. Staph. Sulph-ac. Thuj.
— — his business, Brom. Fluor-ac. Kali-c. Puls. Sep.
— — mental labor, Agar. Chin. Graph. Iod. Kali-b. Nitr-ac. Nux. Oleand. Par. Petr. Plb. Scill. Selen. Spong. Staph. Sulph.
— — others, Amm-m. Calc. Fluor-ac. Stann.
— — friends and society, Anac. Con. Ntr-c. Ntr-m.
— — music, Cham. Phosp-ac. Tabac.
— — play, in children, Bar-c.
— — being spoken to, Ntr-m. Sil.
Autumnal equinox, state of mind worse after, Stram.
Awkwardness, Ambr. Anac. Apis. Bov. Caps. Ip. Ntr-c. Ntr-m. Nux. Puls. Sass. Sulph.
Barking, Bell. Canth.
Bashful, Chin.
Begging, entreating, Ars. Stram.
Bellowing, Bell. *Canth.*
Bewildered, during paroxysms of pain, Acon. Cham. *Coff.* Verat.
Biting, *Bell.* Bufo. Canth. Cupr. Hydroph. Sec-c. *Stram.* Verat.
Blindness, pretended, Verat.
Blood, cannot look at, or a knife, the most horrid thoughts take possession if one does, Alum.
Boldness, Acon. Agar. Alum. Bov. Calad. *Igt.* Merc. *Op.* Puls. Sulph.
Buffoonery, *Bell.* Cic. Croc. Cupr. Hyosc. Igt. Lach. Merc. Op. *Stram.*
Calmness, Op.
Calumniate, desire to, Ip.
Caprice, Acon. Bell. Calc. Caps. Croc. Lyc. Merc. Nitr-ac. Nux. Puls. Sil. Stram. Sulph.
Carelessness, Aur-m. Gels. Op.
Carphologia, picking the bed clothes, Arn. Ars. Bell. Cham. Chin. Cocc. Hep. Hyosc. Iod. Mur-ac. Phosp. Phosp-ac. Rhus. Stram. Sulph.
Cats, imagines, Puls. Stram.
Cautiousness, Graph.
Censoriousness, Ars. Guaj. Nux. Sep. Verat.
Chairs, as if repairing, Cupr.

I. MIND AND DISPOSITION.

Changeable humor, Acon. Agn. Alum. Arn. Ars. Bell. Cannab. Caps. Carb-an. Chin. *Croc* Cupr. Cycl. Ferr. Gels. *Igt.* Iod. Kali-c. Merc-cor. Ntr-m. *Nux-m.* Phell. Phosp. *Plat. Puls.* Sass. Seneg. Stram. Sulph. Sulph-ac. Valer. Zinc.
Cheerful, Brom. Carb-an. Croc. Cupr. Ferr. Gum-gutt. Ox-ac. Verb. Zinc.
Childish behaviour, Acon. Anac. Carb-an. Carb-veg. *Croc. Igt.* Nux-m. Par. Seneg.
Chin feels too long, Glon.
Choler, Acon. Anac. *Aur.* Bar-c. Bry. Cham. Coloc. Croc. Hyosc. Igt. Mez. Ntr-c. *Ntr-m. Nux.* Oleand. *Petr. Phosp.* Plat. Ran-b. Seneg. Sep. Staph. Sulph. Verat.
Clairvoyance, Acon. Phosp. Stann.
Coldness of disposition, Plat. Sabad. Scill.
Company avoided, *Ambr.* Anac. Aur. *Bar-c. Bell.* Calc. Carb-an. Carb-veg. Chin. Cic. Con. Cupr. Cycl. Dig. Eugen. Gels. Graph. Hyosc. *Igt.* Kali-c. Lach. Lyc. Mgn-m. Mang. *Ntr-c.* Puls. Rhus. Sep. Stann.
— desired, Ars. Bism. Bov. Calc. Con. Lyc. Mez. Phosp. Sep. *Stram.*
Comprehension difficult, Agn. Ambr. Cham. Con. Hell. Lyc. Mez. *Ntr-c.* Nux-m. *Oleand.* Zinc.
— of what is heard, Cham. Ntr-c.
— — — read, Agn. Ntr-c.
Conceals himself, *Ars.* Bell. Cupr. *Hell.* Puls. Stram.
Condescension, Ars. Croc. Igt. Lyc. Mosch. *Puls.* Sil.
Confidence, want of self-, Aur.
Conscience alarmed, Amm-c. *Ars. Bell. Cocc.* Coff. *Cupr.* Dig. *Igt.* Merc. Nux. Puls. Ruta. Sil. Stram. *Verat.* Zinc.
Conscientiousness, *Ars.* Cham. Cycl. Hyosc. *Igt.* Lyc. Puls. Sil. *Sulph.*
Contemptuous humor, Alum. *Ars.* Chin. Guaj. Igt. Ip. Lach. Par. Plat. Puls.
— — worse than in open air, or when sun shines in a room, Plat.
Contradiction, Anac. Arn. Aur. Camph. *Caust.* Ferr. Grat. Lach. Lyc. Merc. Ntr-c. Nux. Poth. Ruta.
— intolerable, Aur. Igt. Nicc. *Oleand.*
Contrary humor, everything is disagreeable, Acon. Alum. Ambr. Ant. Ars. Aur. Bell. Calc. Caps. Caust. Con. Croc. Hep. Igt. Ip. Lact. Led. Mgn-c. Mgn-m. *Merc.* Nitr-ac. Nux. Petr. Phosp. Plb. *Puls.* Samb. Sass. Sil. Spong. Sulph.
Course of thinking, slow, Carb-veg. Chin. Ip. Meny. Nux-m. Phosp-ac. Rhus. Ruta. Sep. Thuj.
Cowardice, Bar-c.
Cow-dung eating, Merc.
Creeping about in bed, Stram.
Criticise disposition to, Ars. Guaj. Lach. Nux. Sep. Sulph. Verat.

Cruelty, Anac. Croc. Op.
Crying out, Ant. Arn. Bell. Borax. Cham. Chin. Cina. Ip. Samb. Sep. Verat.
— suddenly, Apis. Ars. Hyosc. Lyc. Stram.
Cursing, *Anac.* Cor-r. Lyc. Nitr-ac. Nux. Puls. Verat.
Dainties desire for, Calc. *Chin.* Ip. Kali-c. Mgn-m. *Ntr-c.* Petr. Rhus.
Dancing, Acon. *Bell.* Cic. Con. Hyosc. Ntr-m. Phosp-ac. Plat. *Stram.* Tabac.
Darkness, state of mind worse in, Calc. Carb-an. Caust. Plat. Rhus. Stram. Valer.
Deafness, pretended, Verat.
Death presentiment of, *Acon.* Ars. *Bell.* Calc. Canth. Cupr. Kali-c. *Lach.* Lyc. Merc. Ntr-m. Nitr. Nitr-ac. *Nux.* Plat. Sep. Staph. Verat. Zinc.
Defiance, Acon. Anac. *Arn.* Canth. Caust. Guaj. *Lyc.* Nux. Spong.
Dejection, Acon. Alum. Anac. Arn. Ars. Aur. Bar-c. Bell. Bov. Brom. *Bry.* Calad. *Calc.* Canth. Caust. Chelid. *Chin.* Colch. Coloc. Creos. Crotal. Cupr. Cycl. Daph. Dros. Elaps. Elat. Graph. Hep. Hydroc-ac. Iris. Iod. Lac-can. Lach. Laur. Lyc. Mang. Merc-jod. Merc-sulph. Merc. Mez. *Ntr-c.* Nti-m. Ntr-nitr. Nicc. Nitr-ac. Nux. Petr. Phosp. Phosp-ac. Plat. Plb. Pod. Psor. Rhus. Rumex. Ruta. Sabin. Sass. *Sep.* Sil. *Sulph.* Sulph-ac. Verat. Viol-tr.
— in the evening, Creos. Mgn-c. Puls. Zinc.
— caused by pain, Sass.
— in open air, Aeth. Sabin.
— after being, angry, Plat.
— when alone, Bov.
Delirium, *Acon.* Aeth. Agar. Anac. Ant. Arn. *Ars.* Aur. *Bell.* Bry. Calc. Camph. Cannab. Canth. Carb-veg. Caust. *Cham. Chin.* Cic. Cina. Coloc. Con. Con. Cupr. Dulc. *Hyosc.* Igt. Iod. Kali-c. Lach. Lachn. Lyc. Merc. Nux-m. Nux. Op. Par. Petr. Phosp. *Plb.* Pod. Puls. Rheum. *Rhus.* Sabad. *Samb.* Sec-c. Spong. Stram. Sulph. Verat.
— cheerful, laughing, Acon. *Bell.* Op. Sulph. Verat.
— frightful, Acon. *Bell.* Calc. Coloc. Hyosc. Nux. *Op.* Puls. Sil. *Stram.*
— furious, Acon. *Bell.* Bry. Colch. Coloc. Op. Plb. Puls. Verat. Zinc.
Delirium, loquacious, *Bell.* Cupr. Lach. Op. Petr. Plat. Rhus. *Stram.* Verat.
— muttering, *Bell.* Crotal. *Hyosc.* Nux. Stram. Tar.
— sorrowful, Acon. Bell. Dulc. Lyc. Puls.
— with eyes open, Cham. Coff. Coloc. Verat.
— sleepiness, Acon. Arn. *Bry.* Coloc. *Puls.*

I. MIND AND DISPOSITION. 5

Delirium of same subject, all the time, Petr.
— periodical, Samb.
— constant, Bapt.
— with coldness, Verat.
— cold feet, Zinc.
— during the pains, Dulc. Verat.
— at night on awaking, Aur. Bry. Cact. Carb-veg. Colch. Dulc. Merc. Ntr-c. Par.
— when falling asleep, Bell. Bry. Calc. Camph. Chin. Gels. Guaj. Igt. Merc. Phosp. Phosp-ac. Spong. Sulph.
— wild, Plb.
— religious, Verat.
Deserted, feeling himself, Carb-veg.
Despair, Acon. Aloe. Alum. Ambr. Arn. Ars. Aur. Bov. Brom. Bry. Calc. Carb-an. Carb-veg. Caust. Chelid. Cupr. Graph. Gum-gut. Hell. Hep. Hydroc-ac. Igt. Iod. Kali-b. Lach. Lyc. Ntr-c. Nitr. Nitr-ac. Petr. Psor. Puls. Sil. Sulph. Tart. Valer. Verat.
— of others, Aur.
— about ruined health, Calc. Staph.
— of recovery, Acon. Bry. Creos. Igt. Kali-c. Nux. Sil.
— — his soul's welfare, Lyc. Puls. Sulph.
Destruction of his things, Merc-jod.
— — clothes (insane), Sulph. Tarant.
— — — cuts them up, Verat.
Dictatorial conduct, Camph. Caust. Ferr. Lach. Lyc. Merc.
Discontentedness, Alum. Amm-c. Amm-m. Ang. Arn. Aur. Bell. Bism. Calc. Carb-an. Caps. Caust. Chin. Cic. Cina. Cinnab. Coloc. Con. Creos. Cupr. Hep. Igt. Kali-c. Ntr-c. Par. Petr. Phosp-ac. Plb. Puls. Rhus. Ruta. Sep. Sil. Spong. Staph Sulph.
Discouragement, Acon. Ambr. Anac. Arn. Ars Aur. Bell. Camph. Canth. Carb an. Carb-veg. Caust. Cham. Chin. Cocc. Coff. Colch. Coloc. Con. Cupr. Dig. Dros. Graph. Hep. Igt. Iod. Ip. Lach. Laur. Lyc. Merc. Ntr-c. Ntr-m. Nitr-ac. Nux. Op. Petr. Phosp-ac. Plb. Pod. Psor. Puls. Tart. Therid. Thuj. Verat. Zinc.
Disesteem of one's self, Agn.
Disobedience, Acon. Amm-c. Amm-m. Arn. Canth. Caps. Caust. Chin. Dig. Guaj. Lyc. Nitr-ac. Nux. Phosp. Spig. Sulph. Viol-tr.
Despise, disposition to, Ars. Ip.
Distrust, Anac. Ant. Arn. Bar-c. Bell. Caust. Cham. Cic. Dros. Hell. Hyosc. Lach. Lyc. Merc. Nux. Op. Plb. Puls. Ruta. Sulph-ac.
— of futurity, Anac. Caust.
Dogmatical, Camph. Caust. Ferr. Lach. Lyc. Merc.
Dogs, afraid of. Chin. Stram.
Doubtful of recovery, Acon. Bry. Calc.

Igt. Kali-c. Lach. Nux. Phosp. Phosp-ac. Puls. Sep. Sulph.
— — his soul's welfare, Ars. Aur. Bell. Croc. Dig. Hyosc. Lach. Nux. Puls. Selen. Stram.
Dreaming while awake, Acon. Ang. Arn. Ars. Bell. Cham. Graph. Hep. Hyosc. Lach. Merc. Op. Phosp. Phosp-ac. Sil. Stram. Thuj.
— about futurity, poetical, Oleand.
Ecstacy, Acon. Agar. Ant. Bell. Lach. Op. Phosp. Stram.
Embarrassed, Hyosc. Sulph.
— in company, Ambr. Carb-veg.
Emotions predominated over by intellect, Viol-od.
Ennui, Alum. Bar-c. Con. Lach. Lyc. Mgn-m. Ntr-c. Nux. Petr. Plb. Zinc.
Envy, Ars. Bry. Calc. Lyc. Ntr-c. Puls. Sep.
Escaping, fleeing from home, Acon. Bell. Bry. Cocc. Coloc. Cupr. Dig. Hyosc. Lach. Merc. Puls. Stram. Verat.
Exaltation, excitement, Acon. Ambr. Anac. Ang. Arn. Asa-f. Bell. Bry. Camph. Chin. Cocc. Coff. Creos. Cub. Cycl. Hydroc-ac. Hyosc. Iod. Kali-c. Kobalt. Lach. Meph. Millef. Ntr-c. Ntr-m. Nitr-ac. Nux-jug. Nux. Petr. Phosp. Phosp-ac. Sabad. Seneg. Stram. Sulph. Sulph-ac. Teucr. Valer. Viol-od. Zinc.
Exaltation of fancy, Alum. Agar. Ang. Bell. Cannab. Chin. Coff. Lach. Mur-ac. Op. Ox-ac. Phosp. Sabad. Stram. Sulph-ac. Valer. Verb. Viol-od.
— in company, Pallad. Sep.
— nervous, Bell. Coff. Nux.
Expression, deficiency of, Con. Crotal. Kali-c. Nux. Puls. Thuj.
Extravagance, Amm-c. Bell. Caust. Chin. Croc. Iod. Petr Phell. Phosp-ac. Plat. Stram. Verat.
Eyes, frivolous closing of, on being questioned, Sep.
Faces, sees, Ambr. Arg-n. Calc. Carb-an. Caust. Op. Sulph.
— — grotesque, Ambr. Calc. Carb-an. Caust. Op. Sulph.
Fancies objects around him will fall, Hyosc.
Fanaticism, religious, Selen. Sulph.
— philosophical, Sulph.
Fatigued, Led. Lyc. Merc. Nux. Sass. Sulph-ac. (compare Fatigue, under Generalities.)
Fatigued by reading. Sil.
— — and writing. Cannab. Sil.
— by the pains, Sass.
— — vexation, Zinc.
Faultfinding, disposed to, Ars. Ip.
Fear of death, Acon. Agn. Alum. Anac. Ars. Asa-f. Ant. Bapt. Bell. Bry. Calc. Cocc. Coff. Cupr. Dig. Graph. Hell.

I. MIND AND DISPOSITION.

Hep. Ip. *Lach.* Lob. *Mosch.* Ntr-m.
Nitr-ac. *Nitr.* Nux. Phosp. *Plat.* Psor.
Puls. Raph. Rheum. Scill. Sec-c. Stram.
Tabac. Tarant. Verat.
Fear of cholera, Lach.
— — disease and misery, Borax. Calc. Iris. Lach.
— — darkness, Bapt. Calc. Lyc. *Puls.* Valer.
— — futurity, Anac. Bar-c. *Bry.* Caust. Chelid. Con. *Dig.* Dros. Dulc. Graph. Grat. Kali-c. Mang. Ntr-c. Ntr-m. Puls. Spig. Staph. Tart.
— — heart disease, Lac-can. Lach.
— — of being devoured, Stram.
— — apoplexy, Fluor-ac. Phosp.
— — being murdered, Op. Phosp. Stram.
— — water, Hyosc.
— — going in a crowd, Acon.
— — mental derangement, Acon. Alum. Ambr. Calc. Lac-can. Lil-tigr. Merc. Phosp. Thuj.
— — misfortune, Ant. Calc. Clem. Fluor-ac. Graph. Lach. Nux.
— — of being poisoned or sold, *Bell.* Bry. *Hyosc.* Rhus.
— — solitude, Ars. Hyosc. Lyc. Stram.
— — spectres, Acon. *Ars. Carb-veg.* Cocc. Dros. Puls. Ran-b. *Sulph.* Zinc.
— — — in evening, *Puls.* Ran-b.
— — — at night, Ars. Carb-veg. Chin. *Sulph.*
— in the evening, Calc. Carb-an. Caust. Dros. Kali-c. Lyc. Merc. Phosp. *Puls.* Ran-b. Valer. Verat.
— at night, Amm-c. *Ars.* Bell. Carb-veg. Caust. *Chin.* Cocc. Con. Dros. Graph. Hep. Ip. Lach. Lyc. Merc. Ntr-c. Ntr-m. Nitr-ac. Phosp. Puls. Rhus. Sil. Stann. *Sulph.* Zinc.
Fearfulness, Aloe. Alum. Amm-c. Ang. *Ars.* Bar-c. *Bell.* Berb. Bry. Calc. *Carb-an.* Caust. Chin. Dros. Igt. Lach. Mgn-c. Nicc. Op. *Phosp.* Plat. Psor. *Puls.* Ran-b. Sec-c. Sep. Spig. Spong. Sulph. Valer. *Verat.*
Fidgety, Aur. Bell. Igt. Puls. Sep. Sil. Sulph.
Fire, wants, to set things on, Hep.
Flinging, throwing himself about, Bell. Canth. Hyosc. Stram.
Fondness, Acon. Anac. Carb-an. Carb-veg. Igt. Nux. Par. Seneg.
Foolish behaviour, Bell. Cic. Croc. Cupr. Hyosc. Igt. Lach. Merc. Nux-m. Op. Stram. Tanac. *Verat.*
Forgetfulness, Acon. Alum. Amm-c. Anac. Bar-c. Bell. Bry. Calad. Calc. Cinnab. Colch. *Con.* Croc. Cycl. Graph. Guaj. Gymnoc. Hell. Hep. Hyosc. *Lach.* Merc. Mosch. Ntr-m. Nux-m. Oleand. Petr. Phosp. Plat. Rhod. Rhus. Sil. Spig. Staph. Stram. Stront. Sulph. Thuj.

Verat. Viol-od. *Zinc.*
— of the word when speaking, Arn.
— — time and place, Merc.
— — what he has said, Mur-ac.
— of dates, Fluor-ac.
— words, Bar-c. Lyc. Pod.
— names, Guaj. Sulph.
— when awake, distinct recollection during half sleep, Selen.
— on awaking, Stann.
— in the morning, Phosp.
Fretfulness, Acon. Aeth. Amm-c. Amm-m. Ang. Arn. *Ars.* Aur. Bell. Berb. *Bry.* Calc. Canth. *Carb-veg. Caust. Cham.* Cinnab. Chin. Cocc. Coloc. Con. Cor-r. Croc. Cycl. Dros. Eugen. Evon. Ferr. *Graph.* Hydroc-ac. *Igt.* Ip. Kali-c. Kali-jod. Led. Lyc. Merc. Mur-ac. Ntr-c. Ntr-m. *Nitr-ac. Nux.* Oleand. Par. Petr. Phell. *Phosp.* Plat. Puls. *Ran-b.* Sabad. Sabin. Scill. Seneg. *Sep. Sil.* Stann. *Staph.* Stram. Sulph. Tart. Teucr. Thea. Verat. Verb. Zinc.
— about trifles, Meph. Ntr-m. Nitr-ac. Scill.
— in open air, Aeth.
— forenoon, Ran-b.
— bad effects from, Cist.
Frightened easily, *Acon.* Alum. Ang. Ant. Arn. Bell. Berb. Borax. *Calc.* Cannab. *Caps. Carb-an.* Caust. Cham. Cic. Cocc. Con. Graph. *Igt. Kali-c.* Kali-jod. *Lach.* Led. Merc. Ntr-c. Ntr-m. Nitr-ac. *Nux.* Op. Petr. Phosp. Plat. Rhus. *Sabad. Samb.* Sep. *Sil.* Spong. Stram. *Sulph.* Sulph-ac. Therid. Verat.
Fury, Aeth. Agar. Ars. *Bell.* Camph. Cannab. *Canth.* Cupr. *Hyosc.* Lyc. Merc. Mosch. Nitr-ac. Plb. Sabad. Sec-c. Seneg. Sol-nig. *Stram.* Verat.
Gestures foolish, Bell. Cic. *Hyosc.* Mosch. *Nux-m. Sep. Stram.* Verat.
Gloominess, Anac. Aur. Bov. Caust. Cham. Chin. *Con.* Dig. Graph. Iod. Meny. Petr. Plb. Rheum. Rhod. Stann. Sulph. Sulph-ac. Tabac. Tar. Verat. Viol-od. Zinc.
Godlessness, want of religious feeling, Anac. Coloc.
Gossiping, Hyosc. Verat.
Gravity, Cannab. Euph. Grat. Led. Nux-m. Sulph-ac.
— at things laughable, Anac.
Grief, Alum. Amm-m. Ars. Bell. Calc. Caust. Coloc. Cycl. *Graph.* Hyosc. *Igt. Lach. Lyc.* Ntr-m. Nux. Op. Phosp-ac. Puls. Sep. *Staph.* Verat.
Grief about his condition, Staph.
— for the future, Ntr-c. Ntr-m.
— undemonstrative, Cycl.
Groaning, *Acon.* Alum. Amm-c. *Bell.* Bry. *Cham.* Cic. Cocc. Colch. *Coff.* Cupr. Graph. Hell. Igt. Merc. *Nux.* Puls.

I. MIND AND DISPOSITION.

Sass. Scill. Sep. Stram. Tart.
Groaning children, Millef.
Growling like a bear, Mgn-m.
— — — dog, Alum. Hell. Lyc.
Hanging, sees persons, Ars.
Happy, Sulph.
Hardheartedness, Anac. Croc.
Hastiness, *Ambr.* Ars. Aur. Bar-c. Bell. Bry. Cannab. Carb-an. Con. Hep. Lach. Laur. Merc. Ntr-c. Ntr-m. Sep. Stram. Sulph. Sulph-ac. Viol-tr.
— in mental labors, Ambr.
— — talking, Bell. Hep.
Hatred of offenders, Agar. Amm-c. Anac. Aur. Calc. Cic. Lach. Led. Mang. Ntr-m. Nitr-ac. Phosp. Stann. Sulph.
Haughtiness, Alum. Arn. Caust. Chin. Cupr. Ferr. Hyosc. Ip. Lach. *Lyc.* Par. *Plat. Stram.* Verat.
Head, believes it to be transparent and speckled brown, Bell.
— foolish shaking of, Bell. Cham.
Help, calling for, Plat.
Hesitation, Aur. Bar-c. Chin. Graph. Mez. Mur-ac. Nux. Puls. Seneg. Sil. Sulph. Thuj.
Hilarity, Acon. Arn. Aur. Cannab. Carb-an. Coff. *Croc.* Ferr. Fluor-ac. Gum-gut. Lachn. Merc-cor. Ntr-m. Nux-m. Sass. Seneg. Spong. Tabac. Tar. Therid. Verb. Zinc.
— at noon, Zinc.
Home, will go, believes himself not to be at, Bell. Bry. *Lach.* Op. Verat.
Homesickness, *Aur.* Bell. *Caps.* Carb-an. Hell. Igt. Merc. Nitr-ac. Phosp-ac. Sacch. Sil.
— with redness of cheeks, *Caps.*
Hopeful, Ferr-m.
Hopelessness, Acon. *Arn.* Ars. Aur. Bar-c. Bell. Bry. Calc. Carb-an. Carb-veg. *Caust.* Chin. Con. Graph. Igt. *Lach.* Lyc. Merc. Ntr-c. Ntr-m. Nitr-ac. Op. Psor. Puls. Rhus. Sep. Sil. Stann. Sulph. Sulph-ac. *Tart.*
Horror, in the evening, Calc. Carb-an. Phosp. (compare Fear.)
Howling, Acon. Arn. Bell. Brom. Cham. Cic. Coff. Ip. Stann. Stram. Verat. (compare Streaming, weeping).
Humor agreeable, Croc. Igt. Lach. Meny. Plat. Sulph-ac. Tart.
Hurry, always in a, Ars.
Hydrophobia, Arg-n. *Bell. Canth.* Hydroph. *Hyosc. Lach. Stram.* Verat.
Hypochondriacal humor, Acon. Agn. Aloe. Alum. Anac. Arn. Ars. Bell. Bry. Cact. *Calc.* Caust. Cham. Chin. Cocc. *Con.* Cupr. Graph. *Grat. Hell. Igt.* Iod. Kali-c. Lyc. Merc. Mez. *Mosch. Ntr-c.* Ntr-m. Nitr-ac. Nux-m. *Nux.* Petr. *Phosp.* Phosp-ac. Plat. *Puls.* Rhus. Sabad. Sabin. Sacch. Seneg. Sep. Stann. Staph. Sulph.

Valer. Viol-od. Zinc.
— with chilliness, Ars. Con. Puls.
— — with coldness, Ars.
— — debility, Ars. Mosch. Nux-m. Plat. Sep. Zinc.
— ears, with noise, Puls.
— face, with heat of, Nux-m.
— — — paleness of, Mosch.
— with fainting, Mosch.
— — fever, Petr.
— — fits, Con.
— — heat, Calc.
— — head with dullness of, Dig.
— hypochondrium, with pains in, Zinc.
— with pulse excited, Plat. Sep.
— — respiratory affections, Lob. Sep.
— stomach, with sickness at, Lyc. Plat.
Hypocrisy, Phosp.
Hysterical humor, Anac. *Asa-f.* Aur. Calc. Cauloph. Caust. *Con.* Croc. Elaps. *Grat. Igt.* Mgn-m. Millef. *Mosch.* Nux-m. Nux. Phosp. Plat. Puls. Sep. Sil Stann. Staph. Sulph. Therid. Valer. *Viol-od.*
Ideas, abundant, Agar. Alum. Ambr. Amm-c. Ars. Aur. *Calc.* Cannab. Canth. Carb-veg. Caust. *Chin.* Cocc. Coloc. Con. Glon. Graph. Hep. Hyosc. Kali-c. Kobalt. Lach. *Lyc. Mur-ac.* Nitr. Nitr-ac. Op. Petr. *Phosp.* Phosp-ac. Plat. *Puls.* Rhus. Sabad. *Sep.* Spong. Stram. Staph. *Sulph.* Tabac. Tereb. Verb. *Viol-od.* Viol-tr. Zinc.
— — in the evening, before going, to sleep, *Chin.* Lyc. *Nux. Puls.* Sabad. Sil. *Staph.* Viol-tr.
— — at night, Borax. *Calc.* Chin. Coff. Graph. Hep. Kali-c. *Lyc. Nux.* Puls. Sabad. Sil. *Staph.* Sulph. Viol-tr.
— confusion of, Camph.
— facetious, Nux-m.
— fixed, Aeth. Carb-veg. Petr. Puls. Sulph. Thuj.
— gay and musical, Sulph.
— of hanging or standing high, Phosp.
— profound, sublime, Lach.
— slowness of, Carb-veg. Chin. Ip. Meny. Nux-m. Phosp-ac. Rhus. Ruta. Sep. Thuj.
— unable to collect, Laur.
— unconnected, on attempt to fix them has a vacant feeling, Gels.
— unsteady, *Acon.* Apis. Lach. Merc. *Puls.* Staph. Tabac. *Valer. Viol-od.* Zinc.
Ill humor, Acon. Aeth. Alum. Amm-m. Ang. *Arg.* Ars. Asa-f. Aur. Bell. Brom. Cact. Calc. Caust. Cham. Chin. Cina. Cocc. Cocc-c. Cor-r. Creos. Cycl. Evon. Fluor-ac. Grat. Hep. Hydroph. Igt. Ip. Kali-b. Kali-c. Lach. Lachn. Led. Lyc. Mgn-s. Mang. Mosch. Ntr-c. Ntr-m. Nitr-ac. Nitr. *Nux.* Petr. *Phosp.* Phosp-ac. Puls. Psor. Sep. Sil. Stann. *Staph.* Stront. *Sulph.* Viol-tr.

I. MIND AND DISPOSITION.

Ill humor in children, *Ant.* Ars. Borax Graph. Puls. Sil. *Tart.*
— in cloudy weather, Aloe.
— in wet weather, Amm-c.
Illness, sense of, in mind and body, Merc.
Illusions, of fancy, Acon. Anac. Ant. *Bell.* Berb. Bry. Calc. Cannab. Canth. Carb-veg. Caust. Chin. Cic. Cocc. Colch. Con. Dulc. Igt. Ind. Hell. Hep. Hyosc. Mgn-m. Mgn-s. Merc. Nux. *Op.* Par. Phosp. *Phosp-ac.* Plat. Puls. *Rhus.* Sabad. Sep. Sil. Stann. *Stram.* Sulph. Verat.
— of hearing, Anac. Bell. Calc. Canth. Carb-veg. Cham. Con. Dros. Mgn-m. Phosp-ac.
— — sight, Bell. Carb-veg. Dulc. Hell. Hep. Hyosc. Kali-c. Mgn-m. Ntr-c. Nitr-ac. Nux. Op. Phosp. Puls. Rhus. Stram. Sulph.
— at night, *Bell.* Cham. Led. Merc. Phosp. Stram.
— of feeling, *Anac.* Bell. Canth. Igt. Iod. Mgn-m. Op. Petr. Phosp. Plat. Rhus. Sabad. *Stram.* Sulph. Tart. Valer.
Imaginations, Anac. *Aur.* Bell. Cham. Chin. Cic. Cocc. Con. Croc. Cupr. Dros. Hyosc *Igt.* Iod. Lach. Mgn-c. Plat. Rhus. Si. S ram. Sulph. Verat.
— abdomen, fancies of reduced, Sabad.
— animals, sees, Ars. *Bell.* Calc. Colch. *Hyosc.* Lac-can. Op. Puls. Stram.
— arrested, as if he would be, Bell.
— of bats, Bell.
— of bees, Puls.
— — body, thinks it covered with brown spots, Bell.
— burned, thinks everything at home is, Bell.
— cancer, of having a, Verat.
— captain, of being a. Cupr.
— of climbing, Hyosc.
— clothes, as if he had on very fine, Aeth. Sulph.
— of crabs, Hyosc.
— criminal of as if he were, Alum. Amm-c. *Ars.* Carb-veg. Caust. Cina. *Cocc.* Coff. Dig. Ferr. Graph. *Hyosc.* Ntr-c. Nitr-ac. Nux. Puls. Ruta. Sil. Stront. Sulph. Verat.
— of corpses, *Anac.* Ars. *Bell.* Canth. Hep. Ntr-c. Nux. Op.
— — ciphers, Phosp-ac. Sulph.
— dead, that is, Apis. Lach.
— of devils, Ars. Bell. Cupr. Dulc. Hyosc. Lach. Plat. Op. Stram. Sulph.
— of disease of his own body, Sabad.
— — dogs, Bell. Puls. Stram.
— double, of being, Anac. Mosch.
— enemies, pursued by, Dros.
— excited, Coff.
— fighting, sees persons, Op.
— of fires, Bell. Calc. Hep. Spong. Sulph.

— — forms, Carb-veg. Cic. Hell. Nitr-ac. Stram. Sulph.
— — — black, Bell. Op. Plat. Puls.
— — — frightful, Bell. Op. Stram.
— — — rising out of the earth, Stram.
— — fowls, Stram.
— — geese, Hyosc.
— — greatness of his own body, *Plat.* Staph.
— — harlequin, Hyosc.
— — headless body, Nux.
— — heads, of having two, Mosch.
— — — hearing footsteps, Canth. Carb-veg.
— — — a bell, Phosp-ac.
— — — some one come in at the door, Con.
— horses, Mgn-m. Zinc.
— humility and lowness of others, Plat. Staph.
— hunts pins, Sil.
— hunter, of being a, Verat.
— insects, sees, Bell. Puls.
— insults imagines, Igt. Nux. Puls.
— island, on a distant, Phosp.
— knocking under the bed, Calc. Canth.
— larger, parts of the body to be, Alum. Op.
— longer, things to be, Berb. Camph. Creos. Dros. Nitr ac. Sulph.
— mice, Calc. Colc. Op.
— people, sees, Hyosc. Mgn-c. Op. *Puls.* Rheum. Sep. Stram.
— presence of others, strangers, Mgn-s.
— proud, Plat. Stram. Verat.
— pregnant, of being, Verat.
— riches, of, Sulph.
— rocks, Mgn-m.
— scorpions, Op.
— scrotum swollen, Sabad.
— soldiers, Bell. Bry. Ntr-c.
— some one in bed, Petr.
— speaks to inanimate objects, Stram.
— thieves, Ars. Merc. Sil.
— transaction of business, Cupr.
— threefold body of having, Ars.
— vexations and offences, Cham. Chin. Dros.
— vivid, Op.
— warts on body, Mez.
— water, Hep. Merc. Tart.
— young girl, imagines herself a, Cic.
Imbecility, Acon. Anac. Ant. Ars. Bell. Hyosc. Laur. Lyc. *Merc.* Ntr-c. *Nux-m.* Op. Par. Phosp-ac. Plb. Sabad. Sil. Sol-n. Stram.
Impatience, Ambr. Ars. Calc. Carb-veg. Dros. Dulc. Hep. Hyosc. Igt. Ip. Lach. Lyc. Ntr-c. Ntr-m. Nitr-ac. Op. Pallad. Phosp-ac. Psor. Puls. Sep. *Sil.* Spong. Sulph. Sulph-ac. Thuj.
Imperious, Arn. Cupr. Lyc. Stront.
Impetuosity, Acon. Anac. *Bry. Carb-veg.* Cham. Croc. Hep. Kali-jod. Led. Ntr-c. Ntr-m. Nitr-ac. *Nux.* Oleand. Phosp. Rheum. Sep. Stront. Zinc.

I. MIND AND DISPOSITION.

Impudence, Bell. Phosp.
Impulsive, Cic.
Inability to express oneself, Bell. Cannab. Lach. Lac-can. Lyc. Nux. Puls. Thuj.
— for mental labor, Acon. *Alum.* Asar. Laur. *Lyc.* Ntr-c. Ntr-m. Phosp-ac. Selen. Sep. Sil. Sol-m. Spig. Spong. Staph. Therid. Thuj.
— — from stupefaction in the head, Acon. Aeth. Asar. Calc. Chin. Nux-m. Nux. Op. Plat. Rhod. Rhus. Sep.
— — fatigue, Calc. Colch. Ntr-c. Nux. Plat. Puls. Sep. Sil.
— to reflect, think, Acon. Alum. Calc. Cycl. Lac-can. Laur. *Lyc.* Ntr-c. Ntr-m. Phosp-ac. Selen. Sep. Sil. Sol-m. Spig. Thuj.
Inattention, Alum. Ang. Amm-c. Amm-m. Bar-c. Bell. Bov. Caust. Cham. Kali-c. Merc. Ntr-m. Nux. Oleand. Phosp-ac. Plat. Puls. Sep. Sulph.
— when learning, reading, etc., Alum. Asar. *Bar-c.* Bell. Caust. Cham. Coff. Kali-c. Ntr-c. Spig. Sulph.
Inciting others, Hyosc.
Inconsolable, *Acon.* Ambr. *Ars. Cham.* Coff. *Nux.* Spong. Stram. Sulph. Verat.
Inconstancy, Asa-f. Bism. Igt. Op.
Indifference, Ambr. Amm-c. Anac. Apis. Arg-n. Arn. *Ars.* Bell. Berb. Bism. Calc. Cannab. Caps. Cham. Chin. Cic. Cina. Clem. Cocc. Con. Croc. Crotal. Cycl. Dig. Euphr. Gymnoc. Hell. *Igt.* Kali-b. Kali-c. Lach. Lyc. Meny. Merc. Mez. Mur-ac. Ntr-c. Ntr-m. Nitr-ac. *Op.* Phosp. *Phosp-ac.* Phyt. Plat. Prun. Puls. Rheum. *Rhod.* Sabin. Scill. Scc-c. *Sep.* Sil. Stann. *Staph.* Veat. Verb. Viol-tr.
— does not complain, Hyosc. Op.
— — — — unless questioned, then says nothing of his condition, Colch.
— says he is well, Arn.
— no desire, no action of will, Hell.
— respecting his business, Arn. Fluor-ac. Sep. *Stram.*
— to relations, Hep. Plat. Phosp. Sep.
— apathetic, Amm-c. Anac. *Bar-c. Bell. Chin.* Con. *Hell. Igt.* Laur. Mez. Ntr-c. *Op. Phosp-ac.* Plat Sep.
— after onanism, Staph.
Indignation, Coloc. Ntr-c. *Staph.*
Indiscretion, Caps. Meny. Puls.
Indolence, Amm-c. Caps. Chelid. Chin. Cocc. Croc. Crotal. Dig. Guaj. Lach. Ntr-m. Nux. Oleand. Phosp. Plat. Rheum. Sep. Sulph. Teucr.
Inhumanity, Anac. Op.
Injuring, mutilating one's self, Ars.
Insanity, madness, Acon. Aeth. Agar. Ant. Arn. Ars. Aur. Bar-c. Bell. Calc. Camph. Cannab. Canth. Cic. Croc. Crotal. Cupr. Dig. ¬Dulc. Hyosc. Igt. **Kali-c.** Lach. Led. Lyc. Ntr-m. Nux-m.

Nux. Op. Phosp. Plat. Plb. Puls. Sabad. Sec-c. Seneg. Sep. Stram. Tart. Tereb. Verat.
— alternating with stupor, Op.
— to dispute, Camph.
— loquacious, Par. Stram.
— with pain in abdomen, Canth. Cupr.
— — appetite with loss of, Verat.
— — blood with discharge of, Merc.
— — breathing with oppression of, Merc.
— — chilliness, with, Calc.
— — coldness of skin, with, Crotal.
— — cough with, Bell. Verat.
— — emaciation, with, Sulph.
— — face with heat of, Verat.
— — — redness, Calc. Op.
— — — paleness, Croc. Merc. Verat.
— — feet, stamping of, Verat.
— — with fright caused by, or anger, Plat.
— — headache, Croc. Verat.
— — heat, Bell. Verat.
— — larynx pains in, Canth.
— — look wild, Cupr.
— — mouth distortion of, Phosp-ac.
— — obscuration of sight, Croc.
— — opthalmia, Croc. Op.
— — perspiration following, Cupr.
— — ptyalism, Verat.
— — pulse quick, Ars. Crotal. Cupr.
— — sleep during, Phosp-ac.
— — trembling, Ars.
— — vomiting, Cupr-ac.
— — vertigo, Nux-m.
— — wantonness, Hyosc. Stram. Verat.
— of drunkards, *Ars.* Bell. Calc. Carb-veg. Chin. Coff. Dig. Hell. Hep. Hyosc. Lach. Merc. Ntr-c. *Nux. Op.* Puls. Stram. Sulph.
Insensibility, mental, *Hyosc.* Phosp-ac. Stram.
Intellect predominates, over feeling, Viol-od.
Irascibility, Amm-c. Arn. Bry. Caps. Carb-veg. Caust. Cham. Graph. Ip. Kali-c. Ntr-c. Ntr-m. Nitr-ac. Nux. Petr. Phosp. Sep. Sil. Sulph. Zinc.
Irresolution, Alum. Ars. Bar-c. Calc. Cham. Chin. Cocc. Cupr. Daph. Ferr. Graph. Hell. Igt. Iod. Kali-c. Lach. Mgn-c. Mez. Ntr-m. Nux-m. Nux. Petr. Phosp. Ruta. Sulph. Tar.
Irritability, *Acon.* Aeth. Amm-m. Anac. Ang. Arg. Arn. *Aur.* Bar-c. Bell. Bry. Bufo. Cact. Cadm. Calc. Canth. *Carb-veg.* Caust. Cham. Chin. Cina. Cocc. Cocc-c. Coff. Colch. Coloc. Con. Creos. Cupr. Dulc. Elaps. Ferr. Graph. Grat. Hep. Hydroph. Hyosc. Igt. *Iod.* Ip. Kali-b. Kali-c. Lach. Lachn. Led. *Lyc.* Mang. Mgn-s. *Merc.* Merc-sulph. Mez. Mur-ac. Ntr-c. Nitr-ac. *Nux.* Petr. *Phosp.* Puls. Ran-b. Rhus. Rumex. Ruta. Sacch. Sang. Seneg. **Sep. Sil.** Stann. Staph.

10 I. MIND AND DISPOSITION.

Stram. Stront. *Sulph.* Sulph-ac. *Teucr.* Valer. Verat.
Irritability nervous, Asar. Lach.
— from contradiction, Igt.
— justifiable, Staph.
— in cloudy weather, Aloe.
— — wet weather, Amm-c.
Jealousy, Apis. Camph. *Hyosc.* Lach. Nux. Puls.
— mocking, Lach.
— with rage and delirium, Hyosc.
Joyfulness, Cannab. Carb-an. Croc. Meny. Zinc. (compare Hilarity.)
— in evening or noon, Zinc.
Joylessness. Acon. Alum. Amm-c. *Anac.* Calc. Cannab Cham. Coloc. *Croc.* Dros. Ip. Laur. Lyc. Ntr-m. *Nitr-ac.* Ol-an. *Phosp.* Prun. Sabin. Sil. Tabac. (compare Dejection.)
Kleptomania, Ars. Bry. Kali-c. Lyc. Nux. Puls Sep. Sulph.
Kneeling and praying, Ars. Stram.
Lamenting, Acon. Arn. Ars. Bism. Brom. Calc. Chin. Cina. Igt. Lach. Mosch. Nux-m. Nux. Phosp. Sulph.
Laughing, Acon. Aloe. Alum. Aur. Bell. Cic. Con. Croc. *Hyosc.* Igt. Ntr-m. Nux-m. Phosp. Plat. Puls. Ran-sc. *Stram.* Sulph. Tar Verat. Verb.
— immoderate, improved, Croc.
— involuntary, Phosp.
— sardonic, Ran-sc. Sec-c. Sol-n. Zinc.
— at serious things, Anac. Ntr-m.
— spasmodic, Acon. Alum. Anac. Asa-f. *Aur.* Calc. Caust. Cic. *Con.* Croc. Cupr. *Igt.* Ntr-m. Nux-m. Phosp. Plat. Stram. Verat. Zinc.
— and weeping alternately, Alum. *Arn.* Borax. Caps. Graph. Lyc. Phosp. *Puls.* Sep. Stram. Sulph. Verat.
— aversion to, Ambr.
— never smiles, Alum.
Locality, errors of, Bry. Lach. Par. Valer. Verat.
Loses his way in well known places, Glon.
Longing for death, Aur-m. Creos.
— — the good, opinion of others, Pallad.
— — light, sunshine and society, Stram.
— — repose and tranquillity, Nux.
— — things rejected as soon as offered, Ars. Bry. Cham. Chin. Dulc. Puls.
Look fixed on one point, staring, Cannab. Cic. Creos. Guaj. Hell. Hyosc. Igt. Mez. Ntr-c. Ran-b.
Looked at, children cannot bear to be, Ant. Ars. Cham.
Loquacity, Aloe. Arg. Ars. Bell. Borax. Bov. Canth. Caust. *Coff.* Croc. Cupr. Eugen. Glon. Grat. Gum-gut. *Hyosc.* Iod. Kali-jod. *Lach.* Lachn. Mgn-c. Meph. Ntr-c. Op. *Par. Selen.* Stann. *Stram.* Tabac. Tar. Teucr. Therid. Thuj. Verat.
— talks to himself, Rhus.

— — about murder, incendiarism, rats, Calc.
Love, disappointed, Hyosc. Igt. Phosp-ac.
— — with jealousy, anger and incoherent talk, H₁osc.
— — silent grief, Igt. Phosp-ac.
Malice, *Acon. Anac.* Ars. *Bell.* Canth. Caps. Carb-an. Chin. Cupr. Guaj. *Hyosc. Lach.* Mosch. Ntr-c. Nitr-ac. *Nux.* Par. Petr. Plat. *Stram.*
Mania á potu, *Ars.* Bell. Calc. Cannab-inb. Coff. Dig. Hell. Hyosc. Lach. *Nux.* Op. Puls. Sep. *Stram.* Sulph.
Meditation, Amm-m. Cannab. Canth. Chin. Cic. Clem. Cocc. Creos. Hell. Hyosc. Igt. Lach. Mez. Ntr-c. Phosp. Phell. Plb. Ran-b. Rhus. Sabad. Sep. Staph. Sulph. *Thuj.*
Melancholy, Acon. Agn. All-cep. Alum. Anac. *Ars.* Asar. *Aur. Bell.* Berb. Cact. *Calc.* Carb-an. *Caust.* Chin. Clem. Cocc. Croc. Cupr. Cycl. Dig. Dros. Graph. *Hell. Hyosc. Igt.* Ind. Iod. Kali-c. *Lach. Lyc.* Merc. Ntr-c. *Ntr-m.* Nitr-ac. Nux-m. Nux. Phosp. Phosp-ac. Plat. *Plb. Puls. Rhus.* Ruta. Sec-c. Selen. *Seneg. Sep.* Sil. Staph. *Stram. Sulph.* Sulph-ac. Tabac. Tilia. *Verat.*
— religious, Ars. Aur. Bell. Igt. Hyosc. Lach. Nux. Psor. Puls. Selen. Sil. Stram.
Memory, acute, Anac. Aur. Bell. Coff. Croc. Cycl. *Hyosc.* Op. Phosp. Seneg.
— loss of, *Anac.* Bell. Bry. Camph. Con. Graph. *Hyosc.* Kali-c. Lac-can. Lach. Laur. Lyc. Ntr-m. Nux-m. Petr. Puls. Selen. Sil Staph. Stram. *Verat.*
— — weakness, of, Acon. *Alum. Anac.* Ars. *Aur.* Bar-c. Bell. Berb. Borax. *Bov.* Bry. Calc. Carb-veg. Caust. Clem. Colch. Con. Creos. Croc. Cycl. Dig. Graph. Guaj. Hell. *Hep.* Hyosc. Igt. *Lach. Laur.* Lyc. Merc. Merc-cor. Mez. Murex. Ntr-c. *Ntr-m.* Nitr-ac Nux-m. Oleand. *Op.* Petr. Plb. Puls. Rhus. Sabin. *Sep.* Sil. Spig. *Staph.* Stram. *Sulph.* Verb. *Viol-od.* Zinc.
— — for business, Creos. Hyosc. Kali-c. Phosp. Sabin. Selen. Sulph.
— — what is heard, Hyosc. Lach. Mez.
— — letters, when reading, Lyc.
— — proper names, Anac. Croc. Guaj. Oleand. Puls. Rhus. *Sulph.*
— — what one has read, Guaj. Hell. Phosp-ac. Staph.
— — has happened, Graph. Ntr-m. Sulph.
— — one has just spoken, Arn. Bar-c. Carb-an. Colch. Hell. Hep. Merc. Mez. Rhod. Sulph. Verat.
Memory, weakness of, sudden and periodical, Carb-veg.

I. MIND AND DISPOSITION.

Memory, weakness of, for things, names, Lyc. Rhus.
— — — — thought, Cocc. Colch. Hyosc. Ntr-m. Staph.
— — — words, Bar-c. Lyc.
Mental derangement from abuse of alcoholic drinks, Ars. Calc. Hep. Nux. Op. Stram.
— dulness, *Alum.* Amm-c. Ant. Ars. Bell. Calc. Cham. Cycl. Graph. *Hell.* Hyosc. *Lach. Laur. Lyc. Mez.* Ntr-c. *Ntr-m.* Nicc. *Nux.* Oleand. Op. *Phosp-ac.* Plb. Puls. *Ran-b.* Rheum. Rhus. Sil. *Staph.* Stram. Sulph. Thuj.
Mental relaxation, prostration, fatigue, Aur. Calc. Colch. Lach. Lyc. Mosch. Ntr-c. Ntr-m. *Nux.* Op. Puls. Rhus. Selen. Seneg. Sep. Sil. Spong. *Stann. Sulph.*
Mild temper, Ars. Calad. Cic. Cocc. Croc. Cupr. Igt. Kali-c. *Lyc.* Mosch. *Puls.* Sil. Stann. Sulph.
Mind, absence of, Acon. Agn. Alum. Amm-c. Anac. Aur. Bar-c. Bell. Bov. Calad. Caust. *Cham.* Chin. Colch. Creos. Daph. Elaps. Hell. Igt. Lac-can. Lyc. Mgn-c. Mosch. Ntr-c. Ntr-m. Nux-m Nux. Oleand. Phosp-ac. Plat. Plb. Puls. Rhus. Ruta. Sep. Verat.
— — periodical attacks of, short lasting, Fluor-ac.
— acuteness, Anac. Asa-f. Aur. Coff. Op. Verat. Viol-od.
— diminished power of, over body, Hell.
— oppression of, Evon. Graph. Iod. Ran-b.
— as if separated from the body, Anac.
Misanthropy, *Amm-c.* Anac. *Aur.* Bar-c. *Calc.* Cic. Hyosc. *Led.* Lyc. Ntr-m. *Phosp.* Plat. Puls. *Stann.*
Mischievous, Cupr. Lach. Nux.
Misplacing words, Alum. Amm-c. Arn. Bov. Calc. Cannab. Caust. Cham. Chin. Cocc. Con. Crotal. Graph. Hep. Hyosc. Kali-c. Lac-can. Lach. Lyc. Merc. Ntr-c. Ntr-m. *Nux.* Puls. Rhod. Sep. Sil. Sulph. Thuj.
Mistakes in calculating, Amm-c.
— — time, Cocc. *Lach.* Nux. Petr. Therid.
— — measure and weight and gives wrong answers, Nux.
— — speaking, *Amm-c. Calc.* Caust. *Cham.* Chin. Con. *Graph. Hep.* Kali-c. Mang. Merc. *Ntr-m. Nux.* Sep. Sil.
— — writing, Amm-c. Bov. Cannab. Cham. Chin. Crotal. Graph. Hep. *Lach.* Ntr-c. Ntr-m. Nux. Puls. Rhod. Sep.
Moaning, Acon. Bell. Cham. Cic. Cina. Coff. Colch. Graph. Hell. Igt. Merc. Mur-ac. Scill. Stram. (compare Groaning.)
Mocking, Ars. Chin. Ip. Lach. Plat. Par.
Monomania, Acon. Carb-veg. *Igt.* Nux-m. Puls. *Sil.* Stram. Thuj.
Moral feeling, want of, *Anac.* Bism. Con. Hyosc. *Laur.* Op. Sabad.
Morose, Acon. Arn. Bell. Bism. Canth. Caps. Caust. Cham. Clem. Colch. Coloc. Creos. Evon. Hyosc. Igt. Ip. Lach. *Led.* Lyc. Mgn-m. Mang. Mur-ac. Nux. Phosp. Prun. *Puls.* Rheum. Rhod. Sang. Sass. Sep. Stann. Sulph. *Thea.* Thuj. Verb. *Viol-tr.* Zinc.
Murder, inclination to, Ars. Chin. *Hep.* Hyosc. Lach. Stram.
Murdered, dread of being, Op. Phosp. Stram.
Murmuring, Apis. Bell. Hyosc. Lach. Lyc. Phosp-ac. Stram.
Muttering, *Bell.* Hyosc. Lach. Nux. Stram.
Naked, desires to be, Hyosc. Phosp.
Obstinacy, Acon. Alum. Amm-c. Arn. Bell. Calc. Caps. Dros. Igt. Kali-c. Lyc. Merc. Ntr-ac. *Nux.* Sil. Spong. Stram. Sulph. Zinc.
Offended humor, Merc.
Offended easily, Acon. Alum. Ars. Aur. Bov. Calc. Caps. Carb-veg. Caust. Cina. Cinnab. Cocc. Lyc. Plat. Puls. Sass. Sep. Sulph. Verat.
Openheartedness, Bov.
Oppression, Carb-veg. Iod. Laur. Tabac.
Overrating himself, Lach. Plat. (compare Pride.)
Peevishness, Acon. Aeth. Agar. Alum. Amm-c. *Amm-m.* Anac. Ant. Ars. Asar. Bar-c. Bell. Bism. Borax. Bov. Bry. *Calc.* Cannab. Canth. Caps. Carb-an. Carb-veg. Caust. Cham. Chin. *Cina.* Clem. Cocc. Colch. Coloc. Con. *Creos.* Cupr. Cycl. Dig. Eugen. *Evon.* Graph. *Grat.* Hep. Hydroc-ac. Igt. Ind. Ip. Kali-c. Lach. Lact. *Led.* Lyc. *Mang.* Merc. Mez. Mgn-c. Mgn-m. Mur-ac. Ntr-c. Ntr-m. Ntr-s. Nitr. Nux. Oleand. Petr. Phosp. *Phosp-ac. Puls.* Rheum. *Rhus.* Sabin. Samb. Sass. Scill. *Sil.* Spong. Stann. *Staph. Stront.* Sulph. *Sulph-ac.* Teucr. Thuj. Tong. Verat. Verb. *Zinc.*
— in evening, Mgn-c. Puls. *Zinc.*
— morning, Amm-c.
— open air, Aeth. Sabin.
Pertinacity, Caps. Dros. Stram.
Petulency, Phell. Spong.
Phlegmatic, Caps. Puls. Sabad. Seneg. (compare Indolence.)
Play, indisposition for, in children, Bar-c.
Pleased with his own taking, Par.
Possessed, condition as if, Anac. Hyosc.
Positiveness, Caust. Lach.
Praying, Aur. Bell. Puls. Stram. Verat.
Precipitation, hurry, Ars. Bov. Calad. Camph. *Igt.* Kali-c. Ntr-m. Puls.
Prediction of day of death, Acon.
Pride, Alum. Arn. Chin. Cupr. Ferr. Hyosc. Ip. *Lach.* Lyc. Par. *Plat.* Stram. Verat.
Projects, forms, Anac. Ang. *Chin.* Coff. Oleand.

Prophecying, Acon. Agar.
Prostration of mind, Cannab. Con. Dig. Graph. Hep. Iod. *Lach.* Laur. Led. Lyc. Merc. Ntr-c. *Ntr-m.* Nitr-ac. *Nux.* Petr. Plat. Sass. Selen. Seneg. Sep. Spong. Stann. Sulph Sulph-ac. Teucr. Zinc.
Pursued, fancies he is, Anac. Bell.
Pusillanimity, *Acon.* Alum. Anac. *Ang.* Aur. *Bar-c. Bry.* Canth. Carb-an. Carb-veg. Caust. *Chin.* Igt. Kali-c. Lyc. Mur-ac. Ntr-m. Nitr. Phosp. *Puls.* Ran-b. Sil. Sulph. Sulph-ac. Tabac. Verb. Zinc.
Quarrelsomeness, Acon. Alum. Arn. Ars. *Aur.* Bell. *Camph. Caust. Cham.* Croc. Crotal. Dulc. Ferr. Hyosc.*Igt.* Kali-jod. *Lach. Lyc. Merc.* Mez. Mosch. Nicc. Ntr-s. *Nux. Ran-b.* Ruta. Sacch. Sep. Verat.
— in afternoon, Dulc.
— — forenoon, Ran-b.
— — evening, Amm-c. Ntr-m.
Questions, declines to answer, Ambr. *Arn.* Coloc. Euphr. Phosp-ac. Verat.
Quiet, wants to be, Gels.
Rage, Ars. Bell. Canth. Cham. Cupr. Hyosc. Nitr-ac. Stram. Verat.
— after insults. Sang. Stram.
Rancor, Nitr-ac.
Rashness, Caps. Meny. Puls.
Reason, loss of, Ambr. Anac. Ars. Asa-f. *Aur.* Bell. Bry. Caps. Caust. Igt. Lach. Merc. Ntr-c. Ntr-m. *Petr.* Phosp-ac. Spong. Sulph. Sulph-ac. Thuj.
Recollection difficult, Berb. Iod. Mez. Thuj. (compare Obstupefaction, in next section.)
— vivid, Croc.
Relations, ignorance of his, Bell. Hyosc. Merc. Verat.
— mocking his, Sec-c.
Religious affections of the mind. Ars. Aur. Bell. Croc. Dig. *Hyosc.* Igt. *Lach. Lyc.* Nux. *Puls.* Selen. Sil. *Stram. Sulph.*
— feeling, absense of, Anac. Coloc.
Repentance, quick, Croc. Oleand.
Reproaches, Acon. *Ars.* Caps. Chin. Igt. *Lach.* Lyc. Ntr-m. Nux. Sep. Verat.
Repugnance, aversion to others, Amm-m. Aur. Calc. Fluor-ac. Stann.
— to his business, Crom. Puls. Sep.
— — music, Acon. Nux. Sabin.
Resentment, long after insults, Nitr-ac.
Reservedness, Alum. Aur. Bell. Bism. Calc. Caps Carb-an. Caust.Cham.Chin. Clem. Coloc. Cycl. Euph. Euphr. Grat. Hell. *Hyosc.* Igt. Ip. Lach. Lyc. Mgn-c. *Mang. Mur-ac.* Ntr-m. Nitr-ac. Nux. Ol-an. Op. Petr. Phosp-ac. Plat. Plb. *Puls.* Rheum.Sabad.Sabin.Spong.*Stann.* Verat.
Resistance, Caps. Nux.
Restlessness, *Acon.* Aeth. Aloe. Ambr.

Amm-c. Apis. Arg. Arn. *Ars. Asa-f.* Aur. *Bell.* Bov. *Bry.* Calc. Camph. Canth. Caps. *Carb-veg.Cham.*Chin.Cina. *Coloc.* Con. Cupr. Dig. Dros. *Dulc. Graph.* Hyosc. Igt. Iod. Ip.Kali-c. Kobalt. Lachn. *Lach.* Lam. *Laur.* Lyc. Mgn-c. Mgn-m. *Merc.* Mez Mosch.*Ntr-c. Nux.*Op.*Phosp.*Phosp-ac.*Plb.*Prun.*Puls.* Rheum. Rhus. *Sabad.* Samb. Sec-c. Sep. *Sil.* Sol-m. Spig. *Stann.* Staph. Stram. Sulph. Sulph-ac. *Tabac. Thuj.* Verat.
— when alone, Mez. *Phosp.*
— with short breathing and dyspnœa, Prun.
— sensation as if everything in abdomen was constricted, Mosch.
— fear of future, Bry.
— hysterical or hypochondrical,Asa-f.Valer.
— ending in rage, Canth.
— in evening, Carb-veg. Laur. Merc.Nux. Phosp.
— at night, (compare Sleep.)
— — driving one out of bed, Graph.
— — with tossing in bed, Acon. Cham. Cina. Ferr. Merc.
— — wants to go from one bed to the other, *Ars.* Bell. *Calc.* Cina. Cham. Hyosc. Mez. Rhus. Sep. Verat.
— during mental occupation, Ambr. Ntr-c.
— in open air, relieved, Laur.
— during a thunder storm, Ntr-c. Ntr-m. Phosp.
Revenge, Agar. Lach.
Rudeness, Ambr Eugen. Hell. *Hyosc.*Lyc. Nux-m. Nux. Op. Phosp. Stram. Verat.
Running about, insane, Bell.Canth.Hyosc. *Nux.* Stram. Verat.
Rhyming. Agar.
Rises sardonicus, Ran-sc. Sec-c. Sol-n. Zinc.
Sadness, Acon. *Agn. Ambr.* Amm-c.Anac. Ars. *Aur.* Bell. Bov. Bry. Cact. *Calc.* Cannab. Carb-an. Caust. Cham. Chelid. Chin. *Clem. Cocc.* Coff. Con. Croc. Dig. Ferr. Graph. Hell. Hep. Hyosc. *Igt.* Ind. Iod. Kali-c. Lact. Lam. Lyc. Mgn-c. Mgn-s. Meny. Mez. Mur-ac. Ntr-c. *Ntr-m.* Ntr-nitr. *Nitr-ac.* Nux. Oleand. *Ol-an.* Petr. Phell. Phosp. *Phosp-ac. Plat. Puls.* Ran-sc. Rhod. Rhus. Sec-c. Sil. Spig. Staph. Stram. Sulph. Tabac. Verat. Viol-od. Vihl-tr. Verat.
— when alone, Bov.
— by consolation, increased, Ntr-m.
— — complaining, relieved, Tabac.
— in the evening. Ant. Ars. Bar-c. Bov. Calc. Carb-an. Cast. Creos. Dig. Ferr. Graph. Hep. Kali-c. Lact. Lyc. Murex. Nitr-ac. Phosp. *Plat.* Ran-sc. Ruta. Seneg. Sep. Stram. Verat. Zinc.
— — bed, Ars. Graph. Stram. Sulph.
— — relieved, Amm-c.
— noon, Zinc.

I. MIND AND DISPOSITION.

Sadness, forenoon, Amm-c. Ant. Cannab. Graph. Phell.
— morning, Alum. Carb-an. Lach. Nitr-ac. Petr. Phosp. Plat.
— of pregnant females, Lach.
— in a room, Plat. Rhus.
— — sunshine, Stram.
— walking in the open air, Ant. Coff. Con. Phosp-ac. Sep. Sulph. Tabac.
Scolding, Bell. Caust. Cor-r. Dulc. Hydroph. Hyosc. Ip. Nux. Petr. Verat. Viol-od.
— without being angry, Dulc.
— with the pains, Cor-r.
Scrupulousness, Aur. Bar-c. Chin. Graph. Nux. Sil. Sulph. Thuj.
— anxious, Ars. Igt. Sulph.
Self-confidence, want of, Anac. Ang. Aur. Bar-c. Bry. Canth. Chin. Igt.Iod. Kali-c. Lyc. Mur-ac. Oleand. Puls. Rhus. Sil. Stram. Tabac. Therid.
— contradiction, Anac.
— control, want of, Lach.
— willed, Calc. Dros.
Senses vanishing of, Acon. Agar. Agn. Alum. Anac. Arn. Ars. Aasa-f. Aur. Bell. Bov. Bry. Calc. Camph. Canth. Caust. Chelid. Cic. Con. Dulc. Hyosc. Kali-c. Lach. Laur. Led. Lyc. Merc. Mosch. Ntr-m. Nux-m. Nux. Oleand. Ol-an. Op. Phosp. Phosp-ac. Plb. Ran-sc. Rhod. Rhus. Sec-c. Sil. Stann. Stram. Staph. Sulph. Tart. Verat. Zinc.
Sensibility of mind, Ang. Ant. Ars. Calc. Cannab. Canth. Coff. Con. Crotal. Creos. Iod. Igt. Lach. Lyc. Nux. Phosp. Plat. Puls. Samb. Seneg. Sep. Sulph. Viol-od.
— excessive, Arn. Cocc. Coff. Nux. (compare in Generalities.)
Sensitiveness, Acon. Alum. Anac. Ang. Ars. Aur. Bell. Bov. Calc. Camph. Canth. Carb-veg. Caust. Cham. Cina. Cocc. Colch. Dros. Iod. Hep. Kali-c. Lach. Lyc. Mgn-c. Mez. Ntr-c. Nitr. Nux. Phosp. Phosp-ac. Plat. Puls. Samb. Sass. Seneg. Sep. Spig. Stann. Staph. Sulph. Viol-od.
Sentimentality, Acon. Calc. Cast. Coff. Igt. Lach.
Serenity, Bell. Coff. Croc. Lach. Laur. Lyc. Ntr-m. Op. Petr. Phosp. Plat. Seneg. Spig. Stram. Verat. Zinc.
Seriousness, Alum. Ambr. Amm-m. Ars. Aur. Bell. Borax. Cham. Chin. Cina. Euphr. Igt. Led. Merc. Nux-m. Phosp-ac. Spig. Staph. Sulph-ac.
Shamelessness, Hell. Hyosc. Mosch. Nux. Op. Phosp. Stram. Verat.
Shrieking, Acon. Arn. Ars. Bell. Borax. Bry. Canth. Caust. Cham. Coff. Cupr. Hyosc. Igt. Ip. Lyc. Nux. Plat. Puls. Rheum. Seneg. Sep. Stram. Verat.

— for aid, Plat.
— in children, Bell. Borax. Cham. Cina. Coff. Ip. Jalap. Rheum. Senna.
Sighing, Bry. Hell. Igt. Lach. Plb. Puls. Rhus.
Silence, Aur. Bell. Carb-an. Caust. Cham. Euph. Euphr. Hell. Hyosc. Igt. Ip. Lyc. Mang. Mur-ac. Nux. Phosp-ac. Plat. Plb. Sil. Verat.
Singing, Acon. Bell. Cocc. Croc. Cupr. Hipp. Hyosc. Mgn-c. Ntr-m. Op. Phosp. Plat. Spong. Stram. Tabac. Teucr. Therid. Verat.
Sits quite stiff, Cham. Hyosc. Puls. Sep. Stram.
— — still, Cham. Puls.
— as if wrapped in deep, sad thoughts and notices nothing, Cocc.
Slanderous disposition, Amm-c. Anac. Ars. Bell. Borax. Hyosc. Ip. Lyc. Nitr-ac. Nux. Petr. Sep. Stram. Verat.
Smaller, things appear, Plat. Stram.
Sobbing, Hell. Lob.
Softness, gentleness, Ars. Igt.
Solicitude, Acon. Alum. Amm-m. Arn. Ars. Aur. Bell. Calad. Calc. Caust. Cham. Chelid. Chin. Cina. Cocc. Dig. Euph. Graph. Igt. Iod. Mgn-s. Meny. Merc. Mur-ac. Nicc. Phell. Ran-c. Rhus. Sep. Sil. Spig. Staph. Stront. Sulph-ac. Tart. Tabac. Verat. Zinc.
— about domestic affairs, Bar-c. Puls. Rhus. Sep. Sulph.
— — — want of, Citr-ac.
— — futurity, Anac. Ant. Arn. Bar-c. Bry. Caust. Chelid. Cic. Con. Dig. Dros. Dulc. Lach. Mang. Ntr-c. Ntr-m. Petr. Phosp. Phosp-ac. Psor. Spig. Stann. Staph. Sulph. Tart. Thuj.
— — health, Acon. Arn. Ars. Bry. Calc. Igt. Kali-c. Lac-can. Lach. Ntr-m. Nitr-ac. Nux. Phosp. Phosp-ac. Psor. Puls. Sep. Staph. Sulph.
— — his soul's welfare, Lyc. Puls. Sulph.
Solitude, aversion to, Ars. Bism. Bov. Cadm. Calc. Clem. Con. Droc. Lyc. Mez. Phosp. Sep. Stram. Verb.
— love of, Aur. Bar-c. Bell. Calc. Chin. Cic. Cinnab. Cupr. Dig. Elaps. Eugen. Graph. Hyosc. Igt. Kali-c. Lach. Led. Lyc. Mgn-m. Meny. Ntr-c. Nicc. Nux. Rhus. Sep. Stann.
Somnambulism, Acon. Alum. Bry. Ntr-m. Op. Petr. Phosp. Rheum. Sil. Stann. Zinc.
Sorrow, Acon. Alum. Amm-c. Amm-m. Anac. Arn. Ars. Bar-c. Caust. Chelid. Cic. Dros. Graph. Igt. Ntr-c. Ntr-m. Nitr. Nux. Op. Phosp-ac. Puls. Spig. Stann. Thuj.
— of futurity, Anac. Arn. Bar-c. Caust. Chelid. Cic. Con. Dig. Dros. Dulc.

I. MIND AND DISPOSITION.

Kali-c. Lach. Mang. Ntr-c. Ntr-m. Phosp. Phosp-ac. Rhus. Spig. Stann. Sulph. Thuj.
Sorrow in evening, Ars. Dig.Graph.Kali-c.
— — — in bed, Ars. Graph.
— — morning in bed, Alum.
— night, Dulc.
— — and day, Caust.
Sorrowful thoughts and reflections at night, Caust.
Spirituous liquors, mental derangements from, *Ars.* Bell. Carb-veg. Chin. Coff. Dig. Hell. Hyosc. Lach. Merc. Ntr-c. Nux. *Op.* Puls. *Stram.* Sulph.
Spitting, Ars. Bell. Cannab. Cupr. Hyosc. Merc. Stram.
Starts, Ang. Con. Kali-c. Ntr-m.
— from least noise, Borax. Kali-jod. Sabad.
— when touched, Kali-c.
Striking, Bell. Canth. Hyosc. Lyc. Ntr-c. Nux. Phosp. Plat. Stram. Stront.
— in children, Cina.
Stubborn, Acon. Arn. Caps. Dig. Dros. Lyc. Nitr-ac. Phosp. Sil. Sulph.
Suicide, disposition to commit, Ambr. Amm-c. *Ars.* Aur. Bell. Carb-veg. Caust. Chin. Creos. Dros. *Hep.* Lach. Merc. Nitr-ac. *Nux.* Psor. *Puls.* Rhus. Sec-c. Sep. Spig. Stram.
— sly disposition for, Aur.
— by drowning, Ant. Bell. Dros. Hell. Hyosc. Puls. Sec-c. Verat.
— — hanging, Ars.
— — shooting, Ant. Aur. Carb-veg. Hep. Nux. Puls.
— — throwing himself from a height, Bell.
Superstitious, Con.
Suspicious, Bar-c. *Bell.* Cham. Dros. Hell. Hyosc. *Lach.* Lyc. Merc. Op. Puls.
Talk, improper, Hyosc. Nux-m.
Talking, slow, Thuj.
— quick, hasty, Ambr. Ars. Bell. Bry. Cocc. Hep. Lach. Merc. Thuj. Verat.
— about the faults of others, Ars. Verat.
— incoherently, Lach. Rhus.
— indistinctly, Hyosc.
— like a drunken man, Lyc.
— nonsense, with eyes open, Hyosc.
— swallows his words when, Staph.
— of animals, battles, Bell.
— to himself, Mosch.
Talk, disinclination to, Acon. Agar. Ambr. Amm-m. *Arg.* Arn. Arn. Ars. *Bell.* Berb. Bry. Cact. Calc. Caust. Cham. Chin. Clem. Cocc. Coloc. Cycl. Dig. Euphr. Grat. Hell. Hipp. Igt. Ip. Lach. Lyc. Mgn-c. Mgn-m. Mgn-s. Meny. Merc. Mez. Murex. Mur-ac. Ntr-m. Ntr-s. Nicc. Nitr-ac. Nux-jug. Nux. Ol-an. Ox-ac. Petr. *Phosp-ac.* Plb. *Puls.* Rheum. Sacch. Sabin. Sil. Spong. Stann. Staph. Sulph-ac. Tabac. Thea.

Thuj. Tong. Verat. Viol-od. Viol-tr. Zinc.
Tearing things, Bell. Hyosc. Stram. Verat.
Teeth, desires to pull out his, Bell.
Temerity, Op.
Tenderness, Croc.
Terror, Acon. Calc. Carb-an. Kali-c. Murex. Phosp. Sabad. Samb.
Thieves, dread of, *Ars.* Con. Igt. *Lach.* Merc. Ntr-m. Sil. Zinc.
Thinking, difficulty of *Alum.* Amm-c. Aur. Bell. Berb. *Calc.* Carb-veg. Cochlear. Con. Dig. *Hell.* Hydroc-ac. *Hyosc.*Lach. Lact. Lyc. Meny. Ntr-c. *Ntr-m.* Nitr-ac. Nux-m. *Nux.* Oleand. Op. Petr. Phosp-ac. Rhus. Sec-c. Sep. Sil. *Staph.* Stram. Sulph. Therid. Thuj.
— — with chronic dulness of mind and sensation as if a board were pressed against the head, Calc.
— — — dullness of head, Sulph.
— inability for, Acon. Alum. Cycl. Hell. Hydroc-ac. Laur. Lyc. Ntr-c. Ntr-m. Phosp-ac. Selen. Sep. Sil. Sol-m. Spig. Thuj.
Thought, confusion of, Amm-c. Ars. Asa-f. Borax. Cannab. Carb-an. *Chin.* Con. Lact. Laur. *Ntr-c.* Ntr-m. Nux. Phosp-ac. Sulph. Verat.
— difficult connection of, Amm-c. Asa-f. Borax. Caps. *Chin.* Lact. Laur. *Ntr-c.* Nux. Phosp-ac. Sulph. Verat.
— flow of, Agar. Alum. Ambr. Anac. Ang. Ars. Borax. Bry. *Calc.* Canth. Caust. *Chin.* Cocc. Coff. Coloc. Con. Graph. Hep. Hyosc. Kali-c. Lach. *Lyc.* Nitr. *Nux.* Oleand. *Op. Phosp.* Phosp-ac. Plat. *Puls.* Rhus. Sabad. *Sep.* Spong. Staph. *Stram. Sulph.* Verb. Viol-od. Viol-tr. Zinc.
— deficiency of, Alum. *Amm-c.* Aur. Calc. Caust. Hell. Hyosc. Ip. *Lach.* Lyc. *Ntr-m.* Nux-m. Oleand. *Phosp-ac.* Rhus. Sep. Sil. Staph. Thuj. Verat.
— instability of, Acon. Berb. Chin. Lyc. Nux-m. Staph.
— vanishing of, Anac. Asar. Borax. Calc. Camph. *Cannab.* Canth. Carb-an. Cham. Coff. Creos. Cupr. Evon. Guaj. Hell. Hep. Iod. Kali-c. *Lach.* Merc. Mez. Nitr-ac. Nux-m. Ol-an. Puls. Ran-b. Rhod. Staph.
— slow flow of, *Alum.* Amm-c. Aur. *Calc.* Chin. Dig. Hell. Hyosc. *Lach.* Lyc. Ntr-c. *Ntr-m.* Nux-m. *Nux.* Petr. Rhus.
— fixed immovable, Iod.
— dwells upon unpleasant subjects, Benz-ac.
Thoughtfulness, profound meditation, Amm-m. Cannab. Canth. Cham. Cic. Cocc. Igt. Lach. Ntr-c. Phosp. Plb. Rhus. Sabad. *Sep. Staph.* Sulph.
Thoughtlessness, Agn. Alum. Ambr.

I. MIND AND DISPOSITION.

Amm-c. Amm-m. Anac. Asa-f. *Bell.* Bov. Cannab. Canth. Caust. Cham. Cic. Clem. Coff. Creos. Croc. Cupr. *Evon.* Guaj. Hell. Igt. Kali-c. *Lach.* Merc. Mez. Ntr-c. Ntr-m. Nitr-ac. *Nux-m.* Phosp. *Phosp-ac.* Rhod. Rhus. Ruta. Sep. Spig. Valer. Verat. Zinc.

Time seems to pass too quickly, Cocc. Therid.

— — — — slowly, Arg-n. Nux. Pallad.

Timidity, Acon. Alum. Anac. Ang. Aur. Bar-c. Bell. Bry. Canth. Carb-an. Carb-veg. Caust. Chin. Igt. Kali-c. Lyc. Mgn-c. Mur-ac. Ntr-m. Nitr-ac. Nitr. Phosp. *Puls.* Ran-b. Sil. Sulph. Sulph-ac. Tabac. Verb. Zinc.

Unconsciousness, Aeth. Apis. *Arn.* Ars. Bar-c. *Bell.* Bry. Calc. *Camph.* Canth. Cham. Cic. Cocc. Colch. Cupr. *Hell. Hyosc.* Kali-c. Lach. *Laur.* Lyc. Mgn-c. Merc. *Mur-ac. Ntr-m.* Nitr-ac. *Nux.* Oleand. *Op.* Phosp. *Phosp-ac. Plat.* Plb. *Puls.* Rhus. *Sec-c. Stram.* Tabac. Tart. Verat.

— sudden, Kali-c.
— from congestion of blood to the head, Bell. Hyosc.
— with deep heavy sleep, preceded by tingling in head and limbs, Sec-c.
— — loss of speech and motion, Laur.
— in forehead, somnolency (eyes closed), Phosp-ac.
— cannot open the eyes, Gels.
— with vertigo, Nux-m.
— in the afternoon, in a warm room, with sleepiness, Puls.
— and drowsiness in head, on rising in the morning, Rhod.
— with tingling in head and pains in limbs, better from motion, Rhus.
— — tingling in head and pains in limbs, worse from motion, Sec-c.
— — pressure in eyes and obscuration of sight, Seneg.
— — vanishing of sight and hearing and convulsive motions of head, Stram.

Verses, writes, Agar. Ant-cr.

Vexation, (compare Fretfulness.)

Vehemence, Aur. Bry. Camph. Carb-veg. Caust. Hep. Hyosc. Led. Lyc. Merc. Ntr-m. Nux. Sep.

Visions, Bell. Berb. Bry. Carb-veg. Dulc. Hell. Hep. *Hyosc.* Kali-c. Mgn-m. Ntr-c. Nitr-ac. Nux. *Op.* Phosp. *Samb. Stram.* Sulph.

— frightful, *Bell.* Bry. Op. Puls. *Stram.*

Vivacity, Alum. Ang. Cannab. Chin. Coff. Crotal. Cupr. Cycl. Gels. Glon. Hipp. Hyosc. Ntr-c. Petr-c. Phosp-ac. Sulph-ac. Verat.

Walks fast, Arg-n.

Wandering talk, Acon. Aeth. Arn. Ars. Aur. *Bell. Bry.* Calc. *Camph.* Canth. Cham. Chin. Cic. Cina. Coloc. Cupr. Dulc. *Hyosc.* Igt. Kali-c. *Lach. Lyc.* Merc. Nux-m. Nux. *Op.* Phosp. *Plat.* Plb. Puls. Rheum. Rhus. Sabin. Sec-c. Spong. *Stram.* Sulph. *Verat.*

— — of business, Bry. Hyosc.
— — at night, Aur. Bell. Bry. Goloc. Dig. Op. Rheum. Sep. Sulph.

Wanting pastime, Plb.

Weariness of life, Ambr. Amm-c. Ant. Ars. Bell. Berb. Carb-veg. Creos. Grat. Lach. Merc. Ntr-c. Ntr-m. Nitr-ac. Phosp. Plb. Sep. Sil. Staph. Sulph-ac. Thuj. Verat.

Wearisomeness, Acon. Aeth. Alum. Amm-m. Anac. Ant. Arn. Ars. Asar. Bell. Bism. Bov. Bry. Calc. Cannab. Caps. Carban. Caust. Cham. Chin. Clem. Cocc. Colch. Coloc. Con. Creos. Cupr. Cycl. Dig. *Evon.* Graph. *Grat.* Guaj. Hep. Igt. Ind. Ip. Kali-c. Lach. Led. Lyc. *Mang.* Merc. Mez. Mur-ac. Ntr-c. Ntr-m. Ntr-s. Nitr-ac. Nux. Oleand. Petr. Phosp. *Phosp-ac.* Plat. Puls. Ran-b. Rat. Rheum. Rhus. Sabin. Samb. Sass. Scill. Sep. Spong. *Staph. Stront.* Sulph. *Sulph-ac.* Teucr. Thuj. Tong. Verb. Viol-tr.

— in the evening, Mgn-c. Puls. *Zinc.*
— — morning, Amm-c.
— — open air, Aeth. Sabin.

Weep, inclination to, *Acon.* Alum. Amm-c. Apis. Arn. Ars. *Aur.* Bar-c. *Bell.* Berb. Borax. Bry. *Calc.* Camph. Canth. Carb-an. Carb-veg. Cast. *Caust. Cham.* Chelid. Chin. Cina. *Coff.* Coloc. Con. Creos. *Dig.* Graph. *Hep. Igt. Iod.* Kali-c. Kali-jod. Lac-can. Lach. Laur. *Lyc.* Mgn-m. Mgn-s. Meny. Merc. Mez. Mosch. Ntr-c. *Ntr-m.* Nitr-ac. Nux. Petr. Phosp-ac. *Plat.* Plb. *Puls.* Rheum. *Rhus.* Ruta. Sep. Sil. Spong. Stann. Stram. Staph. *Sulph.* Sulph-ac. Tart. Verat. Viol-tr.

— when addressed, Staph.
— after rage, Arn.
— in day time, Caust.
— — children, Ars. Bell. Borax. Camph. Caust. Cham. Cina. Coff. Graph. Hyosc. Igt. Kali-c. Lyc. Nitr-ac. Puls. Rheum. Seneg. Sil.
— — — when touched, Ant. Cina. Tart.
— — evening, Amm-c. Calc. Carb-an. Graph. Kali-c. Kali-chl. Lact. Lyc.
— — — relieved, Amm-c. Cast.
— — morning, Amm-c. Borax. Carb-an. Creos. Prun. Puls. Spong.
— at night, Alum. Amm-c. Bar-c. Borax. Calc. Carb-an. Caust. Cham. Cina. Con. Igt. Kali-c. Kali-jod. Lyc. Mgn-c. Merc. *Ntr-m. Nux.* Phosp. Puls. Rhus. Sil. Spong. Stann. Tabac. Thuj.

16   I. MIND AND DISPOSITION.

Weep inclination to, by music excited, Creos. Graph. Ntr-nitr. Ntr-s. Nux. Thuj.
— — during sleep, Alum. Calc. Carb-an. Caust. Cham. Con. Igt. Kali-c. Kali-jod. Lyc. Mgn-c. *Ntr-m. Nux.* Phosp. Puls. Rhus. Sil. Stann. Tabac. Thuj.
Weeping, whining, Alum. Ars. *Bell. Bry.* Canth. *Carb-an. Caust. Cham.* Cic. Cina. Cocc. Coff. Colch. Cupr. *Graph.* Hell. Hyosc. Igt. Ip. Kali-c. Merc. Mez. *Ntr-m.* Phosp. *Plat.* Puls. Ran-b. Rheum. Samb. Scill. *Sep.* Sil. *Staph.* Stram. Sulph. Verat. Zinc.
— and lamentation with hoarse voice, Brom.
— at night, Amm-c. Anac. Arn. Ars. Bry. Caust. Cham. *Chin.* Cina. Hyosc. Igt. Ip. *Lach.* Lyc. Merc. Ntr-m. Nitr-ac. *Nux.* Op. Phosp. Phosp-ac. Rheum. Sulph. Verat.
— during sleep, Caust. Cham. Chin. Igt. Làch. Nitr-ac. *Nux.*
Will, want of control of, Apis.
Wildness, Acon. Mosch. Op. Petr. Phosp. Phosp-ac. Tabac. Tart.
Wit, Caps. Cocc. Croc. *Lach.* Spong.

Words, deficiency of, Anac. Caps. *Cham.* Nux. Phosp-ac. *Thuj.*
Work, inclination to, Cic. Dig. Euphr. Sass. Verat.
— — with heat and tremor, Psor.
— disinclination for, Agar. Aloe. *Alum.* Amm-c. Amm-m. Anac. Arn. Ars. Asa-f. Bar-c. *Bell.* Borax. Cadm. Calc. Calc-ph. Caust. Cham. *Chin.* Clem. Cocc. Coff. Colch. Coloc. *Con.* Croc. Cupr. Cycl. Dig. Dros. Evon. *Graph.* Hyosc. *Igt.* Iod. Ip. Kali-b. Kali-c. *Lach.* Lact. Laur. Mgn-m. Merc. Mez. Mur-ac. Ntr-c. *Ntr-m. Nitr-ac.* Nux-jug. *Nux. Oleand.* Par. Petr. *Phosp.* Plb. Puls. Ran-b. Ran-sc. Rhod. Rhus. Rumex. Ruta. Sabad. Sass. Scill. Sec-c. Sep. Sil. Spong. Staph. Sulph. Tabac. Tar. Teucr. *Therid.* Tong. Verb. Viol-tr. *Zinc.*
— — mental, Agar. Chin. Cinnab. Colch. Kali-b. Iod. Nitr-ac. Par. Petr. Ran-sc. Rumex. Scill. Spig. Staph. Sulph. Teucr.
— — desire for, Brom. Kobalt. Therid.
— — complaints from, Lyc. Ntr-m.
Yielding, pliable mind, Lyc. Puls. Sil.

2. Sensorium.

CLOUDINESS, GIDDINESS, VERTIGO.

Cloudiness, Bell. Bry. Calad. Cocc. Crot. Lact. Laur. Mgn-m. Merc. *Nux. Op.* Phell. Rheum. Samb. Valer.
— dull, Amm-m. Bism. *Calc. Caust.* Cycl. Dig. Iod. *Kali-c.* Lyc. Mgn-m. Mgn-s. Merc. Ntr-m. Ol-an. Pæon. *Phosp.* Ran-b. Samb. *Sil.* Staph. Tart. Verat.
— with cough, Rumex.
— like intoxication, *Agar.* Alum. Ant. *Arg.* Aur. *Bell.* Berb. Bov. Bry. *Camph.* Cannab. *Caps.* Caust. Cham. Cocc. Cocc-c. Con. Cor-r. Creos. Croc. Eugen. Gels. *Graph.* Hydroc-ac. Hyosc. Kali-b. Kali-c. *Laur. Led.* Lyc. Mez. Mosch. Nux-jug. Nux-m. Nux. Op. Phosp-ac. Plb. *Puls.* Rheum. Rhod. *Rhus.* Sec-c. Sil. Spig. Stram. Thuj. Tong. Valer. Verat.
— with diarrhœa, Gels.
— — — delirium, craziness or insensibility, Nux-m.
— in the morning, Agar. Alum. Bell. Bism. *Calc.* Carb-an. Cham. Graph. Iod. Mgn-m. Merc. Phosp. Verat.
— — — evening, Sil.

— after eating and drinking, Bell Cocc. Croc.
— in open air, *Agar.*
— — — relieved, *Amm-m.*
— after scratching behind the ear, Calc.
— in the sun, Ntr-c.
— from tobacco smoking, Alum.
— when walking, Camph.
— from a little beer, Coloc. Con. Kali-chl.
— — — wine, Bov. Con. Cor-r.
— with drowsiness, Arg. Tong.
— — hard stools, Kobalt.
— tremor, Calc.
Dizziness, confusion, indistinctness. Acon. Aeth. Alum. Ambr. Ang. Arn. *Asar.* Bell. Bism. *Bry. Calc.* Caps. Caust. Chin. Cor-r. Croc. Croton. Diad. Dig. Dros. Hipp. Hyosc. Iod. Kali-b. Kali-c. Mgn-c. Mgn-m. Mgn-s. Meny. Merc. Mez. Ntr-m. Ntr-nitr. *Nux-m. Nux.* Ol-an. Op. Par. Phosp. Phosp-ac. *Plat.* Plb. Puls. Ran-b. Rheum. *Rhod.* Rhus. Samb. Sec-c. Selen Seneg. *Sep.* Spig.

2. SENSORIUM.

Staph. Sulph. Sulph-ac. *Tart.* Therid. Thuj. Tong. Valer. Verat. Viol-tr. Zinc.
Dizziness in the occiput, Ambr. Carb-an. Plb. Sec-c. Tong.
— on one side, Sulph-ac.
— like a board before the head, Calc. Cocc. Dulc. Plb.
— as from coryza, Berb.
— — — fatigue, Ntr-m.
— gloomy, Ang. Arg. Calad. Clem. Dig. Meny. Merc. Mez. Ntr-m. Nitr. *Nux.* Op. Phosp-ac. Puls. Rheum. Samb. Thuj. Valer.
— long continued, Calc.
— as if muddled, Agar. Anac. Ant. Ars. Asa-f. Bry. Cor-r. Euphr. Ferr. Meny. Mercurial. Nux Puls. Sec-c. Seneg. Staph. Tabac. Thuj. Verb. Viol-od. Viol-tr.
— — — nailed up, *Acon. Aeth.* Mgn-s. Plat.
— painful, Ang. Arn. Asa-f. *Asar.* Caust. Diad. Dros. *Ntr-m.* Nux-m. Plat. Sec-c. Viol-od.
— as after seminal emissions, Caust. Mez. Phosp-ac.
— like smoke in the brain, Arg. Sulph-ac.
— stunning, Ang. Arg. Asar. Aur. *Cocc.* Croc. Dulc. Kali-c. Mgn-m. Mgn-s. Mez. Par. Rheum. Tart. Verb.
— as if unrefreshed by sleep, Ruta.
— — from watching all night, Ambr. Bry. Chin. *Nux.* Puls.
— in the morning, Clem. Mgn-m. Phosp. *Rhod.* Ruta. Thuj. Zinc.
— — — evening, Euphr. Ruta.
— at night, Psor.
— after dinner, Nux. (compare, after meals.)
— from mental exertion, Cocc.
— in the open air, relieved, Ars. Meny.
— when at rest, Ntr-c.
— in a room, Acon. Ars. Meny. Ntr-c.
— — — warm room, Acon.
— by supporting the head, relieved, Diad.
— when walking, Thea.
— alternating with clearness of ideas, Murex.
— with affections of the eyes, Croc. Op. Rheum. Seneg
— — drowsiness, Rhod. Tart.
— — knocking in the forehead, Ang.
— — nausea, Thuj.
Fatigue of the head, by mental labor, *Aur.* Bar-m. *Calc.* Cinnab. Colch. Graph. Igt. Lyc. Mgn-c. *Ntr-c.* Ntr-m. *Nux.* Petr. Phosp. Plat. *Puls.* Selen. Sep. *Sil.* Sulph.
— in general, Led.
— from nocturnal occupation, Colch. Selen.
Stupefaction, Acon. Agar. Alum. *Arn.* Ars. Asa-f. *Bell.* Bov. Bry. Bufo. Calc. Carb-an. Cina. Cycl. Dulc. Hell. *Hyosc.* Lach. *Laur. Led.* Mgn-m. Merc. Mosch. Nux. Oleand. *Op.* Phosp *Phosp-ac.* *Plb.* Puls. Rhus. Sabin. *Sec-c.* Seneg. Sep. Spig. Stann. Stram. Sulph. Tabac. *Tart.* Valer. *Verat.* Verb. Zinc.
— in the morning, Carb-an. Rhod.
— when reflecting and talking, Borax.
Stupor, Apis. Lach. Phosp-ac. Rhus.
— with sweat, Kali-c.
— — yawning and nausea, Jatr.
— — somnolency without snoring, eyes closed, Phosp-ac.
— — tingling in head and pains in limbs, worse from motion, Sec-c.
— — tingling in head and pains in limbs, better from motion, Rhus.
Vertigo. giddiness, *Acon.* Actea-r. *Aeth. Agar.* Alum. *Ambr.* Anim-c. Amm-m. *Anac.* Ant. Arg-n. *Arn.* Asar. *Bell.* Berb. Borax. Bry. *Calc.* Calc-ph. Camph. Carb-an. Carb-veg. Caust. Cham. Chin. Cic. *Cocc.* Con. Croc. Croton. Cupr. *Dig.* Eugen. Euphr. Ferr. Gels. Glon. Graph. Hell. Hep. *Hyosc.* Igt. Ip. Kali-c. Kali-chl. Lach. Lact. *Laur.* Lob. Lyc. Mgn-c. Mgn-m. Mgn-s. *Merc. Mosch.* Ntr-c. *Ntr-m.* Ntr-s. Nicc. Nitr-ac. Nux-m. *Nux.* Oleand. Ol-an. Op. Par. *Petr. Phosp.* Phosp-ac. Plat. *Plb.* Pod. Prun. *Puls.* Ran-b. Ran-sc. Rhod. *Rhus.* Sabad. Sass. Sec-c. Selen. Seneg. Sep. *Sil.* Spig. Spong. Stann. Stram. *Sulph.* Sulph-ac. *Tabac.* Tar. Tart. Thea. Therid. *Thuj.* Valer. Verat. Verb. Viol-od. Viol-tr. Zinc.
— in cerebellum, Zinc.
— — forehead, Rheum.
— — occiput, Chin. Zinc.
— of almost every kind, *Nux. Phosp. Sec-c. Sil.* Sulph.
— along the back, rising up, *Sil.*
— chronic. Ntr-m. Nux. *Petr. Phosp.* Sec-c.
— in a circular motion, Con.
— with a drawing sensation, Zinc.
— making one fall, *Acon.* Agar. Alum. Ang. Arn. Ars. *Bell.* Berb. Cannab. Caust. *Cic.* Cocc. Coloc. Con. Creos. Croton. Dros. Euph. Ferr. Lact. Led. Mgn-m. Mgn-s. Mez. Ntr-m. *Phell.* Plb. Puls. *Ran-b.* Rheum. Rhod. *Rhus.* Ruta. Sabin. Scill. Sil. Spig. Spong. Tereb. Zinc.
— — backwards, Bell. Led. Rhus.
— — forwards, Arn. Cic. Elaps. Ferr. Lyc. Ntr-m. *Ran-b.* Rhus. Sil.
— — sideways, Benz-ac. Cannab. Con. Dros. Euph. Mez. Rheum. Scill. Zinc.
— — to left side, Anac. Aur. Bell. Cic. Dros. Euph. Lach. Mez. Ntr-c. Spig. Sulph. Zinc.
— — to right side, Ferr.

Vertigo, false, originating in sight and not in the brain, Puls.
— reeling, Bell. Bry. Camph. Caust. Cic. Croc. Ferr. Lyc. Mgn-m. Nux-m.Ol-an. Phosp-ac. Sec-c. Seneg. Spong. Stram. Tabac. Tar. Tereb. Thuj. Verat. Viol-tr.
— as from riding in a carriage, Ferr.
— — rocking, Calad.
— from the stomach proceeding, Kali-c.
— like swimming, Ox-ac.
— — — in bed, Lact.
— — swinging, Calad. Ferr. Merc. Thuj. Zinc.
— turning, Acon. Anac. *Arn.* Asa-f. *Bell.* Bar-m. Berb. Bism. Bry. Calad. Chelid. Cic. Con. Cupr. Euph. Evon. Ferr. Grat. Hydroc-ac. Lact. *Lyc.* Mur-ac. Ntr-m. Ntr-s. *Nux. Oleand. Phosp.* Puls. Ran-b. Rhod. Ruta. *Staph.* Tabac. Tilia. *Valer. Verat. Viol-od.*
— in the morning, *Agar.* Alum. Amm-c. Bell. Bov. Calc. Carb-an. Cham. Graph. Iod. Hipp. Kali-c. Lach. Lact. Lyc. Mgn-c. Mgn-m. Mgn-s. Nicc. Nitr-ac. *Nux.* Ol-an. *Phosp.* Puls. Rhus. Scill. Sep. *Sil. Sulph.* Tellur. Verat. Zinc.
— — bed, Con. Graph. Lach.
— when rising from bed, Mgn-s. Sulph.
— at noon, Arn. Mgn-m. Mgn-s. Ntr-s. Nux. Phosp.
— in the afternoon, Ambr. Benz-ac. Kali-c. Merc. Nux. Phosp. Puls. Rhus. Sep. Sil. Staph.
— — — evening, Amm-c. Apis. Ars. Calc. Carb-veg. Graph. Hep. Kali-c. Mgn-c. Merc. Ntr-s. Nicc. Nitr-ac. *Nux. Phosp. Phosp-ac.* Plat. Puls. Rhus. Spong. Sulph.
— — — — in bed, Lach. *Nux.* Rhus. Staph.
— at night, Amm-c. Calc. Caust. Ntr-c. Phosp. Spong. Sulph. Zinc-ox.
— — different times, *Phosp. Sec-c. Sil. Sulph.*
— after anger, Calc.
— when ascending, Borax.
— — — an eminence, Calc. Con. Sulph.
— — casting down the eyes, Kalm. Oleand. Spig.
— — closing the eyes, Apis. Ars. Calad. Grat. Lach. Thuj. Therid.
— from coffee, Cham.
— in cold stage of intermittent, Caps.
— from congestion of blood, Cact.
— when crossing running water, Ang. Brom. Ferr. Sulph.
— — coughing, Nux.
— — descending, Ferr. Mercurial.
— while eating, Arn. Mgn-m.
— when entering into the open air, Ran-b.
— — exercising, Chin. Cycl. Kali-c.
— — — the arms, Berb. Sep.
— after fright, Op.
— from gaping, Agar.
— when gazing for a long time at some-

thing, Oleand. Sass.
— from indigestion, Sacch.
— when kneeling, Mgn-c.
— — leaning against something, Cycl.
— — — left cheek against hand, Verb.
— from light of sun, Agar. Nux.
— when looking back, Con.
— — — at a height, Cupr. Plb. Thuj.
— — — out of a window, Ox-ac.
— — — up, Calc. Nux. Puls. Sang. Sil. Thuj.
— — — sideways, Thuj.
— — lying down, Ferr. Kalm. Nitr-ac. Nux. Oleand. Ox-ac. Rhus.
— after lying down, Calad. Mgn-c.
— when lying, Apis. Calad. Con. Merc. Rhod. Staph. *Thuj.*
— — relieved, Arn. Cupr. Phell. Stann.
— — on back, Merc. Nux. Sulph.
— during meals, Arn. Mgn-m.
— after meals, Cham. Kali-c. Mgn-s. Merc Ntr-s. Nux. Petr. Phosp. Phosp-ac. Puls. Rhus. Sulph.
— an hour after breakfast or dinner, Selen.
— from mental exertion, Agar. Amm-c. Arn. Borax. Cupr. Grat. Merc-jod. Ntr-c. Sep.
— moving and turning the head, Acon. Aloe. Arn. Calc. Carb-an. Carb-veg. Clem. Cupr. Glon. *Hep.* Kali-c. Meph. Mosch. Pæon. Sang. Selen. Tellur. Therid.
— quickly, Amm-c. *Bar-c.* Calc. Carb-veg. Kali-c. Spig. Staph. Verat.
— after nocturnal emissions, Caust.
— from noise, Therid.
— in open air, *Agar.* Ambr. Ang. Calc. Canth. Croton. Dros. Glon. Laur. Ol-an. Ran-b. Ruta. *Sep.* Sulph. Tar. Thea.
— — — relieved, *Amm-m.* Bell. Mgn-m. Mgn-s. *Phell.* Phosp-ac. Sulph-ac.
— periodical, Ntr-m.
— when pressing the cheek, Verb.
— — raising the body, Acon. *Arn.* Ars. Bell. Bry. Carb-an. Cic. Cocc. Con. Laur. Nux. Op. Puls. Zinc.
— — — the head, Arn. Bry. Chin. Clem. Coloc. Croc. Merc.
— from reading, Amm-c. Arn. Cupr. Grat. Merc-jod. Par.
— — aloud, Par.
— after resting, Lach.
— — head, Sabad.
— when riding in a vehicle, Hep. Sil.
— after rising, Bar-c. Calc. Lyc. Mgn-c. Phosp. Phosp-ac. Sabad. Stann.
— when rising from bed, Bell. Cham. Cinnab. Con. Dulc. Graph. Kali-b. Lyc. Mgn-m. Merc. Ntr-m. Nicc. Nitr-ac. Nux. *Phosp.* Phosp-ac. Puls. Rhus. Ruta. Sep. Sil. Sulph.
— — from sitting, Acon. Asar. Bry. Con. Grat. Kali-b. Kali-c. Laur. Merc-jod. Nicc. Nitr-ac. Ox-ac. Petr. Phosp. Puls. Sabad. Selen. Thuj.

2. SENSORIUM.

Vertigo when rising from stooping, Acon. Arn. Ars. Bell. Berb. Bry. Cic. Puls. Sulph.
— — supine position, Croc. Merc. Oleand. Petr. Puls. Selen. Sil.
— in a room, Amm-m. Lyc. Mgn-m. Staph. Sulph-ac.
— — — warm, Lyc. Phosp-ac.
— — — not in open air, Croc.
— when sitting, Amm-c. Apis. Bell. Calc. Cocc. Croton. Evon. Grat. Lach. Meph. Merc. Nitr-ac. Phosp. *Puls*. Ruta. Sep. Sil. Stann. Staph. *Sulph*. Sulph-ac. Tellur. Viol-od.
— — after walking, Colch.
— when going to sleep, Tellur.
— after sleep, Carb-veg.
— when sneezing, Nux.
— — standing, Apis. Cannab. Croton. Cycl. Euph. Lach. Mgn-c. Merc-sulph. Oleand. Phosp-ac. Rheum. Spig.
— during stool, Kobalt.
— from stooping, Acon. Anac. Bar-c. Bell. Berb. Bry. Calc. Carb-veg. Cinnab. Hell. Kali-b. Kalm. Led. *Lyc*. Meph. Nicc. Ol-an. Petr. Plb. Puls. Sil. Sulph. Therid. Thuj. Verat.
— — with deafness, Merc-cor.
— — not when lying down, Millef.
— — as if falling forwards, Cic. Cupr. Elaps. Sil.
— strong sounds, Therid.
— in sunshine, Agar.
— when supporting the head, relieved, Sabad.
— when talking, Borax. Par.
— after relaxation, Calc. Lach.
— when turning in bed, Con.
— after vexation, Calc.
— when vomiting, Croton.
— — walking, Anac. Arn. Ars. Asar. Cannab. Carb-veg. Cic. Ferr. Ip. Ntr-m. Nitr-ac. Phosp-ac. Ran-sc. Rhus. Spig. Sulph-ac. Tart. Tellur. Viol-tr.
— — in the open air, Agar. Ambr. Ang. Aur. Calc. Cycl. Dros. Euph. Lach. Led. Merc. Mur-ac. Nux-m. Oleand. Ruta. Sep. Spig. Stann. Sulph. Tar. Thea. Thuj.
— — slowly, Millef.
— after walking, Laur.
— — relieved, Amm-c. Staph.
— after wine, Bov. Ntr-c. Zinc.
— when writing, Sep.
— alternately with colic, Verat.
— with anxiety, Bell. Caust. Igt. Merc. Nux-m. Nux. Op. Rhod. Rhus.
— with bellyache, Ntr-m. Spig.
— — brain, sensation of looseness in, Bry.
— — — motion, in, Cycl. Grat.
— — with chilliness, Gels. Merc-cor. Rhus.
— — choking, Sil.
— — coffee, longing for, Nux-m.

— — coldness, icy, of forehead, Lach. Verat
— — constipation, Aloe.
— — death, fear of, Rhus.
— — deafness when stooping, Merc-cor.
— — delirium, Jatr. Nux-m.
— — diarrhoea, Stram.
— — distance of things seeming greater, Anac. Stram.
— — drowsiness, *Aeth*. Arg. Laur. Puls. Stram.
— — ears, buzzing in, Carb-veg. Nux. Puls. Seneg.
— — — ringing in, Sang.
— — epistaxis, Acon. Ant. Brom. Camph. Carb-an. Sulph. Teplitz.
— — eructation, Gymnoc. Ntr-m.
— — sour, Sass.
— — eyes, obscuration of, Acon. Anac. Arg. Bell. Calc. Canth. Carb-an. Cham. Cic. Evon. Ferr. Gels. Gymnoc. Hep. Hyosc. Lact. Laur. Merc. Nux. Oleand. Par. Phosp. Phyt. Puls. Raph. Sabad. Sabin. Seneg. Stram. Sulph. Tereb. Tilia. Zinc.
— — — inability to see printed letters, Lach.
— — — flickering before, Bell. Igt. Mez. Oleand. Tart.
— — — sparks before, Bell. Igt. Mez.
— — — vision, double, Gels.
— — — whirling before, Anac. Laur. Mosch. Ntr-m. Oleand. Sep.
— — — white stars before, Alum.
— — — pain in, Seneg. Tabac.
— — — shut, Arg. Mgn-s.
— — face pale, Croton. Lach. Puls.
— — gout, Sacch.
— — headache, Apis. Arg-n. Ars. Bar-c. Calc. Ferr. Hep. Kali-b. Lach. Lob. Ntr-c. Ox-ac. Phosp. Psor. Puls. Sang. Sep. Stram. Sulph. Tabac. (compare Headache with vertigo).
— — emptiness in head, sensation of, Phosp.
— — head, fulness in, Amm-m. Borax. Lact. Pod. Sabin.
— — heat in head, Puls. Sabin.
— — — which rises to head, body becomes warmer, face becomes red and vertigo ceases, Aeth. Calad. Canth. Plb. Rheum. Rhus.
— — head, humming in, Ntr-s.
— — — jerks in, Ntr-m.
— — — rolling, in Sep.
— — — weakness and heaviness, Bufo. *Camph*. *Caust*. Chin. *Cupr*. *Mgn-m*. Rhod. Spong.
— with' sensation as if the head would fall to the right side, Ferr.
— — hands, trembling of, Puls.
— — hearing, loss of, Nux.
— **heat**, Croc. Merc. Puls.

2. SENSORIUM.

Vertigo with heat, sensation of, in chest and around heart, Lachn.
— — heaviness, Lach.
— — — of lower limbs, Lact.
— — hypochondriacal humor, Phosp.
— — inverted appearance of things, Eugen.
— to lie down, necessity, Ambr. Graph. Merc. Mosch. Nitr-ac. Op.
— motion, before the eyes, Anac. Laur. Mosch. Ntr-m. Oleand. Sep.
— with nape, burning sensation in, Alum.
— — nausea, Acon. Alum. Amm-c. Ant. Apis. Arn. Ars. *Bar-c.* Bell. Borax. Calad. Calc. Calc-ph. Carb-an. Carb-veg. Chin. Cinnab. Cocc. Coloc. Croton. Ferr. Fluor-ac. Graph. Gymnoc. Kali-b. Kalm. Lach. Lob. Lyc. *Merc. Mosch.* Ntr-m. Nicc. Nitr-ac. Petr. *Phosp. Puls.* Sabad. Sang. Sass. Scill. *Sil.* Spig. Spong. Stront. Sulph. Tabac. Tart. Tellur. *Therid.*
— stooping, Millef.
— perspiration cold, Merc-cor. Therid. Verat.
— retching, Sil.
— as if seat were moving, Zinc.
— — — became elevated, Phosp.
— senses, dulness of, Bov. Camph. Chelid. Ntr-m. Nux-m. Plat. Ran-sc. Stann. Stram. Tart. Verat.
— — suspension of, *Camph. Stram.* Tart. Verat.
— shuddering, Chelid.
— sleepiness, Aeth. Arg. Croton. Laur. Puls. Stram.
— speech difficult, Par.
— starting, Aloe.
— stomach pain in, Ambr.
— — — — pit of, Acon.
— — weakness in, Ambr.
— with stupefaction, Bell. Bov. Laur. Psor. (compare Stupefaction).
— syncope, Ars. Berb. Cham. Croc. Hep. Hipp. Lach. Mgn-c. Mosch. Nux. Phosp. Sabad. Sulph.
— torpor, Nux-m.
— tottering, Bry. Cham. Coloc. Ip. Kali-c. Mur-ac. Nicc. Nux-m. Nux. Oleand. Petr. Stram. Tar. Tilia.
— tremor, Dig. Ntr-m.
— unconsciousness, Acon. Ars. Bell. Borax. Canth. Cocc. Jatr. Lach. Laur. Mosch. Nux. Nux-m. Ran-sc. Sep. Tabac.
— momentary, Nux.
— vomit, inclination to, Lach. Ntr-s. Therid.
— vomiting, Tellur.
— sour, Sass.
— wandering talk, Nux-m.
— weakness, Bell. Berb. Croton. Lach. Nicc. Nitr-ac. Sulph. Zinc.
— — head, Caust.
— — and thirst, Ox-ac.

3. Head.

In brain, deep headache, Aloe, Bov. Lam. Therid.
— — as if bruised, Ntr-m.
— — stitches, Alum. Guaj.
— — extending to the ears, Lach. Merc. Puls. Rhus.
Over eyes, pain, Agar. Apis. Arn. Ars. Asa-f. Actea-r. Bar-c. Bell. Berb. Bov. Carb-veg. Cic. Cist. Colch. *Croc.* Croton. Hep. Kali-b. Lach. Lith. Lyc. Meph. Ntr-m. Nux-jug. Nux-m. Nux. Osm. Phosp-ac. Phyt. Puls. Ran-b. Rhus. Selen. Sep. Sulph.
— left eye, Acon. Ars. Brom. Kali-c.

3. HEAD.

Kalm. Lac-can. Nux-m. Nux. Ox-ac. Phosp-ac. Phosp. Plat. Sep. Spig. Tellur. Verat.
Over right eye, Bell. Lac-can. Sang.
— eyes boring, Ol-an.
— — drawing, Agar.
— — fulness of with vertigo, Pod.
— — pressing, Agar. Aloe. Arn. Bar-c. Bov. Brom. Bry. Carb-veg. Chin. Cist. Evon. Fluor-ac. Glon. Gymnoc. Ntr-m. Nux-m. Puls. Sep. Sil. Tabac. Teucr. Zinc.
— rending, Ntr-m.
— shooting from left eye to vertex, Phyt.
— — over left eye, Amm-c. Ant. Berb. Bov. Caust. Kali-b. Ntr-m. Nitr-ac. Phosp-ac. Sep. Zinc.
— squeezing, Asa-f. Colch.
— stinging, stitches, Borax. Ntr-m. Ol-an. Phosp. Phosp-ac. Rhus.
— — — over left eye, Hipp. Kali-jod.
— — — in left eye, Spig.
— stunning, stupefying, Evon.
—*throbbing, Gymnoc. Lach. Nux-m. Spig.
To the eyes, extending, pain, Lach. Spig.
— between the eyes, Lach. Poth.
Behind the eyes, pain, Bad. Daph. Lach. Therid.
To face, extending, pain, Amm-m. Anac. Guaj. Rhus. Thuj.
— drawing, Seneg.
— rending, Amm-m. Anac. Guaj. Lyc. Sil. Thuj.
— stinging, Rhus.
To the jaws, extending, pain, Kali-chl.
To the malar bone, stinging, Ind. Rhus.
To the nape of neck extending, Bar-c. Berb. Jac-cor. Mosch. Nitr. Sabin.
— pressing, Sabin.
— rending, Berb.
— spasmodic drawing, *Mosch*. Nitr.
— alternating with pains, Hyosc.
From nape, proceeding, Bell. Berb. Carb-veg. Ferr. Fluor-ac. Gels. Glon. Puls. Sang. Sil.
— contracting, Puls.
— drawing, Carb-veg. Ferr.
— rending, Berb.
Above root of nose, Acon. Agar. Amm-m. Ars. Asar. Bar-c. Bism. Borax. Camph. Dig. Hep. Igt. Mosch. Nux. Plat Raph. Staph. Tart. Viol-tr.
— boring, Hep.
— compressing, Acon. Mosch.
— constricting, Camph.
— constriction, Acon.
— crampy sensation, as if he would lose his reason, Acon. Igt.
— drawing, Agar. Asar.
— dull, gloomy, making him, Ferr.
— pressing, Amm-m. Asar. Bar-c. Bism. Coloc. Igt. Lod. Raph. Viol-tr. Zinc.

— pricking, stinging, Kali-b.
— squeezing, Acon.
— stinging, Agar. Berb. Chin. Ran-b. Rhus. Sass. Sep.
— stunning, Acon. Asar. Mosch. Tart.
— as if touched by a small metalic body on a small spot, Cinnab.
— throbbing, Ars.
To nose, extending, headache, Ars. Bism. Borax. Croton. Dig. Ferr. Glon. Lach. Lyc. Mez. Ntr-c. Stann.
— root of nose, and eyes, drawing at, Agar.
— nose, boring and digging, Bism.
— contraction, Nitr.
— pressing and throbbing, Mez.
— rending, tearing, Lyc. Ntr-c.
— spasmodic, Ntr-c.
— stinging, Rhus.
— to point of nose, extending, Nitr.
In occiput, Alum. Anac. Bar-c. Carb-an. Elaps. Ferr. Ip. Kali-b. Mosch. Sec-c. Sep. Spig.
— — from binding up the hair, relieved, Nitr.
— — bubbling like boiling water, Ind.
— — burning, Ind. Rhus.
— — coldness, Dulc. Phosp.
— — compressing, Nitr.
— — congestion of blood, Borax, Gl-an.
— — constricting, Camph. Graph.
— — drawing, Arg. Mgn-c. Mosch. Nitr. *Zinc*.
— — dull, Sec-c.
— — fulness, Sulph.
— — heat, Sulph.
— — heaviness, Bry. Carb-an. Lach. Meph. Mur-ac. Ntr-m. Petr. Sulph. Tart. Thuj.
— — jerking, Stann. Thuj.
— — as from a plug, Arg.
— — pressing, Aloe. Ambr. Arg. Bism. Carb-veg. *Colch*. Grat. Igt. Kali-c. Lact. Ntr-s. Ol-an. *Petr*. Zinc.
— — rending, Ambr. Amm-m. Berb. Nitr-ac. Thuj. Zinc.
— — shocks, Cannab.
— — soreness, Eupat. Euph. Nux.
— — spasmodic, *Mosch*. Nitr.
— — squeezing, Ambr. Igt.
— — stinging, stitches, Iris. Petr. Viol-tr. Zinc.
— — tension, Bar-c. *Graph*. Mgn-c. Mosch.
— — throbbing, Aeth. Agar. Alum. Asar. Berb. Bry. Calc. Cannab. Carb-an. Caust. Con. Glon. Hep. Ntr-m. Petr. Puls. Rhus. Sep. Spig.
— — tingling, Rhus.
— — ulcerous pain, Sep.
One-sided, headache, Acon. Apis. Ars. *Asar*. Bell. Calc. *Caps*. *Cham*. *Cic*. *Coff*. *Coloc*. Con. Eugen. Graph. Igt. Ip. Kali-c. Lyc. Ntr-m. Nitr-ac. *Nux*. Petr.

3. HEAD.

Phyt. *Puls*. Ran-b. Sang. *Sep*. Sil. Spig. Spong. Stront. Sulph. Tart. Valer. Zinc.
One side, left side, Acon. Agar. Apis. Arg-n. Brom. Cinnab. Croc. Kali-b. Kalm. Lac-can. Merc. Ntr m. Puls. Selen. Sep. Tellur.
— right side, Agar. Apis. Bell. Bry. Bufo. Cact. Con. Elaps. Gels. Hep. Jac-c. Kali-b. Lach. Merc-jod. Ntr-nitr. Sabad. Sabin. Sacch. Sang. Sll. Spig. Spong.
— ceases on one side becomes more violent on the other, Ntr-m.
— cleaving, Aur.
— coldness, Calc.
— digging, Kali-jod.
— drawing, Acon. *Cham*. Coloc. Sep. Valer.
— numbness, sense of, Ol-an.
— pressing, Agar. *Caps*. Coloc. Mez. Pæon. Verat. Verb.
— rending, tearing, Agar. Ambr. *Anac*. *Cham*. Cocc-c. Colch. *Guaj*. *Merc*. Phosp. Sep. Sil. Thuj.
— squeezing, spasmodic, Coloc. Sass.
— stinging, stitches, Bry. Caps. Cocc-c. Sep.
— stunning, Mez. Verb.
— throbbing, Aur. Croc. Kali-jod. Tart. Tong.
— — from occiput to forehead, Carb-veg. Sil. Spig.
On the side on which one lies, Calad. Graph. Mgn-c. Phosp-ac.
In the sides, pain, Cupr. Mez.
— bursting, Nicc.
— compressing, Asar. Phell.
— drawing, Caps.
— itching, Dig.
— as from a nail, Agar. Coff. Staph.
— as from a plug, *Asa-f*. *Plat*.
— pressing, *Asa-f*. Ntr-s.
— — outwards, Asar
— rending, Caps. Dig. *Guaj*. Millef. Teucr. Zinc.
— in the side, squeezing, Aeth. Scill.
Forehead, pain, Acon. Ant. Apis. Bism. Bufo. Camph. Chin. Cocc. Creos. Diad. Elaps. Hep. Kali-b. Kalm. Kobalt. Led. Ntr-m. Ox-ac. Petr. Phosp. Phosp-ac. Rhod. Rhus. Seneg. Sep. Spong. Staph. Therid. Verb.
— beginning on feft side, Spig.
— like a boil, Hep.
— boring, Ant. *Bism*. Calc. Dulc. Igt. Spig.
— burning, Alum. Bism. Bry. Caust. Dulc. Meny. Merc. Ntr-m. Nux. Phosp. Rhus. Stann. Stront. Spig. Sulph-ac.
— bursting, Amm-c. Ant. Bell. Ntr-c. Ntr-nitr. Oleand. Sil. Spong. Staph.
— by a cold hand, as if touched, Hyper.
— coldness, sense of, Gels. Laur.
— compressing, Apis. Cannab. Lac-can.

Sulph. Verb.
— congestion of blood, Fluor-ac. Mgn-s.
— constricting, Arn. Iris. Par. Valer.
— contracting, Asar. Bism. Graph
— on coughing, Ferr.
— digging, Bism. Dulc.
— drawing, Asar. *Croc*. Guaj. Mgn-c. Ntr-m. *Rhod*. Sabin. Selen. Sil. *Zinc*.
— dulness, Fluor-ac. Gels. Jac-c. Ox-ac. Rumex.
— with chilliness, Aloe.
— emptiness, Sulph.
— empty space between forehead and brain, Caust.
— fall out, as if brain would, in middle of forehead, on straining at stool, Rat.
— fulness, Acon. Amm-m. Nicc. Rhus. Sulph.
— grasping, Con. Ntr-s.
— heat, Chin. Euph. Mgn-s. Phosp. Sil. Viol-od.
— heaviness, *Acon*. Aeth. *Amm-m*. Ars. Bell. *Bism*. Bry. Bruc. *Calc*. Coloc. Creos. Grat. Kali-jod. Laur. Mgn-s. Ntr-c. Nicc. Plb. Rhus. Sabin. *Sil*. *Stann*. Staph. Sulph.
— jerks, Stann. Thuj.
— looseness, Sulph-ac.
— numbness, Fluor-ac. Mgn-m.
— as from a plug, Asa-f. Jac-cor.
— pressing, Aloe. Agar. Alum. Ambr. Amm-m. Apis. Arg. *Arn*. Ars. Asar. Asa-f. Bar-c. Bell. Berb. *Bism*. Borax. *Bry*. Calc-acet. Caust. Chenop. Cic. Clem. *Coloc*. Cor-r. Cycl. Dig. Elaps. Glon. Grat. Guaj. Hydroc-ac. *Hyosc*. Igt. Iod. Ind. Kali-c. Lachn. Mgn-c. *Mgn-m*. Merc. Ntr-c. Ntr-m. Nux. *Ol-an*. Par. Petr. Plat. Psor. Ran-b. *Rhod*. Sabad. Samb. Seneg. Spong. *Stann*. Stram. Staph. *Sulph*. Teucr. Thea. Thuj. Valer. Verb. Viol-tr. Zinc.
— — asunder, Ran-b.
— — outwards, *Amm-c*. *Cor-r*. Dros. Hep. Mgn-s. *Oleand*. Puls. Rhus. Sil. Staph. Thea.
— raging, Cannab.
— rending, tearing, Ambr. Calc. Caust. Cocc c. Hep. Igt. Ip. Lachn. Lyc. Ntr-c. Nitr-ac. Plb. Samb. Thuj. Zinc.
— — with fixed eyes, Spig.
— shocks, Croc. Seneg. Sulph-ac. Thuj.
— soreness, Spig.
— spasmodic pain, Arn. Ntr-c.
— squeezing, Ambr. Asa-f. Igt. Plat.
— stinging, stitches, Acon. Arn. Asa-f. Bell. Camph. Canth. Cocc. Cocc-c. Coloc. Con. Dig. Hyosc. Igt. Laur. Ntr-c. Ntr-m. Rhod. Sep. Sil. Spig. *Sulph*. Tar. Tilia. Valer. Verb. Zinc.
— — in left frontal eminence, Arg-n.
— — like needles in left side, Mang.
— stunning, stupefying, Arg. Arn. Asa-f.

3. HEAD.

Asar. *Bell.* Cic. Cycl. *Hyosc.* Laur. Led. Ntr-c. Oleand. Phosp. Ruta. Sabad. Stann. Valer. Verb.
Forehead tension, Clem. Dig. Merc. Mgn-m. Mosch. Nux. Par. Puls. Sulph. Verb.
— throbbing, Aloe. Amm-c. Ang. Ars. Asar. Creos. Glon. Kalm. Mgn-c. Mgn-m. Merc. Merc-jod. Ntr-m. Phosp. Ruta. Spong.
— — left side of forehead, Acon. Cocc. Kali-c. Nux-m. Par. Verat.
— — from forehead to occiput, Bry.
— tingling, creeping, Arn. *Colch.* Viol-od.
— — ulcerous, Nux.
On a small spot, headache, Ferr-m. Kali-b. Kalm. Lact. Lith. Nux-m. Ox-ac. Ran-sc. Sang. Tellur. Zinc.
To teeth extending, Creos. Graph. Lyc. Merc. Mez. Sil.
— — pressing and throbbing, Mez.
— — rending, tearing, Lyc. Merc.
Temples, boring, Ang. Ant. Clem. Dulc. Hep. Mang. Ol-an.
— burning, Merc.
— compressing, Fluor-ac. Thuj. Verb.
— contracting, Asar. Scill.
— cutting, Lach.
— drawing, Asar. Calc. Guaj. Rhod. Sabin. Seneg.
— fulness, first in right and then left, then to nape, where it disappears, Jac-cor.
— heat with cold cheeks, Berb.
— heaviness, Bism.
— headache, Ambr. Caust. Cina. Creos. Kali-c. Lith. Lyc. Mez. Mosch. Nux-m. Puls. Rhod. Rhus. Verb.
— — right side, Sabin.
— jerking, Arn.
— — left side, Stann.
— as from a nail, Arn. Igt.
— — — plug, *Anac. Asa-f.*
— pressing, Agar. Agn. Anac. Apis. *Asa-f.* Bell. *Bism.* Cinnab. Carb-veg. Cupr. *Cycl.* Dros. Glon. Guaj. Hep. Hipp. Hyosc. Jatr. Kali-c. Lach. Lith. Mang. Ntr-c. Ntr-m. Par. Plat. Ran-b. Ran-sc. *Rhod.* Sabad. Samb. Spig. Stann. Stram. Sulph-ac. Tabac. Teucr. Thuj. Viol-tr. Zinc.
— — inwards, Ran-sc.
— — outwards, Calc. Lob. Ran-sc. Sulph.
— — — with flickering before the eyes, and heat of face, Aloe.
— pushing, Croc.
— rending, tearing, Agn. Alum. Arn. Berb. Cast. Con. Dig. Guaj. Mgn-s. Merc. Phosp. Plb. Puls. Ran-b. Rhus. Samb. Sulph. Zinc.
— — extending to cheek, Lachn.
— shocks, Croc. Lyc. Sulph-ac. Thuj.
— spasmodic pain, Calc.
— stabbing, Alum. Bell. Canth. Cycl. Lac-can. Mgn-c. Phosp. Phosp-ac.

Rhus. Stront. Verb.
— stinging, stitches, Arn. Asa-f. Borax. Cadm. Caust. Cina. Dig. Guaj. Kali-b. Kali-c. Lyc. Mgn-m. Mgn-s. Merc-jod. Phosp-ac. Sil. Sulph. Verb. Zinc.
— — at every step, Aloe.
— stunning, Asar. Sabad. Verb.
— tension, Calc. Cannab. Lith. Mgn-m. Verb.
— throbbing, Cadm. Chelid. Chin. Cocc. Daph. Glon. Ntr-s. Stann. Tabac. Thuj.
— tingling, Plat. Sulph.
— — and coldness of spot, Plat.
— ulcerous pain, Puls.
— vibration, Stront.
To the throat, extending, rending, tearing, Anac. Merc.
To tongue, extending, headache, Ip.
Vertex, Ant. Bufo. Calc. Con. Cupr. Elaps, Kali-b. Lact. Lith. Merc-jod. Ox-ac. Par. Sabad. Scill. Sulph.
— across the top of head from one ear to the other, Pallad.
— boring, Chin. Mgn-s. Spig.
— bruised, Mgn-c. Gum-gut.
— burning, Hyper. Mercurial.
— — in a small spot, Graph.
— bursting, Ntr-s.
— coldness, Laur. Sep. Valer. Verat.
— compressing, Graph.
— cracking, Coff.
— cutting, Con. *Lach.* Verat.
— digging, Samb.
— drawing, *Calc.*
— fulness, Psor.
— heat, Calc. Eupat. Sulph.
— as from a nail, Evon. Hell. Nux. Staph. *Thuj.*
— — staying in a room thick with smoke Ang.
— pressing, Aloe. Ambr. Cact. Calc. Cannab. Chin. Croc. Ferr. Hep. Hipp. Igt. Iod. Kali-b. Lac-can. Lach. Lith. Lyc. Nicc. Ol-an. Ran-b. Rheum. Tabac.
— — to spine, without pain, Benz-ac.
— — asunder, Carb-an. Ran-b.
— outwards, Par.
— pulled out, as if a cluster of hair was, Ind.
— rending, tearing, Ambr. Ind. Lachn. Nitr-ac.
— soreness, Spig.
— stinging, stitches, Carb-veg. Chelid. Con. Ip. Raph. Rat. Sabad.
— tension to upper jaw, Stront.
— throbbing, Agar. Alum. Cocc. Glon. Hyper. Lach- Ntr-c. Sil. Stram. Sulph.
— tingling, Cupr. Sulph.
— ulcerous pain, Cast. Zinc.
Agitation, waving in head, Acon. Caust. Dig. Hep. Ind. Mgn-m.
Like air passing through the head, Aur. Cor-r. Puls.

3. HEAD.

Like something alive in the head, Petr. Sil.
Arthritic headache, Arn. Ars. *Asar.* Aur. Bell. Benz-ac. Bry. *Caps.* Caust. Cham. Cic. Chin. *Coloc.* Con. *Eugen.* Graph. Guaj. Hyosc. Igt. Ip. Mang. Ntr-c. *Ntr-m. Nitr-ac. Nux.* Petr. Phosp. Plat. Puls. Rhus. Sabin. Sep. *Verat.* Zinc.
— in the afternoon, Aur. Coloc.
— — — evening, Eugen.
— periodical, Bell.
— Like a ball, rising up, Acon. Plb. (compare Hysterical headache).
— — — from naval, Acon. Plat. Plb.
Bend the head backwards, necessity to, Nitr.
Blows in the head, Aeth. Caust. Ind. Ntr-m. Phosp-ac. Ran-b. (compare Jerks and shocks).
Boiling water in the head, like, Acon. Ind.
Boring, Agar. Ang. Ant. Aur. Bism. Calc. Chin. Clem. Dulc. *Hep.* Graph. Igt. Lach. Merc. Ntr-m. *Ntr-s.* Oleand. Ol-an. Pæon. Petr. Plat. Puls. Sabin. Sep. Spig. Stann. Staph. Sulph. Zinc.
— on right side, changing to stitches in the evening, Bell.
— pressing, Chin.
— rending, tearing, Igt.
— stinging, stitches, Igt. Merc. Puls.
Bruised, pain as if, Agar. Amm-m. Anac. Ang. Ars. *Aur.* Bov. Camph. Caust. Cham. Chin. Coff. Con. Cupr. *Euph. Euphr.* Gels. Glon. Gymnoc. *Hell.* Hipp. Igt. Iod. Ip. Kobalt. Lach. Merc. Mur-ac. *Nux.* Op. Phosp. Puls. Staph. Sulph. Sulph-ac. *Verat.* Zinc.
— as if in the brain, Ntr-m.
Bubbling in head like water, Bell. Berb. Par. Sep. Sulph.
Burning in head, Acon. *Arn.* Ars. Aur. Aur-s. Bell. Bism. Bry. *Canth.* Caust. Chin. Dulc. *Eugen.* Hell. Lact. Mang. *Merc.* Nitr-ac. Nux-jug. Nux. Phosp. Plb. Rhus. Stann. Tar. Verat.
— rest of body cool, Arn.
— in brain, Acon.
— contracting, Bism.
— pressing, Mang.
— rending, tearing, Merc.
Bursting, as if, Amm-c. *Amm-m.* Ant. Bell. Bry. Calc. *Caps.* Cast. Cham. *Chin.* Creos. Daph. Dolich. Euphr. Igt. Kobalt. Lach. *Merc.* Merc-jod. Ntr-c. *Ntr-m.* Ntr-s. Nicc. Nux. Oleand. Phosp. Phosp-ac. Psor. Puls. *Rat.* Sep. Sil. Spig. *Spong.* Staph. Sulph. Sulph-ac. (compare Pressing asunder and outwards.)
Chronic headache, *Amm-c.* Con. Sulph.
— — of old people, Iod.
Cleaving headache, Aur. Phosp.
Coldness in head, Ambr. Arn. Bell. Calc.
Dulc. Kali-c. Laur. Merc. Phosp. Phyt. Sabad. Sep. Tilia. Valer.
— especially on right side, Calc. Verat.
— sensation as if a cold spot, Sulph.
Colic alternating with headache, Cina.
Compressing sensation, *Aeth. Alum.* Arg. Arn. Asar. Bov. *Bry.* Cannab. Caust. Cic. Coloc. Creos. Daph. Graph. Ind. Kali-jod. Lact. Lam. Laur. Mgn-m. Mgn-s. *Meny.* Merc. Mosch. Ntr-m. Ntr-s. Nitr. Nux-m. Ol-an. Phell. Phosp-ac. *Plat.* Puls. Rhus. Sabin. Selen. Spig. Spong. *Staph.* Stront. Tart. Thuj. Zinc.
— as from a band, Iod. Plat.
Concussion of brain, Arn. *Cic.* Led. Rhus. Sulph-ac.
— — when moving, Mang.
Congestion of blood, Acon. Aloe. *Ambr.* Amm-m. Anac. *Ant.* Apis. Arg-n. *Arn.* Asa-f. *Aur. Bell. Borax.* Bry. Calc. *Cannab.* Canth. Carb-an. Carb-veg. Caust. *Cham.* Chin. Cinnab. Cocc-c. Coff. Coloc. Creos. Cycl. Dulc. Elaps. *Ferr.* Glon. Graph. Hyosc. Igt. *Iod. Kali-c.* Kali-chl. *Lach.* Laur. *Lyc.* Mgn-c. Mgn-m. *Mgn-s. Mang.* Merc. *Millef. Mosch.* Ntr-c. Ntr-m. *Nitr-ac. Nux.* Ol-an. *Op.* Phell. *Phosp.* Plb. Psor. Puls. Ran-b. Rhus. Sang. Seneg. *Sep. Sil. Spong. Stram. Sulph. Tabac.* Tar. Tellur. *Thuj.* Verat. Viol-od. Zinc.
— when bending forewards, Cor-r. Elaps.
— with menses suppressed, Apis.
— in morning in bed, Lyc.
— from music, Ambr.
— at night, Amm-c. *Psor.* Puls. Sil.
— periodical, Ferr.
— protruding the eyes, Aloe.
— when stooping, Acon. Bell. Cor-r. Lach. Seneg. Sep. Verat.
— — talking, Coff.
— from tobacco-smoking, Mgn-c.
— with unconsciousness, Hyosc.
— from abdomen, Croton.
— — chest, Sulph.
Constricting, sensation, Acon. Anac. Arn. Asa-f. Cadm. Camph. Cocc. Graph. *Hyosc.* Stann. Sulph-ac. *Tart.* Verat.
— — concentrates at the top of nose, Nitr.
Contracting, Ang. Asar. Eugen. Grat. Hyosc. Nitr. Plat. Puls. Scill. Sep. Tar. Valer.(compare Cramping and spasmodic).
— in brain, Laur.
Cracking when walking, Acon. Ars. Cham. Dig. Puls.
— — sitting quietly, Coff.
Cramping, Acon. *Ambr.* Ang. Colch. *Coloc.* Eugen. Igt. Nux. *Phosp-ac. Plat.* Ran-sc. Rheum. Scill. Teucr.
— tightening, Nux.

3. HEAD.

Crawling, Arg. Arn. Colch. Cupr. Hyosc. Plat. Puls. Rhus. Sulph.
Cry out, pain compelling to, Cupr. Sep.
Cutting, Arn. Lach. Ntr-m. Verat.
— as with knives, followed by sensation of coldness, Arn.
— as if split open with a wedge, body icy cold, thirst, Lachn.
Daily headache, Bell. Calc. Con. Lach. Mgn-c. Ntr-m. Nux. Sep. Sil. Sulph.
Day, every other, headache, Ambr.
Dampish room, headache as if in, *Agn.*
Deep in brain, Therid. (compare In brain deep.)
Digging, Agar. Anac. Bar-c. Bism. Bry. Caust. Clem. Coloc. Dulc. Kali-jod. Merc. Nux. Phell. Sabin. Samb. Spig.
— up, incisive pain, in the whole left hemisphere, Arg-n.
— outwards, Dulc.
Diminution of brain, sense of, Grat.
Distention sense of, Bell. Par. *Ran-b. Ran-sc.* Therid. (compare Enlargement, Fulness, Pressing asunder.)
Drawing pain, Acon. Agar. Asar. *Calc.* Caps. *Carb-veg. Cham.* Cina. Coloc. Con. Croc. Cupr. Ferr. Guaj. Kali-c. *Mgn-c.* Mang. *Mosch.* Ntr-m. Nitr. Nux. Ol-an. Petr. Puls. Ran-sc. *Rhod.* Rhus. ,Sabin. *Scill.* Seneg. Sep. Stann. *Sulph.* Sulph-ac. Tart. Tong. Valer. *Zinc.*
Drawn forward, head feels as if, Sang.
Dull pain, Agar. All-cep. Ant. Chelid. Cina. Glon. Lachn. Lact. Meny. Meph. Tereb. Teucr. Thuj. Verb.
Enlargement of head, sense of, Arg-n. Apis. Berb. Bov. Cor-r. Dulc. Gels. Glon. Ind. Kali-jod. Kobalt. Lachn. Lith. Mang. Meph. Nux. Ran-b. Ran-sc. Stront. Tar. Therid.
— — occiput, Dulc.
— elongated, Hyper.
Falling forwards, sense in brain, Berb. Bry. *Dig.* Hipp. Laur.
Flattened, sense in forehead as if, Cor-r.
Fluctuating, waving in the brain, Bell. Chenop. Hep. Hyosc. Mgn-m. Par.
Fulness, *Acon.* Actea-r. All-cep. *Amm-m.* Apis. Bell. Berb. *Borax.* Bruc. *Bry.* Calc. Calc-ph. Caps. Cast. Chin. Cinnab. Clem. Con. Creos. Crot. Daph. Elaps. Gels. Glon. Graph. Grat. Guaj. Igt. Iris. Jac-cor. Kobalt. Meph. Merc. Merc-jod. Merc-sulph. Ntr-c. *Nicc.* Nitr-ac. Petr. Phell. Phosp. Psor. Ran-b. *Ran-sc. Rhus.* Spong. *Sulph.* Sulph-ac. Tellur. *Tereb.*
Gnawing, Pæon. *Ran-sc.*
Grasping, Con. Mgn-m. Ntr-s.
Gurgling, Sep. (compare Bubbling).
Hammering, *Amm-c.* Aur. Calc. Clem. Ferr. Lach. Mez. Ntr-c. Phosp-ac. (compare Throbbing).

Heat, Acon. Actea-r. *Ambr.* • Amm-c. Amm-m. *Arn. Aur. Bell.* Benz-ac. Berb. Borax. Bry. Carb-an. Carb-veg. Caust. Chin. Cycl. Daph. Euphr. Grat. Hell. Hyosc. Jatr. Ind. Kali-chl. Kali-jod. Kalm. Lach. Lact. *Laur.* Mgn-c. Mgn-m. Mgn-s. Merc. Ntr-c. Ntr-m. Nicc. Nitr-ac. Nux-m. Ol-an. Pæon. Phell. Phosp. Phosp-ac. Plb. Psor. Ran-b. Rat. Rheum. Sep. Sil. Stram. Stront. *Sulph.* Tabac. Tart. Therid. Tilia. Viol-od.
— in the morning in bed, Berb. Lyc.
— — — afternoon in walking, Stront.
— at night, Camph. *Sil.*
— with cold body, Arn. Chin. Hyosc. Nux.
— from tobacco-smoking, Mgn-c.
— flushes of, from abdomen to head, Ind.
— rising up, Calad. Canth. Gum-gut.
— — from chest, Sulph.
— — — spine, Phosp.
— in forehead, Alum. Bell. Canth. Coloc. Euphr. Grat. Merc. Viol-od.
Heaviness, *Acon* Agar. Alum. *Amm-m. Arn. Ars.* Aur. Bar-m. Bell. Berb. Bov. Bry. Cact. *Calc. Camph.* Carb-an. *Carb-veg.* Cast. *Cham.* Chin. Cic. Clem. Con. Creos. Croton. Cupr. Dulc. Euphr. Ferr. Gels. *Hell.* Hipp. Hyper. Igt. *Ip.* Iris. Jatr. *Kali-jod.* Lac-can. Lach. Lachn. Lact. *Laur.* Lob. Mgn-c. *Mgn-m.* Mgn-s. Mang. *Meny.* Meph. Merc. Merc-cor. Mosch. Murex. Mur-ac. *Ntr-m. Nicc.* Nitr-ac. Nitr. Nux-m. Nux. Oleand. *Op.* Pæon Petr. *Phell.* Phosp. *Phosp-ac. Plb.* Prun. *Puls.* Ran-sc. Rat. *Rheum. Rhus. Sabin.* Sang. Scill. *Sep. Sil.* Spig. Spong. *Stann.* Staph. *Sulph.* Sulph-ac. *Tabac.* Tellur. Tereb. Thea. *Tong.* Verat. Verb. Viol-od. Viol-tr.
— painful, Hell. Nicc. Oleand. Sabad. Verb.
— pressing, Bism. Nux. *Rhus.* Scill. Tereb.
— with bleeding of nose, Ntr-sulph.
— and pressure as if the head would fall forward, Agn.
— with drowsiness and pain in back, Gum-gut.
— stunning, as after intoxication, Nitr.
— in the morning, Agar. Amm-m. Clem. Con. Croc. Nicc. Nitr. *Nux.* Petr.
— — in the evening, Sep.
— daily, Ntr-m. Sil.
— exercise, increased by, Calc.
— when moving body, Calc.
— eyes, Nux.
— when looking sideways, Agn.
— in open air, relieved, Ars.
— — in a room, Ars.
— when stooping, Acon. Berb. Petr. Rhus. Senna. Sulph-ac.
— after stopping, Tong. Viol-tr.

3. HEAD.

Heaviness, after vexation, Mgn-c.
— when walking, Thea.
Hollowness, Arg. Cina. *Cocc.* Cor-r. Cupr. Ntr-m Ox-ac. Phosp. *Puls. Seneg.* Sulph.
Hoop around head, Aeth. Merc. Sulph. Therid. (compare As if screwed together).
Humming, Sulph.
Hydrocephalus, Acon. Apis. *Bell.* Borax. Cham. Con. Cupr. Dig. *Hell. Hyosc.* Lact. Merc. Nux. Rat. Samb. Stram. Valer. Zinc.
Hysterical, Aur. Bry. Valer.
Increasing pains, slowly decreasing, Plat. Stront.
— — suddenly disappearing, Sulph-ac.
Inflammation of brain, *Acon. Bell. Bry. Camph.* Canth. *Cupr. Hell. Hyosc.* Merc. Phosp. Stram.
— sense of, Daph.
— after exertion in the winter season, Hyosc.
— from heat of sun, Camph. Therid.
— nervous, Bry. *Hyosc.*
Intoxication, as from, Ambr. Bry. Carb-an. Chin. Nitr. Nux. Puls. Samb. Sulph.
Itching, Dig.
Jerking pain, Anac. *Arn.* Bry. *Chin.* Ign. Mgn-c. Mgn-m. Mur-ac. Pæon. Phosp. Phosp-ac. *Puls.* Rat. Sep. Sulph. Teucr. Thuj.
Jerks, (compare Shocks).
Knocking, Amm-c. Ang.
Lightness, unpleasant sensation of. Hipp. Stram. (compare Hollowness).
Looseness of brain, sensation of, Acon. Amm-c. Bar-c. Bry. Carb-an. Cic. Croc. Hyosc. Mgn-s. Ntr-s. Nux-m. *Rhus.* Sep. Staph. *Sulph-ac.* Verat.
— without pain, Laur.
— when exercising, Acon. Carb-an. Croc. Mgn-s. Nux-m. Nux.
— — stepping, Acon. Kobalt. Nux. Rhus. Staph. Sulph-ac. Verat.
Motion, shaking of the brain, *Acon.* Amm-c. Ars. Bar-c. Bell. Calc. Carb-an. Chin. Croc. Dig. Hyosc. Kali-c. Kobalt. *Laur.* Mgn-s. Ntr-m. Nux-m. Nux. Rheum. Rhus. Staph. Sulph. Sulph-ac. Verat.
— when drinking and talking, Acon.
— — exercising, Acon. Bry. Carb-an. Croc. Led. Mgn-s. Ntr-m. Nux-m. Nux. Sulph.
— — making a false step, Led.
— — stooping, Bry Dig. Laur. Rheum.
Move the head, necessity to, caused by the pains, Chin. Cor-r.
Nail pierced into brain, as from a, Agar. Arn. Coff. Evon. Hep. *Ign.* Lyc. *Nux.* Staph. Thuj. (compare As from a plug).
— — in the left side, Agar. Ntr-m.
— — — right side, Agar. Hep. Thuj.

Night watching pain, as from, Ambr. Bry.
Numbness, Apis. Carb-an. Con. Fluor-ac. Graph. Mgn-m. Meph. Ol-an. Plat. Tart Thuj.
Out-pressing, Acon. Amm-c. Calc. Creos. Hep. Mgn-s. Par. Rhus. Sil. Staph. Thuj. (compare As if bursting).
Paralysis of brain, incipient, Ars. Lyc. Op. Phosp. Zinc.
Periodical headache, Aloe. Ambr. Arn. Ars. Bell. Benz-ac. Calc. Ferr. Kali-b. Mur-ac. Ntr-c. Ntr-m. Ntr-s. *Nux.* Puls. Sang. Sep. Sil.
— — 4 P.M. to 3 A.M., Bell.
— — every other day, Actea-r. Ambr.
— — — fortnight, Nicc.
— — seven days, Sacch. Sulph.
— nervous, Arn. Bell. Ferr. Nux. Spig. Sulph.
Piercing pain, Creos.
Pinching, Mez. Petr. Verb.
Plug, as from a, *Anac.* Arg. Asa-f. Con. Jac-c. Plat. Prun. Ruta. Sulph-ac. (compare As from a nail).
Pressing, Aloe. Alum. *Ambr. Amm-m. Ang.* Arn. Ars. *Asar.* Bar-c. Bell. Berb. *Bism. Bov.* Bry. Calad. Calc. Cannab. Caps. *Carb-an. Carb-veg. Caust.* Cic. *Chin.* Cina. *Colch.* Cor-r. Crot. Cupr. Diad. *Dig. Dros.* Dulc. Eugen. *Euph.* Euphr. *Evon.* Ferr. *Grat.* Guaj. Hell. *Hep. Hyosc. Ign.* Iod. Kalm. Kali-c. Lach. Lam. Led. *Lyc. Mgn-c. Mgn-m.* Mgn-s. Mang. Meny. *Mez. Mur-ac.* Ntr-c. Ntr-m. Nitr-ac. *Nitr.* Nux. *Oleand.* Par. *Petr.* Phosp. Phosp-ac. *Plat.* Puls. Ran-b. *Ran-sc.* Rheum. *Rhod. Rhus. Ruta. Sabad. Samb.* Sass. Scill. *Seneg.* Sep. *Sil. Spig. Spong. Stann. Staph. Sulph.* Sulph-ac. Tabac. *Tar. Tart.* Tereb. Thuj. Tong. *Valer. Verat.* Verb. Viol-tr. *Zinc.*
— asunder, Aloe. *Bell. Bry.* Caps. Cocc. Ign. Kali-jod. Mez. Ntr-m. Nux-m. Nux. Ran-b. Rhus. Samb. *Sep.* Spig. *Staph.* Tar. Zinc.
— burning, Aloe. Lact. Mang. Sep. Sulph-ac. Tar.
— constricting, Graph.
— cramp-like, Ars. Colch. Phosp-ac. Plat. Ran-sc. Zinc.
— digging, Bry. Clem.
— downwards, Ambr. Cina. Cupr. Laur. *Phosp.* Senna.
— drawing, Agar. Ang. Ant. Arg. Ars. Asa-f. Aur. Carb-veg. Caust. Coff. Hell. Hep. Ign. Iod. Kali-c. Mosch. Ntr-c. Nitr-ac. Ol-an. Ran-b. Ran-sc. *Rhod.* Rhus. Sabad. Sass. Spig. Stann. Staph. Tart. Tar. Thuj.
— gnawing, *Ran-sc.*
— heavy, like a stone, *Bism.* Cannab. *Cina.* Led. Meny. Merc-jod. *Nux. Rhus.*

3. HEAD.

Pressing, jerking, Dig. Thuj.
— inwards, *Anac.* Hell. *Plat. Ran-sc.*
— outwards, Acon. Asar. *Asa-f.* Bell. Bry. *Cor-r.* Creos. Dros. Hep. Igt. Kali-jod. Kobalt. Nitr-ac. *Oleand.* Phosp. Prun. Ran-sc. Spong. Sulph.
— rending, tearing, Agar. Anac. *Chin. Samb.* Stann. Staph.
— semi-lateral, Amm-c. Meny. Nux. Rhus.
— as if the head would split, with pupils contracted, voice faint, Bell.
— squeezing, Ambr. Coloc. Eugen. Igt. *Phosp-ac. Plat.* Ran-sc.
— stinging, Canth. Caps. Euph. *Petr. Sabin. Sass.* Staph. Valer.
— throbbing, Mez. Nux-m.
— tightening, Clem. Lyc. Mgn-m. Merc. Op. Therid.
Prickling, Amm-m. Hydroc-ac. Lachn. Viol-od.
Pulled, as if the hair were, Alum. Mgn-c. Mgn-m.
Pulsation. Alum. Asar. *Bell.* Carb-veg. Chelid. Chin. Croc. Creos. Daph. Ferr. Lact. Led. Nux. Oleand. Op. Plb. Puls. Rhus. Sabad. Spong. Thuj. (compare Throbbing).
Raging, Aur. Caust. Cinnab. Ind. Led. Mgn-m. Millef.
Rasping pain, Sabin.
Remitting pains, Plat. *Valer.*
Rending, tearing, Aeth. Agar. Alum. Ambr. Amm-m. *Anac.* Ant. Arg. *Arn.* Ars. Aur. Bell. Berb. Bov. Bruc. Bry. Calc. *Canth.* Caps. Carb-veg. Cast. *Cham. Chin.* Cina. Cocc. Coff. Colch. Coloc. Con. Croton. Dig. Graph. *Guaj. Igt.* Ind. Iod. Ip. Kali-c. Lact. Led. *Lyc.* Mgn-c. Mgn-m. Mgn-s. *Merc.* Millef. Mur-ac. Ntr-c. Ntr-m. Nicc. Nux. *Ol-an.* Phosp. Phosp-ac. Plat. Plb. *Puls.* Ran-b. Rat. Rheum. Rhus. Ruta. *Samb.* Sass. Sep. *Sil.* Spig. Stann. Staph. *Sulph.* Sulph-ac. Tart. Tereb. Teucr. Thuj. *Tong.* Zinc.
— crazy, crazy feeling runs up the back, Lil-tigr.
— digging, Coloc. Spig.
— drawing, Caps. Cina. Guaj. Kali-c. Nux. Puls. Rhus.
— jerking, Anac. Arn. *Chin.* Mgn-c. Mur-ac. Ntr-nitr. Pæon. Puls. Rat. Teucr. Thuj.
— stinging, Caps. Cocc. *Igt.* Mgn-m. *Ntr-m.* Nicc. Puls.
— tearing asunder, Agar. Amm-m. Coff. *Mur-ac.* Ntr-s. Op. *Puls.* Staph. Sulph-ac. *Verat.*
— with vomiting when raising the head, Ars.
— extending to face, Amm-m. Anac. Bry. Guaj. Lyc. Thuj.

— — drawing, Seneg.
— — stinging, Rhus.
Rigidity of brain, sensation of, Phosp.
Roaring, buzzing, humming, Ars. Aur. Calc. Caust. Creos. Ferr. Graph. Hep. Kali-c. Lact. Mgn-m. Ntr-s. Nux. Plat. Puls. Rhus. Sass. *Sulph.* Zinc.
— in evening and after meals, Cinnab.
— — hysterical persons, Aur.
Rolling in head, Eugen. Graph. Sep.
Screwing pain, Sabad.
— — behind the ears, Ox-ac.
Screwed in, as if, Mgn-s. Ntr-m. Puls. Ran-b. Sass. Stann. Sulph., (compare Spasm, tension.)
— — a vice, Aeth. Arg-n. Bry. Carb-veg. Glon. Mgn-c. Merc. Nitr-ac. Oleand. Petr. Plat. Rat. Sabad. Spig. Tart.
Sensitiveness of brain, Con. Merc. Nitr-ac. Phosp., (compare Aggravations).
Shaking of the brain, Elaps. Hyosc. Lact. Verat.
— — when coughing, Lact.
— — — exercising, Mang. Spig.
— — — stepping false, Led.
— — — treading on the ground and walking Lyc. Nux. Sep. Sil. Spig. Viol-tr.
Shocks, jerks, Acon. Ars. Bell. Caust. Carb-veg. Clem. *Croc.* Ip. Lact. Lyc. Mur-ac. Ntr-c. Ntr-m. Ntr-s. Nux. Phosp. Phosp-ac. Rhus. Samb. Sang. Seneg. Sep. *Spig.* Stann. *Sulph-ac.* Thuj.
— when walking in the open air, Spig.
— — — rapidly and ascending steps, Ant. Arn. Bell. Par. Phosp-ac.
— relieved by external pressure, Bell.
— or jerks, pains coming on, in, *Dig.* Mur-ac. Thuj.
Sleeping tco much, as after, Bov. Thuj.
Small, as if too, Coff.
Smarting pains, Sabin.
Smoke in the brain, as from, Arg. Sulph-ac.
Softening of brain, Lach.
Soreness, sense of, Camph. *Canth.* Daph. Glon. Phyt. Spig. Zinc.
Spasmodic pain, Acon. Ambr. Ang. Arn. Ars. Calc. Carb-veg. Colch. Coloc. Croton. Igt. Mosch. Murex. Ntr-c. Nicc. Petr. Phosp-ac. Plat. Ran-b. Rheum. Scill. Stann.
— — drawing, *Mosch.* Petr.
— — tearing, Ntr-c.
Stinging, stiches, *Acon.* Aloe. *Aeth. Alum.* Amm-c. Anac. Arg. *Arn.* Ars. Aur. Bar-c. Bell. Berb. *Borax.* Bov. Bruc. Bry. Camph. Canth. Caps. Carb-veg. *Caust.* Cham. Chelid. Chin. *Cic.* Cinnab. Cocc-c. *Con.* Croton. Cycl. Daph. *Dig.* Elaps. Euphr. *Evon.* Ferr. Gels. Grat. Guaj. *Hep.* Hipp. Hydroc-ac. Hyosc. *Igt.* Ind. *Ip. Kali-c.* Lach. Lact. Lob. *Lyc. Mgn-c.* Mgn-m. *Mgn-s.* Mang. Millef. *Mur-ac.* Ntr-c. *Ntr-m.* Nitr-s.

3. HEAD.

Nicc. *Nitr-ac*. *Nitr*. Nux. Ol-an. *Par*.
Petr. Phosp. Phosp-ac. Plb. *Puls*. Raph.
Rat. Rhod. *Rhus*. *Sabin*. Sabad. *Sass*.
Scill. Selen. Sep. Sil. Spig. Stann.
Staph. *Stront*. *Sulph*. *Sulph-ac*. Tabac.
Tar. *Tart*. Thuj. Tong. *Valer*. Verb.
Viol-tr. Zinc.
Stinging, drawing, Mang. Scill.
— jerking, *Ntr-m*. Nux. Puls.
— as from knives, Bell. Lach.
— inward, Coloc.
— outwards, Asa-f. Bry. Con. Ntr-c. Sep.
Stomach, headache rising as from, Con.
Straining in the head, Rheum.
Stunning, stupefying pain, Acon. Anac.
Ant. Arg. Arn. Ars. *Asa-f*. Asar. *Bell*.
Bov. Calc. Cic. Cina. Cinnab. Con.
Croton. Cupr. Cycl. Dros. Dulc. Iod.
Kali-c. Hell. *Hyosc*. Lac-can. *Laur*. Led.
Lyc. Mgn-m. Mosch. Mez. *Nitr*. *Oleand*.
Phosp. Puls. Rheum. Ruta. Sabad. Sabin.
Stann. *Staph*. Sulph. Tart. Thuj. Valer.
Verb.
— compressing, *Mosch*.
— drawing, Asar.
— pressing, Arg. Arn. Ars. *Asar*. Calc.
Cic. Cina. *Croton*. Cupr. *Dros*. Dulc. *Evon*.
Hell. *Hyosc*. Mez. *Ruta*. *Sabad*. *Stann*.
Sulph. *Tart*. Verb.
Stupefying, stinging, Verb.
— throbbing, Sabin.
— tightening, Asa-f. Oleand.
Suddenly originating headache, Sabin.
Valer.
Sunstroke, Camph. Glon. Therid.
— from having slept in the sun, Bell.
Swelling sensation of, Bell. Par. Ran-b.
Ran-sc. Therid.
Thick, head feels, Therid.
Throbbing, *Acon*. Actea-r. Aeth. Aloe. Alum.
Arn. Ars. Asar. Aur. *Bell*. *Borax*. Bov.
Bry. Cact. Calc. *Camph*. *Cannab*. *Caps*.
Carb-veg. *Cast*. *Cham*. Cocc. Colch.
Creos. Croc. Croton. Dros. Eupat.
Euphr. Ferr. Ferr-m. Gels. Glon. Graph.
Grat. Hipp. *Igt*. Ip. Iod. Kali-c. Kali-jod.
Lach. *Laur*. Led. Lith. *Lyc*. Mgn-m.
Mang. Merc. Mez. Millef. Ntr-c. Ntr-m.
Nitr-ac. Nux-m. Oleand. Ol-an. Op. Par.
Petr. Phell. Phosp. Plb. *Puls*. *Rheum*.
Rhod. Rhus. Sabad. Sabin. Sang. *Sass*.
Scill. Seneg. *Sep*. *Sil*. Spong. Stann.
Stram. *Sulph*. Tabac. Tart. Therid.
Thuj. *Tong*. *Verat*. Zinc.
— from abdomen preceding, Rheum.
— when breathing, Carb-veg.
— gnawing, Par.
— without heat or coldness, Laur.
— intermittent, Ferr-m.
— jerking, Bry. Igt. Phosp.
— painless, with fear to go to sleep, Nux-m.
— stinging, Puls.
— tearing, Mgn-m.

— ulcerous, Cast. Mang.
Tightening pain, Asa-f. Bar-c. Calc. Cannab.
Carb-veg. Clem. Dig. *Graph*. Gymnoc.
Hep. Kali-chl. Lyc. Mgn-c. Mgn-m.
Mang. Merc. Meny. *Mosch*. Ntr-c. Nitr-ac.
Nux. Oleand. Op. Par. Petr. Rhod.
Sabad. Samb. *Stront*. Sulph. Therid.
Verb.
— drawing, Mang. Mosch.
— stinging, Mang.
— as from a tape, Gels.
Tingling, Arg. Arn. Chelid. *Colch*. *Cupr*.
Plat. Puls. *Rhus*. Sec-c. Sulph.
Tired, brain feels, Apis.
Turning in the head, Sabad. Sil.
Ulcerous pain. Amm-c. Bov. Cast. Caust.
Hep. Mang. Merc. Nux. Puls.
Vibration, Grat. Lyc. Nux. Sass. Sil. Stront.
Verb.
— in the evening, Stront.
— when stepping out, Lyc. Nux. Sil.
— — talking, Sass.
— — walking, Verb.
Violent pains, Bell. Coloc. Lach. Merc.
Water in the brain, sense like, Acon. Bell.
Dig. Ind. Phosp-ac. Samb.
— — — boiling, like, Acon. Ind.
Wind blowing through skull, like, Aur.
Puls.
— — — on rocking, Cor-r.
Weakness in the head, *Ambr*. Phosp. Ran-b.
Rhus. Stram. Sulph-ac. Thuj.
— on the side on which one rests, Mgn-m.
— disabling, Iod.
— as if a headache were coming on, Ambr.
Iod. Lac-can. Phosp. Stram. Thuj.
Weariness, Ntr-m.
Whirling, Ars. Fluor-ac. Glon. Sil.
Conditions.
— every other day, Actea-r. Ambr.
— day and night, Rhus. Viol-tr.
— in the morning, *Agar*. Ambr. Amm-c.
Amm-m. Anac. Ars. Aur. Benz-ac Berb.
Bov. Bry. Cadm. Calc. Calc-ph. Carb-an.
Caust. Cham. Cina. Clem. Con. Croton.
Croc. Euph. Ferr. *Graph*. *Hep*. Igt. Jatr.
Kali-b. Kali-c. Kalm. Kobalt. Lach.
Lith. Lyc. Mgn-c. Mgn-m. Murex. Ntr-c.
Ntr-m. Nitr-ac. Nitr. Nux-m. *Nux*.
Pallad. Petr. *Phosp*. *Phosp-ac*. Phyt. Pod.
Psor. Puls. Rheum. Ruta. Sang. *Scill*.
Sep. Sil. Spig. Stann. Staph. *Sulph*.
Thuj. Zinc.
— 3 A. M., Thuj.
— 5 A. M., Kali-jod.
— 10 A. M. to 6 P. M., Apis.
— at same hour, Kali-b.
— every alternate morning, Eupat.
— in bed, *Agar*. Anac. Berb. Bov.
Bry. Calc. Calc-ph. *Cham*. Con. Creos.
Lach. Lact. Mgn-s. Murex. Nitr-ac.
Ntr-m. Nux. Puls. Rheum. Rhod.
Rhus. *Scill*. Staph. Thuj. **Zinc-ox**.

— — with nausea, Calc. Graph. Ntr-m.
  Nux. Sep. Sil. Stram. Sulph.
— after breakfast, Lyc. Nux-m.
— when rising, Amm-m. Apis. Arg-n.
  Croton. Cycl. Lact. Nux. Puls.
— — — relieved, Murex.
— in forenoon, Hepar. Kali-b. Sabad. Sep.
  Selen. Sil.
— — — 10 A. M. Borax.
— at noon, Arg.
— — — to evening, Sil.
— in the afternoon, Acon. Aeth. Asar. Bell.
  Berb. Coloc. Graph. Kali-b. Lac-can.
  Lach. Lact. Lyc. Pallad. Selen. Sil.
  Stront.
— 4 P. M. to 8 P. M. Hell. Lyc.
— 4 P. M. to 3 A. M. Bell.
— 3 P. M. Thuj.
In the evening, twilight, Ang.
In evening, Alum. Amm-c. Anac. Ang.
  Apis. Bry. Caps. Carb-veg. Cham.
  Cinnab. Croc. Crot. *Eugen.* Euphr.
  Ferr. Kali-chl. Kalm. Lach. Lob. Lyc.
  Mgn-m. Meph. Mosch. Petr. Phosp.
  Puls. Rhus. Ruta. Sep. Stront.
  Sulph. Tart. Therid. Thuj. Valer. Zinc
— 1 to 10 P. M. Mgn-c. Plat. Sil.
— — bed, in Ars. Lyc. Mgn-m. Phosp.
  Puls. Sep. Sulph. Zinc.
— continued to the next evening, Cist.
  Nitr.
At night Amm-c. Ars. Berb. Bov. Cact.
  Calc. Camph. Canth. Carb-veg. Caust.
  Cham. Chin. Con. Creos. Eugen. *Hep.*
  Lyc. Mgn-c. Mgn-s. *Merc.* Ntr-s. Nitr.
  ac. Par. Phosp-ac. Phosp. Puls. Raph.
  Rhus. Sil. *Sulph. Tart.* Zinc.
— augmented and continued, Puls.
— by nausea in the evening preceded,
  Phosp.
Midnight, after, Ferr. Hep. Phosp-ac.
— 1 A. M. Pallad.
— 3 A. M. Thuj.
Draft of air, from Acon. Bell. Benz-ac.
  Cadm. Calc. Chin. Coloc. Nux-m. Nux.
  Phosp. Selen. Sil. Valer. Verb.
Angry, after being, Lyc. Mgn-c. Ntr-m.
  Petr. Phosp. Rhus.
Arms, from exerting, Ferr-magn. Ntr-s.
Arms moving, the, Rhus.
Ascending steps, Ant. Arn. Bell. Calc.
  Ferr-mgn. Glon. Lach. Meny. Par.
  Phosp-ac. Sil. Sulph.
Bathing, from, Ant.
— relieved, from Lact-ac.
Beer, from Rhus.
Bending head, by backward. Clem. Dig.
  Mang.
— — — relieved, from, Apis. Bell. Cupr.
  Murex. Rhus. Thuj. Valer. Verat.
Bending forwards, by Acon. Asar. Bell.
  Cor-r. Igt. Kobalt. Nux. Spig. Thuj.
  (compare When stooping.)

Binding anything around head, Calc.
  Cham. Lach. Rhus. Thuj.
— — relieved, *Arg-n.* Bell. Bry. Hep.
  Mgn-m. Nux. Psor. Puls. Rhod.
  Sil.
Binding up the hair relieves, Nitr.
Bleeding of nose relieves, Bufo. Mgn-s.
Blowing of nose,, Sulph.
Bodily, exertion, Calc.
Breakfast, after, Bufo. Lyc. Nux-m.
Change of temperature in, *Ran-b.* Verb.
Coffee, from, Cham. Cocc. Igt. Nitr. Nux.
— relieved, from, Coloc.
Cold, from a, Bell. Calc. Carb-veg. Cham.
  Puls.
Cold suppressed from a, Acon. Ars. Bell.
  Calc. Carb-veg. Cham. Chin. Cina. Lach.
  Lyc. Nux. Puls. Sulph.
Cold in the head, when getting, Aur. Dulc.
Coldness, from external, Verb.
Cold air, from, Camph. Carb-an. Caust.
  Ferr. Grat. Ntr-m. Nux-m. Puls. Rhod.
  Rhus.
— — relieved, Dros. Euphr. Nitr-ac.
  Phosp. Seneg. Tart.
Cold, applications, relieved by, Aloe. Ars.
  Asar. Bell. Bry. Cham. Cycl. Glon.
  Lac-can. Spig. Tart. Zinc.
Company, in a large, Mgn-c.
Compressing the head, relieved when,
  Cinnab. Puls.
Concussions, from, Arn. Bell. Cocc. Hep.
  Phosp-ac.
Contradiction, from, Lyc. Mgn-c. Ntr-m.
  Petr. Phosp. Rhus.
Coughing, Bell. Ferr. Kali-c. Spig. Sulph.
  (compare Cough with headache).
Covering the head from, Led.
— — — coldness felt, Valer.
— — — better from, Hep. Lob. Psor. Sil.
Drinking, after, Acon. Cocc. Merc.
— — something cold, Dig.
Entering into cold air when, *Ran-b.* Verb.
— — warm air when, Ran-b.
— — a room when, Spong. Tong.
Evacuations too small from, Con.
Eructations relieved from, Lach.
Exercising when, *Acon.* Agn. Amm-c.
  Amm-m. Arn. Bell. *Bry,* Calc. Calc-ph.
  Carb-an. Chin. Croc. Dulc. Grat. Kali-c.
  Lob. Mgn-s. Mez. *Ntr-m. Nux-m. Nux.*
  Phosp-ac. Plat. Samb. *Spig.* Staph.
  Sulph. Therid.
— — relieved, Guaj. Mgn-m. Mur-ac. Tar.
  Tart.
Eyes, opening the, when, Bry. Chin. Gent.
  Fatigue, from, Sil.
Flatus, by emissions of, relieved, Cic.
Forehead wrinkling up, the, when, Ntr-m.
Moving or turning the eyes, when, Bell.
  Bry. *Caps.* Croton. Cupr. Dig. Hep.
  Mgn-s. Mur-ac. Nux. Puls. Rhus. Sep.
  Spig. Sulph. Valer.

3. HEAD.

Hair cut, from getting the, Bell. Glon.
Stove, near a hot, Actea-r. Bar-m.
Looking at something, when intently, Mur-ac. Spong.
— — relieved, Agn.
Looking downwards, when, Oleand. Spig.
— upwards, relieved, when, Thuj.
Laughing, when, Phosp, Tong.
Lead and tin working in, from, Sulph.
Leaning on the head, relieved when, Bell. Brom. Diad. Kali-c. Meny. Merc.
Lemonade, from, Selen.
Lifting wrong, from, Calc. Phosp-ac. Rhus.
Light of a candle, from, Bufo. Croc. Sang.
— of day, from, Sep.
Looking at anything, when, Cupr. Lith. Plb. Thuj.
Lying down, when, Ambr. Bell. Camph. Coloc. Euphr. Gels. Igt. Lith. Lyc. Mgn-c. Mgn-m. Nux. Phosp. Puls. Ran-b. Therid.
— on left side, Cinnab.
— on painful side, when, Calad. Graph. Mgn-c. Phosp-ac.
— on back, when, Cinnab. Coloc.
— — relieved, Caust. Spong.
Lying, relieved when, Alum. Amm-m. Calc. Calc-ph. Camph. Canth. Colch. Con. Cupr. Dulc. Hell. Igt. Lach. Ntr-m. Nux. Oleand. Phosp. Spig.
Lying with head high, relieved, when, Caps. Ntr-m. Spig. Stront. Sulph.
Lying after, Calad. Ox-ac.
Masticating, when, Phosp. Sulph.
Meals, during, Graph. Ntr-s. Ran-b.
— — relieved, Phell.
Meals, after, Amm-c. Ant. Ars. Calc. Carb-an. Carb-veg. Cinnab. Cocc. Evon. Graph. Lyc. Ntr-s. Nux-m. Nux. Pæon. Rhus. Sil. Zinc.
— relieved, after Lith. Phosp. (compare During and after meals).
Mechanical injuries, from, *Arn. Cic.*
Meditation, from Asar. Calc. Chin. Colch. Igt. Lyc. Ntr-c. Nux. Petr. Puls. Sabad. Sil.
Mental exertion, *Anac.* Arn. *Asar. Aur.* Calc. Chin. *Cina.* Colch. Daph. Dig. Graph. Igt. Lach. Lact. Lyc. Mgn-c. Ntr-c. Ntr-m. *Nux.* Ol-an. *Par.* Petr. Phosp. Phosp-ac. *Sabad.* Sil. Sulph.
Menses, from sudden suppression of, Lith.
Mercury, from Puls. (compare generalities).
Moist weather, during, Carb-an. Rhod.
Mouth, when opening the, Spig.
Moving head, Acon. Bell. Berb. Calc. Camph. Caps. Chin. Cic. Con. Cor-r. Dros. Gels. Glon. Graph. Hell. Hep. Kali-c. Lach. Lyc. Ntr-c. Ntr-m. Nux. jug. Nux-m. Nux. Phosp-ac. Puls. Sang. Sec-c. Sep. Sil. Spig. Spong. Therid.
— head relieved, when, Euphr. Mur-ac. Plat. Rhod. Rhus. Stann. Sulph.
From music, Ambr. Phosp.
— noise, Anac. Bell. Bufo. Cact. Hyosc. Igt. Iod. Merc. Nitr-ac. Phosp-ac. Spig. Therid.
— strong odors, Igt. Selen.
In open air, Alum. Arg-n. Bell. Bov. Cadm. *Calc.* Calc-ph. Cham. Chelid. Chin. Cina. Coff. Cocc. Con. Eupat. Ferr. Hep. Kali-c. Kalm. Lach. *Mang.* Mez. Mur-ac. Nux. Ran-b. Spig. Sulph. Valer.
— — relieved, Acon. Actea-r. All-cep. Alum. Ant. Ars. Cannab. Coloc. Croc. Crot. Diad. Hell. Jatr. Kobalt. Laur. *Mang.* Meny. Mgn-m. Mosch. Ntr-m. Nicc. Nitr. Phell. Phosp. Plat Puls. Seneg. Sep. Stann. *Tabac.* Thuj. Viol-tr. Zinc.
From overheating, Carb-veg. Sil.
By perspiration preceded, Ferr.
From perspiration suppressed, Cham.
— perspiration relieved, Ntr-m. Thuj.
When pressing upon head, Agar. Arg. Bry. Cast. Chin. Cupr. Lach. Lact. Mez. Phosp-ac. Sass. Valer. Verb.
— — — relieved, Amm-c. Apis. Bell. Bry. Cinnab. Con. Glon. Guaj. Meny. Nicc. Nux. Par. Puls. Sep. Spig. Stann. Staph. Sulph. Verat.
— — — hard pressure relieved, Chin. Nux-m.
— raising head, Bov. Scill. Seneg. Sulph. Viol-tr.
— — — relieved, Kali-c.
By rattling noise of vehicles, Nitr-ac.
From reading, Agn. Apis. Arg. Arn Calc. Caust. Cina. Croton. Igt. Lach. Ntr-s. Par.
By rest relieved, Bry. Colch. Hell. Sep.
From rich food, Carb-veg. Colch. Cycl. Ip. Ntr-c. Ntr-m. Puls. Sep. Thuj.
When riding in a carriage, Cocc. Graph. Iod. Kali-c. Meph.
— — — — relieved, Nitr. Nitr-ac.
— rising from sitting, Bell. Grat. Lam. Lyc. Mur-ac. Ox-ac.
— — stooping, Acon. Cor-r. Daph. Lam. Mur-ac. Nux. Tong. Viol-tr.
— — — relieved, Con.
— rising up relieved, Cic. Mgn-c.
In a room, Arn. Ars. Croton, Jatr. Kobalt. Laur. *Mang.* Mosch. Nicc. Ntr-c. Plat. Seneg. Sep. Zinc.
— — relieved, Bell. Bov. Chin. Cocc. Coff. Eupat. Hep. Mang. Merc. Nux. Spig. Sulph-ac.
From running, Ntr-m.
— shaking head, Bell. Hep. Phosp-ac.
In sitting, Agar. Canth. Guaj. Puls. Rat. Ruta. Spong.

3. HEAD.

— — relieved, Gels. Lam. Merc. Sulph.
— — erect, Caust.
— — — relieved, Cic. Tart.
— — up from lying, Cor-r. Mur-ac. Nux.
— — — — relieved, Aloe. Bell. Lith. Mgn-c. Scill.
In sleep, Cham. Mgn-c.
— — relieved, Hell. Pallad. Sep.
After sleeping, Cocc. Glon. Merc. Ox-ac. Psor. Sulph.
— — relieved, Lac-can. Phosp. Puls. Thuj.
When sneezing, Kali-c.
From spirituous liquors, Ant. Calc. Carb-veg. Igt. *Nux*. Ran-b. *Rhod*. Ruta. *Selen*. Verat. Zinc.
When standing, Arg. Canth. Guaj. *Tar*.
— stepping hard, Bell. Bry. Calc. Chin. Con. Hell. Kali-c. Lyc. Nitr-ac. Nux. Phosp. Rhus. Sil. Spig. Sulph.
— — wrong, Anac. Led.
— stooping, Acon. Alum. Asar. Bar-c. Bell. Berb. Borax. Calc. Calc-ph. Camph. Chelid. Cic. Coloc. Cor-r. Creos. Cycl. Dig. Dros. Ferr. Gels. Glon. Hell. Hep. Igt. Kali-c. Kobalt. Lach. Laur. Ntr-s. Nicc. Nitr. Nux. Petr. Phosp. Plat. Puls. Rheum. *Rhus*. Sang. Senna. Seneg. *Sep*. Sil. Spig. Staph. Sulph-ac. Thuj. Verat.
— — relieved, Cina. Hyosc. Igt. Mang. Mez. Nux. Viol-tr.
— exposed to the sun, Acon. Bell. Bruc. Cadm. Camph. Glon. Hipp. Igt. Lach. Ntr-c, Nux. Selen. Therid. Valer.
From talking, Acon. Cact. Chin. Coff. Con. Dulc. Igt. Iod. Mgn-c. Mez. Phosp. Sil. Sulph.
— — of others, Igt.
— tea, Selen,
When thinking of the pain, relieved. Camph. Cic.
From tobacco smoke, Acon. Ant. Gels. Igt. Mgn-c. Par.
— — — relieved, Diad.
By touching, pain altered. Asa-f.
— — — increased, Agar. Anac. Arg. Bell. Bry. Calc. Camph. Cast. Chin. Con. Cupr. Ip. Lact. Lyc. Merc. Mez. Nux-m. Phosp. Phosp-ac. Staph.
— — — relieved, Asa-f.
When treading on the ground, Chin. Lyc. Nitr-ac. Nux. Phosp. *Rhus*. Sep. Sil. Spig. Sulph.
— turning in bed, Meph.
— uncovering the body, relieved, Cor-r. Glon.
Urination frequent, relieved by, Gels.
From veal, Nitr.
— vexation, Lyc. Mgn-c. Ntr-m. *Petr*. Phosp.
By vomiting, increased, Eugen.

— — relieved, Glon. Hipp. Sang. Raph.
When walking, Aloe. Arn. Caps. Chin. Glon. Iod. Lyc. Nitr-ac. Nux. Phosp. Puls. Sep. Spig. Stront. Sulph. Thea. Viol-tr.
— — relieved, Canth. Cham.
— — in cold air, Caps.
— — in open air, Alum. Cina. Coff. Con. Grat. Kali-c. Mur-ac. Nux. Spig. Spong. Sulph-ac.
— — — relieved, Alum. Ant. Ars. Canth. Coff. Coloc. Cor-r. Diad. Glon. Hep. Hyosc. Lith. Phell. Ran-b. Rhus. Thuj.
After walk in the open air, Amm-c. Calc. Hep. Mur-ac. Nicc. Petr. Sabad.
When walking rapidly, Bell. Bry. Iod. Sep.
— — in the wind, Chin.
In warm air, Acon. Amm-c. Arn. Bar-c. Bell. Bry. Carb-veg. Caps. Cocc-c. Euph. Igt. Iod. Ip. Mosch. Seneg. Sil. Spong.
Warmth relieves, Bell. Caps. Caust. Cinnab. Cocc. Colch. Kali-c. Mgn-m. Nux-m. Nux. Rhus. Stront. Sulph.
In the warm room, All-cep. Apis. Arn. Bar-c. Croc. Laur. Ntr-c. Phosp. Puls. Sulph. Zinc.
When exposed to the wind, Cham. Chin. Mur-ac.
— — cold wind, Aur. Lac-can. Nux. Rhus.
From cold water, applied relief, Ars. Bell. Bry. Cycl. Glon. Lac-can. Zinc.
From change of weather, Lach. Ran-b. Verb.
From wine drinking, *Nux*. Ox-ac. *Rhod*. *Selen*. Zinc.
Wrapping up the head, Calc. Carb-veg. Chin. Glon.
— — — relieved, Mgn-m. Sil.
When writing, Igt. Ntr-m. compare mental exertion.
When yawning, Agar.
Accompanied by, pain in abdomen, Con.
— agitation, Lyc,
— — of the blood. Phosp.
— anorexia, Phosp. Ran-b. Rheum. Stront.
— arms, jerking of, Verat.
— asthma, Coloc.
— back pain in small of, Kobalt.
— — lassitude, Lob.
— — weakness of, Coloc.
— to bend the head backwards, necessity, Nitr.
— breath, fetid, Apis.
— alternating with oppression of chest, Glon.
— chilly sensation, Hell.

3. HEAD.

— chills, Aloe. Arg-n. Cadm. Evon. Jatr. Mgn-s, Mez. Sil. Thuj.
— coition desire for, Sep.
— colic, Acon. Aloe. Cocc. Cupr-acet. Tereb.
— constipation, Aloe. Con. Nux.
— coryza, Acon. All-cep. Euphr. Hell. Kali-chl. Kali-jod. Lach. Sabad.
— — if it stops, headache, Kali-b.
— cranium, as if too small, Bell.
— cries, extorting, Coloc. Cupr. Sep.
— dejection, Berb. Lact. Ran-b. Therid.
— delirium, Nux. Verat.
— diarrhoea. Aloe. Apis. Jatr.
— dolefulness, Selen.
— ears, hardness of hearing, Dulc. Grat. Stram.
— — buzzing in, Acon. Ars. Dulc. Lact. Murex. Puls. Sulph.
— — hammering, Spig.
— — heat of, Lyc.
— — stinging, Borax. Croton. Merc. Rhus.
— epilepsy, after, Cina. Cupr.
— epistaxis, Alum. Ant. Bry. Cadm. Carb-an. Coff. Dulc. Sep.
— eructations, Arg-n. Calc. Graph. Lyc. Ntr-c. Nux. Phosp. Sil. Sulph.
— evening, fever, Led. Lob.
— eyes, bloatedness, Rheum.
— — congestion of blood, Alum.
— — contraction of lids, Agar. Bell. Nitr. Ntr-m. Oleand. Sep. Sulph. Tart.
— — dazzling in sun, Euphr.
— — downward pressure, Carb-an.
— — heat, burning, Ambr. Bov. *Eug.*
— — obscuration, dulness, Arg. Cycl. Gels. Grat. Igt. Kali-b. Meph. Mur-ac. Ntr-c. Ntr-m. Puls. Raph. Sass. Sil. Stann. Sulph. Zinc.
— — pain, Ambr. Bism. Bry. Carb-an. Cina. Cocc. Croc. Croton. Eugen. Kali-c. Hipp. Led. Lyc. Ntr-c. Nitr-ac. Psor. Puls. Seneg. Sil. Stam.
— — — as if torn out, Cocc.
— — — with the pain, the eyes become smaller, Aloe.
— — — in back part of eyes, Kobalt.
— — pressing the eyes out, Acon. Lachn.
— — running with water, lachrymation, Eugen. Igt. Osm. Puls. Spong.
— — sparks, Eugen. Lach. Psor. Spong. Viol-od.
— — spasm, Viol-od,
— — stinging, Puls.
— — drawing of, Bell. Creos.
— eyelids, twitching of, Millef.
— face, heat of, Aloe. Ang. Calc. Calc-ph. Cannab. Chenop. Creos. Diad. Ferr. Gels. Lob. Ntr-m. Nux. Rhus. Stront.
— — pain, Lyc. Sil. Tong.
— — pale, Acon. Ambr. Alum. Hell. Phosp. Verat.
— — redness, Acon. Bry. Calc. Cannab.

— — Creos. Ferr. Glon. Igt. Kali-jod. Mgn-s. Plat. Rhus. Spong. Stront. Thuj.
— — yellow, Lach.
— feet, cold, Bufo.
— fingers, coldness of, Hell.
— — paleness, Verat.
— — tearing, occasional, Nitr.
— flatulency, Calc-ph.
— forgetfulness, Caps.
— fretfulness, Kali-c. Kali-jod. Sil. Stann. Thuj. Tong.
— giddiness, vertigo, Acon. Anac. Arg-n. Ars. Calc. Canth. Cupr. Cycl. Ferr. Gels. Hep. Hipp. Hydroc-ac. Kali-b. Kali-chl. Kalm. Lach. Lob. Lyc. Mgn-m. Mgn-s. Meph. Merc. Ntr-c. Nicc. Nitr-ac. Nux. Phosp. Prun. Psor. Puls. Sang. Sep. Spig. Stram. Stront. Sulph. Tabac. Tart.
— after headache, Merc-sulph.
— hands cold, Benz-ac.
— heat, general, Calc. Cor-r. Merc. Ntr-s.
— heaviness of limbs, Sil.
— hunger, Elaps.
— jaws, tremor of, Carb-veg.
— impulse to run hither and thither, with, Ars. Coloc.
— indifference, Puls.
— indolence, Calc-ph. Lact.
— insanity, fear of, Ambr.
— irritability, Bell. Berb. Calc-ph. Creos. Kali-c. Kali-jod. Lac-can. *Meph. Nux. Stann. Thuj. Tong.
— lie down necessity to, Bell. Bry. Calc. Con. Ferr. Lach. Lyc. Mosch. Ntr-c. Ntr-m. Nitr-ac. Petr. Phosp-ac. Rhus. Sass. Selen. Sil. Sulph.
— — unable to remain, Coloc.
Accompaind in limbs, pains as if beaten in, Acon.
— low spirits, Agar.
— moaning, with, Ars. Bell.
— nape, numbness in the, Spig.
— pain, Puls. Verat.
— — when raising the head. Senna.
— — stiffness, Arg. Graph. Lach. Mgn-c. Nitr. Spig. Verat.
— nausea, Acon. *Alum. Amm-c.* Ant. Arg. Arn. Benz-ac. Borax. Bry. *Calc.* Camph. Caps. *Carb-veg.* Caust. Cic. Chin. Cocc. *Coloc.* Con. Cor-r. Croc. Dros. *Eugen.* Eupat. Glon. Graph. Hep. Igt. *Ip.* Iris. Kali-b. Kali-c. Lac-can. Lach. Mgn-c. Meph. *Mosch.* Ntr-c. *Ntr-m. Nitr-ac. Nux.* Petr. Phosp. Phyt. Plat. Puls. Ran-b. Sang. Sass. Sep. Sil. *Stann.* Stram. Stront. *Sulph. Tabac.* Therid. *Verat.* Zinc.
— with inclination to vomit, *Alum.* Arg. Ars. *Calc.* Camph. Cocc. Con. Grat. Igt. Tabac.
— — and vomiturition, Stann.
— — vomiting, Arn. Bar-m. Bry. Cadm.

3. HEAD.

Caps. Chin. Cimex. Cocc. Con. Creos. Eugen. Graph. Iris. Ip. Jatr. Kali-c. Lach. Mez. Mosch. Ntr-m. Nitr-ac. Nux. Phosp. Plat. Puls. Sang. Sass. Sep. Therid. Verat. Zinc.
— — of bile, Nicc. Sang.
— — sour, Nux. Sass.
— olfactory nerves sensitiveness of, Phosp.
— pains in heart extend to head, Lith.
— palpitation of heart, Bufo. Hep. Tart.
— perspiration, general, Merc. Ntr-s.
— — cold, Graph.
— — in forehead warm, Glon.
— — — cold, Verat.
— — on head, Acon.
— precedes headache, Ferr.
— photophobia, Euphr. Kali-c. Puls.
— restlessness, Cadm. Cor-r. Lyc. Par. Prun. Ruta.
— rheumatic pains and stiffness of limbs. Sang.
— pain in right shoulder-joint, Lach.
— shuddering, Berb. Evon. Hell. Jatr. Lach Mgn-s. Mez. Nux. Puls. Sil.Thuj.
— sleepiness, Bruc. Creos. Gels. Hipp. Lach. Ntr-s. Nitr. Ran-b. Stann. Stront.
— sneezing, Gels. Kali-chl.
— stomach, burning in, Jatr. Sang.
— — pain at, Benz-ac. Verat.
— — — pit of, Arg.
— — vitiated, Nux-m. Puls. (compare Generalities.)
— talk, to, disinclination, Thuj.
— taste bitter, Creos.
— thirst, Cadm. Cham. Cupr. Eugen. Hipp. Nicc.
— toothache, Rhus.
— trembling of body, Borax.
— unconsciousness, Arn. Bell. Carb-veg. Cocc. Cycl. Kali-b. Puls. Sabin. Sil.
— urinal discharge, increased, Cinnab. Eugen. Gels. Selen. Verat.
— weakness, Agar. Alum. Chin. Creos. Lob. Lyc. Nux. Sil. Sulph.
— — in back, Pallad.
— weariness, Berb.
— weep, disposition to, Ars. Creos. Plat. Ran-b.

4. Scalp.

Adhesion, sensation of, Arn. Berb.
Ascending steps, pain when, Hell.
Baldness, Bar-c. Fluor-ac. Lyc. Zinc.
Beaten, sense on head, as if, Hell. Ip. Petr. Ruta.
— — on occiput, *Hell.*
Bent forward, the head, Lach.
— — — when walking, Sulph.
Biting (see itching).
Blood vessels distention of, Bell. Sang. *Thuj.*
Boils, Hell. Led. Merc. Nux. Petr. Puls. Ruta. Sep. Sil.
— painful, Hell. Hep. Kali-c. Merc. Mez. Nux. Puls.
— — to touch, Ars. Hep. Kali-c. Ruta.
— by tearing on the spot, preceded, Ruta.
— burning, biting, sensitive to touch and cold, Ars.
— suppurating, Calc. Kali-c.
Bones, pain in, Acon. Ant. *Arg. Aur.* Canth. Cina. Cinnab. Ip. Kali-b. Mez. *Nitr-ac.* Phosp-ac. Rhod. Ruta, Staph.
— — as from air blowing, Acon.
— — as if beaten, Ip.
— — as if constricted by a tape, Nitr-ac. Sulph.
— — drawing, Canth. Nitr-ac. Phosp-ac. *Rhod.* Ruta.
— — when lying, Aur.
— — pressing, *Arg.* Nitr-ac. Rhod. Staph.
— — as if separated, with increased temperature, Arg-n.
— — stinging as from a sharp needle, Kali-b
— — as from swelling, Ant.
— — tearing, *Arg.* Merc. Rhod.
— — tension and stinging, Merc. Ruta.

4. SCALP.

Bones, pain when touched, compelling one to cry out, Cupr.
— — — — pain in, increased, Mez.
— swelling of, Aur. Sulph.
Boring pain, Lyc.
— with the head in the pillows, Apis. Bell. Hell. Sulph.
Bruising pain, Ars. Bar-c. Ferr. Hell. Ip. Mez. Petr. Rhod. *Ruta.*
Burning, Ars. Bry. Coloc. Croton. Cupr. Lyc. Merc. Ol-an. Ran-b. Sabad. Staph. Tabac. Viol-tr.
— to eyes extending, Spig.
— on forehead, Clem. Coloc. Cupr. Diad. Meny. Sabad. Spig.
— on temples, Croton. Cupr. Spig.
— on vertex, Cupr. Ntr-m.
Caries, Aur. Nitr-ac. Staph.
— with burning pains, Phosp-ac.
Chills on the scalp, Agn. Ambr. Merc-cor. Sep. Stann. Stront. Sulph. Verat.
— on the part effected, Kali-jod.
— commence on scalp. Mosch.
Circumference of the head, great in children, Calc. *Sil.*
Coldness on scalp, Agar. *Calc.* Iris. Sabad. Sep. *Sulph.* Verat.
— sense of, Acon. Agar. Ambr. Arn. Bell. Calc. Cannab. Chelid. Lach. Laur. Mosch. Phosp. Verat.
— — on forehead, Cinnab. Merc.
— one sided, Ruta.
— circumscribed parts, in, Sulph.
— from nape proceeding, Chelid.
— from vertex down to sacrum, when headeach is over, Laur.
Contraction of scalp, Ntr-m. Plat. Ran-sc. Rhus.
— in skin of forehead, Gels.
— sense of, Carb-veg. Chin. Plat. Sulph.
Covering is intolerable, Led.
— relieves, Hep. Psor. Sil.
Creeping, sensation of, Arg-n. Bar-c. Cannab. Staph.
Cutting pain, Clem. Sass.
Daily pain of scalp, Ntr-c.
Dandruff, Ars. Alum. Calc. Graph. Kali-c. Lac-can. Lach. Mez. Oleand. Phosp. *Staph.* Thuj.
— itching, Alum. Mgn-c. *Staph.*
— — in rainy weather, Mgn-c.
Distortion of head, Camph. Cupr.
From draft of air, pain, Acon.
Drawing pain, Canth. Chenop. Chin. Graph. Lact. Mgn-m. Meny. Nitr-ac. Petr. Phosp-ac. Puls. *Rhod.* Rhus. Ruta. Sass. Sep. Staph. Thuj.
— to face extending, Mgn-m.
— to glands of throat, Graph.
— — to teeth, Graph. Mgn-m. Petr.
— on temples and forehead, Petr.
Like drops of water, falling on the head, Cannab.

Enlargement sense of, Arg-n. Berb. Bov. Cor-r. Daph. Dulc. Ind. Mang. Meph. Ran-sc. Therid.
— — in occiput, Dulc.
Eruption in general, Arg. *Bar-c.* Cic. Hep. *Lyc.* Merc. Mez. Nitr-ac. *Petr.* Puls. Seneg. Sulph. Sulph-ac.
— burning, Cic. Merc. Oleand.
— — after scratching, Hep. Oleand. Vinca.
— crusty, Dulc. Ferr-m. Lyc. Mez. Rhus. Sil. Thuj.
— dry, Ars. *Bar-c.* Merc. Psor. Rhus. Sep. Sil. Sulph.
— eating away the hair, Dulc. Merc. *Rhus.*
— fetid, offensive, Hep. Lyc. Merc. Psor. Rhus. Sep. Sil. *Staph.* Sulph. Vinca.
— herpetic, dry, *Rhus.* Thuj.
— itching, Ars. Clem. Ferr. Hep. Merc. *Mez.* Oleand. *Rhus.* Sil. *Staph.* Sulph.
— itching at night, Oleand. *Rhus.*
— knots, lumps, Graph. Hep. Sil.
— thick leather like crusts, thick and white pus under hair glued up, elevated white scabs looking chalky, Mez.
— moist, humid, Alum. Bar-c. Clem. Creos. *Graph.* Hell. Hep. Lyc. *Merc.* Mez. Nitr-ac. *Oleand.* Psor. Rhus. Ruta. Sep. *Sil. Staph.* Sulph. Vinca.
— painful, Arg. Bar-c. Clem. Graph. Hep. Lac-can. Lachn. Merc. Mez. Ruta.
— periodical every year, Rhus.
— like pimples, Arg. Clem. Creos. Hep. Lac-can. Led. Mez. Psor. Sep.
— with pus filled, Ars. Berb. Clem. Puls.
— scaly, Clem. Oleand.
— sore, smarting, Hep. Ruta.
— suppurating, Bar-m. *Cic. Lyc. Rhus.*
— — greenish, Rhus.
— — yellowish, Merc.
— tinea, Alum. *Ars. Bar-c.* Brom. *Calc. Carb-an.* Chelid. Cic. Creos. *Graph.* Hell. Hep. Kali-c. Lyc. Merc. Ntr-m. *Oleand.* Petr. *Rhus.* Ruta. Sep. *Sil. Staph. Sulph.* Vinca.
— — with liquid stools, Psor.
— — dry, *Dulc.* Mez.
— — moist, *Sil.*
— — white, Thuj.
— — to touch painful, *Hep.* Ruta.
Erysipelas, Ars. Bell. *Euph.* Lach. Rhus.
Fontanels open, in children, Calc. Calc-ph. Cupr. Merc. Sep. *Sil.* Sulph.
— fall in, Apis.
Formication, *Arn. Chelid.* Colch. Led. Ranb. Rhus. *Sabad.* Tabac.
Furrows on forehead, Cham. Hell. Lyc. Rheum. Rhus. Sep. Stram.
Furuncles, Bar-c. Bell. Calc. Kali-c. Led. Mgn-m. Mur-ac. Nitr-ac Rhus.
Gnawing sensation, Bar-c. Berb. Meny.
Hair, bristling, Arn. Canth. Dulc. Lachn. Spong. Zinc.
— dry, Alum. Hipp. *Kali-c.* Plb. Psor.

4. SCALP.

Sulph.
Hair flabby, Phosp-ac.
— flaxen, Phosp-ac.
— gray, Graph. Lyc. Phosp-ac. Sulph-ac.
— greasy, Bry. Phosp-ac.
— falling out, *Ambr*. Amm-c. *Ant*. Ars. Aur. Bar-c. Bov. *Calc*. Carb-an. Carb-veg. Con. Creos. Cycl. Ferr. Ferr-m. Fluor-ac. *Graph*. Hell. *Hep*. Hipp. Igt. Kali-c. Lyc. Mgn-c. *Merc*. *Ntr-m*. Nitr-ac. Nitr. Osm. Par. Petr. Phosp-ac. *Phosp*. *Plb*. Sass. *Sec-c*. Selen. Sep. Sil. Staph. *Sulph*. Sulph-ac. Zinc.
— — from the eyebrows, Kali-c. Plb. Selen.
— — mustaches, Plb. Selen.
— — whiskers, Graph. Kali-c. Ntr-m. Phosp-ac. Plb.
— — sides of head, Calc. Graph. Merc. Phosp.
— — occiput, Carb-veg.
— — in lying in women, Calc. Lach. Ntr-m. Sulph.
— painfulness of, Alum. Ambr. Asar. Calc. Caps. Chin. Ferr. Mez. Par. Sulph. Thuj. *Verat*
— — when brushed backwards, *Puls*. Rhus.
— — after scratching, Caps.
— — as if pulled, Acon. Alum. Canth. Chin. Ind. Rhus. Selen.
— — to touch, Ambr. *Chin*. Cinnab. Ferr. Mez. Sep. Sulph.
Heat, *Acon*. Aloc. Alum. Arn. *Bell*. Borax. Bry. Calc. Camph. *Canth*. Carb-an. *Carb-veg*. Coloc. Con. *Dig*. Dros. Graph. *Lach*. Laur. Mgn-c. Merc. Ntr-c. Ntr-m. Nitr-ac. *Phosp*. Sep. *Sil*. Stram. Stront. *Sulph*. Tart. Verat.
— on forehead, Cham. Diad. Euphr.
— — with cold cheeks, Bell.
— of part affected, Kali-jod.
Immobility, Arn. Berb.
Itching, Agar. Agn. Amm-c. Amm-m. Alum. Anac. Ant. Arg-n. Bar-c. Berb. Bov. Calc. Calc-ph. Caps. Cham. Coloc. Con. Cycl. Dros. Fluor-ac. Gels. *Graph*. Grat. Kali-c. Kobalt. Lach. Laur. Led. Lyc. Merc. Mez. Nitr. Nitr-ac. *Oleand*. Ol-an. Phosp. Puls. Ran-b. *Rhod*. *Ruta*. Sabad. Selen. Seneg. *Sep*. Sil. Spong. Staph. Sulph. Sulph-ac. Thuj. Vinca. Zinc.
— on forehead, Graph. Sep. Sulph.
— in evening, Agn. Berb. Carb-veg. Rhod.
— at night, Oleand. *Rhus*.
— biting, Agn. Led. Mez. Puls. Ran-b. Ran-sc. Rhod. Tnuj.
— burning, Ars. Berb. Hep. Lyc. Merc. Mez. Sabad. Sil.
— gnawing, Agn. Bar-c. Caps. Oleand. Rhod. Rhus. Ruta. Staph. Thuj.
— after scratching increased, Merc. Phosp. Thuj.
— — with pain, Caps.

— — changing the place, Berb. Cycl.
— — rasping, Oleand.
— in sleep, Agn.
— stinging, Berb. Cycl. Sep.
Jerking painful, Agar. Bry. Cham. Croton. Hell.
Knitting the brows, Rheum. Viol-od.
Lice, *Psor*. *Sabad*.
Lumps, tubercles, Calc. Daph. Hell. Igt. Petr. Puls. Rhus. Ruta. Sep. Sil.
— painful, Hell. Nux. Puls. Ruta.
— suppurating, Calc. Kali-c.
In lying pain, Aur. Thuj.
When masticating pain in temples, Thuj.
Motions convulsive, Camph. Cupr. Lyc. Sep. *Stram*.
— distortion, Cupr.
— drawn to one side. *Camph*. Cina. Cupr. Hyosc.
— jerks, *Alum*. Cic. Cina. Samb. Sep.
— opisthotonos, Bell. Camph. Cic. Dig. Hep. Igt. Nux. Sep. Stram.
— shocks, Cic. Kali-c. Sep.
— involuntary when writing, Caust.
— sinking of head backwards, Chin. Dig.
— on turning head, cannot easily turn it back again, Cic.
When opening the mouth, pain in temples, Ang.
Movememt of scalp, Evon. Ntr-m. Sang. Sep.
When moving the head, pain, Cupr Hell.
Muscles twitching of, Arg. Lach.
Nocturnal pain, Led. Ntr-s. Thuj.
— — with chilliness and chattering of teeth, Ntr-s.
Numbness, sense of, Ang. Berb. Caust. Mercurial. Mez. Petr. Plat.
Painfulness of scalp, Ars. Bar-c. Bell. Carb-a. Carb-veg. Caps. Chin. Creos. Ferr. Lith. Ntr-s. Nitr-ac. Nitr. Nux. Petr. Rhus. Sass. Selen. Sil. Staph. Tart. Thuj.
— from pressing of hat, Agar. Carb-a. Carb-veg. Crot. Nitr-ac. Sil-
— from scratching, Bar-c. Caps.
— in small spots, Aloe.
— from strain in loins, Ambr.
— from touch, Agar. Ambr. Arg. Ars. Bar-c. Bov. Bufo. Chin. Cinnab. Cupr. Ferr. Merc. Mez. Ntr-m. Ntr-s. Nitr-ac. Nux-m. Nux. Par. Petr. Rhus. Selen. Sil. Sulph. Thuj. Zinc.
Perspiration, Acon. Anac. Ang. Ars. Bell. Berb. Bry. Bufo. *Calc*. Carb-veg. *Cham*. Chin. Cina. Coloc. Dig. Graph. Guaj. Gum-gut. Hep. Kali-c. Lach. Led. Merc. Mez. Mosch. Ntr-c. Ntr-m. Nitr-ac. Nux. Petr. Phosp. Pod. Puls. Raph. Rheum. Rhus. *Sep*. Sil. Staph. Sulph. Tart. Valer. Verat.
— in evening, *Calc*. *Sep*.

4. SCALP.

Perspiration at night, Coloc. Ntr-m.
— on forehead, Chin. Croton. Hep. Lachn. Led. Nux. Sabad. Stann. Tart.
— clammy, Cham. Merc. Nux.
— cold, Benz-ac. Bry. Cina. Cocc. Colch. Croc. Dig. Hep. Lachn. Merc Op. Puls. Verat.
— — on forehead, Acon. Carb-veg. Chin. Cina. Dros. Ip. Kali-c. Staph. Verat.
— hot, with the pains, Cham. Glon.
— — on forehead, Croton. Tart.
— when walking, Led.
— — in open air, Graph. Guaj. Nux.
— half of head and face, cold to touch, Nux.
— only, hair wet, Rheum.
— all over except head, Thuj.
— and side on which he does not lie, Nux. Sil.
— oily greasy, sour smelling, Bry.
— only, and palms of hands, and much turbid urine, Phosp.
— semilateral, Nux.
— in sleep, Calc. Merc. Pod. Sil.
— during sleep, with coldness of flesh in dentition, Pod.
— sour smelling, Bry. Merc Sil.
— stooping, when, Berb.
Plica Polonica, Bov. Creos. Lyc. Psor. Vinca.
Pressing pain, Arg. Nitr-ac. Oleand. Phosp-ac. Rhod. Sass.
— on forehead, Cic. Chin.
— on temples, Agar. Thuj.
From pressure external, pain, Agar. Arg. Carb-an. Carb-veg. Croton. Nitr-ac. Sil.
Prickling, Croton. Hell. Sabad.
Pulsation, Chelid. Guaj.
Like pulled by the hair, pain, Acon. Alum. Canth. Chin. Iod. Rhus. Selen.
Quivering between the eyebrows when reading, Ang.
Raising frequently the head from the bed, Stram.
Rending, tearing, Arg. Bry. Carb-a. Carb-veg. Chenop. Graph. Lyc. Ntr-c. Ntr-s. Ol-an. Rhod. Rhus. Sass. Sep. Viol-tr.
— on forehead, Carb-veg; Ntr-c.
— from limbs originating, Carb-veg.
— on occiput, Carb-veg.
— on the side, Carb-a. Kali-b.
— to teeth and glands of throat, extending Graph.
— on vertex, Ntr-c.
Rhagades after scratching, Oleand.
Rheumatic pain, Graph. Guaj. Staph.
Rolling of head, Bell.
— — — in difficult dentition, Pod.
With a rough, wind pain, Nux.
Rubs the forehead, Verat.
Scabs, scrufs, on scalp, Ars. Bar-m. Bov. Bry. Calc. Carb-a. Chelid. Graph. Hep. Ntr-m. Oleand. Petr. Rhus. Ruta. Sil.
Sulph.
Scraping sensation, Lyc.
Shuddering, Seneg.
Smarting after scratching, Oleand.
Soreness, sense of, Alum. Ambr. Arg. Bell. Bry. Dros. Ntr-m. Nux. Ol-an. Par. Petr. Rhod. Staph. Zinc.
Sore spots on head, Bov.
Spasmodic pain, Bell.
Stiffness of muscles of forehead, Jatr.
Stinging, stitches, Agn. Berb. Caust. Chin. Cinnab. Daph. Dig. Euphr. Guaj. Ol-an. Phosp-ac. Phosp. Prun. Ran-b. Sass. Staph. Thuj.
— at 3 P. M. Staph.
— in forehead, Chin. Euphr.
— on sides of heads, Phosp.
— in temples, Dig. Euphr. Guaj. Thuj.
When stooping pain on head, Hell.
Straining, Caust.
Swelling sense of, Aeth. Berb. Guaj. Dig. compare Enlargement.
— — when entering a room, Aeth.
— of scalp, Ars. Bell. Bov. Cham. Cupr. Daph. Lach. Merc-cor. Rhus. Sep.
— — painful, Daph.
— — purplish red, with redness of face, Cupr.
— — semilateral, Daph.
— inflammatory, suppurating. or becoming carious, pain on external pressure or when lying on them, Nitr-ac.
To take cold liability, Bar-c. Calc. Carb-veg. Hyosc. Kali-c. Led. Lyc. Ntr-m. Nux. Phosp. Rhus. Sep. Sil.
— — from having the hair cut, Bell. Glon.
Tenderness, sensitiveness of scalp, Agar. Ars. Bov. Calc. Carb-a. Carb-veg. Chin. Crot. Iod. Merc-sulph. Nitr-ac. Nitr. Nux-m. Petr. Phosp. Rhus. Sass. Selen. Sil. Spong. Stann. Tar. Tong. Zinc. compare painfulness.
— of temples, Nux-m.
— — vertex, Scill.
Tension, Agn. Ang. Apis. Arn. Asar. Berb. Caust. Lach. Lam. Merc. Nitr-ac. Ol-an. Phosp. Ran-sc. Ruta. Spig. Stront. Tar. Viol-od.
— on forehead, Carb-an. Evon. Par. Phosp.
— — with wrinkles, Grat.
— — temples, when masticating, Ang.
— — vertex, Carb-an.
Throbbing in temples, Guaj. Pod.
Tightness of scalp, Carb-an. Caust. Hell. Merc. Lam. Spig.
— sense of, Agn. Bell. Berb. Bry. Caust. Viol-od.
Thinness of skull, sense of, Bell.
To touch painfulness, Agar. Ambr. Arg. Ars. Bov. Chin. Cinnab. Cupr. Ferr. Mez. Ntr-m. Nitr-ac. Nitr. Nux-m. Nux. Par. Petr. Puls. Sil. Spig. Thuj. compare Pressure.

To touch painfulness, increased by, Agar. Bry. Mez. Sass.
When touching the hair pain, Agar. Ambr. Chin. Cinnab. Ferr. Mez. Puls. Rhus.
Tremor of head, Alum. Aur. Bell. Calc. *Cocc.* Hyosc. Igt. Kali-chl. Lith. Lyc. Sep. Tabac. *Tart.*
Tumors, Calc. Hell. Nux. Petr. Puls. Ruta. Sep. Sil.
Twitching, on scalp, Agar. Bry. Hell.
Ulcers small, Ruta.

Ulcerous pain, Petr. Rhod. Rhus. Sulph-ac. Zinc.
By walking pain increased, Graph. Sass.
Warmth sense of, Verat.
Weakness of head, Arn. *Caust.* Chin. Cupr. Rhod. Spong. Viol-od.
— — — with falling backwards, Camph. Chin. *Dig.* Rhod. Viol-tr.
— — — — forwards, *Cupr.* Viol-od.
— — — — sideways Spong.
From wrong lifting pain, Amb.

5. Eyes and Sight.

Aching pains in orbits, Bov. Cupr. Par. Ph.
Agglutination, Agar. *Alum.* Apis. Bar-c. Bell. *Bry.* Calc. Cham. *Dig.* Euph. Graph. *Igt. Kali-c.* Led. *Lyc. Mgn-c.* Nux. *Phosp. Puls.* Rhod. Rhus. Spig. Spong. *Staph.* Sulph. Thuj.
— in the morning, Caust, *Chelid.* Dig. Graph. Kali-b. *Kali-c.* Mgn-c. Mang. Millef. Nicc. Nux. Phosp. Psor. Sass.
— at night, *Alum.* Amm-c. Ang. Ant. Ars. Bar-c. Bell. Bov. Bry. Calc. *Carb-veg.* Cast. Cham. Chelid. Cic. *Croc.* Creos. Dig. *Euph.* Euphr. Ferr. Graph. Gum-gut. Hep. Igt. Kali-c. Led. *Lyc.* Mgn-c. *Mgn-m.* Merc. Ntr-c. Ntr-m. Nitr-ac. Nux. Ol-an. Phosp. Plb. Puls. Rat. Rhod. Rhus. Sass. Sep. *Sil.* Stann. Staph. Stram. Sulph. Tar. Thuj. Verat.
Amaurosis, *Aur.* Bell. Calc. Caust. Chelid. Cic. Con. Dig. Dulc. Euphr. Gels. Guaj. Hyosc. Ntr-m. Op. Phosp. Plb. Puls. Sec-c. Sep. *Sil.* Stram. Sulph. Zinc. (compare Paralysis of optic nerve.)
— incipient, Bell. Calc. Cannab. *Caps. Caust. Chin.* Hyosc. *Merc. Ntr-m. Puls. Rhus.* Ruta. Spig. *Sulph. Tart.*
Anxious look, Aloe. Arn. Nux.
Arthritic affection, Ant. Ars. Bell. Bry. Cham, Coloc. Dig. Hep. Merc. Nux. Puls. Rhus. Spig.
Beaten, pain around eyes, as if parts were, Ntr-s.
Biting, Berb. Carb-veg. Caust. Chin. *Clem.* Creos. Euphr. Graph. Kali-c. Kali-jod. Lact. Lyc. *Merc. Nux.* Ol-an. Petr. Rheum. Rhus. Sabad. Sep. Sil. Stann. Staph. Sulph. Sulph-ac. Tabac. *Teucr.* Thuj. Valer. Viol-tr. Zinc.
— below the eyes when rubbing, Con.
— in the lids, *Clem.* Creos. Lyc. Sep. Spig.

Sulph. Zinc.
— in the canth, Carb-veg. Con. Mez. Mur. ac. Ran-b. *Ran-sc.* Ruta. Sil. *Staph. Sulph.* Tart. Teucr. Zinc.
— as from dust Rheum.
Blear-eyedness, Acon. Asar. Bry. Elaps. *Euphr.* Merc. Par. Puls. Sep. Spig. Tart. Teucr.
Bleeding from eyes, Bell. Calc. Carb-veg. *Cham.* Lach. *Nux.*
— — lids, Arn. *Bell.*
Blindness paroxysms of (in the day), Acon. Con. Meny. Nitr. Nux. Phosp. Sil. Stram. Sulph.
— — in the evening, Bell.
— — at night, *Bell.* Cadm. Chelid. *Hyosc.* Meph. Merc. Puls. *Verat.*
— — in sunlight, Con.
— followed by headache, sight returns with increasing headache, Kali-b.
— momentary, as from fainting, Agar. Aur. Bell. Calc. Caust. Cic. Dros. Ferr. Hep. Hyosc. Mang. Merc. Ntr-m. Nitr. Oleand. Phosp. Puls. Spig. Stram.
— periodical, Chelid. Chin. Dig. Euphr. Hyosc. Merc. Ntr-m. Phosp. Puls. Sep. Sil. Sulph. Tart.
— sudden, Mosch.
Bloatedness of lids, Psor. Spong.
Blood, congestion of to eyes, Alum. Bell. Kali-ch. Phosp. Plb. Seneg.
— — when stooping, Seneg.
— oozing of from, Calc. Crotal.
— specks on eyeball, Nux.
Blueness of eyes, Verat.
— lids, Dig. Dros.
— canthi, Sass.
Boil on canthus, Bell. Bry. Calc. Ntr-c. Petr. Puls. Sil. Stann.
Bones of orbits, pain in, Phosp.
Boring sense in eyes, Puls. Spig.

5. EYES AND SIGHT.

Too bright seeming, everything, Camph. Nux.
Bright appearances, Amm-c. Aur. Bar-c. Bell. Borax. Bry. Camph. Cannab. Croc. Con. Dig. Graph. Iod. Kali-c. Nux. Puls. Spig. Stront. Tart. Valer. Verat. Zinc.
— brightness, clearness, Kali-c. *Valer.*
— circles fiery, Puls.
— fire, Amm-c. Aur. Bell. Bry. Cannab. Caust. Con. Croc. Dig. Dulc. Elaps. Hyosc. Kali-c. Kali-chl. Lach. Merc. Ntr-c. Ntr-m. Nux. Puls. Sec-c. Sep. Sil. Staph. Stram. Sulph. Verat. Viol-od. Zinc.
— fiery zig-zags around everything, Ntr-m.
— flakes fiery, Zinc.
— flashes of light, lightenings, Croc. Kali-c. Ntr-c. Nux. Sec-c. Spig. Staph.
— flickering zig-zags, Igt.
— glittering, Aloe. Alum. Amm-c. Bell. Borax. Carb-veg. Caust. Cham. Chin. Cic. Cina. Con. Dig. Fluor-ac. Gels. Graph. Hep. Igt. Iod. Led. Lyc. Nux. Petr. Plat. Seneg. Sep. Staph. Stram. Stront. Tabac. Tart. Therid. Verat. Viol-od.
— red spots, Hyosc. Lac-can.
— shining spots, Seneg.
— sparks, Ars. Aur. Bar-c. Bell. Caust. Cycl. Dig. Dulc. Glon. Iod. Kali-c. Kali-chl. Lach. Merc. Mez. Ntr-c. Ntr-s. Nux. Petr. Phosp. Sep. Sil. Staph. Valer. Verat.
— streaks of light, Amm-c. Glon. Ntr-m. Sep.
— luminous rays from light to eyes, Cham.
— red bar before the eyes on opening them, Elaps.
— in the evening, Kali-c.
— after blowing the nose, Ntr-s.
— with closed eyes, Alum; Kali-c.
— when coughing or sneezing, Kali-chl.
— in the dark, Bar-c. Lyc. Staph. Thuj. *Valer.*
— when raising the eyes, Zinc.
— when rising from lying, Verat.
— — from sitting, Tart. Verat.
As if bruised pain, Cocc. Gels. *Hep.* Lyc. Nux. Sulph. Tart. *Verat.*
— — in lids, Hep.
— — sockets, Cupr.
Burning, Acon. Agn. All-cep. Alum. Ambr. *Amm-c. Ang.* Ars. *Asa-f. Asar.* Aur. *Bar-c.* Bell. Berb. Borax. *Bry.* Calad. *Calc. Canth. Caps. Carb. veg. Cast.* Caust. Cham. Chin. Cic. *Coloc.* Con. Cor-r. *Croc.* Creos. Croton. Cycl. Elaps. *Eugen.* Euphr. *Ferr.* Fluor-ac. Graph. Grat. Gum-gut. Hep. Hipp. Kali-b. Kali-c, Kali-jod. Lach. Lachn. Laur. Led. *Lyc.* Mgn-c. Mgn-s. *Mang.* Meph. *Merc.* Merc-cor.
Ntr-c. Ntr-m. *Ntr-s.* Nicc. Nitr-ac. *Nitr.* Nux-m. *Nux.* Ol-an. Osm. Pæon. Par. Petr. Phell. Phosp-ac. *Phosp.* Phyt. Puls. Rat. *Rhod.* Rhus. Ruta. Sabad. Sass. Seneg. Sep. Sil. Spig. Spong. Stann. Staph. Stront. *Sulph.* Sulph-ac. *Tabac.* Tar. Tart. *Thuj. Tong.* Valer. Viol-od. Zinc.
— in the morning, Amm-c. Graph. Mgn-s. Nicc. Nitr-ac. Nitr. Phell. Rat. Rhod. Sass. Seneg. Sep. Stront. Zinc.
— at twilight disappears at candlelight Amm-m.
— below the eyes when rubbing, Con.
— on the brows, *Dig.*
— in canthi, Agar. *Amm-m.* Calc. Carb-veg. Cinnab. Ntr-m.Nux. Petr. *Phosp-ac.* Phosp. Ran-b. Scill. *Sulph.* Thuj.
— — edges, Meph. Nux.
— — the lids, Ars. Aur. Bell. Berb. Bry. Calc. Caust. Chenop. Clem. Colch. Croc. Kali-b. Lact. Lyc. Nux. Oleand. Phell. Phosp-ac. Phyt. Sass. Seneg. Stann. Sulph. Zinc.
Candle light seeming too dark, Euphr.
— — flaring, Anac. Euphr.
— — by a halo surrounded, Alum. Anac. Bell. Dig. Ferr. Lach. Mgn-m. Nitr. Phosp. Puls. Ruta. Sass. Sep. Stann. Stront. Sulph.
— — — blue, Lach.
— — — green, Phosp. Sep.
— — — rainbow-colored, Ferr. Nitr. Stann.
— — — red, Ruta.
Cataract. *Amm-c.* Bar-c. Bell. Calc. *Cannab. Caust.* Chelid. Chin. Con. Dig. Euphr. Hep. Hyosc. Lyc. *Mgn-c.* Merc. Ntr-m. Nitr-ac. Op. Phosp. Puls. Rhus. Ruta. *Sil.* Tellur.
— after contusion, Con.
— incipient, Puls.
— reticularis, Caust. Plb.
— viridis, Phosp. Puls.
Ciliary neuralgia with iritis, Mez.
Close the eyes, disposition to, Ox-ac.
Clouds, before the eyes, Berb. Cast. Croton. Kalm. Lact. Ol-an. Sabin.
— — the right eye, Ferr-m.
Coldness in eyes Alum. Amm-c. Asa-f. Calc. *Con.* Lachn. Lyc. *Plat.*
— — edges of lids, Kali-c. Phosp-ac.
— — canthi, Asar.
— — in evening, Lyc.
— — when walking in the open air, Alum. Con.
Colors before the eyes, Agar. Amm-c. Anac. Arn. Bell. Calc.Caust. Chin. Cic. Cocc. Con. Dig. Euphr. Hep. Kali-c. Mgn-c. Merc. Ntr-c. Nitr-ac. Nitr. Phosp. Ruta. Sass. Sep. Sil. Stram. Stront. Sulph. Thuj.
— blue, Bell. Hipp. Kali-c. Lyc. Nicc. Stram. Stront.

5. EYES AND SIGHT.

Colors blue before right eye, Nicc.
— gray, Nitr-ac. Nux. Phosp. Sep. Sil. Stram.
— green, *Dig.* Kali-c. Merc. Phosp. Ruta. Sep Stront. Sulph. Zinc.
— red, Bell. Cact. Con. Croc. Elaps. Hyosc. Sass. Stront. Sulph.
— striped, Amm-c. Bell. Con. Ntr-m. Puls. Sep.
— variegated, Bell. Cic. Con. Dig. Kali-c. Nicc. Nitr. Phosp-ac. Phosp. Stram.
— white, Amm-c. Kali-c.
— yellow, Alum. Ars. Bell. *Canth. Dig.* Kali-b. Kali-c. Sep. Sil. Stront. Sulph.
— in the evening, Nitr. Sass.
— around the candle, Calc. Nitr. Sep. Stann.
— in the dark, Stront.
— when reading, Cic. Croc.
— in a room, Con.
— after rubbing the eyes, Stront.
Compression of the eyes, Aur. Bell. Cannab. Chin. Cor-r. Hep. Plat. Tabac. Verat. Viol-od. Zinc.
— — of lids, Asa-f. Euphr.
Condylomata of eyebrows, *Thuj.*
Confusion of letters when reading, Bry. Chin. Daph. Dros. Graph. Lach. Lyc. Meph. Ntr-m. Seneg. Sil. Stram.
Congestion of blood to eyes, Aloe, Alum. Bell. Plb. Seneg.
— — when stooping, Seneg.
— — to lids, Gels.
Conjunctiva, brown spots on, Kali-b.
— pustules, on Merc.
— swollen, Bell. Bry. Sulph.
Contracting sensation, Croton. Euphr. Plb. Rat. Ruta. Scill. Verb.
— — in lids, Croton. Euphr. Nux. Plb. Rhod. Tabac. Viol-tr.
Contraction, spasmodic of lids, Acon. Alum. Ars. Bell. Calc. Cham. Croc. Cupr. Hep. Hyosc. Merc. Ntr-m. Sil. Spong. Staph. Stram. Sulph. Tart. Viol-od.
— in morning, Calc. Spong. Sulph.
— in evening, Hep. Ntr-m.
— of eyes, when putting on spectacles, Borax.
Convulsions of eyes, *Bell.* Canth. Cocc. Cupr. Hyosc. *Igt.* Spig.
— — lids, Berb. Igt. Lach. Rheum.
— — — when reading, Berb.
— occasioned by light, Bell.
Cornea, fungus hœmatodes, Calc. Lyc. Sep. Sil.
— granular pustules, Kali-b.
— inflammation, *Euphr.* Spig.
— irritation, Croton.
— opacity, Agn. Apis. Arg-n. Cadm. Calc. Cannab. Chelid. Chin. Croton. Euph. Euphr. *Mgn-c.* Nitr-ac. Op. Puls. Sacch. *Seneg.* Sulph. Zing.

— bluish, Euphr.
— as from dust on it, Sulph.
— from wounds, Euphr.
— painless, Dig.
— pellicle from wounds, Euphr.
— specks, spots, Apis. Ars, *Aur. Bell.* Cadm, Calc. Cannab. Chelid. Con. *Euphr. Hep.* Lyc. *Nitr-ac.* Nux. Sep. Sil. Ruta. Sulph.
— — scars from, *Euphr.* Sil.
— vesicles, on, Sulph.
Cuting pain in eyes, Calc. Coloc. Merc. Puls. Verat. Viol-tr.
— — lids, Calc. *Merc.*
— — and heat after operations, Croc.
Dark, black, bodies before the eyes, Bell. Calc. Canth. Chin. Cocc. Dros. Euphr. Hep. Kali-c. Lyc. Mgn-c. Mosch. Mur-ac. Petr. Phosp. Plb. Rhus. Sep. Sil. Staph. Stram.
— clouds, Cast. Ol-an. Sabin.
— — when lying on left side, Merc-jod.
— flies, Agar. Amm-m. Aur. Bell. Calc. Caust. Chin. Cocc. Coff. Con. Dig. Dulc. Lact. Merc. Ntr-m. Nitr-ac. Phosp. Rhus. Ruta. Sep. Sil. Stram. Sulph.
— black mote before left eye, Agar. Merc.
— network, Anac. Bar-c. Caust. Ntr-ac.
— points, Amm-c. Amm-m. Con. Chin. Elaps. Kali-c. *Merc.* Ntr-c. Ntr-m. *Nitr-ac.* Nux. Sep. Sulph. Tabac. Tereb. Thuj.
— spots, Acon. Agar. Amm-c. Amm-m. Anac. Aur. Bar-c. Bell. Calc. Cast. Carb-veg. Chin. Cocc. Con. Euphr. Evon. Glon. Kali-c. Lact. Lyc. Mgn-c. Merc. Ntr-c. Ntr-m. Nitr-ac. Nux. Petr. Phosp-ac. Phosp. Ruta. Sec-c. Sep. Sil. Sulph. Tabac. Thuj. Verat.
— — when stooping, Lact.
— very near, Lyc.
— stars, Cast.
— streaks, Phosp-ac.
— in the daytime, Amm-m.
— with candle light, evening, Amm-m.
— when gazing at anything, Amm-m.
— when looking down, with nausea and eructations, Kalm.
— when reading, Calc. Kali-c.
— when rising from sitting or lying, Verat.
— in a room, Con.
Darkness, cloudiness, before the eyes, Acon. Ambr. Ang. Arg-n. Arn. Ars. Asa-f. Asar. Aur. Bell. Berb. Bry. Calc. Camph. Cham. *Cic.* Chin. Cupr. Dig. *Evon.* Graph. Hep. Hyosc. Lach. Lact. Laur. Lyc. Meny. Mosch. Ntr-m. Nitr-ac. *Nitr.* Oleand. Op. Phosp. Puls. Scill. Sec-c. *Stram.* Sulph. *Thuj.*
— evening, Puls.

5. EYES AND SIGHT.

Darkness from smell of camphor, Nitr.
— from candle light, Phosp.
— with deafness, alternating, Cic.
— when looking sideways, Oleand.
— — — at anything white, Cham.
— after meals, Calc.
— when reading, Calc. Dros. Hep. Meny. Ntr-m. Sulph. Thuj.
— on one side only, Cham.
— with sleepiness, Thuj.
— when stooping, Graph. Ntr-m.
— — walking, Cic. Ntr-m.
— — writing, Asa-f.
Day blindness, Con. Sulph.
Duzzled eyes, Con.
— in evening, Lyc.
— by bright light, Bar-c. Bry. Calc. Camph. Caust. Cham. Clem. Con. Dros. Euphr. *Kali-c.* Igt. Lith. Lyc. Merc. Nitr-ac. Phosp-ac. Phosp. Sil. Sulph.
— light of a candle, Phosp.
— gazing at anything bright, Phosp-ac.
— when reading, Seneg.
— spot before eyes, Chelid.
Detached as if eyeballs were, Carb-an.
Diffusion of light, Bell. Puls.
Digging pain, Colch. Spig.
Dilated lids, Ant.
Dimness of eyes, Arn. Ars. Bell. Bov. Bry. Con. Cupr. Cycl. Ferr. Kali-jod. Lyc. Merc. Mosch. Sang. Spig. Spong. Stann. Stram.
Dimsightedness, Acon. *Agar.* Alum. Amb. Amm-c. Amm-m. Anac. Ang. Arn. Ars. Aur. Bar-c. Bell. Berb. Bov. Bry. Cact. Calc. *Cannab.* Caps. *Caust.* Chelid. Chin. *Cina.* Clem. Cocc. Coloc. *Con.* Creos. Croc. Cycl. Dig. Dros. Dulc. *Euph.* Evon. Ferr. Gels. Glon. Hœmatox. *Hep.* Hydroc-ac. *Hyosc.* Ip. Iod. Kali-b. Lact. Laur. Led. *Lyc.* Mgn-c. Mang. Meph. Merc. Ntr-c. Ntr-m. Ntr-s. Nitr-ac. *Ol-an.* Op. Phosp-ac. *Phosp.* Plat. *Plb.* Psor. *Puls.* Rhus. *Ruta.* Sacch. Sang. *Sass. Seneg.* Sep. *Sil.* Spig. Stann. Staph. Stram. *Sulph. Tabac. Tart.* Thuj. Valer. Verb.
— frequent, Sang.
— with increased brightness alternating, Hep.
— like cuticle before the eyes, Caust. Daph. Puls. Rat.
— like feathers before the eyes, Calc. Creos. Lyc. Ntr-c. Ntr-m. Sulph.
— like gauze, Berb. Bufo. Calc. *Caust.* Creos. Croc. Dros. Dulc. Hydroc-ac. Lach. Lact. Laur. Ntr-m. Petr. *Phosp.* Plat. Puls. Rhus. Sec. *Sep.* Sil. *Sulph.* Tabac. Tilia. Thuj. Verb.
— — blue, Lach.
— — gray, Phosp.
— glittering, Alum. Amm-c. Led. Seneg. Tart.

— misty, Acon: Agar. Alum. Ambr. Amm-m. Ang. Arn. Asa-f. Bar-c. Bell. Bism. Bry. *Calc.* Caust. Con. Creos. Croc. Croton. *Cycl.* Diad. Dig. Euphr. Evon. Grat. Igt. Lachn. Lact. Laur. Lyc. Merc. Meph. Ntr-c. Ntr-m. Nicc. Nitr-ac. Petr. Phell. Phosp-ac. *Phosp. Plb.* Puls. *Ruta.* Sabin. Sass. Sec-c. Sep. Sil. Spig. Staph. Stram. Sulph. Tart.
— smoky, Gels.
— like water in eyes, Staph.
— to wipe compelling, Creos. Croc. Laccan. Ntr-c. Plb. *Puls.* Rat.
— by wiping relieved, Cina. Caps. Croc. Plb. Puls.
— by wiping increased, Seneg.
— in the morning, Caps. Cham. *Chelid.* Puls.
— in the evening, Cham. Croc. Ferr. Hep. Lachn. Puls. *Tabac.*
— with candle light, Croc. Hep.
— sunlight, Bry.
— after eating, Calc.
— after exertion of the eyes, *Ruta.*
— with inclination to vomit, Puls.
— when looking at a distance, Cast. Gels. Ruta.
— — intently, Calc. Phell.
— during pregnancy, Gels.
— when reading, Bar-c. Calc. Cina. Croc. Grat. Hep. Meny. Ntr-m. Ox-ac. Rhod. Sep.
— after reading. Cocc. *Ruta.*
— when rising from a seat, Puls.
— after sleep at noon, Puls.
— with sleepiness, Mgn-s.
— when writing. Asar. Grat. Kobalt. Ntr-m. Ol-an. Rhod. Sep.
— worse after every headache, Caust.
Diplopia, Agar. Amm-c. Aur. Bell. Cannab. *Cic,* Clem. Con. Cycl. Dig. Eugen. Euph. Gels. *Hyosc.* Iod. Lith. Lob. Lyc. Merc-cor. Ntr-m. N!cc. Nitr-ac. Oleand. Petr. Puls. Rhus. Sec-c. Sep. Spig. Spong. Stram. Sulph. Thuj. Verat.
— of one eye, Cham.
— horizontal, Oleand.
— on looking in light, Therid.
Distance of objects seeming greater, Anac. Carb-an. Cic. Lyc. Ntr-m. Nicc. Nux-m. Ox-ac. Phosp. Stann. Stram. Sulph.
Distension sense of, Caust. Con. (compare Enlargement).
Distortion of eyes, Acon. Ars. Bell. *Camph.* Canth. *Cham.* Cic. *Cupr.* Dig. Hydroc-ac. *Hyosc.* Lach. *Laur.* Op. Petr. Phosp-ac. Plat. Plb. Ran-sc. Sec-c. Spig. Stann. Stram. Sulph. Verat.
— upwards, Verat.
Downcast eyes, Ang. Arn. Asar. Bell. Bov. Chin. Con. Creos. Cycl. Ferr. Hyosc. Iod. Kali-c. Lach. Merc. Nitr-ac. Phosp-ac. Rheum. Rhus. Sabin.

5. EYES AND SIGHT. 41

Spig. Spong. Stann. Valer. Verat.
Downward pressure in eyes, Hell. Seneg.
— — in lids, Chelid.
Drawing sensation in eyes, Cannab. Colch. Ol-an.
— — about eyes, Fluor-ac. Plat.
— — in lids, Colch. Rheum. Seneg. Tong.
Drawing up of eyebrows, upper lids, looks fixed, Lachn.
Dryness of eyes, Ars. Asa-f. Bell. Berb. Bry. Caust. Clem. Croc. Elaps. Euphr. Kali-c. Laur. Lyc. Mgn-c. *Mang.* Ntr-m. Ntr-s. Nicc. Nux-m. Pæon. Pallad. Phell. *Puls. Rhod.* Rumex. Seneg. Spig. *Staph.* Sulph. Tong. Verat. Zinc.
— in room lachrymation, Phell. Sulph.
— of lids, Acon. Ars. Cocc. Daph. Euph. Hipp-m. Merc-cor. Puls. Verat.
— — edges, Ars. Cham.
— canthi, Euph.
— in light, Ars.
— when reading, Aur.
— in room, Sulph.
— when sleeping, Puls.
— sense of, Asar. Asa-f. Bar-c. Bell. Berb. Lachn. Lith. *Nux-m.* Nux. Pæon. Sil.
— — in lids, Bar-c. Berb. Graph. Pallad.
— — of canthi, Arg. Nux. Thuj.
Dulness of eyes, Aeth. All-cep. Ang. Arn. Ars. Asar. Bell. Berb. Bov. Bry. Chin. Con. Creos. Cycl. Ferr. Glon. Kali-c. Kalm. Hyosc. Iod. Lach. Merc. Mosch. Nitr-ac. Phosp-ac. Rheum. Sabin. Spig. Spong. Stann. Valer. Verat.
— — — after little exertion, Ferr.
— — — after meals, Valer.
— — — while reading, Grat.
Dull letters appear when reading, Chin. Dros. Sil.
Like dust in the eyes, Acon. Lach. Lachn. Rheum. Sulph.
— — on cornea, Sulph.
Ectropion, Bell. Igt.
Enlargement of eyes, sensation of, Ant. Calad. Caust. Con. Lach. Mez. Op. *Par.* Phosp-ac. *Plb.* Spig.
Eruption, rash, about eyes, Sulph.
— below eyes, Hep.
— on eyebrows, Guaj. Selen. Thuj.
— on lids, Hep. Sil.
— on eyebrows yellow crusty, Spong.
— fine, around eyes, Euphr.
— pimples in eyebrows, Kali-c.
— scaly herpes on lids, Creos.
— scrufs around eyes, Merc.
Eye gum, Amm-c. *Ant.* Bism. Graph. Ip. Nux. *Seneg.* Staph. (compare Mucus).
— on lids, Agar. Amm-c. Graph. *Seneg.*
— — in morning, *Seneg.*
— in canthi, *Ant.* Bism. Nux. Staph.
Falling down of lids, Acon. Bell. Croc.

Graph. Merc. Ntr-c. Op. Phell. Sep. Spig. Spong. Sulph. Tart. Viol-od. *Viol-tr.* Zinc.
— — of upper lid, Acon. Bell. Caust. Cham. Chelid. Graph. Nux. Sep. Sil.
False sight, Bell. Hyosc. Kali-c. Plat. Stram.
— — confused, Con. Graph. Plat. Selen. Stram.
Fatigue, drowsy, Acon. Asa-f. Phell. Plat. Plb. Tart. Thuj. Viol-od. Viol-tr.
— pain as from, Meph. Oleand.
— — as from study, Oleand.
Feverish sight, Sol-m.
Flashes of light before eyes, Brom. Croc. Ntr-c. Spig. Staph.
Flow of tears, Acon. *Euphr.* Merc. *Par.* Puls. Rhus. *Spig.*
As from foreign bodies pain, Acon. Arn. *Calc.* Caps. Cocc-c. Euphr. Igt. Kali-b. Meph. Ruta. Sil. *Sulph.*
Like fire sparkling from eyes sensation, Clem. Dulc.
Fire glare of intolerable, Merc.
Fixed look, Acon. Aeth. Ang. Arn. Ars. Asar. Bar-m. Bell. Camph. Cic. Cupr. Hell. Hydroc-ac. Hyosc. Igt. Kali-c. Lach. Laur. Lyc. Merc. Mosch. Nux. Op. Puls. Rhus. Ruta. Scill. Sec-c. Seneg. Stram. Tart.
Fullness sense of in eyes, Apis. Nux-m.
— — in lids, Gels.
Fungus medullaris of eye, Bell. Calc. Lyc. Sep. Sil.
Glassy appearance of eyes, Bry. Cocc. Elaps. Op. Phosp-ac. Sep.
— — in morning, Sep.
Gnawing pain, Agn. Plat.
— eyelids, Agn. Berb.
Green color of eyes, Canth.
— — ring around, Verat.
Haggard eyes, Ars. Bell. Cupr. Op. Sec-c.
Hair falling off from eyebrows, Alum. Plb. Selen.
— before the sight, Sang.
— sense of one in eye, Tabac.
— as one pulled out, sensation, Prun.
Heat in eyes, Ang. *Bell.* Carb-veg. Cham. Chin. Clem. *Cor-r.* Creos. *Diad.* Glon. Graph. Kali-b. Lach. Lyc. Mang. Meph. Merc. Nicc. Phosp. Plat. Psor. Sabin. Sil. Spig. Sulph. *Tabac. Verat.* Verb. Viol-od.
— in canthi, Carb-veg. Phosp. Thuj.
Heat and lacerating pains after operations, Croc.
Heat when closing the eyes, Cor-r.
— in evening with candlelight, Graph.
Heaviness in eyes, *Hell.* Hipp-m. Lachn. Plb. Sulph.
— of lids, Acon. Apis. Bell. Berb. Caust. Cham. Chelid. Gels. Graph. Kali-b. Lac-can. Lach. Lyc. Mercurial. Ntr-c.

5. EYES AND SIGHT.

Ntr-s. Nux. Phell. Rhus. Sep. Sil. Spong. Sulph. Viol-od.
Heaviness in morning, as if they could not be kept open, Nitr-ac. Sep.
Hemiopia, Aur. Calc. Caust. Lith. Lob. Lyc. Mur-ac. Ntr-m. Spig.
— horizontal, Aur.
— perpendicular, Caust. Lyc. Mur-ac. Ntr-m.
— of right half of an object, Lith.
Herpes on lids, Bry. Creos. Sulph.
Hordeolum on lid, Amm-c. Bry. Con. Ferr. Graph. Lyc. Merc. Phosp-ac. Phosp. Puls. Rhus. Sep. Stann. Staph. Sulph. Thuj.
— — upper lid, Ferr. Puls.
— — lower lid, Rhus.
— — left eye, Elaps.
— — left lower lid, Hyper.
Illusions of sight, Bell. Calc. Camph. Canth. Carb-veg. *Dig.* Dulc. Hell. Hep. Hyosc. Kali-c. Mgn-m. Nitr-ac. Nitr. Nux. Op. Phosp. *Stram.* Sulph.
— things seeming larger, Euph. Hyosp. Laur. Ntr-m. Nicc. Osm. Ox-ac. Phosp.
— — smaller, Hyosc. *Plat. Stram.*
— — — before the right eye, Thuj.
Immobility of eyes, Amm-c. Ang. Bar-m. Camph. Op. Hydroc-ac. Rat.
Increased vision, can read small print distinctly, Coff.
Indistinct vision, Kali-jod. Osm. Stram.
For infants, affections of eyes, Acon. Bell. Borax. *Bry.* Calc. *Cham. Euphr.* Nux. Puls. Sulph.
Inflammation of eyes, *Acon.* All-cep. Alum. *Amb. Ant.* Apis. Arg-n. *Ars.* Asar. Aur. *Bar-c. Bell.* Borax. Brom. *Bry.* Cadm. Calad. *Calc.* Camph. Cannab. Canth. Caps. *Caust. Cham. Chin.* Cinnab. *Clem.* Coloc. Con. Creos. Croton. Cupr. Daph. Dig. Dulc. Elaps. Eugen. *Euph. Euphr.* Ferr. *Graph. Hep.* Hyosc. Igt. Iod. Ip. Kali-b. Kali-c. Kalm. Lach. *Led. Lyc.* Mgn-c. Mgn-m. *Merc. Mez.* Ntr-c. Ntr. m. *Nitr-ac. Nux.* Op. Petr. Phosp-ac. *Phosp.* Plb. *Puls.* Ran-b. Rat. Rhus. Sacch. *Sep.* Sil. *Spig. Staph.* Stram. *Sulph.* Sulph-ac. Tar. Teucr. Thuj. *Verat.* Zinc.
— of upper part of eye ball as far as covered with the lid, Igt.
— rheumatic of left eye, conjunctiva red, swollen, looks like raw meat, redness from eye over whole cheek, Apis.
— with suggilation after injuries, Arn.
— of lids, *Acon.* Ant. *Ars.* Bar-c. Bell. Bry. Calc. Cannab. *Caust.* Cham. Chelid. Chin. Cocc. Con. Creos. Dig. Euphr. *Hep.* Hyosc. Iris. Kali-b. Kali-c. Lach. Lyc. Merc. *Ntr-c. Ntr-m.* Nux. Phosp-ac. Psor. Puls. *Rhus.* Rumex. Sass. *Sep. Spig.* Stann. Staph. *Sulph. Thuj.* Verat.

Zinc.
— edges, Bell. *Cham.* Clem. *Dig.* Euphr. Hep. Lach. Merc. Nux. *Puls. Staph.* Stram.
— canthi, Borax. Calc. Zinc.
— curuncles, Berb.
— conjunctiva, Arg-n. Ars. Dig. Hep. Merc. Sulph.
— cornea, Euhprc. Spig.
— internal surface of lids, Ars. Bell. Merc. Nux. Phosp. Puls. Rhus. Sil. Sulph.
— — preventing opening, Ars.
— iris, Clem. Merc-cor. Mez. Plb. Sulph.
— meibomian glands, Gham. Dig. Euphr. Puls. Staph. Stram.
— pupil, Plb.
— acute, Acon. Bry. Cham. Merc. Nux. Puls.
— arthritic, Ant. Ars. Bell. Bry. Cham. Coloc. Dig. Hep. Merc. Nux. Puls. Rhus. Spig.
— catarrhal, after a cold, Acon. Bell. Calc. Cham. Dulc. Euphr. Iod. Nux. Puls. Sulph.
— chronic, Apis.
— erysipilatous, *Acon. Hep.*
— after suppressed gonorrhoea, Puls.
— scrofulous, Ars. *Aur.* Bell. *Calc.* Cannab. *Caust.* Chin. Cist. Dig. Dulc. Euphr. Ferr. Hep. Igt. Mgn-c. Merc. Ntr-m. *Nux. Puls.* Rhus. *Sulph.*
— syphilitic, *Merc. Nitr-ac.*
— in the evening increased, Chin.
— from foreign bodies, Acon. Arn. *Calc. Sulph.*
— with headache, Led. Verat.
— in infants, Acon. Arn. Bell. Borax. *Bry. Calc. Cham. Euphr.* Nux. Puls. Sulph.
— from sand and dust, Sulph.
Injuries, thrusts in the eye, Symph.
— from a needle, Led.
Inverted, objects appear, Bell.
Irritation of eyes in evening with candle light, Lyc.
Itching in eyes, *Agar.* All-cep. Alum. Ant. Apis. Arg. Bell. Berb. Borax. Bruc. Bry. Bufo. Calc. Carb-veg. Caust. Creos. Kali-b. Kalm. Lach. Lob. Merc. Mosch. Mur-ac. Ntr-c. Ntr-m. Nicc. Nux. Ol-an. Pæon. Petr. *Phell.* Phosp. Puls. Ran-b. Ruta. Sep. Sil. *Sulph.* Viol-tr. Zinc.
— on left eye, Elaps.
— about eyes, Agn. Berb. Con.
— in eyebrows, Agar. Agn. Alum. Caust. Con. Fluor-ac. Laur. Par. Selen. Sil. Sulph.
— on lids, *Agn.* Ambr. Bell. Bry. Calc. Caust. Con. Croc. Cycl. Euphr. Grat. Kali-b. Lob. Mez. Nux. Pæon. Phosp. Rhus. Sep. *Sulph.* Zinc.
— — edges, Carb-veg. Creos. Jatr. Nux.

5. EYES AND SIGHT. 43

Prun. Staph.
Itching canthi, Arg. Bell. Benz-ac. Berb. Borax. Bruc. Calc. Carb-veg. Cinnab. Clem. Con. Euphr. Ferr-m. Fluor-ac. Gum-gut. Led. Lyc. Mosch. Mur-ac. Nux. Prun. Ruta. Staph. *Sulph.* Zinc.
— eyelashes, Grat.
— in evening, Cupr. Gum-gut. Pallad.
— by rubbing relieved, Oleand.
Lachrymal fistula, Calc. Chelid. Fluor-ac. Ntr-c. Nitr-ac. Puls. Sil. Stann. Sulph.
— discharging pus on pressure, Puls.
— suppurating, Calc.
Lachrymation, Acon. All-cep. Aloe. Alum. Amm-c. Apis. Arg-n. Arn. Ars. Asar. Bell. Brom. Bry. Calc. Caps. Carb-veg. Caust. Chin. Cinnab. Cina. Clem. Coloc. Creos. Croc. Croton. Daph. Dig. Eugen. *Euph. Euphr. Ferr. Graph.* Grat. Hep. Igt. Iod. Ip. Kali-b. Kali-c. Kali-jod. Lach. *Led. Lyc.* Mgn-c. Mgn-s. *Merc.* Mez. Millef. Mosch. Ntr-m. Ntr-s. Nicc. Nitr-ac. Nitr. Nux-m. Nux. Oleand. Ol-an. Osm. *Par.* Petr. Phosp-ac. *Phosp.* Phyt. Puls. Ran-b. Ran-sc. Rheum. *Rhus.* Ruta. *Sabad.* Sabin. Selen. *Seneg. Sep. Sil. Spig.* Spong. Staph. *Stram.* Sulph. *Sulph-ac.* Tar. Teucr. *Thuj. Verat.*
— from right eye, Brom. Sang.
— in morning, Calc. Creos. Lachn. Mgn-c. Merc. Ntr-m. Nitr. Phell. Phosp. Rat. Staph. Sulph.
— in evening, Asar. Eugen. Mgn-m. Merc. Phosp. Rhus. Sep.
— in cold air, Dig. Lyc. Phosp. Puls. Sil. Sulph.
— when coughing, Sabad.
— when gaping, Sabad. Staph. Viol-od.
— when gazing at anything, Cinnab.
— — — bright, Chelid. Mgn-m. Sabad.
— from light, Creos. Dig. Puls.
— of sun, Bry. Igt.
— in open air, Arn. Bell. Bry. Calc. Caust. Colch. Euph. Kobalt. Merc. Nitr-ac. Phell. Phosp. Puls. Rheum. Ruta. Sabad. Seneg. Sep. *Sil.* Staph. Sulph. Thuj. Verat.
— — relieved, Phyt.
— with the pains, Sabad.
— when reading, Croc. Grat. Nitr-ac. Sulph-ac.
— in room, Asar.
— — not in open air, Croc.
— in wind, Euphr. Phosp. Puls. Rhus. Sil. Sulph.
— after writing, Ferr.
— when writing, Calc.
Light longing for, Acon. Amm-m. Bell. Stram.
Loosness of eyes in sockets, sensation of, Carb-an.
Lumps in lids, Staph. Sulph. Thuj.

Lustrelessness, Arn. Asar. Bell. Bov. Bry. Daph. Ferr. Merc. Phosp-ac. Sabin.
Like a membrane drawn over the eyes, sensation, Caust. Daph. Puls. Rat.
Moist spot on canthus, Ant.
Motion of eyes difficult, Arn. Hep.
— — lids, difficult, Arn. Mercurial. Nux-m.
— of lines when reading, Bell. Cic. Con. Merc.
Motionless eyes, Aeth. Ang. Arn. Bar-m. Bell. Camph. Cic. Dolich. Tart. (compare Staring.)
Movement before the eyes, as from a swarm of insects, Caust.
— of objects before the eyes, Cic. Con. Euphr. Laur. Lyc. Mosch. Nux. Oleand. Par.
Mucus secreted, Agar. Amm-c. Ant. Arg-n. Bar-m. Bism. Calc. Cham. Dig. *Euphr.* Graph. Ip. Kali-jod. Lachn. Lact. Lyc. Ntr-m. Nux. Seneg. Staph. Sulph.
— — in eyes drying up and forming scurfs, Arg-n.
— — in lids, Graph. Lact. Sulph.
— — canthi, Euph. Kali-b. Kali-c. Ntr-m.
— — thick mucus, Puls.
— sensation as if hanging over eyes which must be wiped away, Croc. Puls.
Myopia, *Agar.* Amm-c. Anac. *Ang.* Berb. Cact. Calc. *Carb-veg.* Chin. *Con.* Cycl. Euph. Graph. Grat. Hep. Hyosc. Lach. Lyc. *Mang.* Meph. Mez. Ntr-c. Ntr-m. Nitr-ac. Ol-an. Petr. Phosp-ac. *Phosp. Plb.* Puls. Ruta. Spong. *Stram.* Sulph. Sulph-ac. Tart. *Thuj. Valer.* Viol-od. Viol-tr.
— when reading, Grat.
As if a nail stuck in the orbital margin, pain Hell.
Narrowing of intervals between eyelids, Agar. Euphr. Ntr-m. Nux. Rhus.
Nearer, everything seems, Bov. Cic. Stram.
Like needles darting through eyes, Eupat.
Nervous affections of eyes, *Cic.*
Night blindness, Bell. Cadm. Hyosc. Stram. Verat.
Nodosities, (see Hordeolum.)
Obliquely drawn lids, Seneg.
To open the lids difficulty, Ambr. Arg. Ars. Caust. Hydroc-ac. Hyosc. Kali-c. Merc. Ntr-c. Phosp. Spig. Sulph-ac.
— in morning, Ambr. Nicc. Nitr-ac.
— at night, *Cocc.* Rhus. *Sep.*
Openness, spasmodic, Ang. Arn. Bell. Dolich. Guaj. Hyosc. Laur. Lyc. Op. Stram.
— — in sleep, Bell. Bry. Ferr. Ip. Op. Phosp-ac. Samb. Sulph. Tart.
Outwards, pressure in eyes, Guaj. Mgn-s. Mez. Seneg. (compare Enlargement.)
As if overshadowed everything appears, Seneg.

5. EYES AND SIGHT.

Pain in eyeball, Ox-ac. Pod.
— — and behind left eye, Pallad.
Pale appearance of things, Puls. Rhus.
— — when reading, Chin. Dros. Sil.
Paralysis of lids, Alum. Bell. Cocc. Gels. Graph. Hydroc-ac. Nitr-ac. Op. Plb. Rhus. Sep. Spig. Stram. Verat. Zinc.
— upper, Caust. Dulc. Nitr-ac. Op. Plb. Spig. Verat.
— — right, Alum.
— optic nerve, Anac. Aur. Bar-c. Bell. Bry. Calc. Cannab. Caust. Chin. Cocc. Con. Croc. Dig. Dros. Dulc. Euphr. Ferr. Hyosc. Kali-c. Laur. Lyc. Merc. Ntr-c. Ntr-m. Nitr-ac. Oleand. Op. Petr. Plb. Phosp. Puls. Rhus. Ruta. Sec-c. Sep. Sil. Spig. Staph. Sulph. Verat. Zinc.
Photophobia, Acon. All-cep. Alum. Amm-c. Amm-m. Anac. Ant. Apis. Arn. Ars. Arum-trif. Asar. Bell. Berb. Bry. Calc. Camph. Cannab-ind. Cast. Caust. Cham. Cic. Chin. Cina. Clem. Coff. Con. Croc. Dros. Elaps. Eupat. Euphr. Graph. Hell. Hep. Hyosc. Igt. Kali-b. Kali-c. Kali-jod. Lach. Lyc. Mgn-s. Merc. Mercurial. Mosch. Ntr-c. Ntr-m. Ntr-s. Nitr. Nux. Phosp-ac. Phosp. Psor. Puls. Rhus. Seneg. Sep. Sil. Spig. Staph. Stram. Sulph. Sulph-ac. Tabac. Tar. Therid. Verat. Zing.
— without inflammation of eyes, Con. Hell.
— at candlelight, Borax. Calc. Cast. Con. Dros. Gels. Merc. Phosp.
— in day time, Acon. Ant. Bell. Bry. Camph. Con. Euphr. Graph. Hell. Hep. Igt. Merc. Ntr-c. Nux. Phosp-ac. Phosp. Psor. Sep. Sil.
— light of fire, Merc.
— in morning, Amm-c. Amm-m. Ntr-s. Nitr. Nux.
— after onanism, Cina.
— from sunlight, Asar. Berb. Cast. Euphr. Sulph.
— in warm weather, Sulph.
Presbyopia, Alum. Amm-c. Bell. Bry. Carb-an. Caust. Con. Dros. Hyosc. Lach. Led. Mgn-m. Mez. Mosch. Ntr-c. Ntr-m. Petr. Phosp. Sep. Spig. Sulph.
Pressing asunder sensation, Ang. Arn. Asar. Laur. Op.
— inwards sensation, Aur. Bell. Cannab. Chin. Cor-r. Daph. Tabac. Zinc.
— outwards sensation, Asar. Bry. Daph. Guaj. Gymnoc. Lach. Mgn-s. Mez. Seneg.
Pressure, Acon. Agar. Aloe. Alum. Ambr. Anac. Ang. Arn. Ars. Bar-c. Bell. Berb. Bism. Borax. Bry. Calc. Carb-veg. Cast. Caust. Cham. Chin. Cinnab. Clem. Cocc. Coloc. Con. Croc. Cupr. Dig. Dulc. Euphr. Ferr-m. Fluor-ac. Glon. Graph. Grat. Hep. Igt. Ind. Kali-c. Kali, chl. Kalm. Lach. Lact. Led.

Lob. Lyc. Mang. Meny. Meph. Merc. Merc-cor. Mez. Mosch. Ntr-s. Nicc. Nitr-ac. Nux. Oleand. Ol-an. Petr. Phosp-ac. Phosp. Plat. Plb. Psor. Puls. Ran-b. Ran-sc. Rhod. Rhus. Ruta. Sabad. Sass. Seneg. Sep. Sil. Spig. Spong. Staph. Stram. Stront. Sulph. Sulph-ac. Tabac. Tart. Thuj. Valer. Verat. Zinc.
— in right eye in evening, Kalm.
— behind right eyeball, Fluor-ac.
— as from a plug, Anac.
— round the eyes, Arn.
— in brows, Dig.
— in canthi, Alum. Carb-veg. Mosch. Stann. Staph. Tar.
— from face upwards, Rhod.
— downwards, Hell.
— in lids, Bry. Cham. Croc. Cupr. Euphr. Graph. Meph. Rheum. Seneg. Sil. Spong. Stann. Staph. Stram. Sulph.
— — upper, Chelid. Igt.
— in orbits, Aloe. Bov. Con. Cor-r.
— in orbital bone, Bov. Par.
— — orbital ridge, Chin. Rhod.
Prickling in evening at candlelight, Sep.
Protrusion of eyes, Acon. Aeth. Aloe. Ang Arn. Ars. Aur. Bell. Brom. Canth. Caps. Chin. Cocc. Con. Cupr. Dros. Glon. Guaj. Hydroc-ac. Hyosc. Laur. Merc-cor. Op. Spong. Stann. Thuj. Verat.
— sensation of, Par.
Pulsation in eyes, Asar.
Pupils contracted, Anac. Ars. Bell. Camph. Cham. Chelid. Cic. Cocc. Croton. Daph. Dros. Hœmatox. Igt. Lact. Mang. Merc-cor. Mez. Nux-m. Nux. Plb. Puls. Rheum. Samb. Scill. Sec-c. Sep. Sil. Sulph. Thuj. Verat. Zinc.
— one, the other dilated, Rhod.
— to contract, difficulty, Nitr-ac.
— angular, Merc-cor.
— dilated, Acon. Aeth. Agn. Bar-c. Bar-m. Bell. Brom. Calc. Carb-an. Cic. Cina. Chin. Cocc. Croc. Cycl. Dig. Gels. Guaj. Hell. Hydroc-ac. Hyosc. Hyper. Igt. Ip. Lach. Lact. Laur. Led. Mang. Mercurial. Ntr-c. Nitr. Nux. Op. Phosp-ac. Puls. Raph. Samb. Sec-c. Scill. Spig. Staph. Stram. Verat. Zinc.
— insensible, Aeth. Bar-m. Carb-veg. Chin. Cupr. Dig. Euphr. Hydroc-ac. Merc-cor. Op. Stram.
— motionless, Bar-c. Bell. Cainca. Cupr. Hydroc-ac. Hyosc. Laur. Nitr-ac. Op. Stram.
— unequal, Merc-cor. Sulph.
Pustules on conjunctioa, Merc.
— around eyes, Euphr. Hep. Staph. Sulph.
— — eyelids, Hep. Mosch. Selen.
Quivering of eyes, Amm-m. Hyosc. Petr. Rat. Rhus. Stann.
— of brows, Ol-an. Ruta.
— of canthi, Phosp.

5. EYES AND SIGHT.

Quivering of lids, *Agar.* Asaf. Calc. Carb-veg. Croc. Grat. Ind. *Ol-an.* Par. Petr. Phell. Rhosp. *Plat. Rat.* Rhod. Rhus. Sabin. Sep. Stront. *Sulph.* Tongo. (compare twitching).
To read small print, inability, Cadm. Meph. *Ntr-c.*
Redness of eyes, Acon. All-cep. Aloe. Ang. Apis. Arn. Aur. Bell. Bry. Bufo. Calc. Caps. Chin. Cinnab. Clem. Coff. Creos. Croton. Dros. Elaps. Euphr. *Ferr.* Glon. Hœmatox. *Hyosc.* Igt. Ip. Kali-c. Kali-chl. Kali-jod. Lach. Mgn-c. Mgn-m. Merc. Nicc. Nux. *Op.* Phosp. Psor. Raph. *Rhus.* Sep. *Sil. Spig.* Spong. *Stram.* Sulph. Sulph. Snlph-ac. Tabac. Tart. *Thuj.* Verat.
— of lids, Acon. *Ant.* Apis. Ars. Aur. Bell. Berb. Bry. Calc. Cannab. Cham. Creos. Ferr. Graph. Kali-b. Merc. Mur-ac. Nicc. Ntr-m. Nux. *Puls Sep.* Sulph. Teucr. Zinc.
— — edges, Creos.
— canthi, Bell. Brnc. Bry. Iris. Kali-b. Nux. Tabac. Teucr. Zinc.
— conjunctiva, Apis. Ars. Bell. Berb. Dig. Lach. Lact. Meph. Merc. Nux. Phosp. Puls. Sulph.
— — of old people, Lact.
— iris, Sulph.
— of veins of eyes, Acon. Aeth. Ambr. Apis. Bell. Elaps. Graph. Igt. Kali-b. Meny. Spig. Sulph.
Red spots on lid, Camph.
Reflection before sight, black, Phosp.
— — — blue, Lach.
— — varigated, around objects, Cic.
— around candle, Anac. Bell. Nitr. Sep. Stann. Staph.
— before sight, green, Sep.
— — rainbow colored, Nitr. Stann.
Rending, tearing, in eyes, Asar. Aur. Berb. Bry. Coloc. Euph. Hyper. Kali-c. Kobalt. Lyc. Nux. Prun. *Puls.* Scill. *Verat.* Zinc.
— on brows, Thuj.
— in lids, Berb. Plb.
— outwards, Sil.
Resetting or refixing of eyeball, sensation of, Sec.
Retraction, sense of, Hep.
Rub the eyes, need to, Croc. Ntr-c. Plb. Puls. Rat.
Rubbing or friction, sense of in eye, Puls. Sulph.
Running together, the letters when reading, Bell. Bry. Clem. Chin. Dros. Graph. Hyosc. Lyc. Meph. Ntr-m. Seneg. Sil. Stram. Viol-od.
Sad look, Stram.
As from sand in the eyes, pain, Alum. Asaf. Berb. Bruc. Bry. Caps. Caust. Chin. Cina. Cor-r. Creos. Dig. Euphr. Fluor-ac. Grat. Graph. Hep. Igt. Kobalt. Lach.
Lith. Merc. Ol-an. Phosp. Puls. Sil. Stront. Sulph. Tar. Teucr. Thuj. Viol-tr.
Scabs around eyes, *Merc.* Sulph.
— on brows, Sep.
— — lids *Merc.* Sep.
Sclerotica, distention of, Bell. Bry.
Scraping pain in eyes, Puls.
Scrofulous affections, Acon. Ars. *Aur.* Bell. Calc. Cannab. *Caust.* Chin. Cist. Dig. Dulc. *Euphr.* Ferr. Hep. Igt. Mgn-c. Merc. Ntr-m. *Nux.* Puls. Rhus. *Sulph.*
Shade, all objects appear to be in the, Seneg.
Shining eyes, Aeth. Bell. Cupr. Nux. (compare Sparkling.)
Shooting pain, Apis. Berb. Cinnab.
Sideways, turned, eyes, Dig.
Smaller letters appear, Glon. Merc-cor.
Smallness and inexpressiveness of eyes, Lach.
Left eye smaller than the right, Scill.
Smarting, Calc. Carb-veg. Caust. Chin. Clem. Creos. Euphr. Iod. Kali-c. Lact. Lyc. Merc. Ntr-m. Nux. Ol-an. Petr. Phosp. Plat. Pod. Rheum. Rhod. Rhus. Sabad. Sabin. Sep. Stann. Staph. Stront. Sulph. Sulph-ac. Tabac. Teucr. Thuj. Thuj. Tong. Valer. Viol-tr. Zinc.
— in canthi, Carb-veg. Con. Kali-b. Lact. Mez. Mur-ac. Nux. Phosp. Ran-b. Ransc. Ruta. Sil. Staph. Sulph. Tart. Teucr. Zinc.
— in lids, Aur. Calc. Clem. Lyc. Rhus. Sep. Spig. Sulph. Zinc.
— as from salt, Clem. Merc. Nux. Sulph. Teucr. Valer.
Smoky back ground of eyes, Chin.
In the sockets, pain, Bell. Iod. Selen. Spig.
Softening of sclerotica, Bell.
— of eyelids, Sulph.
Soreness sense of, Ant. Bar-c. Bry. *Canth.* Cham. Cor-r. Croc. Glon. Gymn. Hep. Lith. Lyc. Stann. Sulph. *Zinc.*
— — of lids, Bar-c. *Canth.* Cor-r. Croc. Hep. Spig. Sulph. *Zinc.*
— — — edges, Arn. Nux. Valer.
— — canthi, Ang. Apis. Cham. Nux. *Ran-b.* Zinc.
— — in caruncles, Ferr-m.
— — — right, Kali-b.
— — orbital ridge, Plat.
Sparkling eyes, Acon. Aeth. Arn. Bell. Bry. Cainca. Canth. Cupr. Hyosc. Lach. Lachn. Merc-cor. Millef. Mosch. Nux. *Stram.* (compare Shining.)
Spasms of eyes, Acon. Bell. Canth. Kali-chl. (compare Convulsions.)
— — lids, Alum. Bell. *Cham.* Croc. *Hep.* Hydroc-ac. *Hyosc.* Rhod. Ruta. Seneg. Viol-od.
— in light, Berb.

5. EYES AND SIGHT.

Spasms at night, Croc. Ntr-m.
Spasmodic pain, Cannab.
— — on orbital ridge, Plat.
Specks, running, oozing, in canthus, Ant.
Staring look, Acon. Aeth. Alum. Ang. Arn. Ars. Asar. Bar-m. Bell. Bry. Camph. Canth. Cic. Cocc. Con. Cupr. Dig. Glon. Hell. Hep. Hyosc. Igt. Kali-c. Lachn. Laur. Merc. Merc-cor. Mez. Mosch. Mur-ac. Nux. Op. Phosp-ac. Rhus. Scill. Sec-c. Seneg. Sep. Stram. Sulph. Verat. Zinc.
Stiffness of eyes, Berb.
— — lids, Kalm. Meny. Rhus. Spig.
Stinging, stitches, Acon. All-cep. Alum. *Ant*, Apis. Ars. Bell. Berb. Bry. Calc. Cham. Cic. Cinnab. Cist. Coloc. Croton. Cycl. Dig. Euph. Euphr. Ferr. Glon. Graph. Hep. *Kali-c.* Kali-chl. Kalm. Lach. *Lyc.* Mgn-c. Mgn-s. Meph. Ntr-c. Ntr-m. *Nitr-ac.* Nux. *Ol-an.* Petr. Phell. Phosp. Phyt. *Puls. Sass. Sep.* Spig. *Spong.* Staph. Sulph. Tar. Thuj. Viol-tr. Zinc. Zing.
— — in right eye, Hyper. Lith.
— — left eye, Brom. Cist.
— lids, Aur. Brom. Cinnab. Cycl. Lyc. Nicc. Pæon. Stann. Sulph.
— — lower, Euphr.
— canthi, Asar. Bell. Calc. Clem. Con. Croton. Ferr-m. Phosp.
— on orbital ridge, Rhod.
— outwards, Dros. *Mur-ac. Ntr-c.* Sil.
— inwards, Coloc.
— without redness, Lyc.
Strabismus, *Alum.* Apis. *Bell.* Cycl. *Hyosc.* Meny. Puls. Sec-c. Spig. Stram.
Suggilation, Bell. Cham. Lach. Nux.
— in lids, Arn.
Sunken eyes, Anac. *Ars.* Berb. Calc. Camph. Cic. Chin. Colch. Coloc. Cupr. Dros. Ferr. Glon. Iod. Kali-c. Lyc. Nitr-ac. Op. Phosp. Phosp-ac. Raph. Sec-c. Spong. *Stann. Staph.* Teucr. Verat.
Suppuration of eyes, Bry. Caust. Nitr-ac.
— in canthi, Bell. Kali-c. Led. Nux. Zinc.
Swelling, of eyes, *Acon.* Ars. Bar-c. Bry. Bufo. Ferr. Guaj. *Kali-c.* Mgn-c. Nux. Plb. *Rhus. Stram.*
— around eyes, All-cep.
— in morning, Bar-c.
— evening, Sep.
— of lids, Acon. Alum. Apis. Arg. Arn. *Ars.* Bar-c. Bell. Berb. Bry. Calc. Caust. Cham. Colch. Creos. Croton. Cycl. Dig. Euphr. Ferr. Graph. Igt. Iod. Kali-b. Kali-c. Lach. Lyc. Mang. Merc. Mur-ac. Ntr-c. Nitr-ac. Nux. Phosp. Psor. Puls. Rhus. Ruta. Scill. Seneg. Sep. Stram. *Sulph. Thuj.* Valer. Verat.
— hard and red, *Acon. Thuj.*
— between lids and brows, Kali-c.

— under eyes, Apis. Phosp.
— upper lids, Bry. Cycl. Igt. Kali-c. Ntr-c.
— lower lids, Dig. Op. Raph.
— erysipelatous of eyes and around them, Acon. Hep. Rhus.
— oedematous, Ars. Croton. Kali-b. Kali-jod. Puls. Raph. Rhus. Sacch. Teucr.
— purple colored, Phyt.
— watery white, Iod.
— of conjunctiva, Apis. Bell. Bry. Nux. Sep.
— of lachrymal caruncle, Bell. Brom. Sil.
— of canthus, Bell. Sass.
— meibomian glands, Nicc.
Swelling, sensation of, Cocc-c. Croc. Guaj. Par. (compare Enlargment.)
— — of eyelids, Caust.
— as after weeping, Croc.
Swimming eyes, Bry. Sep. Tart. Teucr. (compare Watery.)
Syphilitic affections of eyes, Merc. Nitr-ac.
Tears acrid, Ars. Bell. Bry. Coloc. Creos. Dig. Euphr. Gum-gut. Led. Merc. *Ntr-m.* Puls. Spig.
— — during the day, agglutination at night, Igt.
— biting, Creos. Dig. Eugen. *Euph. Euphr.* Led. Sabin. Spig. Teucr.
— burning, Apis. Arn. Bell. Cadm. Creos. Eugen. Euphr.
— cold, Lach.
— greasy, Sulph.
— mild, All-cep.
— salty, Bell. Creos.
— shining, Dig. Euph. Euphr. Led. Sabin. Spig.
Tenderness of lids, Bad.
Tension in eyes, Aur. Hyper. Lach. Nux. Plat. Sabin. Stram.
— around eyes, Nux-m.
— in lids, Acon. Nux-m. *Oleand.* Stram. Sulph-ac. Tong.
— in sockets, *Plat.*
Thread as if in eye, Tabac.
— as if tightly drawn through eyeball and backwards into the middle of the brain, Par.
Throbbing in eyes, Asar. Aur-s. Rheum.
Tickling about eyes, Amb. Aur-s.
Tingling, crawling around eyes, *Arn.*
— in eyes, Spig.
— in eyebrows, Croc.
— in canthi, Plat.
— in lids, Chin. Seneg.
Torn out pain as if eyes were, Cocc.
Torpor, of eyelids, Rhus. Spig.
Tremor of eyes, Op. Sulph.
— — lids, Carb-veg. Iod. Mercurial. Op. Plat. Verat.
Tremulous look, Con. Plat.
Turning in of eyelashes, Graph. Puls.

5. EYES AND SIGHT.

Turning in of eyelashes especially external canthus, Borax.
— back of eyelids, Apis. Bell.
— around in eyes sensation of, Bov. Cist.
— before eyes, Scill.
— of letters when reading, Cic. Con.
Turned up eyes are, Cupr. Mosch. Op.
— — upper lid, Igt.
Twitching, *Agar*. Amm-m. Apis. *Cham*. Croton. Glon. Mez. Nicc. Petr. *Rat*. Rhus. Selen. Stann.
— right eye, Rat.
— left eye, Selen.
— of eyebrows, Cic. Cina. Ol-an. Ruta.
— of lids, Agar. Asar. Calc. Carb-veg. Caust. Cham. Creos. Croc. Croton. Dulc. Grat. Hell. Hydroc-ac. Ind. Iod. Ip. Kali-b. Lyc. Meny. Merc. Nux. Ol-an. Par. Petr. Plat. Puls. Rat. Rheum. Rhod. Rhus. Sabin. Seneg. Sep. Spig. Stront. Sulph.
— — upper, Lachn. Ntr-m.
— — — left, Jatr.
— — lower, Amm-c. Iod. Kali-jod. Graph. Seneg. Sep. Sulph.
— canthi, Phosp.
— in cold air, Dulc.
— in sleep, Rheum.
Ulceration of eyes, *Caust*. Nitr-ac. (compare Suppuration.)
— of canthi, Kali-c. Zinc.
Ulcers of lids, Merc. Ntr-m. *Spig. Stram.*
— of margins, Clem. Colch. Croton. *Euphr.* Lyc. *Merc.* Phosp. Puls. Sil. Spig. Staph. *Sulph.*
Ulcerous pain above eyes, Hep.
Unanimated eyes, *Aeth*. Kali-c. (compare Dimness, lustreless.)
Unsteady look, Aloe. Bell. Par. Stann.
Upward, eyeball turned, Verat.
Vanishing of sight. *Cic*. Dros. Merc. Ntr-m. Nicc. Puls. Spig. Tabac. Verat.
— when exerting eyes, Nicc.
— — looking at anything white, Tabac.
— — reading, Dros. Ntr-m.
— — walking, Cic.
— — writing, Ntr-m.
— with vertigo, perspiration and epistaxis, Ox-ac.
Veil, gray before the eyes, Berb. *Phosp.* Sil.
Veins distention of, Ambr. Bell. Kali-b. Kali-c. Spig.
— blueness of, Igt.
— redness of, Acon. Aeth. Ambr. Bell. Graph. Igt. Kali-b. Meph. Merc. Phosp-ac. Spig. Sulph.
— — in external canthus, Merc.
Vice, as if eyes were compressed in, Rat.
Viscous matter in canthus, Agar. Ntr-m.
Warts on eyebrows, Caust.
As from water in eyes, sensation, Staph.
Watery appearance of eyes, Bry. Creos.

Daph. Sep. Tart. Teucr. Verat. (compare Swimming.)
Wavering look, Bell. Ntr-m.
Weakness of sight, *Agar. Anac.* Apis. Ars. Bar-c. Bell. Calc. Cannab. Caps. Carb-an. Carb-veg. Cast. Chelid. Chin. Cic. Cina. Con. Creos. Croc. Daph. Dig. Dros. Euphr. Gels. Hep. Hyosc. Igt. Iod. Kalm. Lach. Lact. Lam. Led. Lyc. Mang. Merc. Ntr-m. Ntr-s. Nicc. Nux-m. Osm. Par. Phosp. Plat. Rheum. Rhus. Ruta. Sabad. Sec-c. Sep. Sil. Spig. Staph. Stram. Stront. Sulph.
— in morning, Phosp.
— — evening, Cast. Nicc.
— chronic, from onanism, Cina.
— of eyes, they remain in what ever direction turned, Spig.
— — lids, Grat.
As after weeping pain, Croc. Tabac. Teucr.
Wheels, circles, rings colored, before eyes, Nitr. Stront.
— — fiery, Puls.
Whirling sensation in eyes, Bov. Cist.
— before eyes, Scill.
White spots before eyes, Ars. Camph. Chin. Cocc. Nux. Op. Sulph. Rat.
Wild look, Arg-n. Ars. *Bell*. Con. Cupr. Glon. Hyosc. Op. Sec-c.
Winking, Croc. Euphr. Ferr-m. Mez. Spig.
To wipe the eyes, inclination, Croc. Creos. Lac-can. Lyc. Ntr-c. Plb. *Puls*. Rat.
Yellowness of whites of eyes, Ars. Bell. Bry. Calc. *Canth*. Carb-an. Caust. Cham. Chelid. Chin. Clem. Cocc. Con. Corn-c. Crotal. Dig. Gels. Graph. *Iod*. Kali-b. Lach. Lyc. Mgn-m. Ntr-c. Nitr-ac. Nux. Op. Phosp. *Plb*. Sec-c. Sep. Verat.
— of lower part of eyeball, Nux.
— brown rings around eyes, Nitr-ac.
— spot on white of eye, Phosp-ac.
— spots before eyes when sewing, Amm-m.
In the morning pain, Acon. Amm-c. Berb. Bry. Mgn-s. Meph. Ntr-s. Nitr. Nux. Par. Phell. Sep. Sil. Sulph-ac.
— — afternoon, Eugen.
— — evening, Agn. Alum. Amm-m. Apis. Asar. Berb. Bry. Cast. Chin. Con. Croc. Daph. Hep. Iod. Kalm. Led. *Lyc.* Mgn-s. Meph. Ntr-s. Nicc. Ol-an. Phell. Phosp-ac. Puls. Rat. Sass. Seneg. Tong. Zinc.
— — twilight, pain relieved by light, Amm-m.
At night, Apis. Kobalt. Nux.
From candle light, pain, Calc. Cina. Croc. Cor-r. Kali-c. Lyc. Mgn-s. Mang. Mez. Ntr-s. Nux-m. Sep.
— a cold, Acon. All-cep. Bell. Calc. Cham. Iod. Lact. Nux. Puls. Sulph.
— day light pain, Agn. Ars. Calc. Euphr. Hep. Kali-c. Kobalt. Ntr-s. Puls. Rhod.

Ruta. Seneg. Sulph.
From sun light, pain, Asar. Chin. Sulph.
— dust, Sulph.
While exerting the eyes, Bar-c. *Carb-veg.*
    Cina. Mang. Merc. Phyt. Plat. Rheum.
    Rhod. Ruta. Staph. Sulph-ac.
After exerting the eyes, Ruta.
When looking at anything bright, pain,
    Mgn-m. Nux.
— — at a distance, Cast.
— — sideways, Mgn-s.
— — upwards, Carb-veg. Plb. Sabab.
From mechanical causes, Arn. Croc. Led.
When moving or turning eyes, pain, Acon.
    Ars. Bell. Berb. Bry. Caps. Cham.
    Chin. Con. Cupr. Hep. Hipp. Igt. Lach.
    Meph. Mur-ac. Op. Ran-sc. Rhus. Spig.
    Sulph.
— — lids, Hep.
— — head, pain in eyes, Cham.
When blowing the nose, momentary blindness, Caust.
— opening the eyes, pain, Alum. Bry.
    Canth. Nux. Therid.
— — widely, Cochlear.
— closing the eyes relieved, Bry. Calc.
Con.
In the open air, Berb. Kalm. Merc. Ol-an.
    Sulph-ac. Teucr.
— — cold air, relieved, Asar.
When reading, Asar. Berb. Calc. Cina.
    Con. Croc. Cycl. Dulc. Kali-c. Lith.
    Ntr-c. Ntr-s. Oleand. Phyt. Seneg.
    Sulph-ac.
— — pain, in the day, Calc.
— — — in candle light, Agn. Calc. Kali-c.
    Ntr-c. Ruta. Sass. Seneg. Tong.
In a room, Asar. Dig.
When rubbing, Creos.
From sand and dust, Acon. Calc. Sulph.
— sharp air, pain, Thuj.
When shutting the eyes, pain, Clem. Croc.
— touching the eyes, pain, Agar. Aur.
    Caust. Cupr. Dig. Hep. Kali-c. Nux.
    Sang. Tart.
Warm room worse, Arg-n.
Water, cold, causes tension in eyes, and
    redness, Nicc.
From wine drinking, pain, Zinc.
— wind, Asar. Lyc.
— writing pain, Kobalt. Ntr-c. Seneg.
    Staph.

6. Ears and Hearing.

Agglutination of auricle to head, Oleand.
Like air passing into ears, sensation,
    Graph. Mez.
Blisters on ears, Meph.
Blood, congestion of, Lyc. Phosp. Puls.
    Sulph.
Blows on ears, sensation of, Arn. Ntr-m.
    Nux. Pæon. Plat.
Boils before and behind the ears, Bry.
    Sulph.
— on ear, Sil. Sulph.
Bones, swelling of, Puls.
Boring, sensation of, Amm-m. Bell. Cupr.
    Euphr. Hell. Hydroc-ac. Kali-jod. Lact.
    Mgn-m. Merc-jod. Ntr-m. Ol-an. Phell.
    Plb. Ran-sc. Rhod. Sil.
— about ears, Rhod.
— behind ears, Cupr.
— with fingers in ears, Mez.
Bruising pain, *Arn.* Cic. *Ruta.*
Burning sensation, Agar. All-cep. Alum.
    Ars. Caust. Clem. Creos. Igt. Jac-cor.
    Mercurial, Sang. Spig. Tabac.
— on the lobes, Nitr. Sabad.
— inside, Aur-s. Canth. Croton. Jatr.
— — right ear, Brom.
— outwards, Berb. Sulph.
— is if frostbitten, Agar.
Caries of mastoid process, *Aur.* Nitr-ac.
    Sil.
In children, affections of ears, Zinc.
Coldness sense of, Lach. Meny. Plat.
— — — right, burning of left ear, Ntr-nitr.
— — internally, Merc.
— with sense of heat, alternating, Verat.
Compressing pain, Cannab. Spong. Thuj.
Contracting pain, Bry. Dig. Sass. Spong.
Coroding pain, Arg. Berb. Plat.
Cutting pain, Ars. Dros. Gum-gut.
Digging pain, Ant. Hell.
Drawing, sense of, Lact. Mgn-m. Oleand.
    Ran-sc.
— inside, Colch. Creos. Cycl. Ferr. Merc.
    Mez. Phosp-ac. Sil. Stann. Sulph. Valer.
— when swallowing, Ferr-m.
— outwards, Con.

6. EARS AND HEARING.

Dryness in ears, Colch. *Graph.* Lach. Nitr-ac. Petr.
— — — sensation, Petr. Phosp.
Earwax, accumulation of, *Con.* Cycl. Hep. Selen. Sil. Zinc-ox.
— discharge of, Amm-m. Anac. Kali-c. Lyc. Merc. Mosch. Ntr-m. Nitr-ac. Phosp. Puls.
— dry, Lac-can. Petr.
— fluid, Con. Lach. Merc. Selen. Sil.
— hard, Elaps. Lach. Puls. Selen.
— moist, Sil.
— like rotten paper, Con.
— slimy, Con.
— wanting, Carb-veg. Lach.
— black, Elaps. Puls.
— pale, Lach.
— red, Con.
— white, Con. Lach. Sep.
Eruption on ears, Amm-m. *Bar-c.* Bov. Calc. Carb-veg. *Cic.* Chin. Hep. Lyc. Mosch. Mur-ac. Petr. *Psor.* Puls. Sep. Tellur. Verb.
— in front of ears, Berb. *Cic.* Oleand.
— behind, *Bar-c.* Calc. Carb-veg. *Cic.* Graph. *Hep.* Lach. Lyc. Mez. Oleand. Psor. Sep. Sil.
— on the lobes, Puls. Sass. Tellur. Teucr.
— pimple in concha, Creos.
— biting, Puls.
— burning, Cic. Mosch. Puls. Sass.
— itching, Mez. Pallad. Puls. Sass.
— moist, Bov. Calc. Creos. Graph. Lyc. Mez. Psor.
— pimples, Merc.
— purulent, Cic. Cycl. Psor. Sep.
— pustules, Carb-veg.
— scaly, Psor. Teucr.
— scurfy, Aur-m. Bov. Calc. Graph. Hep. Lach. Lyc. Mur-ac. Psor. Puls. Sass. Sil.
— — in right external ear, Cinnab.
— vesicular, Tellur.
Erysipelas, Meph. Puls.
Excoriation behind ears, *Graph.* Kali-c. Lach. Nitr-ac. Petr. Psor. Sulph.
— pain of, Cic. Mgn-m.
— — inside, Borax. Caust. Merc. Sep.
Exostosis, Puls.
False hearing, misunderstanding, Bov. Phosp.
Fetid smell of ears, Graph.
Formication, Ars. Colch. Merc. Plat.
— right ear, Osm.
— inside, Ambr. Calc. Caust. Laur. Nitr. Puls. Samb.
From freezing, Agar. Colch.
Gland, parotid, boring pain in, Sabad.
— hardness, Amm-c. Con. Sil.
— inflammation, Amm-c. Bell. Brom. Calc. Cham. *Kali-c.* Merc. Nux. *Rhus.* Sass.
— pressing, Merc.
— rending, tearing, Bell.
— stinging, stitches, Asa-f. Bell. Bry. Calc.

Igt. Kali-b. Merc. Phosp. Sep. Spong. Sulph.
— swelling, *Amm-c.* Aur. Bar-c. *Bell.* Brom. *Calc.* Carb-an. *Carb-veg.* Cham. *Chin.* Cist. Cocc. Con. Dig. *Igt. Kali-c.* Lach. *Merc.* Nitr-ac. Nux. Puls. *Rhus.* Sil.
— on right side, swelling, Amm-c. Merc.
— — — left side Brom. Kali-b. Rhus.
— after measles, or Scarletina, Iod. Mgn-c.
— ulceration, Bar-c. Rhus. Sass. Sil.
— — in scarlet fever, Rhus.
— about ears affections of, Amm-c. Arn. Bar-c. *Bell.* Calc. Carb-an. Carb-veg. *Cham.* Chin. *Con.* Igt. Kali-c. Hyosc. *Merc.* Nitr-ac. Phosp. Puls. *Rhus.* Sep. Sil. Staph. Sulph.
Hearing acute, Coff. Mur-ac.
— — in evening in bed, Kali-c.
Deafness, Ant. Aur. Bar-c. Bell. Carb-veg. Chlorum. Croton. Elaps. Hydroc-ac. Hyosc. Lachn. Lach. Mgn-m. Merc. Merc-dulc. Ntr-c. Nicc. *Nitr.* Phosp-ac. Plb. Psor. Raph. *Sec-c.* Stram. Sulph.
— when vomiting, Bar-m.
Diminished hearing, *Amb. Ang.* Bov. Con. Cor-r. Cycl. *Kali.* Laur. Par. Plb.
Hearing, difficult Aeth. Agn. All-cep. Ambr. *Amm-c.* Amm-m. *Anac.* Ant. *Arn.* Ars. *Asar.* Asa-f. Bar-c. *Bell.* Borax. Bry. *Calc.* Carb-an. Carb-veg. Caps. Caust. Chin. Cic. Cocc. Con. Creos. Dig. Dros. Dulc. *Graph.* Hep. Hydroc-ac. Hyosc. *Iod. Kali-c.* Lach. Laur. *Led. Lyc.* Mgn-c. Mgn-m *Mang. Merc.* Mez. Mosch. *Mur-ac. Ntr-m. Nitr-ac.* Nux. Oleand. Op. *Petr. Phosp. Phosp-ac.* Plb. Psor. Puls. Rheum. Rhus. Ruta. Sabad. Sabin. *Sec-c.* Sep. *Sil.* Spig. *Spong. Staph. Stram. Sulph. Sulph-ac.* Tar. Tellur. Thuj. *Verat. Verb.*
— after previous burnings and stingings, Caps.
— in left ear, Arg-n.
— in right, Led.
— with discharge of pus, Asa-f.
— like a leaf or membrane, sensation, Acon. Ant. Calad. Galc. Cannab. Mgn-m. Nitr-ac. Sabad. Sulph-ac. Verb.
— obstruction of ears, Bry. Carb-veg. Chelid. Con. Iod. Lyc. *Mang.* Meny. Nitr-ac. Selen. Sep. Sil. *Spig. Sulph.* Verat. Verb.
— — sense of, Aeth. Ang. Arg. Ars. *Asar.* Borax. Bry. Calc. Carb-veg. Caust. Cham. Cist. Cocc. Colch. Cycl. Glon. Hipp. Lach. Led. Mang. Merc. Meny. Ntr-c. Nitr-ac. Puls. Sep. Sil. Spig. Sulph. Verat. Verb.
— — occasional, Calad. Nitr-ac. Sulph. Verb.

6. EARS AND HEARING.

Hearing difficulty of, right side, Cocc.
— left side Jac-cor.
— left to right, Sulph.
— right to left, Elaps.
— in the evening, Nicc. Tar.
— after a cold, Merc.
— — in the head, Bell. Led. Puls.
— during cough, Chelid.
— after cutting the hair, Bell. Led. Puls.
— at a distance, Phosp-ac.
— from elongation of tonsils, Aur. Merc. Nitr-ac. *Staph.*
— with full moon increased, Sil.
— to human voice, Ars. Phosp. Sil. Sulph.
— except for speech, Igt.
— from induration and swelling of tonsils, Nitr-ac.
— after suppressed intermittents, Calc. Carb-veg. Hep. Puls. Sulph.
— — measles, Arg-n. Asar. Puls. Sil. Spig. Sulph.
— after mechanical injuries, Arn.
— after abuse of mercury, Asa-f. Nitr-ac. *Staph.*
— — nitric acid, Petr.
— from paralysis of auditory nerves, Nitr.
— periodical, Sec. *Spig.*
— when reading aloud, Verb.
— in a room, Mgn-c.
— by stooping increased, Croc.
— sudden, Gels. Nicc. Plb. Sec-c. Sep.
— in changeable weather, Mang.
— before wind and rain, Nux-m.
— alternating with obscuration of sight, Cic.
— — otorrhoea, Puls.
— relieved when blowing the nose, Mang. *Merc.* Sil. Sulph.
— — with a crack, Sil.
— — after earwax is removed, Con.
— — when riding in a carriage, Graph.
— — when swallowing, Merc.
— illusions of, as if air were passing into ear, Graph.
— — sound of a bell, Ars. Chin. Clem. Sass. Valer.
— — buzzing, Agar. Ambr. Amm-c. Amm-m. Ars. *Aur. Bar-c.* Cact. Calc. *Carb-an.* Carb-veg. Cast. *Chin.* Cocc. Croc. Dros. Hep. Iod. Kali-c. Mgn-c. Mang. Merc. Mur-ac. Ntr-m. Nicc. *Petr.* Phosp. Puls. Sec-c. *Sep.* Stront. *Sulph.* Sulph-ac. Tart. Therid. Zinc.
— — right ear, Elaps. Mgn-c.
— chirping, Puls. Sil. Sulph.
— clashing, *Mang.* Sabad. Sil.
— crackling, Alum. *Bar-c.* Calc. Kali-c. Lach. Meny. Mosch. Nitr-ac. Sulph.
— crying, Phosp-ac. Stann.
— detonation, snapping, Calc. Mang. Sabad. Sil. Sulph.

— — like a cannon. with a few drops of blood, Mosch.
— drum, sounds of, Lach.
— fluttering, Bell. Calc. Cham. Graph. Mgn-c. Plat. Puls. Sil. Spig.
— hammering, Spig.
— hissing, Dig. Graph. Sil. Teucr.
— humming, Acon. Aloe. Alum. Amm-c. Anac. Ant. Arn. Bell. Bry. Calc. Casc. Caust. Chin. Con. Croc. Dros. Dulc. Graph. Lyc. Hyosc. Iod. Mur-ac. Ntr-m. Nicc. Nitr-ac. *Nux.* Ol-an. Puls. Psor. Sabad. Spig. Sulph.
— music, Calc. Ntr-c.
— — sounds shrill, Coff.
— ringing, Ambr. Arg-n. Ars. Calc. Cast. Chin. Clem. Elaps. Glon. *Led.* Mgn-s. Merc. Ntr-m. Ntr-s. Nitr. Psor. Sang. Sass. Sil. Sulph-ac.
— roaring, Acon. Agn. All-cep. Anac. *Ant.* Arn. Ars. Aur. Bell. Berb. Borax. Bry. Cannab. Carb-an. Carb-veg. *Caust.* Chin. Cinnab. Colch. Con. Croc. Cupr. Daph. Dros. Evon. Ferr. Hep. Hydroc-ac. Kali-c. Lac-can. Led. Lyc. Mgn-c. Mang. Merc. Ntr-m. Nicc. *Nitr-ac.* Nux. Ol-an. Op. Petr. *Plat.* Puls. Rheum. Rhod. Sep. *Sulph.* Therid. Verat.
— — in left ear, Borax.
— — with every attack of pain, Ars.
— rolling, Graph. *Plat.*
— rushing, Dulc. Phosp.
— rustling, Bell. Borax. Caust. Mang. Merc. Phosp. Puls. Sil. *Therid.* Viol-od.
— shocks, as of distant artillery, Bad.
— singing, Glon. Graph. Kali-c. Ol-an. Petros.
— sounds mixed together, Carb-an.
— squashing, Calc. Mang.
— striking of a clock, Tereb.
— throbbing, Hep.
— thundering, Calc. Caust. Chelid. Lach. Oleand. Petr. Plat. Rhod.
— tinkling, Agn. Aloe. Amm-c. Amm-m. Bar-c. Bell. Carb-veg. Cham. Chin. *Con.* Ferr-m. Graph. Kali-c. Lyc. Mgn-c. Meny. Mur-ac. Ntr-m. Nitr. Nux. Oleand. Ol-an. Op. Par. Petr. Puls. Sass. Stann. Staph. Sulph. Tereb. Valer. Viol-od.
— voices, Cham. Elaps.
— water boiling, Dig. Thuj.
— — rushing, Cocc.
— wind, strong, Igt.
— — whizzing, like, Chelid.
— whistling, Creos. Elaps. Graph. Mur-ac. Nux. Sil. Teucr.
— in evening, buzzing, Sulph-ac.
— — tingling, Croc. Lact. Merc.
— at night buzzing, roaring, Amm-c. Graph.
— — singing, tingling, Rat.
— — voices, Cham.
— when blowing the nose, crying, Phosp-

6. EARS AND HEARING.

ac. Stann.
Hearing, illusions of, when gaping, squashing, Mang.
— when masticating, crackling, Alum. Calc. Graph. Mang. Meny. Ntr-m. Nux.
— by noise increased, Ol-an.
— when reading aloud, cracking, Aloe.
— — rising from sitting, buzzing, Verat.
— in a room, roaring, Mgn-c.
— when sneezing, crackling, Bar-c.
— — stooping, roaring, Croc.
— — swallowing, crackling, Alum. Bar-c. Elaps.
— — — detonation, Cic.
— — — roaring, Mgn-c.
— — — squashing, Calc-c.
— — talking, hissing, Teucr.
— — walking crackling, Bar-c. Meny.
— relieved by leaning on head, buzzing, Kli-c.
— — — boring in the ear, Cast.
— sensitiveness of, Acon. Arn. Ars. Aur. Bell. Bry. Calad. Calc. Cham. Chin. Coff. Con. Graph. Iod. Lyc. Mur-ac. Ntr-c. Nux. Petr. Phosp. Phosp-ac. Plb. Puls. Seneg. Sep. Sil. Spig. Sulph. Therid. *Viol-od.*
— — too great, Coff. Lyc. Mur-ac. Phosp. Sep. Sil. Sulph. Therid.
— — in evening, Kali-c.
— — to music, Acon. Cham. Coff. Lyc. Phosp-ac. Sep. Sulph. Viol-od.
— — — noise, Acon. Apis. Ars. Bry. Chin. Igt. Iod. Ip. Kali-c. Lyc. Mgn-c. Mgn-m. Mur-ac. Ntr-c. Phosp-ac. Plb. Sil. Therid. Zinc.
— — — organs, Lyc.
— — — sounds, Lyc. Therid.
— — — talking of other people, Ars. Phosp-ac. Verat.
— — — violin playing, Viol-od.
— — when falling asleep, Calad.
— — in bed, Kali-c.
Heat of ears, Aloe. Alum. Ang. Ant. Asar. Camph. Carb-veg. Casc. Chin. Clem. Creos. Hep. Hipp. Igt. Jatr. Kali-c. Meph. Ntr-m. Puls. Sabin. Tabac.
— and redness of one ear, Alum.
— of left ear, Jac-cor.
— — lobes, Camph. Chin.
— inside, Calc. Canth. Casc. Puls.
— one sided, Alum. Carb-veg. Igt.
— in evening, Alum. Carb-veg.
— with coldness alternating, Berb. Verat.
— streaming from ears, Aeth. Par.
Herpes in front of ears, Oleand.
— behind, Cist. Graph. Mgn-m. Oleand. Sep.
— on lobes, Caust. Cist. Sep. Teucr.
— inside, Creos.
Jerking pain, Ang. Fluor-ac. Petr. *Puls.* *Rhod.* Spig. Valer.
— — on ears, Cina.
— — in front, Ang.

— — on lobes, Nitr.
Inflammation of ears, Bell. Borax. Bov. Bry. Cact. Canth. Creos. Kali-b. Kali-c. Mgn-c. Merc. Merc-cor. Puls.
— right ear, Bell.
— left ear, Puls.
— of edges, Sil.
— lobes, Creos. Nitr.
— inside, Acon. Bell. Borax. Bov. Bry. Calc. Canth. Hep. *Kino.* Mgn-m. Merc. Nux. Puls. Sil. Spig.
— of petrous bone, tender to touch, Caps.
Irritation sense of, Arg. Plat.
Itching, *Agar.* Alum. *Amm-c.* *Arg.* Bar-c. Berb. Bov. Carb-veg. Caust. Con. Fluor-ac. Graph. Grat. *Hep.* Igt. Kali-c. Meph. Phosp. Raph. Sep. Sil. Spig. Sulph. Tellur.
— left ear, Benz-ac. Tellur,
— behind the ears, Mgn-m. Mez. Ntr-m. Nitr-ac. Therid.
— of lobes, Arg. Kali-b. Sabad. Sulph.
— — at night, Nux.
— inside, Anac. Caps. Cupr. Cycl. Elaps. Ferr-m. Fluor-ac. Kali-c. Laur. Nux. Puls. Rat. Rheum. Ruta. Samb. Sep.
— — deep, Rumex.
— — right side, Cinnab.
— — left side, Cocc-c.
— burning and redness as if frozen, Agar. Hep.
Moist, humid, behind ears, Graph. Kali-c. Nitr-ac, Ol-an. Petr. *Psor.*
— on edges, Sil.
Numbness, sense of, *Plat.*
Open sensation as if ears were, Aur-m.
Otalgia, spasmodic, All-cep. Aloe. *Anac. Ang.* Asar. Bell. Bry. Cainca. Cannab. *Caust. Cham.* Colch. Croc. Croton. Dros. Dulc. Euph. *Guaj.* Kino. Lyc. Mang. Meph. *Merc.* Mez. Mur-ac. Ntr-c. Nitr. Nux-m. *Nux.* Par. Petr. Phosp. *Plat.* Prun. Psor. *Puls.* Ran-sc. Rheum. *Rhod.* Rhus. Sabin. Sep. *Sil.* *Spig.* Spong. Stann. Teucr. Thuj. Valer. Zinc.
— right ear, Bell. Lac-can. Ran-sc. Rhod.
— left ear, Calend. Guaj. Lac-can. Lith. Puls.
— behind left ear, in bone to neck, Lith.
From other parts to the ear extending, pains, Mang.
Otorrhoea, Alum. Amm-c. Amm-m. Anac. Asa-f. Bar-c. Bell. Borax. Bov. Calc. Calend. Caust. Carb-an. *Carb-veg.* Cham. Cist. Colch. Con. Graph. Hep. Kali-c. Kino. Lach. Lyc. Meny. Merc. *Ntr-m.* Nitr-ac. Petr. Phosp. Puls. Rhus. Selen. Sep. *Sil.* Spig. Sulph. (compare Running.)
— bloody, Bar-c. Bell. Bry. Calc. Caust. Cic. Con. Elaps. Graph. Lyc. Merc. Mosch. Nitr-ac. Petr. Puls. Rhus. Sep. Sil. Sulph.

6. EARS AND HEARING.

Otorrhoea brownish, Anac.
— offensive, Aur. Bov. Carb-veg. Caust. Cist. Kali-b. Hep. Merc. Merc-cor. Thuj. Zinc.
— — like fish brine, Tellur.
— purulent, All-cep. Alum. Amm-c. Amm-m. Arn. *Asa-f.* Aur. Bell. *Borax. Bov. Calc.* Carb-an. Carb-veg. Caust. Cham. Cist. *Con.* Gels. Graph. *Hep.* Kali-b. Kali-c. *Kino.* Lach. Lyc. *Merc.* Ntr-m. Nitr-ac. Petr. Psor. *Puls.* Rhus. Sacch. Sep. Sil. Sulph. Zinc.
— — after abuse of mercury, Asa-f.
— thin, Cham. Merc. Sep. Sil.
— watery, Cist. Tellur.
— yellow, alternating with difficulty of hearing, Phosp.
— yellowish green, Elaps.
— after measles, Colch.
— after scarlet fever, Kali-b.
Paralysis auditory nerve, *Bell.* Calc. Caust. Chelid. Dulc. Graph. *Hyosc.* Lyc. Merc. Nitr-ac. Nux. Op. *Puls.* Sec-c. *Sil.*
Periosteum behind ear swollen, Carb-an.
Pinching behind ear, Pæon. Sabin.
— inside, Bell. Ferr-m.
Like a plug, sensation in ear, Anac. *Spig.*
Polypus, *Calc.* Staph.
Pressing in ear, Anac. Asar. Asa-f. Bell. Camph. Caps. Creos. Cupr. Fluor-ac. Hydroc-ac. Mur-ac. Oleand. Rheum. Ruta. Sabad. Sass. Seneg. Spig. Spong. Verat.
— behind, Thuj.
— forward in ears, *Cannab.* Caust. Ntr-s. Nux. Par. *Puls.* Spong.
— — in right ear, Prun.
Pulsation, *Calc. Mgn-m.* Spig. (compare Throbbing.)|
Pustules in ear, Berb.
Redness of ears, Agar. Ant. Apis. Camph. Chin. Creos. Igt. Hipp-m. Mgn-c. Meph. Puls. Tabac.
— bluish, Tellur.
— in evening, Alum. Carb-veg.
— behind, Oleand. Petr. Tabac.
— of lobes, Camph. Chin.
— one sided, Alum. Carb-veg. Igt.
Rending, tearing, in ears, Acon. Aeth. Agar. Ambr. *Anac.* Arn. Bell. Berb. Caps. Cast. Cham. Chenop. Colch. Con. Cupr. Dulc. Grat. Guaj. Ind. Iod. Kali-jod. Kalm. Lachn. *Merc.* Meph. Mez. Mur-ac. Nux. Ol-an. Par. Phell. *Phosp. Plumb. Puls. Rhod.* Scill. Spig. Stann. Stront. Sulph. Sulph-ac. *Thuj. Verb.* Zinc.
— right ear, Kali-jod.
— left ear, Acon. Puls.
— left to right, Aloe.
— right to left, Sulph.
— about the ears, *Con.* Rhod.
— — behind, Dig. Ind. Nitr.

— in front, Ang.
— on ears, Chin. Dulc.
— from ear down to neck, Tar.
Retraction, sense of, Verb.
Reverberation of every sound, Caust. Hydroc-ac. Lach. Nitr-ac. Nux. Phosp. Phosp-ac.
— of words, Nitr-ac. Phosp-ac. Phosp.
Rough epidermis in ears, Oleand.
Like a rough body in Eustachian tube, sensation, Nux-m.
Running ears, Amm-m. Anac. *Kali-c. Lyc.* Ntr-m. *Nitr-ac.* (compare Otorrhoea.)
— of mucus, Calc. Lyc. Merc. Phosp. Puls. Sulph.
— after inflammation, Kino.
Scratching sensation, Ruta.
Screwing pain, Bell.
Sensitiveness of ears, Kali-jod.
— to wind, Lach.
— want of, Mur-ac.
Spasmodic pain, Cina. Merc. Murex. Oleand. Ran-b. Spig. *Thuj.*
— inside, *Ang.* Creos. Croc. Ferr. Merc. Mur-ac. Petr. Phosp-ac. *Plat.* Ran-b. Samb. Thuj. Valer.
— behind Murex.
Steatoma at lobe, Nitr-ac.
Stench from ears, Graph.
— behind ears, Oleand.
Stinging, stitches, Acon. Aeth. *Alum. Anac.* Ant. Arg. *Arn.* Ars. Aur. Bar-c. Bell. Berb. Borax. Bry. Calc. Camph. Caust. *Cham.* Chelid. Chin. Colch. *Con.* Creos. Croton. Dros. Ferr. Gels. Graph. Grat. Hell. Hep. Hyper. Kali-b. Kali-c. Kali-jod. Kino. Lob. Mgn-s. Mang. Meny. *Merc.* Merc-cor. Ntr-c. Ntr-m. *Ntr-s.* Nicc. *Nitr-ac. Nitr. Nux. Phosp. Phosp-ac. Puls.* Ran-b. Raph. Rat. Ruta. Samb. Sass. Sep. *Staph. Sulph.* Tabac. Tar. Teucr. *Thuj.* Verat. Verb. *Viol-od.* Zinc.
— in right ear, Acon. Aeth. Caust. Creos. Kalm. Kino. Ntr-m. Nitr-ac. Nux-m. Phyt. Ran-b. Zinc.
— in left ear, Mgn-c. Mgn-m. Mgn-s. Sang. Sep. *Staph.* Sulph.
— — to roof of mouth, same side of head and neck, sore to touch, glands swollen, Kali-b.
— through left ear from roof of mouth, Kobalt.
— sudden in left ear, extending to left side of neck and sternum, Cocc-c.
— first in left then right, Aloe.
— first in right then left, Sulph.
— on ears, Caust. Dulc. Ferr-m. Mgn-m. Ran-sc.
— behind ears, *Arn.* Bell. Berb. Nitr. Sulph. Tabac.
— — right ear, Kalm.
— about the ears, *Con.*

6. EARS AND HEARING. 53

Stinging on the lobes, Sabad.
— inwards, Lob. Ntr-s.
— outwards, *Amm-c.* Berb. Con. *Kali-c.* Ntr-s. Sil.
Strokes, blows, in ears, Arn. Ntr-m. Nux. Pæon. Plat.
Swelling of ears, *Acon* Alum. Anac. Ant. Apis. Bell. Calc. *Caust.* Cist. Creos. Kali-c. Ntr-m. Nitr. Psor. Puls. Rhus. Sep. Sil. Spong. Tellur. Zinc.
Swelling in front, Bry. Cist.
— behind, Berb. Bry. Caps. Carb-an. Tab-ac.
— in ears, Cist. Lach. Nitr-ac.
— of lobes, right, Nitr.
— around ears, Phyt.
— of periosteum, behind ears, Carb-an.
— of petrous portion, Caps.
— sense of, inside, Thuj.
Tension, Ambr. Creos. Lact.
— inside, Asar. Aur. Cham. Dig. Lact.
— behind, Nitr-ac. Nitr.
Throbbing in ears, Aloe. Bar-c. Berb. Cact. Calc. Cannab. Carb-veg. Coloc. Graph. Lach. Mgn-m. Merc-jod. Mez. Mur-ac. Ntr-c. Ntr-m. Nitr-ac. Phosp. Rheum. Rhus. Sil. Spig. Tellur. Thuj.
— on lobes, Ferr-m.
— disappearing on stooping, Cannab.
Tickling, Acon. Kalm. Spig.
— inside, Ambr. Kali-c.
Tingling, Bell. Calc. Caust. Con. Kali-c. Lyc. Nux. Puls. Sulph.
Tumor, small in ear, Berb.
— on lobe, Merc.
Tympanum, as if relaxed, Rheum.
Ulcer in ear, Bov. *Camph.* Kali-c.
— right ear, Bov.
— left ear, Camph.
Ulcerousness of ears, (suppuration,) Amm-c. Merc. Lyc. Oleand. Spong. Stann.
— inner ear, Carb-veg.
Ulcerous pain, Anac. Ferr. Mgn-c.
Wen on lobe, Nitr-ac.
Whimpering tune in ear, Ant.
Like water in left ear, Graph.
Like water passing out of ears, Calc. Spig. Sulph.
— wind passing out of ears, *Bell.* Chelid.

Stram.
As if wind passing into or blowing at, Caust. Mang. Meny. Plat. Staph.
Like a worm in ear, sensation, Rhod.
In the morning in bed, pain, Nux.
In the evening, earache, Carb-veg. Ran-b. Thuj.
— in bed, Thuj.
At night, pain, Alum. Bar-c. Nitr. Nux.
— when lying on the ear, Bar-c. Nitr.
Day and night, earache, Hell.
When blowing the nose, pain, Hep. Phosp-ac.
— — — relieved, Mang.
From cold air, pain, Agar. Colch.
— a cold, pain, Dulc. Merc.
— — in the head, *Bell.* Led. Puls.
While eating, earache, Verb.
With the full moon worse, Sil.
From laughing, earache, Mang.
When leaning on the head, earache, Arn. Lac-can. Lach. Nitr.
— masticating, earache, Nux. Seneg.
From suppressed measles, otorrhœa, Puls.
— mechanical injuries, pain, Arn.
— abuse of mercury, Asa-f. Nitr-ac. Staph.
— music, pain, Ambr. Cham. Creos. *Phosp-ac.* Tabac.
In the open air, earache, Bry. Con. Euph. Lachn. Lyc. Tabac.
When speaking, earache, Mang.
— swallowing, earache, Anac. Bov. Dros. Ferr-m. Mang. Nux.
After vexation, earache, Sulph.
When walking, earache, Bry. Con. Mang.
— — in open air, Benz-ac. Bry. Con.
After a walk in the open air, pain, Bry.
From warmth of bed, aggravation, Merc.
When the weather changes, Mang.
Before wind and rain, pain, Nux-m.
With headache, earache, Merc. Phosp. Psor. Ran-sc.
— cold legs, Thuj.
— faceache, Merc. Phosp-ac.
— micturition, profuse, Thuj.
— nausea, Dulc.
— toothache, Meph. Phosp-ac. Ran-sc.
Pains which extort cries, Nux.
— — almost deprive one of reason, Puls.

7. Nose and Smell.

As of air, pain passing through posterior nares, on coughing or talking, Mgn-s.
Anosmia, loss of smell, *Anac.* Calc. Hep. Hyosc. Ip. Mgn-m. *Ntr-m.* Phell. Phosp. Plb. Rhod. Sang. Sep. *Sil.* Zinc.
As if beaten, pain, Bell. Hep.

Biting in nose, Ang. Aur. Bry. Euph. Ran-sc. Sabad. Spig.
Black pores on nose, Dros. Graph. Sabin. *Sulph.*
— — sweaty, Graph.
Blackish nose, Merc.

7. NOSE AND SMELL.

Bleeding of nose, (see Epistaxis).
Blood, congestion of to nose, Amm-c. Cupr. Samb.
— — when stooping, Amm-c.
— discharged from nose, acrid. Nitr. Sil.
— — black, Ant. Arn. Asar. Bism. Bry. Canth. Cham. Cinnab. Creos. *Croc.* Cupr. Lach. Lyc. Mgn-c. Nitr-ac. Nux-m. Nux. Phosp-ac. Plat. Puls. Sec-c. Selen. Sep. Stram. Sulph. Sulph-ac.
— — bright, Acon. Creos. *Dulc.* Hyosc. Lach. Led. Sabad.
— — clotted, Acon. Bell. Cham. *Chin.* Croc. Ferr. Hyosc. Igt. Ip. Plat. Puls. Rhus. Sabin. Stram.
— — coagulating quickly, Merc. Nitr-ac.
— — nose continuously full of coagulated blood, Ferr.
— — pale, Arn. Bell. Dulc. Hyosc. Lachn. Led. Phosp. Rhus. Sabin. Sec-c.
— — and thin but soon coagulates, Chin. Creos. Dig. Dulc. Tilia.
— — viscid, Croc. Cupr. Sec-c.
— — warm, Dulc.
— — discharged by blowing the nose, Agar. Alum. Amm-c. Ant. Aur. Borax. Calc-ph. Canth. Caust. Dros. Ferr. Graph. Lach. Lyc. Merc. Mez. Ntr-m. Nitr-ac. Nux. Par. Phosp. Puls. Rhus. Sep. Stront. Sulph. Thuj.
— — in the morning, Caust.
— — in evening and at night, Graph.
Bloody crusts in nose, Ambr. Amm-c. Ferr. Nux. Stront.
Blueness of, alæ-nasi, Hydroc-ac.
Body sensation as if a foreign body in nose, Calc-ph.
Bones, pain in, *Aur.* Carb-an. Colch. Ind. Merc. Ntr-m. Nitr. Sil. Thuj. Verat.
Boring pain, Ntr-m. Spig. Sulph.
— with fingers in nose, Cina. Ph-ac. Seneg.
— — until it bleeds, Arum-trif.
— picking at the nose, Arum-trif. Hyper.
Bruising pain, Arn. Bell. Cic. Cina. Hep. Puls. Viol-od.
Burning sensation, Aur-m. Bell. Cist. Kali-c. Mercurial.
— inside, *Ars.* Aur-m. *Canth.* Cina. Cist. Hep. Kali-c. Mgn-m. Mez. Nicc. Nitr-ac. Nitr. Phosp. Stann. Sulph. Tab-ac.
— in nostrils, Bov. Chenop. Kali-jod. Mgn-m. Phell. Rat.
— on point, Carb-an. Nicc. Ol-an.
— spot on nose, Iod.
Cancer of nose, Ars. *Aur.* Calc. Carb-an. *Sep.* Sulph.
— epethelial, on right, alæ-nasi, Creos.
Caries, Aur.
Coldness of nose, Aloe. Arn. Bell. Chin. Cist. Cycl. Dros. Igt. Mang. Murex. Nux. Plb. Sulph. Verat.
— in nose when inhaling air, Ant. Hipp.

Compressing pain, Acon. Verat.
— as from a claw, Nitr.
Condylomatous excresences, Nitr-ac.
Contracting pain, Sabad.
Corrosion in nostrils, Berb.
— in upper part of nose, Sil.
Convulsive motion (fan like) of nasal muscles, Lyc.
Coppery redness of nose, *Cannab.*
Crackling in nose, Sulph.
Cracks in nostrils, *Ant.* Graph.
— on point, Carb-an.
Cramping pain in alæ, Plat. Zinc.
— — in root, Arn. Hyosc. Zinc.
Crawling, Arn. Borax.
— in nostrils, Agar. Aur-m. Berb. Carb-veg. Gran. Ol-an. Ran-sc. Sabad. Spig. Tabab. Teucr.
— in point, Musch. Pæon. Rheum.
Cutting pain in nasal bones, Iod. Merc-jod.
Deadness of skin, Ntr-m.
Desquamation, Ars. Aur. Canth. Carb-an. Croton. Ntr-c.
— furfuraceous, Ars. Aur.
Digging pain, Coloc. Nitr.
Drawing pain, Rheum. Thuj.
Epistaxis, *Acon.* Agar. All-cep. Aloe. *Ambr. Amm-c.* Anac. Ant. *Arg. Arn.* Ars. Aur. *Bar-c. Bell.* Berb. Borax. *Bry.* Cact. Calc. *Cannab.* Canth. Caps. Carb-an. *Carb-veg.* Caust. *Chin. Cina.* Cinnab. Coff. Con. Cor-r. *Creos. Croc.* Croton. *Dros. Dulc.* Euphr. Ferr. Graph. *Hep.* Igt. Iod. *Ip.* Kali-c. *Kali-jod.* Lach. Lachn. *Led. Lyc.* Meph. *Merc. Millef. Mosch.* Mur-ac. Ntr-c. Ntr-m. *Nitr-ac.* Nitr. Nux-m. *Nux.* Petr. *Phosp.* Phosp-ac. Plat. *Puls. Rat. Rhod. Rhus.* Ruta-Sabad. Sabin. Sass. *Sec-c.* Scill. *Sep. Sil. Spong.* Staph. Stram. *Sulph.* Sulph-ac. Tereb. *Thuj.* Tilia. Verat. Zinc.
— in plethoric persons, Acon.
— in putrid fevers, Arn.
— in morning, Agar. Ambr. Amm-c. Ant. Bell. Bov. Bry. Calc. Canth. Caps. Carb-veg. Creos. Croc. Hep. Hipp. Hyosc. Kali-c. Lach. Mgn-c. Merc. *Nitr-ac. Nux.* Puls. Rhus. Sabin.
— in bed, Caps.
— afternoon, Lyc.
— 3 P. M, Sulph.
— evening, Ant. Colch. Dros. Ferr. Graph. Phosp. Sulph.
— night, Ant. Bell. Calc. Carb-veg. Cor-r. Croc. Graph. Hyosc. Kali-chl. Mgn-s. Merc. Nitr-ac. Puls. *Rhus.* Sabin. Verat.
— after blowing the nose, Agar. Bar-c. Bry. Chin. Cinnab. Ntr-c. Nitr-ac. Nux. Spong. Sulph.
— from one nostril at a time, Cor-r. Croc.
— — right nostril, Kali-b. Kali-chl.
— from congestion to head, Alum. Graph.
— with the cough, Merc. Ntr-m.

7. NOSE AND SMELL. 55

Epistaxis from a dry, hot nose, Cannab.
— from exertion, Carb.-veg.
— with face, heat of, Graph.
— with fainting, Calc.
— with giddiness, Carb-an. Sulph.
— after hawking, Rhus.
— with head, pain in, Alum. Carb-an. Dulc.
— after headache, Ant.
— relieves headache, Bufo.
— after meals, Amm-c.
— from being overheated, Thuj.
— with loss of sight, Ind.
— after singing, Hep.
— in sleep, Bov. Bry. Merc.
— during stool, Carb-veg. Phosp.
— when stooping, Dros. Ferr. Ntr-m. Rhus. Sil.
— after washing, Amm-c.
— after weeping, Nitr-ac.
— with amenorrhoes, Bry. Cact. Puls.
— with dry coryza, Ars. Puls.
— with fainting, Cannab. Croc. Lach.
— with face, heat of, Graph.
— — paleness of face, Carb-veg.
— with hœmmorrhoids, Sep.
— with heaviness of head, Coff.
— with profuse menstruation, Acon.
— during pregnancy, Sep.
— with vanishing of sight, Ind.
— with vertigo, Carb-an. Sulph.
— followed by sore nostrils, Bry.
— sneezing followed by, Ind.
Eruption on nose, Alum. Amm-c. Ant. Aur. Bell. Brom. Carb-an. Carb-veg. Caust. Clem. Euphr. Kali-c. Lach. Mgn-c. Merc. Ntr-c. Nicc. Nitr-ac. Petr. Phosp-ac. Plb. Puls. Rhus. Sep. Sil. Spig. Sulph. Tar. (compare Herpes, scabs).
— inside, Mgn-c. Phell. Sil.
— on corners, Plb.
— on point, *Caust.* Carb-veg. Clem. Nitr-ac. Sep. Sil. Spong.
— on septum, Ol-an. Psor.
— below nose, Caps. Scill.
— on alæ, Euphr. Rhus. Thuj.
— bleeding on touch, Merc.
— burning, Alum. Graph. Ntr-m. Ol-an.
— herpetic, Nitr-ac. Spig.
— knobby tip of nose, Aur.
— itching, Nitr-ac. Palad. Phell. Scill.
— lupus on left side of nose, Creos.
— moist, Ol-an. Scill. Thuj.
— painful, Caps. Mgn-c.
— — to touch, Clem.
— pimples, Amm-c. Caps. Caust. Clem. Euphr. Kali-c. Lach. Ol-an. Ox-ac. Pallad. Petr. Plb. Sil.
— — filled with pus. Clem. Euphr. Petr. Plb.
— red, Aur. Croton. Lach. Thuj.
— sore, smarting, Spig.
— stinging, stitches, Scill.

— vesicles, Clem. Mgn-m. Nitr-ac. Phell. Plb. Sil.
Exhalatious from nose fetid, *Aur. Bell.* Calc. Con. *Graph.* Kali-b. Ntr-c. *Nitr-ac.* Nux *Phosp.* Phosp-ac. Puls. Rhus. Sulph.
— putrid, Bell. Graph.
— sickly sweetish, Nitr-ac.
— like urine, Graph.
Exostosis, Merc.
Freckles, Phosp. Sulph.
Fulness sense of in nose, Par.
— — at root extending to neck and clavicles, Gels.
Furuncles, boils, Alum. Amm-c. Carb-an. Mgn-m. Sil.
Gnawing sense in nose, *Sil.*
Grasping pain, Nitr.
Hardness of alæ-nasi, Thuj.
Heat in nose, Cannab. Canth. Chin. Clem. Cor-r. Hep. Mgn-m. Nux. Sang.
— air feels hot in nose, Kali-b.
Heaviness, Amm-c. Colch. Merc. Samb. Sil. Stann.
— when stooping, Amm-c. Sil.
— sense of in bones, Colch.
Herpetice ruption on alæ-nasi, Nitr-ac. Spig.
— — across nose, Sep. Sulph.
Inflammation of nose, Arn. Aur. *Bell.* Bry. *Calc.* Cannab. Canth. Cist. Croton. *Hep.* Lach. Mang. Merc. Ntr-m. Nux. Phell. Phosp. Plb. Ran-b. Rat. *Rhus. Sep. Sulph.* Verat.
— chronic, Fluor-ac.
— inside Agar. *Bell.* Bry. Canth. Cham. Cist. Cocc. Con. Mang. Merc. *Nux.* Phosp. Ran-b. Rhus. Sil. Stann. *Sulph.* Verat.
— after mercury, Con. Sil.
— one sided, left, Cist. Ntr-m.
— of tip, Borax. Bry. Kali-c. Lyc. Merc. Nicc. *Nitr. Sep.* Sulph.
— of septum, Psor.
Itching of nose, *Agar.* Amm-c. Arg-n. Aur-s. Borax. *Carb-veg.* Chelid. Cina. Grat. Igt. Jatr. Lac-can. Merc. Nux. Oleand. Rat. Samb. Sep. *Spig.*
— inside, *Agar.* Caust. Cina. Hyper. Lac-can. Nux. Ol-an. Rat. *Sabad.* Selen. Seneg.
— of point, Caust. Ol-an. Sil.
— of wings, Caust. Ntr-s. Selen.
Nocturnal pain, Bell. Cor-r. Lach.
— — with sleeplessness, Cor-r.
Nodosities in nostrils, Ars.
Odors in nose, on one side only, Ntr-m.
— acid, Alum. Bell.
— agreeable, Agn. Puls.
— as of blood, Nux. Psor. Sil.
— brimstone, Ars. Nux.
— burnt horn, Sulph.
— — sponge, Anac.
— candle snuffs, Nux.

7. NOSE AND SMELL.

Odor, cheese, Nux.
— coffee, Puls.
— fetid things, Aur. Bell. Calc. Creos. Elaps. Graph. Kali-b. Lac-can. Meny. Nitr-ac. Nux. Par. Phosp-ac. Phosp. Plb. Puls. Sep. Verat.
— — with anorexia, Creos.
— — when breathing through the nose, Nitr-ac.
— fish brine or fermented beer, Agn. Bell. Thuj.
— herrings, Agn. Bell.
— horse-radish, Raph.
— manure, Anac. Calc. Mgn-c. Verat.
— as from mucus from coryza, Graph. Merc. Puls. *Sulph.*
— musk, Agn.
— nauseous, Canth. Meny.
— pus, Seneg. Sulph.
— putrid, Aur. Bell. Calc. Creos. Graph. Kobalt. Meny. Nitr-ac. Par. Phosp. Sep. Verat.
— — eggs, Aur. Bell. Calc. Meny. Merc. Phosp. Sep. Sulph.
— — smell of bread and milk, Par.
— sickly, Aur. Nitr-ac. Nux. Sil.
— smoke, Sulph.
— sulphurous, Anac. Ars. Calc. Graph. Nux. Plb.
— sweetish, Aur.
— of tallow, Valer.
— of tar, Ars. Con.
— of tobacco, Puls.
— of wiskey, Aur.
Paleness around nose, Cina.
— of nose, Ntr-m.
Pinched as if nostrils were, Lachn.
Plugs of dried mucus in nose, Kali-b. Sep. *Sil.*
Polypus, Calc. Merc-cor. Phosp. Sang. Sep. Sil. Staph. Teucr.
Pressing pain in nose, Asa-f. Colch. Grat. Mgn-c. Merc. Oleand. Ran-b.
— — on root, Agn. Cannab. Dulc. Kali-b. Kalm. Hipp-m. Hyosc. Prun. Ruta.
Prickling in point, Berb. Ran-sc.
Puffiness, Bell. Caust. Kali-c. Merc. Ntr-c. Phosp-ac. Puls. Rhus. Sep.
Pulsation in nose, Cor-r.
Purulent discharge from nose, Alum. Amm-c. Arg. *Asa-f. Aur.* Calc. Cic. Cina. Con. Graph. Lach. Lyc. Merc. Nux. Petr. Phosp-ac. Puls. Rhus. Sulph.
— acrid, excoriating, Ars. Lyc. Merc.
— bloody, Arg. Arg-n. Phosp-ac.
— fetid, Asa-f. *Aur.* Graph. Lyc. Merc. Nitr-ac. Nux. Rhus.
— green, Asa-f. Aur. Kali-b. Lac-can. Nux. Puls. Rhus. Sep.
— thick, Alum.
— yellow, Alum. Aur. Cic. Graph. Lac-can. Merc. Nitr-ac. Puls.
— with clots of blood, Arg-n.

— nightly closing of nostrils with pus, Lyc.
Quivering on nose, Chelid. Stront.
Red spots on nose, Iod. Phosp-ac. Sil.
Redness of nose, *Alum.* Aur. *Bell. Calc.* Cannab. Canth. Carb-veg. Chin. Fluor-ac. Hep. Iod. Kali-c. Kali-jod. Lach. Lith. Mgn-c. Mang. *Merc.* Merc-cor. *Phosp.* Plb. Psor. *Ran-b.* Rhus. Stann. Sulph. Thuj.
— inside, Bell. Bry. Merc. Nux. Phell. Phosp. Sulph.
— of the corners, Plb.
— of nostrils, Cocc. Kali-b. Lach. Phell.
— of tip, Calc. Carb-an. Carb-veg. Lach. Nicc. Nitr-ac. Rhus. Sil.
— — on getting angry, Vinca.
— in open cold air, Aloe.
— in warm weather, Bell.
— with white pimples on it, Ntr-c.
Rending, tearing pain, Ind. Kali-jod. Nicc.
Scabs on nose, (scurf) Carb-an. Carb-veg. Caust. Chin. Mang. Ntr-m. Nitr-ac. Phosp-ac. Sass. Sep. Sil. Spong.
— below nose, Bar-c. Sass.
— inside, Alum. Aur. Borax. Brom. Cic. Cocc-c. Croton. Graph. Hep. Kali-b. Lach. Mez. Nitr-ac. Phosp. Ran-b. Rat. Sass. Sep. Sil. Staph. Sulph. Thuj.
— — right side, Iod.
— on and in nostrils, Ant. Aur. Borax. Bov. Cic. Kali-c. Lyc. Mgn-m. Merc. Rat.
— on point, Carb-an Carb-veg. Nitr-ac. *Sep.* Sil.
— discharge of large scab from gathering high up in nose, Arum-trif.
— — thick heavy yellow crusts from high up, Croton.
Smelling, sensitiveness of, Acon. Aur. Bar-c. *Bell. Cham.* Chin. Cocc. *Colch.* Graph. *Hep.* Kali-c. *Lyc.* Nux. Phosp. Plb. Sabad. Sep. *Sulph.* Tabac.
— — to acids, Dros.
— — bread and meat smell, like putrid meat, Par.
— — eggs and fat, *Colch.*
— — flowers, Graph.
— — garlic, Sabad.
— — syrup, Sang.
— — tobacco, Bell.
— — wine, Tabac.
Smelling too acute, Acon. *Agar.* Alum. Anac. Arn. Aur. *Bell* Calc. Cham. Chin. Cocc. *Coff.* Colch. Con. Cycl. Graph. Hep. Kali-c. Lyc. Mez. Nux. Phosp. Sabad. Sep. Sulph. Tabac.
— diminished, Alum. Anac. Bell. *Calc.* Cycl. Hep. Hyosc. Kali-c. Lyc. Mez. Ntr-m. Nux. Op. *Plb. Puls.* Rhus. Sec-c. *Sep. Sil.* Tabac. Zinc.
— wanting, Alum. Amm-m. *Anac.* Aur. Bell. Calc. Camph. Caps. Caust Hep.

7. NOSE AND SMELL. 57

Hyosc. Ip. Kali-b. Kali-jod. Lyc. Mgn-m. Mang. Mez. *Ntr-m.* Op. Phell. Phosp. Plb. Psor. Puls. Rhod. Rhus. Sang. Sec-c. Sep. *Sil.* Sulph. Zinc.
Soreness in the nose, Agar. Alum. Amm-m. Ang. Ant. Bov. Brom. Camph. Cocc. Euphr. Graph. Igt. Kali-b. Kali-c. Lac-can. Lach. Lact. Lith. Mgn-m. Mgn-s. Mang. *Mez.* Mur-ac. Nitr-ac. Nux. Ol-an. Rhus. Sil. *Thuj.* Zinc.
— of corners, Ant. Phosp.
— of nostrils, Ant. Graph. Kali-c. Puls.
Soreness sensation of, Ars. Cic. Euphr. Hep. Kali-b. Merc. Mez. Psor. Puls. Scill. Sil. Staph.
— — inside, Amm-m. Camph. Cocc. Colch. Graph. Hyper. Igt. Kali-c. Kali-jod. Mgn-s. Ntr-m. Nux. Puls. Rhus. Sil.
— — of nostrils, Amm-c. Chenop. Mgn-m. Scill.
— — of point, Borax. Cist. *Rhus.*
Spasm in, aloe-nasi, *Amb.*
Spasmodic pains, Plat. Zinc.
— at root, Arn. Hyosc. Zinc.
Splinter, pain, as from a, Nitr-ac.
Spots on nose, red, Iod. Phosp-ac. Sil.
— — yellow, Sep.
Stinging, stitches, Bell. Mur-ac. *Nitr-ac.* Spig.
— in point, Nitr.
— on right side on blowing the nose, as if the bones rubbed, Kali-b.
— upper part nasal cavity, Teucr.
— at root, Nicc.
Stupefying pain, Acon. Oleand. Rheum.
Suffocating pain, Euph.
Summer freckles, Phosp. Sulph.
Swelling of nose, Alum. Amm-c. *Arn.* Ars. Asa-f. *Aur. Bell.* Borax Bov. Brom. *Bry. Calc.* Cannab. *Canth.* Carb-an. Caust. Cham. Cist. Cocc. Cocc-c. Cor-r. Fluor-ac. Graph. Hep. Igt. Kali-c. Kali-jod. Lach. Lith. Lyc. Mgn-m. *Merc.* Merc-cor. Ntr-m. Nicc. Nitr-ac. Nitr. Petr. *Phosp.* Phosp-ac. Puls. Ran-b. Rat. Rhus. *Sep. Sulph.* Thuj. *Zinc.*
— red shining, commencing on right side to tip, Ox-ac.
— inside, Amm-c. Bell. Canth. Cist. Cocc. Igt. Lach. Nitr. Zinc.
— one sided, Cocc. Croc. Zinc.
— — left side, Cist. Ntr-m.
— — right, Cocc. Lith. Merc-jod. Ox-ac.
— of point, Borax. Calc. Merc-s. Nicc. Ox-ac, *Sep.* Sulph.

— of ridge, Kali-b. Phosp-ac.
— of wings, Lach. Mgn-m. Ntr-m. Ox-ac. Phell. Thuj.
— of a spot on right lachrymal bone which throbs, Kali-b.
— of the bones of nose, Merc.
Tenderness of nose, Agar. Amm-m. Kali-b. Ntr-m.
— inside, Agar. Amm-m. Croton. Kali-jod.
— to touch, pressure, Amm.m. Croton. Sil.
Tension on nose, *Asa-f.* Merc. Ran-b.
— inside, Graph.
— in the bones, Thuj.
— on the root, Meny.
— in the wings, Thuj.
Throbbing, Coloc. Cor-r. Mgn-m. Sil.
Tickling, Arg. Carb-veg. Hydroc-ac. Kali-b. Kalm. Ol-an. *Spig.*
Tingling, *Arn.*
— inside, Arg. Berb. Carb-veg. Colch. Ol-an. Ran-b. Ran-ac. Rat. *Sabad.* Spig. Tabac.
— on point, Mosch. Pæon. Rheum.
Torpor sense of, Asa-f. Plat. Samb. Viol-od.
Tremulous sensation at point, Chelid.
Hard tumor in nose, Ars.
Ulceration of nose, Cham. *Staph.* Sulph. (compare Scabs.)
— inside, Ars. Cor-r. Jatr. Kali-b. *Kali-c.* Merc. Ntr-m. Nitr. *Sil.*
— of nostrils, Alum. Arn. Aur. *Calc.* Cham. Cor-r. *Graph.* Igt. Kali-b. *Kali-c.* Lyc. Mgn-m. Merc. Ntr-c. Nitr-ac. Nitr. Petr. Phosp. Puls. *Sep.* Sil. Sulph.
— — right with burning, Gum-gut.
— of wings, Puls.
— — external, emitting a watery humor, Puls.
— of root, visible, Mez.
Ulcerous pain, Mgn-s. Puls.
— — inside, *Amm-m.* Ars. Aur. Bell. Borax. Bry. Hep. Nux. Puls. Sil. Verat.
Warmth, sensation of, Rheum.
Warts, old on nose, Caust. Thuj.
Wrinkled skin of nose, Cham.
From abuse of Mercury, Aur. Con. Sil.
When pressing on nose, pain relieved, Agn.
When touched, pain, Aur. Bell. Bry. Colch. Hep. Merc. Led. Mgn-m. Mgn-s. Ntr-c. Ntr-m. Nitr-ac. Nitr. Phosp. Rhus. Sil.

8. Face.

LIPS AND LOWER JAW.

Aged expression, Hydroc-ac.
Altered face, Aeth. Ars. Caust. Cham. Colch. Cupr. Lyc. Op. Sacch. Stram. Verat.
Anxious expression, Aeth *Bell.* Cupr.
Apthæ on lips, Ip.
Arthritic pains in lower jaws, *Caust.*
As if beaten in zygoma, Cor-r. Sulph-ac. Zinc.
— — — bones of face, Kali-b.
— — — malar bones, Ntr-m.
Bewildered appearance, Plb. Stram. Zinc.
Biting in face, like salt, Cannab.
Blackish face, *Chin.* Cor-r.
— lips, Acon.*Ars.* Bry. *Chin.* Merc. Phosp-ac. Psor. Rhus. Scill. Tart. *Verat.*
Black pores on face, Dig. Graph. Hep. Ntr-c. Nitr-ac. Sabad. Sabin. Selen. Sulph.
— on chin, Dros.
— — — and upper lip, Sulph.
— — ulcerating, Dig.
Bleeding lips, Aloe. Ars. Arum-trif. Bry. Carb-an. Igt. Kali-c. Kobalt. Ntr-m.
Bloatedness of face, Acon. *Amm-c.* Apis. Arn. *Ars.* Aur. Bar-c. *Bell.* Bry. Cact. Calc. Cham. *Chin.* Cina. Cocc. Colch. Con. Dig. Dros. Dulc. Elaps. Hell. Hipp-m. Hydroc-ac. *Hyosc.* Hyper. Ip. Kali-b. *Kali-c.* Lach. Laur. Led. Lyc. Mgn-c. Meph. Merc. Merc-cor. Mez. *Ntr-c.* Op. *Phosp.* Plb. Puls. Sacch. *Samb.* Sang. Sep. *Spig.* Spong. Tart. Thuj. Vinca.
— glossy, Aur.
— about eyes, Apis. Ars. Ferr. Elaps. Merc. Nitr-ac. Phosp. Rhus.
— under eyes, Apis. Ars. Bry. Kali-c. Oleand. Phosp. Puls.
— over eyes, Lyc. Ruta. Sep.
— between the eyes, Lyc.
— — lids and eyebrows, Kali-c.
— lower lip, heavy and burns, Mur-ac.
Blood blisters on upper lip, Ntr-m.
Blue color of face, Acon. Agar. Ang. Arg-n. *Ars.* Aur. Bad. Bell. Bry. Camph. *Cina.* Con. Creos. Croc. Cupr. Dig. Dros. Hep. Hydroc-ac. Hyosc. Igt. Ip. Lach. Lachn. Laur. Lyc. Merc. Ntr-m. Nux. Op. Ox-ac. Puls. *Samb.* Sang. Spong. Staph. Verat.
— of cheeks, *Cham.*
— of lips, Ang. Arg-n Ars. Berb. Caust. Chin. *Cupr. Dig.* Lachn. Lyc. Mosch. Phosp. Verat.
— about mouth, *Cina.* Cupr.
— under eyes, Ars. Chin. Ip. Oleand.

Rhus. Sec-c.
— around eyes, Canth. Chin.
— pale bluish, Hydroc-ac.
Bluish red face, Bell. Bry. Calc. Cupr. Merc. Op. Puls.
— — bloated, Acon. Ang. Bry. Hep. Merc. Op. Phosp.
Blue spots on face, Ferr.
— circles around eyes, Anac. Ars. Bad. Berb. Bism. Calc. *Chin.* Cina. Cocc. Corn-c. Cupr. Ferr. Graph. Hipp-m. Igt. Ip. Jatr. Kali-c. Lach. Lyc. Merc. Mez. Ntr-c. Nux-m. Nux. Oleand. Pallad. *Phosp.* Phosp-ac. Rhus. Sabad. Sabin. *Sec-c.* Sep. Stann. Staph. Sulph. Verat.
Boils on face, Alum. Ant.
— — forehead, Sep.
— — lips and chin, painful, Hep.
Bones, inflammation, *Aur. Staph.*
— pain, Aeth. *Caps.* Hell. *Hep.* Merc-jod. Ntr-m. Nitr. Nux. Zinc.
— — when touched, Hep.
— swelling, Aur. Sil.
— swelling of chin, Aur.
— — forehead, Aur.
— — lower jaw, Aur. Sil.
— — temples, Spig.
Boring pain, Bell. Euph. *Mgn-c. Thuj.*
— in cheek bones, Bov. Ind. *Stront.*
— — lower jaw, Bov. Ind. Sabad.
Break, sensation as if lower jaw would, Phosp-ac.
Brown, the face becomes, Iod.
— red face, Bry. Hyosc. Nitr-ac. *Op.* Puls. Samb. Sep. Stram. Sulph.
— — when angry, Staph.
— streak (thin) along upper lip at junction with lower, Ars.
— lips, Ars. Bry. Oleand. Op. Phosp. Psor. Staph. Tart.
Bruising pain, *Ruta.*
— in left malar bone, Cor-r. Sulph. Sulph-ac. Zinc.
— — right malar bone, and right side of head, a small spot pulsates and burns like fire, Merc-jod.
Burning pain, Arg-n. *Ars.* Bell. Coloc. Euphr. Graph. Rhus. Stann. Thuj.
— — in cheeks, Agar. Asar. Caust. Clem. Daph. Ol-an. Phosp-ac. Puls. Rhus.
— — cheek bone, Caust. Cist. Grat. Ol-an. Par. Spig. Staph. Thuj.
— — in left zygoma, then right, Gels.
— — in chin, Anac. Caust.
— — in jaws, Anac. Daph.
— — below eyes, Dros.

8. FACE.

Boring pain, in lips, Amm-c. Amm-m. Arn. Ars. Asa-f. Aur-m. Berb. Borax. Bry. Caps. Carb-an. Cic. Croton. Laccan. Mgn-s. Merc. Mez. Mur-ac. Ntr-s. Rhod. Sabad. Spig. Sulph. Tabac. Tart.
— — — upper, Brom. Mez. Sulph.
— — — lower, Clem. Coloc.
— — — in corners of mouth, Mez.
Cancer in face, *Ars.* Sil.
— on lips, *Ars.* Clem. *Con.* Sil. Sulph.
— — lower lip, Ars. Clem. Sil.
— — — from smoking, Con.
Changing color of face, Acon. Alum. Ars. Bell. Borax. Bov. Camph. Caps. Cham. Chin. Cina. Croc. Ferr. Hyosc. Igt. Kali-c. Laur. Led. Mgn-c. Mgn-s. Nux. Oleand. Op. Phosp. Phosp-ac. Plat. Puls. Scill. Spig. Sulph-ac. Verat. Zinc.
— appearance, Scill.
Chewing motion, Acon. Bell. Bry. Cham. Lach. Mosch. Verat.
Closed, disposed to keep the jaws tightly, Kobalt.
Coldness of face, Ars. Bell. Bism. Camph. Cic. Cina. Cupr. Hyosc. Iris. Lyc. Oxac. Plat. Sec-c. Verat.
— painful, Lyc.
— one sided, Puls.
— of cheeks, Bell. Cham. Lyc.
— on left cheek to ear, Lob.
— of lips, Ars. Cupr. Verat.
— sense of, Merc. *Plat.* Ran-sc.
— — about chin and mouth, *Plat.*
Congestion of blood to the face, Bar-c. Cocc-c. Ind. *Stram.*
Contraction in cheek, Laur. Rhus.
— in frontal muscles Rheum.
— sudden fierce, of muscles of right cheek. Eupat.
— facial muscles especially around mouth, Gels.
— sensation of, Bell. Mosch.
Convulsions of face, Bell. Calc. Canth. *Cham.* Dig. *Igt. Ip.* Lyc. Ntr-c. Op. Phosp. Stram. Sulph.
— of mouth, Bell. Cham. Dulc. Igt. *Ip.* Lyc. Merc. Oleand. Op. Stram.
— one sided, left, Dig.
Coppery eruption on face, Ars. Aur. Carban. Rhus. Ruta. Verat.
— — about chin and mouth, Verat.
— color, Calc. Creos. Sec.
Copper colored spots, Benz-ac.
Cracks on skin of face, Nicc. Sil.
— in lips, Agar. Aloe. Alum. *Amm-c. Amm-m. Arn.* Arum-trif. *Ars.* Aur. Barc. Bell. Bov. *Bry.* Calc. Caps. Carb-an. Carb-veg. Cham. Chin. Colch. Con. Cor-r. *Croc.* Cupr. Dros. Graph. *Igt.* Iris. Jatr. Kali-c. Kali-jod. Kalm. Lach. Mgn-m. *Merc.* Ntr-c. *Ntr-m.* Nicc. Nitr-ac. Nux. Ol-an. Par. Phosp. Phosp-ac. Plat. Puls. Sabad. Scill. Selen. Sulph. Tabac. Tar. Tart. *Verat.* Zinc.
— upper lip, Hell. Mez. Ntr-c.
— lower lip, Apis. Mez.
— — middle of, Cham. Hep. Puls.
— corners of mouth, Amm-c. Ant. Arumtrif. Cinnab. Merc. Mez.
— ulcerating, Merc. Phosp-ac.
Cracking in maxillary joint when chewing, Amm-c. Meny. Rhus. Thuj.
— — — when opening the mouth wide, Sabad.
Cramp like pain in left malar bone to eye. Coloc.
Crawling, creeping, (see Tingling.)
Crustea lacta, *Ars.* Bar-c. Bell. *Calc.* Carbveg. Caust. *Cic.* Cycl. *Dulc.* Graph. Hep. Lyc. *Merc.* Ntr-m. Phosp. Rhus. *Sass.* Sep. *Sulph. Viol-tr.*
Cutting pain in face, *Bell.* Rhus. Staph.
— — from root of nose to ear, Elaps.
Cystic tumor on cheek, Graph.
Dark red face, *Bar-c. Camph.* Coloc. Gels. Op. Sec-c. *Verat.*
— — lips, Bar-c. Bell.
Death like appearance, Ars. Canth. *Plb.* Verat.
Despairing appearance, Canth. Hœmatox.
Despuamation of skin, Apis. Canth. Phosp. Puls. Thuj.
— — lips, Acon. Aloe. Alum. Amm-m. Arum-trif. Berb. Canth. Caps. Cham. Con. Creos. Kali-c. Kobalt. Lac-can. Mez. Mosch. Ntr-m. Ntr-s. *Nux.* Plb. Puls. Sep. Sulph-ac. Thuj.
Digging pain, Bov. Euphr.
— — in cheek bones, *Mgn-c. Thuj.*
— — — rami of lower jaw, Kali-b.
Dirty color of face, Iod. Mgn-c. Merc. Phosp. Sec-c.
Discolored face, *Mgn-c. Sec-c.*
— spots on face, Sec-c.
Disfigured face, Aeth. *Ars.* Bism. Colch. Iod. Phosp-ac. Rhus. *Spig.*
Dislocation, easy of maxillary joint, Petr. Staph.
— — in morning in bed, Petr.
— sense of, Con. Rhus.
Distortion of face, Acon. Amm-m. Ang. Ars. Bell. Bism. Camph. Caust. Cham. Cic. Cocc. *Cupr.* Graph. Hydroc-ac. Hyosc. Igt. Ip. Lach. Laur. Lyc. Merccor. Op. Plat. Plb. Rhus. Scill. Sec-c. Sol-n. *Stram.* Verat.
— of lips and mouth, *Bell.* Dulc. Lyc. Nux. Op. Sec-c. Stram.
— of mouth, spasmodic, Bell. Bry. Cupr. Graph. Lach. Merc. Nux. Op. Phospac. Plat. Sec-c. Stram.
— corners of mouth, Hydroc-ac.
— one sided, Dulc. Graph.
Drawing pain in face, Aloe. Ars. Bar-c. Cham. Colch. Creos. Hep. Kali-c.

8. FACE.

Mgn-m. Nux. Ol-an. Phosp-ac. *Ran-sc.* Sep. Verat.
Drawing in cheek bones, Alum. Bell.Carb-veg. Colch. DigGraph. Hyper. Kali-chl. Phosp. Stann. Staph. Sulph. Tart. Valer. Viol-od.
— — left, Chelid.
— on chin, Agar. Caust.
— — jaws, Aur. Cham. Mez. Phosp-ac. Puls. Sil.
— in orbits, Stann.
— back of lips, Bell. Merc-cor.
Dry, parched lips, Acon. Aloe. Alum. *Amm-c. Amm-m.* Ang. Ant. Arg-n. Ars. Bar-c. Bell. Berb. *Bry.* Chenop. *Chin.* Con. Creos. Croton. Dig. Dros. Ferr. Gels. Hyosc. Hyper. *Igt.* Iris. Kali-jod. Kalm. Lach. Mgn-s. Merc. Mercurial. Ntr-m. Ntr-s. Nux.' Oleand. 'Phosp. Phosp-ac. Plat. Psor. Rhod. Rhus. Sang. Sep. Stram. Sulph. Tabac. *Tart.* Verat. Vinca. Zing.
— — — morning, Chenop.
— — — evening, Mgn-s.
— — — and black, Acon. Phosp.
— and tongue, Ars. Cham. Lach. Lyc. Phosp.
— upper lip peels off, Ntr-s.
Dull, heavy expression, Corn-c. Gels. Merc.
— pain in right malar bone, Hell.
Earth colored face, Ars. Bism. Borax. Bry. *Chin.* Cic. Creos. *Croc. Ferr.* Igt. Iod. Ip. Lach. *Laur. Lyc.* Mgn-c. Mgn-s. *Merc.* Mez. Mosch. Ntr-m. Nitr-ac. *Nux.* Ol-an. Op. Pallad. Phosp. Sacch. Sil. Zinc.
Emaciation of face, Ars. Calc. Mez. Selen. Sep. Tabac.
Eruption in the face, Alum-ambr. *Amm-c.* *Amm-m.* Ant. *Ars. Bar-c.* Bell. Bov. Bry. *Calc.* Carb-an. Carb-veg. *Caust.* Cic. Cist. Clem. Coloc. Con. Dulc. Euph. Gels. *Graph. Hep.* Igt. Ip. Kali-Iod. Lach. Led. *Lyc. Mgn-m. Merc.* Mez. Mur-ac. Ntr-m. *Nitr-ac.* Nux. Petr. Phosp. Phosp-ac. Rhus. Sabad. *Sass.* Sep. Sil. *Staph. Sulph.* Thuj. Valer. Verat. Viol-tr.
— on cheeks, Amm-c. Ant. Bell. Bov. Calc. Caust. Cic. Creos. Dig. Dulc. Kali-jod. Lach. Lyc. Merc. Ntr-m. Sep. Sil. Staph. Verat.
— — chin, Amm-c. Ant. Bell. Carb-veg. Cic. Clem. Creos. Dig. Dulc. *Graph.* Lyc. Merc. Ntr-m. Ntr-s. Nux. Par. Phosp-ac. Rhus. *Sep.* Sil. Sulph. Thuj. Verat. Zinc.
— — — painful, Merc. Rhus. Sass. Sulph.
— on forehead, Alum. Ambr. Ant. Aur. Bell. Bov. *Calc.* Caps. Cauloph. Caust. Cic. Clem. Creos. Dulc. Hep. Led. Mgn-m. Mur-ac. Ntr-c. Ntr-m. Nitr-ac.

Par. Phosp. Phosp-ac. Psor. Rhus. Sass. Sep. Sulph.
Eruption on lips, Alum. *Amm-c.* Arg-n. Ars. Bell. Berb. Borax. Bry. *Calc.* Caps. Carb-an. Carb-veg. Caust. Cham. Cic. Clem. Con. Dig.Graph.Hell.Hep.Igt.Ip. Lach. Lyc. Mgn-m. Merc. *Mur-ac.* Ntr-c. Ntr-m. Ntr-s. Nicc. Nux. Par. Petr. Phosp. Phosp-ac. Plat. Rhod. Ruta. Sass. *Scill.* Seneg. *Sep. Sil.* Spong. Staph. Sulph. Thuj.
— upper lip, Ars. Bell. Cic. Creos. Kali-c. *Lyc.* Mang. Ntr-c. Ntr-m. Par. Phyt. Rhus. Scill. Staph. Sulph.
— lower lip, Bry. Calc. Igt. Ntr-m. Phosp-ac.
— on red part of lips, Ant. Ars. Sep. Sil.
— about mouth, Amm-c. Anac. Ars. Borax. Bov. Bry. Calc. Caust. Creos. *Graph.* Lach. Laur. Lyc. *Mgn-m.* Ntr-c. Ntr-m. Nux. Par. Phosp. Rhus. Sep. Sil. Staph. Sulph.
— on corners of mouth, Ant. *Bell.* Bov. Calc. Carb-veg. Caust. Creos. Hep. Igt. Lyc. *Mang.* Merc. Ntr-m. Nux. Petr. Phosp. Phosp-ac. Psor. Seneg. Senna. Sep Sil. Tabac. Verat.
— about eyes, Agn. Arn. Ars. Con. Hep. Staph. Sulph.
— — eyelids, Bry. Creos. Sulph.
— — eyebrows, Caust. Kali-c. Par. Selen. Staph.
— — nose, Ant. Bell. Caust. Clem. Par-Rhus. Sulph. Tar.
— on temples, Alum. Ant. Arg. Bell. Calc. Dulc. Lyc. *Mur-ac.* Ntr-m. Nitr-ac.
— in whiskers, Ambr. Calc. Graph. Lach. Nitr-ac.
— acne rosacea, Ars. Aur. Calc-ph. Carb-an. Caust. Creos. Lach. Led. Rhus. Ruta. Sep.
— — around chin and mouth, Verat.
— biting, Bry. Merc. Ntr-m. Plat. Sil.
— blackish, Spig.
— bleeding when scratched, Merc. Par. Rhus.
— blotches hard, Arg-n.
— brownish, Dulc.
— burning, Ant. Calc. Euphr. Mgn-m. Merc. Ntr-m. Rat. Rhus. Seneg. Senna. Staph. Viol-tr.
— — when scratched, Ntr-s. Sass.
— — when wetting the face, Euphr.
— confluent, Carb-veg. Cic.
— corrosive, Dig.
— dry, Psor.
— excoriating, Mez.
— raw, fat pustules, Mez.
— impetigo, Ars. Calc. Graph. Lyc. Rhus. Sep.
— — on forehead, Ant. Creos. Led. Rhus. Sep. Sulph.
— jerking, painful, Rhus.

8. FACE. 61

Eruptions, itching, Amm-c. Calc. Caust. Con. Dig. Euphr. Lyc. Mgn-m. *Merc.* Ntr-c. Nitr-ac. Ol-an. Sass. Staph. Thuj. Zinc.
— — in warmth, Euphr.
— leaving livid spots, Ferr. Lach. Thuj.
— like measels especially on face, Gels.
— miliary, Cham. Euphr. Ip. Par. Verat.
— millet like, Par.
— moist, Ant. Ars. Calc. Clem. Cic. Dulc. Lyc. *Merc.* Mez. Ntr-c. Psor. Rhus. Sep. Sil. Viol-tr.
— — fetid, Cic. Merc.
— — yellow, Rhus. Viol-tr.
— at night painful, Viol-tr.
— in open air disappearing, Calc.
— painful, Eugen. Sulph.
— — at night, Viol-tr.
— — to touch, Bell. *Hep.* Led. Par. Valer. Verat.
— pimples, red, Ambr. Carb-an. Eugen. *Mur-ac.* Ntr-m. *Nitr-ac.* Petr. Phosp. Phosp-ac. Sep.
— — on chin, Ferr-m. Merc. Phosp-ac. Rhus. Thuj.
— — on forehead, Ambr. Clem. Ferr-m. Hep. Led. *Mur-ac.* Ntr-m. Nitr-ac. Par. Sep.
— — on lips, Ferr-m. *Mur-ac.* Par. Petr. Phosp-ac. Ruta. Thuj.
— — — upper, Ant. Spig.
— red, on lower maxilla, Par.
— — about mouth, Phosp. Rhus.
— — on corners of mouth, Petr.
— — on temples, Arg. *Mur-ac.* Nitr-ac.
— — in whiskers, Amb.
— pustules, Carb-veg.
— rasping, Bry. Ntr-m. Sil.
— raw, as if skin were, Graph.
— red, Ant. Aur. Calc-ph. Caust. Cham. Cic. Euphr. Led. Nitr-ac. Par. Sep.
— — blotches on bloated face, Elaps.
— like roughness of skin, Sep.
— scaly, Ant. Ars. Aur. Sep. Sil.
— scurfy, Ant. Calc. Cic. Graph. Hep. Merc. Mur-ac. Petr. Phosp-ac. Psor. Rhus. Sep. Sil. Thuj. Viol-tr.
— — with large humid eruption on head, Psor.
— sore smarting, Cic. Ip. Rhod. Verat.
— stinging, stitches, painful, Clem. Led. Plat. Staph.
— suppurating, Ant. *Cic.* Lyc. Rhus.
— tinea facies, Ars. Bar-c. Calc. Cic. Cycl. Dulc. Merc. Sass. Sulph. Viol-tr.
— vesicular, comes out in cold air, Dulc.
— clear vesicles on upper lip, Mang.
— large water blisters on margin of lower lip, Mgn-m.
— white, Clem. Hell. Valer.
— yellow, Ant. Cic. Creos. Dulc. *Euph.* *Merc.* Ntr-c. Phosp-ac. Sep.
— — blister, secreting a thick yellow fluid, Euph.

— with scanty menstruation, Graph.
Erysipelas, Acon. Ars. Apis. *Bell.* Borax. Bufo. Calc. Camph. *Canth.* *Carb-an.* Cham. *Euph.* Gels. *Graph.* Gymnoc. *Hep.* Lach. Meph. Puls. *Rhus.* Sep. Stram. Sulph. *Sulph-ac.* Thuj.
— on forehead, Ruta.
— one sided, Borax. Sep. Stram.
— — right to left, Apis. Graph. Sulph.
— — left to right, Rhus.
— — beginning on right ear, Sulph.
— — from root of decayed tooth, Sep.
— on hands and neck, Hydrast.
— after toothache, Cham.
— spreading in rays, Graph.
— vesiculous, Ars. Bell. Cist. *Euph.* Graph. Hep. Lach. *Rhus.* Sulph.
— chronic, Tereb.
Fatigued expression, Aur. Sulph.
Fear expression of, Stram.
Flushes of heat, Alum. Ambr. Bufo. Chenop. Cist. Cocc. Cocc-c. *Graph.* Kali-c. Kali-chl. *Lyc.* Phosp. Pod. Tellur. Teucr. Thuj.
— — on cheek, Clem. Cocc.
— — from chest, Sulph.
Freckles, Amm-c. Ant. Calc. Dulc. Graph. Kali-c. *Lyc.* Mur-ac. Ntr-c. Nitr-ac. Nux-m. Phosp. Puls. Sep. Sulph. Thuj.
Fretting (corrosion) sense of, *Agn.* Ambr. Ruta.
— — in bones, Arg. Ind. Samb.
— — in chin and lips, Plat.
— — on forehead and whiskers, Amb.
Fulness, sense of, Sang.
Furuncles, boils, on cheek, Alum. Amm-c. Arn. Bar-c. Bell. Bry. Calc. Carb-veg. China. Cina. Laur. Led. Mez. Mur-ac. Ntr-c. Ntr-m. Nitr-ac. Sil.
— small blood boils on face, Iris.
— on chin, Hep. Nitr-ac. Sil.
— — under, Carb-veg.
— — right side, Kobalt.
— on lips, Ntr-c. Petr.
— boils, in front of ears, Carb-veg.
— on forehead, Led.
— on temples, Mur-ac.
— glands of lower jaw, Parotid (compare under Ears.)
— boring pain in, Sabad.
— bruising, Ars.
— hardness, Bar-c. Calc. Carb-an. Clem. Cocc. Graph. Merc. Rhus. Sec-c. Staph.
— inflammation, Bar-c. Bell. Calc. Canth. Kali-c. *Merc.* Nitr-ac. Plb. Rhus. Sass. Sec-c. Staph. Verb.
— lumps, Clem.
— pain in general, Amm-c. Arn.* Aur. Calc. Cic. Chin. Cor-r. Igt. *Nitr-ac.* Rhus. Sep. Stann. Staph. Verat.
— — when swallowing, Cor-r. Nux. Stram.
— — touched, Clem. Sil. Sulph.
— — moving the neck, Igt.

5

8. FACE.

Furuncles, pressing pain, Ars. Igt. Stram.
— stinging, stitches, Bell. Merc. Mez. Nux. Sulph.
— swelling, Amm-c. Amm-m. Arn. Ars. Arum-trif. Asa-f. Aur. Bar-c. Bell. Bov. Brom. Bry. Calad. Calc. Carb-an. Cham. Chin. Cic. Clem. Cocc. Cor-r. Croton. Dulc. Graph. Hep. Iod. Kali-c. Kali-jod. Led. Lyc. Merc. Ntr-c. Ntr-m. Nitr-ac. Nux. Petr. Phosp. Plb. Puls. Rhus. Sep. Sil. Spig. Spong. Stann. Staph. Sulph. Sulph-ac. Thuj. Verat.
— — painful, hard, Bar-c. Calc. Hell. Iod. Mur-ac. Petr. Sil. Staph. Sulph.
— tension, Clem. Spong.
— throbbing, Amm-c. Bov. Clem.
— with pain extending to teeth, Ind.
Gloomy expression, Ntr-c. Zinc.
Gnawing in facial bones, Arg. Eugen. Ind.
— — lower maxilla, Ind.
— about mouth, Puls.
Grasping sensation between nose and eye, Mang.
Grayish color, Berb. Carb-veg. Creos. Gels. Hydroc-ac. Lach. Laur. Mez.
Greasy face, Ntr-m. Plb. Selen. Thuj.
— lips, Amm-m.
Greenish color, Ars. Carbo-veg. Verat.
— ring around eyes, Verat.
Half opened mouth, Ang. Bell. Camph. Hyosc. Samb.
Hanging down of lower jaw, Ars. Lyc. Mur-ac. Op.
— — lower lip, Hipp-m.
Hardness of cheeks, Cham. Merc-cor.
Heat in the face, Acon. Amm-c. Amm-m. Anac. Ang. Ant. Arg-n. Arn. Asa-f. Asar. Aur. Bell. Berb. Bov. Brom. Bry. Cannab. Canth. Cham. Chin. Cinnab. Cocc. Coff. Colch. Con. Cor-r. Corn-c. Creos. Croc. Diad. Dros. Ferr. Fluor-ac. Gels. Glon. Grat. Hell. Hep. Hydroph. Hyosc. Hyper. Jatr. Lach. Lact. Mang. Meny. Merc. Mez. Mosch. Mur-ac. Ntr-c. Ntr-m. Nux-m. Nux. Op. Ox-ac. Pæon. Petr. Phosp-ac. Plat. Psor. Ran-b. Rat. Rhus. Rumex. Sabad. Samb. Sang. Scill. Seneg. Sep. Sil. Stront. Sulph. Tabac. Tart. Thuj. Tilia. Verat. Zing.
— on cheeks, Ant. Bov. Chin. Cocc. Cocc-c. Daph. Merc. Oleand. Rhus. Valer.
— on that which is exposed to air, Phosp-ac. Viol-tr.
— of right cheek, and chilliness over whole body, Puls.
— and redness of one cheek, Igt.
— — — left cheek, Borax.
— — — right cheek, Ntr-m. Nicc.
— — — first in right later in left, Brom.
— and paleness of one cheek, redness and coldness of the other, Mosch.
— in forehead, Cham. Diad. Euphr.
— on lips, Aloe. Arn. Gels.
— semi-lateral, Arn. Benz-ac. Igt. Murex. Spong. Viol-tr.
— flushes of, Alum. Ambr. Chenop. Cist. Cocc. Graph. Kali-c. Kali-chl. Lyc. Phosp. Pod. Teucr. Thuj.
— — on cheeks, Cocc.
— burning, Amm-m. Apis. Arn. Bell. Bry. Caps. Croc. Diad. Grat. Igt. Iod. Ntr-c. Nux. Pæon. Plat. Rhus. Sabad. Sang. Stront. Sulph. Tabac. Thuj. Verat.
— — heat and redness of left side, Asa-f. Lac-can. Murex. Ntr-m. Ol-an. Phosp-ac. Spig.
— — of malar bones, Cist.
— in morning, Croc.
— in afternoon, Anac. Carb-an.
— in evening, Ang. Arn. Plat. Thuj.
— at night, Hep.
— by bending forward increased, Cor-r.
— after drinking wine, Sabad.
— when excited, with headache, Aloe.
— from exercise and talking, Scill.
— intellectual labor, Amm-c.
— in open air, Mur-ac. Val.
— when sleeping, Meny.
— with dryness of mouth, Plat.
— with nausea, lassitude, Anac.
— with thirst, Petr. Plat.
— with yawning, Daph.
— without redness, Thuj.
— sensation of, Ang. Euphr. Hyper. Tar.
— — in evening, Ang.
Heaviness sense of, Alum. Nicc.
Hemiplegia, Caust. Graph.
Herpes, Amm-c. Anac. Ars. Bar-c. Calc. Carb-an. Carb-veg. Cic. Con. Creos. Dulc. Graph. Hep. Led. Lyc. Merc. Nitr-ac. Rhus. Sabad. Sep. Sulph. Thuj.
— on cheek, Amm-c. Creos. Dulc. Kali-jod. Nicc. Phosp-ac.
— on chin. Amm-c. Carb-veg. Chelid. Dulc. Nux. Sil.
— about eyes, Bry. Creos. Sulph.
— on forehead, Caps. Dulc.
— on lips, Caust. Ntr-c. Phosp-ac. Sass.
— corners of lips, Carb-veg. Phosp-ac. Sulph.
— about mouth, Amm-c. Anac. Ars. Borax. Creos. Mgn-c. Ntr-c. Ntr-m. Par. Phosp. Rhus. Sep. Sulph.
— about nose, Rhus. Sulph.
— in whiskers, Lach. Nitr-ac.
— burning, Led. Rhus.
— dry, Ars. Kali-jod. Led.
— jerking, painful, Rhus.
— itching, Caps. Kali-jod. Nicc. Nitr-ac. Rhus. Sulph.
— mealy, Ars. Bry. Cic. Creos. Lyc. Merc. Nitr-ac. Sulph. Thuj.
— moist, Carb-veg. Con. Dulc. Ntr-c. Phosp-ac. Sulph.
— rough, Led.

8. FACE.

Herpes, scurfy, Calc. Creos. Graph. Led. Lyc. Sep. Sulph.
— chronic, Led.
— thick brown or yellow crusts, Dulc.
— red from corner of right nostril to cheek, Elaps.
Hippocratic face, *Ars.* Canth. Carb-veg. *Chin.* Ferr. Lach. Lyc. *Phosp. Phosp-ac.* Plb. *Sec-c.* Stann. Staph. Tart. *Verat.*
Jerks in jaws, *Cham.*
Jerking pain, Colch.
— in cheek bones, Cina. Colch. Mang. Spig. Stront.
Induration of lips, Bell. Sil.
— — schirrus, Sil.
— — sense of, Cycl.
Inflammation of face, Sep.
— of chin, Caust.
— of lips, Ars. Canth.
— of penostrum, lower jaw, Merc-cor.
Inflammatory pain, *Acon.* Arn. *Aur.* Bar-c. Bry. Euph. *Staph.*
Inspired expression, Hydroc-ac.
Irregular features, Phosp-ac.
Itching, *Agn.* Alum. Ambr. Amm-c. Bell. Berb. *Calc.* Cannab. Chelid. Colch. Con. Dolich. Fluor-ac. Gels. Glon. Hipp-m. Lach. Lyc. Ntr-c. Ntr-m. Ntr-s. Nux. Phosp. Phosp-ac. Rhus. Ruta. Sass. Sep. Sulph-ac. Verat.
— — at night, Kalm.
— on cheeks, Agar. Agn. Ang. Ant. Bell. Ruta. Spong.
— on cheek bones and nose, Bell. Hyper.
— on forehead, Alum. Ambr. Caps. Chelid. Led. Ntr-m. Sulph.
— on lips, Ol-an. Sabad.
— — upper, Bar-c.
— about mouth, Anac. Hep.
— in whiskers, Agar. Ambr. Calc. Kobalt. Ntr-m. Sil.
— biting, burning, lower jaw, Par.
— itching as if frostbitten, Agar.
Lameness, facial muscles, Seneg.
—pain as of, Evon. Sabin.
Leaden color, Ars. Lach. Merc.
Lumps indurations in face, Bry. Mgn-c. *Led.* Oleand. Puls.
— in forehead, Cic. Con. Led. Oleand.
— — lower jaw, Graph.
— temples, red, Thuj.
Lupus, extending to mouth and throat, Cist.
Miliary eruption, Cham. Euphr. Hep. Lach. Verat.
Morose expression, Mgn-c.
Mucus, viscid, on lips in the morning, Kali-jod.
Mouth, difficult to open, Caust. Colch. Lach. Merc-dulc. Nux. Psor.
— open, Ang-spur. Bell. Camph. Hyosc. Op. Ox-ac. Puls. Samb. Scill.
Muscles, tension of, Ang.
Net work of small veins on chin, *Plat.*

Nocturnal pains, Con. Led. Mgn-c.
— in lower jaw, Sil.
Numbness, sensation of, Asar. Plat. Samb. (compare Stunning pains.)
— cheek bones, Asa-f. *Caps. Mez. Oleand.* Plat.
— chin, Asa-f. Plat.
— lips, Ambr. Cic. Ntr-m.
— — upper, Cycl. Oleand.
— about mouth, Plat.
Old, face looks, Hydroc-ac.
One sided pain, Acon. Amm-c. Caust. Cham. Colch. Creos. Evon. Grat. Kali-b. Kalm. Mez. Nux. Ol-an. Phosp. Tong. Verat.
Pain, features denoting, Aeth. *Colch.* Lact. *Puls.* Raph. Stram.
Paleness, *Acon.* Aeth. Ambr. Amm-c. Anac. Apis. Arg-n. *Arn.* Ars. Bad. Bell. Berb. Bism. Borax. Bov. Brom. *Calc. Camph.* Cannab. *Canth.* Caps. Carb-veg. *Cham.* Chenop. *Chin.* Cic. *Cina.* Clem. Cocc. Colch. Coloc. Con. Croc. *Cupr.* Cycl. *Dig.* Dros. Dulc. Ferr. Gels. Glon. *Graph.* Hœmatox. Hell. Hydroc-ac. Hyosc. Igt. *Iod. Ip.* Jatr. Kali-c. Kali-jod. Kalm. Lach. Lact. *Laur.* Led. *Lyc. Mgn-c. Mgn-m. Mang. Merc.* Merc-cor. Mez. Mosch. Ntr-c. Ntr-m. Ntr-s. *Nitr-ac.* Nitr. Nux-m. *Nux. Oleand.* Ol-an. *Op.* Ox-ac. Petr. Phell. *Phosp.* Phosp-ac. Phyt. *Plat.* Plb. *Puls.* Rhus. Sabin. Sacch. *Sec-c. Sep.* Sil. *Spig.* Spong. *Stann.* Stram. *Sulph.* Sulph-ac. *Tabac. Tart.* Tereb. Teucr. *Tong.* Valer. *Verat.* Zinc.
— one sided, Acon. Arn. Bell. Cham. Coloc. Igt. Mosch. Nux. Tabac. Verat.
— around eyes, Ars.
— of lips, Caust. Ferr. Hipp-m. Lyc. Thuj.
— in morning, after rising, Bov.
— — evening, Lyc.
— when rising from lying, Acon. (Verat the reverse).
— with red spots, Sulph.
— during cloudy weather, Aloe.
Paralysis one sided, of face, Caust. Graph.
— upper lip, Cadm. Graph.
— lower jaw, Ars. Dulc. Lach.
Perspiration of face, Alum. Amm-m. Ars. Calc. Carb-veg. Cham. Coff. Fluor-ac. Glon. Igt. Lyc. Merc. Mosch. Nux. Psor. Puls. Rhus. Samb. Sep. Spig. Sulph. Tart. Tellur. Valer. *Verat.*
— on cheek on which one lies, Acon.
— — — does not lie, Thuj.
— — upper lip, Acon. Kali-b.
— about mouth and nose, Rheum.
—on face only, Igt.
— — — during sleep, Prun.
— — and scalp, Puls. Valer. Verat.
— — right cheek, Puls.
— cold Benz-ac. Cact. Cadm. Camph.

8. FACE.

Cina. Dig. Merc-cor. Nux. Ox-ac.
Rheum. Rhus. Ruta. Spong. Sulph.
Verat.
Perspiration, cold face only, Cocc.
— clammy, Cham.
Pewter like color, Zinc.
Pimples on face, Nitr-ac. Nux. Ol-an. Pallad. Psor. Vinca. (compare Eruption.)
— suppurating, Tar. Verat.
— on chin, Clem. Hep. Kali-chl. Merc. Ntr-s. Par. Phosp-ac. Rhus. Sass. Thuj.
— on lips, Bufo. Carb-veg. Kali-chl. Merc. Nux. Phosp-ac.
— — border of upper lip, sore and smarting, Hep.
— — corners of mouth, Petr. Tar.
— about nose, Par. Tar.
— on forehead, small red, Ambr. Clem. Hep. Led. Mur-ac. Ntr-m. Nitr-ac. Par. Phosp. Sep.
— — itching in evening, Mgn-m.
— small painless, Ant. Bar-c. Calc. Carb-veg. Cic. Creos. Graph. Lyc. Merc. Ntr-m. Phosp-ac. Sep. Sulph.
— with sticking, pricking sensation, Dros.
Pinching pain, Verat.
Pointed appearance, Ars. Chin. Nux. Phosp-ac. Rhus. Staph. Verat. (compare Hippocratic face.)
Pressing pain, Bry. Rhus. *Staph.* Tar. *Verb.*
— — in cheek bones. Anac. *Arg.* Bell. Berb. *Bism. Caps.* Hyosc. Kali-chl. Merc. *Mez. Oleand. Plat.* Sabin. Samb. Spig. Stann. Staph. Sulph. Tart. Teucr. Verb. Viol-od.
— — on chin, Asa-f.
— — — lower jaw, Berb. Cupr Spig.
— in orbits, Stann.
— asunder in facial bones, *Colch.*
— — face, Asa-f. Dros.
— — lower jaw, Ambr.
Prickling in face, Caust. Ferr-m. Hep. Nux-m.
— — right malar bone, Ind.
— below eyes, Dros.
— on lips, Ferr-m. Sabad.
Prosopalgia, *Acon.* Agar. Alum. Ambr. Amm-c. Amm-m. *Arn. Ars.* Asa-f. Asar. *Aur.* Bar-c. Bell. Berb. Borax. Bov. Bry. *Calc.* Cannab. *Caps.* Caust. Cham. Chin. Coloc. *Con.* Creos. Dig. Dros. Euph. Euphr. Evon. Ferr-m. Gran. Grat. Guaj. Hep. Hyosc. Kali-c. Kali-jod. Kalm. Lach. Led. Lyc. Mgn-c. Mgn-m. Mang. Merc. Mez. Ntr-s. Nitr-ac. Nux. Ol-an. Pæon. Phosp. Phosp-ac. Plat. Ran-b. Ran-sc. Rhus. Ruta. Sabad. Sabin. Sec-c. Sep. Spig. Spong. *Stann. Staph.* Sulph. Tereb. *Thuj. Verat.* Verb. Viol-od. (compare the different pains.)
— left side, Colch. Spig. Thuj.

— right side, Doryanth. Kalm.
— nervous, *Bell. Caps.* Chin. Mgn-m. Nux. *Verb.*
— neuralgic, from abuse of tobacco, Sep.
— periodical, Spig.
— with cutting pains, Bell. Chin. Clem. Rhus. Staph.
Puffiness of cheek, Arn. Cham. Puls.
Pulsation, Agar. Arn. Bell. Cannab. Caust. Cham. Clem. Creos. Croc. Staph.
— jaws, Plat.
— cheek bones, Mgn-c. Sulph.
Purple colored lips, Ars. Bar-c.
— — net like appearance on chin, Plat.
— — face, Apis. Con. Op. Puls.
Pustules on face, Ant. Arn.
— — scurfy with large red areola. Nitr-ac.
Quivering in face, Agar. Phell.
— — lips, Cast. Lact.
Redness of face, *Acon.* Aeth. Arg. Arn. Ars. Aur. Bar-c. *Bell. Bov. Bry.* Cact. Calc. Canth. *Caps.* Cham. Chelid. Chin. Cic. *Cocc.* Cocc-c. Coff. Creos. Croc. Cupr. Eupat. Euphr. *Ferr.* Ferr-m. Glon. *Grat.* Guaj. *Hep.* Hydroph. *Hyosc.* Igt. Iod. Ip. Kali-c. Lach. Lyc. Mgn-c. Meny. Merc. Mur-ac. Ntr-c. Nicc. Nitr. *Nux. Op.* Ox-ac. Phosp. *Plat.* Psor. Puls. Ran-b. Rhus. *Sabad.* Samb. Scill. Sil. Spig. Spong. Stann. Staph. *Stram.* Stront. Sulph. *Tabac.* Tar. Tart. Thuj. Valer. Verat. Zing.
— of cheeks, Acon. Agar. Alum. Ars. Calc. Cannab. Cham. Chin. Cocc. Coff. Colch. Coloc. Creos. Ferr. Kali-c. Lach. Merc. Mercurial. Mosch. Nitr-ac. Nux. Oleand. Puls. Ran-b. Rhus. Sang. Spig. Spong. Tong. Valer.
— right side, Elaps. Puls.
— and paleness, alternately, Acon. Amm-c. Bell. Borax. Bov. Caps. Cham. Chin. Cina. Croc. Ferr. Kali-c. Hyosc. Igt. Led. Nux. Op. Phosp. Phosp-ac Plat. Puls. Scill. Sulph-ac. Verat.
— one sided, Acon. Arn. Bell. Cham. Coloc. Ip. Nux. Mosch. Rheum. Tart. Verat.
— of right cheek, without heat, paleness of left with heat, Mosch.
— of left cheek, Ntr-m.
— blood red, Stram.
— blue, Ang. Bell. Puls. Staph.
— brown, Bry. Op.
— circumscribed, Acon. Benz-ac. Calc. Chin. Croc. Dulc. Ferr. Iod. Kali-c. Lach. Lyc. Op. Phosp. Puls. Sabad. Samb. Stram. Sulph. Thuj.
— — 1 to 8 A. M. Lachn.
— — during delirium. Lach.
— coppery, Alum.
— dark, *Bar-c.* Bell. Bry. *Camph.* Coloc. Creos. Op. *Sec-c.* Stann. Sulph. *Verat.*
— glowing, Bell. Bry. Cocc. Croc. *Ferr.*

8. FACE.

Hep. Mur-ac. *Plat. Sabad.* Sil. *Stram.* Tabac. Thuj.
Redness after anger, Staph.
— even if skin is cold, Ol-an.
— when lying, pale on rising, Verat. (Acon. reverse).
— of chin, Zinc.
— — lips, Aloe. Arum-trif. Bar-c. Bell. Lac-can. Merc-cor. Spig. Sulph.
— dark of lips, Bell. Gins. Mez.
— around mouth, Ip.
Red points on face, Caps.
— skin around mouth, Ip.
— spots, Alum. Ambr. Bell. Bry. Carb-an. Croc. Ferr. Lyc. Merc. Op. Poth. Samb. Sil. Sulph. Tabac.
— spots on forehead, Sass.
— — burning, Samb. Sil.
— — after meals, Sil.
Relaxation of facial muscles, *Coloc. Op.*
Rending, tearing pains, Alum. *Agar.* Amm-c. Amm-m. Arg. Bell. Berb. Borax. Bry. Carb-veg. *Colch.* Coloc. Con. Evon. Grat. Hep. Kali-jod. Led. Lyc. Merc. *Ntr-s.* Nitr-ac. Phosp. Plb. Staph. Sulph. Tong. Viol-od.
— in cheek bones, *Aeth.* Agar. Alum. *Amm-m. Arg.* Berb. Borax. Calc. Carb-veg. Cina. Graph. Ind. Kali-c Lyc. *Mgn-c.* Mgn-s. Merc. Mur-ac. *Ntr-s.* Nitr-ac. Nitr. Nux. *Phosp.* Ruta. Sep. Spig. Staph. Stront. Sulph-ac. Tabac. Teucr. Zinc.
— — chin, Agar.
— — front of jaw, Bov.
— — jaw, *Agar.* Bell. Berb. Merc. Plb. *Rat.* Tong.
— — — lower, Bov. Ind. Kalm. Puls. Viol-od.
— — upper lip, Caust.
— between nose and eye, Mang.
Rheumatic pain, *Acon.*
Risus sardonicus, Bell. Ran-sc. Sol-n.
Rough spots on forehead, Pallad. Rhus. Sass. Sep. Sulph.
Roughness of skin of face, Alum. Rhus. Sep. Sulph.
— — every summer, Kalm.
— lips, Merc. Sulph. Tabac.
— sense of, Mgn-m.
— about mouth, Anac. Ars.
— red, Sep. Sulph.
Sad expression, Ant. Colch. Cupr.
Scabs, scurfs on face, Alum. Ant. Ars. Calc. Cic. Coloc Dulc. Graph. Hep. Lach. Lyc. Merc. Mez. Mur-ac. Nitr-ac. Petr. Rhus. Sass. Sep. Sil. Sulph. Thuj. Verat. Viol-tr.
— on cheeks, Bell. Cic. Creos. Lach.
— — chin, Dulc. Cic. Creos. *Graph.* Merc. Sep.
— — forehead and temples, Dulc. *Mur-ac.*
— — lips, Bell. Berb. Borax. Calc. Cham.

Cic. Igt. Merc. Mur-ac. Ntr-m. Nux. Petr. Phosp. Phosp-ac. Scill. *Sep.* Sil. Staph. Sulph.
— about mouth, Calc. *Graph.*
— in corners of mouth, Igt. Petr.
— in whiskers, Calc. Lach.
Shining face, Aur. Ntr-m. Plb. Rheum.
— lips, Amm-m.
Shocks, blows in zygoma, Hep.
Sickly color, Amm-c. Borax. Chin. *Cina.* Clem. Con. Kali-c. Lachn. Mgn-c. *Mang.* Ntr-s. Nitr. *Nux.* Phosp-ac. Psor. Sil. Rhus. *Sulph.* Teucr.
— — about eyes, *Cina.*
Silly expression, Stram.
Slimy lips, Kali-jod. Stram. Zinc.
— — in morning, Kali-jod.
Smarting as if caused by salt, Cannab.
Soreness of lips, Arum-trif. Canth. Caust. Cham. Cupr. Graph. Kobalt. Lac-can. Lyc. Mez. Ntr-m.
— — corners of mouth, Ant. Caust. Eupat. Hell. Lyc. Mez.
— sensation of in face, Con. Graph. Puls.
— — on jaw, right side, around ear, could not open the mouth, Psor.
— — — lips, Igt. Ip. Phosp-ac. Plat. Sabad.
— — — inner surface, lower lip, Igt.
— — — upper, Kali-c. Mez. Scill. Sil.
— — chin, Aur. Plat.
— — about mouth, Puls.
— — right corner of mouth, Pallad.
— in corner of mouth, Sulph-ac.
Spasm, cramp, of face, Nitr-ac. Ol-an. Rhus.
— cheek bones, *Ang.* Cina. Cocc. Dig. Hyosc. Mgn-m. Mez. Ruta. Sep. Val.
— left, Ol-an. *Plat.*
— lips, *Ambr.* Caust. Kali-c. Ran-b.
— masseters, Ang. Cocc. Cupr. Mang.
— maxilla, Agar. Asa-f. Coloc. Kali-c. Mang. Ran-b.
— maxillary joint, Colch. Kali-c. Nicc. Ol-an. Rhus. Sil. Spong. Stann.
Spider-web, sensation of, on face, Bar-c. Borax. Graph. Ran-sc.
Spotted skin of face, Sabad.
Stiffness of cheeks when speaking and chewing, Euphr.
— — face sense of, Sang.
— — masseters, Sass.
— — jaws, Bell. Caust. Cocc. Daph. Euphr. Gels. Glon. Graph. Hydroph. Hyosc. Merc. Ntr-s. Nux. Petr. Rhus. Sass. Sep. Therid. Thuj.
— in morning in bed, Therid.
— of lips, Kalm.
— — upper, as if made of wood, Euphr.
Stinging, stitches, pain, Amm-c. Ars. Asar. Bell. Cham. Coloc. Con. Euphr. Fluor-ac. Graph. Guaj. Hœmatox. Kali-chl. Mang. Merc-jod. Nitr-ac. Puls. Rhus. Sep. Spong. Stann.

8. FACE.

Stinging, stitches, cheek bones, Aeth. Alum. Ars. Berb. Carb-an. Evon. Guaj. Merc. Par. Phosp. Psor. Sabin. Sil. Staph. Verb.
— — — left, Kali-jod. Merc-jod.
— — — right, Guaj.
— hot, in left malar bone, Par.
— chin, Agar. Euphr. Lact.
— lips, Asa-f. Bell. Hipp-m. Sabad.
— jaw, Acon. Berb. Carb-an.
— — lower, Euphr. Kali-chl. Kalm. Lact. Mang. Sabin. Sil. Thuj.
— maxillary joint, Bell. Hep. Tabac.
Stunning pain, *Mez. Plat. Verb.*
Stupid expression, Stram.
Suffering expression, Cham. Plat.
Sunken face, Aeth. Apis. Arg-n. *Arn. Ars.* Bell. Berb. Canth. *Chin.* Corn-c. Cupr. Dros. *Ferr.* Ferr-m. Gels. Hydroc-ac. Laur. *Lyc.* Mang. Oleand. Ol-an. *Op. Phosp.* Phosp-ac. Plat. Scill. Sec-c. *Stann. Staph. Tart.* Tereb. *Verat.*
— — pale, Bell. Lyc. Mang. Nux. Verat.
— — — with distorted countenence, Ars. Bell. Cham. Hydroc-ac. Igt. Lach.
— — — — and anxious, Ars. Bell. Cham. Laur. Stram.
— eyes, Anac. Ars. Berb. Camph. Cic. Colch. Coloc. Cupr. Cycl. Dros. Ferr. Iod. Kali-c. Lach. Lyc. Nitr-ac. Nux. Op. Ox-ac. *Phosp.* Phosp-ac. Puls. *Sec-c.* Spong. Stann. *Staph.* Sulph. Verat.
Suppuration, pain like in malar bone, Ntr-m.
Swelling of face, *Ars.* Arum-trif. *Bar-c.* Bell. Borax. Bov. Bry. Calc. Canth. Carb-veg. Cic. Cinnab. Coloc. Graph. Guaj. Gymnoc. *Hep.* Hipp-m. Hydroc-ac. Hyosc. Kali-c. Kali-jod. Lach. Lachn. Lyc. Mgn-c. *Merc.* Ntr-m. Nux. Op. Rhus. Sacch. Sec-c. *Stram.* Verat.
— — upper half, Bry.
— — left side, Arg-n.
— — after pains in face, Calc.
— cheeks, Amm-c. Apis. *Arn.* Ars. *Aur.* Bell. Bov. Bry. Carb-veg. Caust. *Cham.* Dig. Euph. *Kali-c. Kali-jod.* Merc. Merc-cor. Ntr-c. Nitr-ac. Nux. Puls. Sep. *Spong.* Stann. Staph. Sulph.
— of one cheek, with face-ache and pain bones, Nux.
— — right cheek, extending to right side of nose, Elaps.
— — cheek-bones, Mgn-c.
— — chin, Caust.
— above the eyes, Lyc.
— between eyes and brows, Kali-c.
— under the eyes, Ars. Bry. Merc. Nux. Oleand.
— lips, Alum. Arn. Arum-trif. Ars. Asa-f. Aur. *Bell.* Bry. Calc. Canth. Caps. Carb-an. Carb-veg. Chin. Dig. Hell. Hep. Kali-c. Kali-chl. Kalm. Lach. Lachn. Lyc. Merc. Merc-cor. Mez. Ntr-

c. Nitr-ac. Op. Puls. Rhus. Sep. Sil. Staph. *Sulph.* Thuj.
— — upper lips, Apis. Arg. Bar-c. Bell. Bov. Calc. Canth. Grat. Kali-c. Lyc. Merc-cor. Ntr-c. *Ntr-m.* Phosp. Rhus. Staph. Sulph. Vinca.
— — lower lip, Alum. Asa-f. Calc. Caust. Lyc. Mez. Mur-ac. Ntr-m. Puls. Sep. Sil.
— of lymphatics, Lact.
— — maxilla, upper, Alum. Stann.
— — — lower, Acon. Calc. Caust. Kali-c. Merc. Phosp.
— about mouth, Carb-an. Nux.
— — — corner of, Oleand. Vinca.
— around nose, Nux.
— root of nose, Bry.
— above nasal bone, red, making a saddle painful to touch, Poth.
— one-sided, Arn. *Ars.* Bell. Bry. Canth. *Cham. Merc.* Nux. Plb. Puls. Sep. Staph.
— right side, *Merc.*
— — — with sore throat, Nicc.
— temples, Cham.
— bulbous, Alum.
— dropsical, Apis. Colch. Euph. Hell. Merc-cor. Sacch. Thuj.
— elastic, Ars.
— erysipelatous, Acon. Bell. Euph. Graph. Hep. Lach. Rhus. Sulph.
— hard, hot and shining, Amm-c. *Arn.* Ars. Bell.
— painful, Bell. Borax.
— pale, *Bov.* Euph. Hell. Nux. Sep. Sulph.
— red, *Arn.* Ars. Bell. Borax. Cic. Coloc. Euph. *Kali-c.* Lach. Merc. Ntr-c. Nux. Oleand. Rhus. Sulph.
— shining, Arn. Spig.
— with syncope, Ars.
— — vertigo, Ars.
— of temporal arteries, Chin. Ferr. Thuj.
— — veins, Sang. Thuj.
— sense of, in face, Aeth. Alum. Bar-c. Daph. Grat. Gynmoc. Nicc. Nux-m. Puls. Sulph-ac.
— — cheeks, Acon. Samb.
— — — lips, Lact.
— — — upper, Glon.
— — — jaw, Daph.
— — when entering room from open air, Aeth.
Tenderness of skin of face, Puls.
Tension in skin of face, Alum. *Bar-c.* Graph. Grat. Hep. Hyper. Kali-c. Lach. Lyc. Mgn-c. Merc. Mercurial. Mosch. Nitr. Phell. *Phosp. Phosp-ac.* Puls. Rheum. Rhus. Samb. Viol-od. Viol-tr.
— forehead, Viol-tr.
— around mouth and nose, Nux.
— on chin, Verb.
— below the eyes, Nux. Viol-od.
— semi-lateral, Phosp.
— as if muscles were drawn to one side, Cist.
— with desire to sneeze, Kali-chl.

8. FACE.

Terror, expression of, Canth.
Thick skin of face, Bell. Viol-tr.
— spots, Carb-an.
Throbbing pain, *Arn.* Staph.
— — in cheek bones, Mgn-c.
Tickling about cheek, bone and nose, Bell.
Tightening, tensive pain, Amm-c. Asa-f. Coloc. Kali-chl. Lach. Mgn-m. *Ol-an.* Verat. *Verb.*
— cheek bones, Caust. *Chelid.* Kali-chl. *Plat. Verb.*
— lips, Sep. Spig.
— masseters, *Sass.* Verb.
— maxilla, *Aur.* Caust.
— maxillary joint, Amm-m. Bell. Daph. Sass. Verb.
Timid expression, Stram.
Tingling, Acon. Alum. Ambr. Bell. Cannab. *Colch.* Grat. Lach. Lachn. Lact. Laur. Nux. Ol-an. Pæon. Plat. Ran-b. Rhus. Sabad. Sec-c.
— cheeks and lips, Agn. *Arn.* Ars. Berb.
— right cheek, Elaps. Gymnoc.
— left cheek, Evon.
— chin and nose, Ran-b. Verat.
— lips, Ntr-m.
— upper lip, Pæon.
— forehead, and whiskers, Ambr.
Tremor of facial muscles, *Ambr. Op.*
— — lips, Aloe. Lach. Lact. Ran-sc. Stram- Sulph.
— under lip, Con. Sulph.
Trismus, Ang. Arn. Bell. Bry. Calc. Camph. Canth. Caust. Cham. Cic. Con. Gels. Hydroc-ac. Hyosc. Igt. Lach. Laur. Merc. Nux. Op. Phosp. Plat. Plb. Rhus. Sec-c. Sil. Stram. Sulph. Verat.
— with widely open lips, Ang.
— — teeth tight together, Cic.
Twitching in facial muscles, Agar. *Ambr.* Arn. Ars. Bar-c. Bell. Cannab. *Cham.* Graph. Hell. Hyosc. *Igt.* Iod.*Ip.* Kali-c. Lach. Lyc. Meny. Merc. Mez. Nitr-ac. Nitr. Nux. *Op.* Phosp. Puls. Ran-sc. Selen. Stront. Sulph. Tart. Thuj. Valer. Verat.
— — left side, Puls.
— — morning in bed, Nux.
— — right cheek, Agar.
— above eyes, Mez.
— in lips, Carb-veg. *Cham.* Ip. Lact. Sulph. *Thuj.*
— — — lower, Hipp.
— — — upper, Nicc.
— — — in morning in sleep, Ol-an.
— — — in cold air, Dulc.
— — corners of mouth, Borax. *Igt.* Oleand. *Op.* Rheum.
Turburcles on face, Alum. Mgn-n.
Typical, periodical, pains in face, Spig.
Ulcers in face, Ars. Con. Iod. Psor.
— on left cheek, Iod. Ntr-m.

— — chin, Merc. Ntr-m.
— — lips, Amm-m. Ars. Bell. Caps. Cham. Chin. *Cic.* Con. *Graph.* Hep. Kali-b. Kali-c. Lyc. *Merc.* Mez.Ntr-c. Ntr-m. *Nitr-ac.* Nux. Phosp-ac. Psor. Sep. *Sil. Staph.* Sulph. Zinc.
— — border of lower lip, Lyc.
— about mouth. Ntr-c. Nitr-ac.
— — corners of mouth, Amm-m. Ant. Bell. *Bov.* Calc. Carb-veg. Graph. Hep. Igt. Ip. *Mang.* Merc. Mez. Ntr-m. Nitr-ac. Nux, *Phosp.* Psor. Sil. Thuj. Zinc.
— burning and stinging, Nux.
— with hard edges, smarting, on mucus surface of lips, Kali-b.
— eating, Con. Nux.
— putrid smelling, Merc.
Ulcerous pain, Acon.
Veins distended in face, Ferr. Op.
— — nets as if marble, Calc. Carb-veg. Lyc. Thuj.
— — red, Lach.
Vesicles, Ant. Cist. Clem. *Euph.* Graph. Hep. Lach. Ol-an. Rhus. Sulph. Valer.
— on chin, Hep. Sass.
— — lips, Carb-an. Clem. Con. Hell. Hep. Merc. Mgn-m. Ntr-c. Ntr-m. Plat. Rhod.
— — — lower, Ntr-s. Par.
— — — upper, Rat. Seneg. Valer.
— — — sanguineous, Ntr-m.
— — white, Hell.
— — corners of mouth, *Seneg.* Senna.
— — forehead, Seneg.
— white as if sunburned, Clem.
— full of yellowish humor, Euph.
— — — — followed by desquamation, Hipp-m.
Wandering expression, Plb. Stram. Zinc.
Warmth, sense of, Asar.
Warts on face, Caust. Dulc. Kali-c. Sep.
Waxy look, Sil.
White of egg, sensation of, *Alum.* Mgn-c. Phosp-ac. Sulph-ac.
Wretched expression, Mez.
Wrinkles in forehead, Hell. Rheum. (compare Scalp).
— — face, Calc. Hell. Lyc. Stram.
— — lips, Amm-c.
Yellow color, Acon. *Ambr.* Arn. *Ars.* Bell. Bry. Calc. *Canth.* Carb-an. *Caust.*Cham. Chenop. Chin. *Con.* Corn-c. Croc. Crotal. Dig. Ferr. Gels. *Graph.* Hell. Hep. Hipp-m. *Iod.* Ip. Kali-b. *Kali-c.* Lach. Lachn. Laur. *Lyc. Mgn-m. Merc.* Merc-cor. Ntr-c. Ntr-m. Nitr-ac.*Nux.*Op. Petr. Phosp. *Plb. Puls.* Rhus. *Sec-c.* Sep. Spig. Sulph. Verat.
— about eyes, Nitr-ac. Nux. Spig.
— — mouth, Agar. Ars. Gina. Mgn-m. Sep.
— — — and nose, Nux. Sep.

Yellow across above nose and cheeks, Sep.
— on temples, Caust.
— trace on lips, Stram.
— color brownish, Iod.
— granulations on skin, Ant.
— grayish, Carb-veg. Chin. Laur.
— greenish, Carb-veg.
— in intermittents, Amm-c. *Con.* Ferr. Ntr-c. Ntr-m.
— spots on face, Ambr. Colch. Ferr.
— — on cheek and nose, Sep.
— — forehead and upper lip, Ntr-c.
— — upper lip, Sulph.
— streaks on upper lip, Stram.
In evening, pain in face, Caps. Phosp. Plat.
— — — lips, Mgn-s.
At night, pain, Con. Led. Mgn-c. Sil.
— — relieved, Ang.
— — lower jaw, Sil.
— — in lying, Phosp.
— — when at rest, intolerable, *Mgn-c.*
— — with toothache, succeeded by shuddering and sleep, Led.
When biting the teeth together, pain, Ntr-m. Verb.
— — — — — in maxillary joint, Cor-r.
From a cold, pain, Phosp.
— cold temperature, Agar. Colch.
When laughing, pain, Borax. Mang. Tabac.
— — in maxillary joint, Tabac.
— masticating, pain, Alum. Ang. Phosp. Plat. Verb.

— — — in maxillary joint, Amm-m. Cor-r.
After meals pain in jaw, Mang.
When moving the jaws, pain, Alum. Amm-c. Borax. Cor-r. Mang. Ntr-m. Phosp. Spig. Verb.
— — — — relieved, Ang.
— opening mouth, pain, Phosp.
— — — in maxillary joint, Amm-c. Cor-r. Hep. Nicc.
— shutting mouth, pain in maxillary joint, Bar-c.
— sleeping, pain, Caps.
— speaking, pain, Phosp.
By pressure, pain increased, Cina. Dros. Verb.
— — relieved, Bry.
When at rest, pain, Ang. Mgn-c.
By rubbing, pain relieved or altered, Plb.
When touched, pain. Caps. Chin. Cina. Cor-r. Cupr. Dig. Dros. *Hep.* Phosp. Puls. Spig.
— — in lips, Bry. *Hep.* Merc. Mez.
— — relieved, Thuj.
From warmth of bed, faceache worse, Glon.
After washing, a rasping pain in face, Con.
Desire to wash the face in cold water, Fluor-ac.
During bad weather, pain, Bell.
With anguish at heart, Spig.
— tears, Phosp-ac.
— vomiting, Lach.

9. Teeth and Gums.

Aching, Ars. Bism. Borax. Chin. Euph. Guaj. Iod. Ntr-m. Nux-m. Oleand. Staph. Tar. Verat.
— in sound teeth, Arn. Bry. Hyosc. Rhus. Sulph.
— — left side, Brom.
To arms and fingers, pain extending, Sep.
Arthritic toothache, Cycl. Nux. Rhus. Staph.
Black covered teeth, Chin. Merc.
— — gums, Merc.
—, teeth turn, Merc. Plb. Scill. Staph.
Bleeding of gums, Agar. Alum. Ambr. Amm-c. Anac. Ant. Arg. Arg-n. Ars. Arum. Aur. Bar-c. Bell. Berb. Borax. *Bov.* Calc. Carb-an. *Carb-veg.* Caust. Cist. Con. Croton. Creos. Euphr. Ferr-m. Graph. Hep. Iod. Kali-chl. Lyc. Mgn-c. *Mgn-m.* Merc. Merc-cor. Ntr-m. Nitr. Nitr-ac. Nux-m. *Nux. Phosp.*

Phosp-ac. Ran-sc. Rat. Ruta. *Sep.* Sil. *Staph. Sulph.* Sulph-ac. Tereb. Tong. Zinc.
— when cleaning them, Kali-chl.
—, blood coagulates quickly, Creos.
— teeth, Ambr. Ant. Bar-c. Carb-veg. Croton. Phosp. Rat. Sulph. Tar. Tong. Zinc.
— at night, Bov.
— when pressed upon, Ferr-m. Merc.
— — sucking them, Bell. Bov. Rat.
Blood, which comes out of teeth black, Graph.
— — — — — sour, Graph. Rat. Tar. Tong.
Blows on teeth, sensation of, Tar.
Bluish gums, Oleand. Sabad.
— red, Con.
Boils on gums, Arn. Kali-jod. Lyc. Ntr-s. Nux-jug. Phosp-ac. Plb. *Staph.*

9. TEETH AND GUMS.

Boring toothache, Alum. Bell. Bov. Calc. Con. Cycl. Grat. Kali-c. *Lach*. Mgn-c. Mez. Ntr-c. Ntr-m. Nux. Phosp. Selen. Sil. Sulph.
Breaking off of teeth, Plb.
Broken, pain as if, in teeth, Ntr-m.
Bruised, pain as if, in teeth, Igt.
— as if, between gums and teeth, Hyosc.
Burning in teeth, Bar-c. Dulc. Mgn-c. Mez. Nux. Phosp-ac. Sulph.
— — gums, Bell. Cham. *Merc*. Mur-ac. Ntr-s. Nux. Petr. Puls. Rhus. Sep. Stront. Tereb.
Caries of teeth, Amm-c. Calc. Carb-an. Creos. Euph. Merc. Mez. Phosp. Plb. Sabad. *Sep*. Sil. Staph.
— — roots, Mez. Thuj.
To cheek bone, pain extending, Chenop.
In children, toothache, Calc. Cham. Igt. Rheum.
As from cold air blowing on teeth, sensation, Cocc-c.
Coldness, sense of in teeth, Asar. Diad. Grat. Ol-an. Rat. Rheum.
— at points of incisors, Gum-gut.
— daily, Diad.
As from congestion of blood, toothache, Calc.
Contracting pain, Carb-veg.
Corrosive pains, Cacl. Carb-veg. Cham. Con. Kali-c. Nicc. Phosp. Puls. Staph. Sulph-ac. Thuj.
Cracking of teeth when rubbing them, Selen.
Cracks in gums, *Plat*.
Crawling in teeth, Mur-ac. Rhus.
— — gums, Arn.
Crumbling teeth, Borax. Creos. *Euph*. Lach. Plb. Staph. Thuj.
Crushed pain as if, in molars, Igt.
Cutting pain in gums, Par.
— — teeth, Graph. Oleand. Ran-b.
— — roots, Camph.
Decayed, hollow, teeth, pain in, Acon. Aloe. Alum. *Ambr*. Amm-c. Ang. *Ant*. Bar-c. Borax. Bov. Bry Cham. *Chin*. Cocc. Coff. Con. Creos. Fluor-ac. Hep. Ip. *Lach*. Meph. *Merc*. *Mez*. Ntr-m. Ntr-s. Nitr-ac. Nitr. Nux. Ox-ac. Par. Phosp-ac. Plb. Puls. Rheum. Sang. Sil. Spig. *Staph*. Sulph. Tabac. Tar. Thuj.
Decay of teeth suddenly, Mez.
— — — as soon as they appear, Creos.
— — molars, Clem.
— — lower molars, right side, Aloe.
Dentition difficult in children, *Calc. Cham.* Cic. Creos. Cupr. Hyosc. *Igt. Rheum*. Sil.
Digging pain, Ant. Borax. Bov. Calc. Cham. Kali-c. Ntr-c. Nux. Plat. Puls. Rat. Rheum. Ruta. Seneg. Sil. Sulph-ac.
Dirty, livid color of gums, Merc.

Drawing pains in gums, Ars. Caps. Nux. Staph. Tabac.
— — teeth, *Ambr*. *Amm-c*. Anac. Ang. Bar-c. Bell. Bism. *Bov*. *Bry*. *Calc*. Canth. Caps. Carb-an. *Carb-veg*. Caust. Cham. Chin. *Clem Cocc-c*. *Con*. Creos. *Cycl*. Daph. Graph. Guaj. Hep. Iod. Kali-c. Lach. Lyc. Mgn-c. Meph. Mez. Ntr-s. Ntr-m. Nitr-ac. Nitr. Nux. Ol-an. Oleand. Par. Phosp. Phosp-ac. Plat. *Puls*. Ran-b. *Ran-sc. Rhod.* Sabad. Sabin. Sass. *Sep*. Sil. *Staph*. *Sulph*. Tabac. Tar. Tereb. Thuj. Verat. Zinc.
— — nerves, Coloc. Puls.
— — roots, Staph.
Dulness of teeth, as if set on edge, Amm-c. Ars. Aur. Berb. Caps. Ferr-m. Kali-chl. Lach. Lyc. Merc. Mez. Ntr-m. Nitr-ac. *Nux-m*. Phosp. Phosp-ac. Sep. Sil. Spong. Sulph. *Sulph-ac. Tar.* Tart-ac.
— as if covered with lime, Nux-m.
— on left side, Cor-r.
— with sour vomiting, Sacch.
From the ear, toothache originating, Ol-an.
To the ear, extending, Alum. Amm-c. Anac. Ars. Bell. Borax. Bry. Caust. Cham. Chenop. Chin. Creos. Ind. Lach. Mgn-c. *Merc*. Meph. Mez. Ntr-m. Nicc. Nux-m. Nux. Ol-an. Puls. Rat. Rhus. Sep. Staph. Sulph. Viol-od.
— right ear, Nicc.
Elongation of teeth, Arn. Caust. Sulph.
— sensation of, Arn. Ars. Bell. Berb. Bry. Calc. Camph. Caps. Caust. Clem. Creos. Hyosc. Kali-jod. Lach. Lachn. Mgn-c. Mgn-m. Merc. Merc-cor. Mez. Ntr-m. Ntr-s. Nicc. Nitr-ac. Phyt. Rat. Stann. Sulph.
— — in hollow teeth, Hep.
— — gums, Nitr-ac.
Excrescences on gums, Staph.
Exfoliation of teeth, Lach. Staph.
To eyes extending, toothache, Bell. Cham. Creos. Lach. Merc. Ntr-m. Nicc. Puls. Tar.
— face extending, toothache, Alum. Amm-c. Hyosc. Merc. *Mez*. Nux. Puls. Rhus. Sulph.
Falling out of teeth, *Merc*. Nux. Plb. *Sec-c*.
— — — — sensation as of, Stram.
In females, toothache, Bell. Cham. Mgn-c. Mgn-m. Puls.
Fistula of gums, Calc. Canth. Caust. Fluor-ac. Lyc. Mgn-c. Ntr-m. Nitr-ac. Petr. Sil. Staph. Sulph.
— — upper incisors, Canth.
— near right eye tooth, Fluor-ac.
Gnawing toothache, Berb. Calc. Carb-veg. Con. Nicc. Phosp. Rhus. Staph. Sulph-ac. *Thuj*.
Grinding of teeth, Acon. Ant. Apis. Arn.

9. TEETH AND GUMS.

Ars. Aur. Bar-c. Canth. Caust. Cham. Cic. Cina. Coff. Con. *Hyosc.* Igt. Lyc. Merc. Phosp. Plb. Pod. Sec-c. *Stram.* *Verat.*
Grinding of teeh when sleeping, Ars.
— — — — in a sitting posture, Ant.
Into head extending, toothache, Ant. Ars. Bar-c. Borax. Cham. Clem. Cupr. Mgn-c. Merc. Mez. Nux-m. Nux. Puls. Rhus. Sulph.
Heaviness, sense of, in teeth, Fluor-ac. Verat.
Hollowness of teeth, *Creos.* Mez. Phosp. Plb. Sabad. *Sep. Staph.*
Jerking toothache, *Amm-c.* Anac. Ant. Bell. *Bry. Calc.* Cast. Cham. *Chin. Clem. Cocc-c.* Coff. Con. Creos. Kali-c. Mgn-c. Mgn-s. Merc. Mez. Nitr-ac. Nux. Phosp. Plb. *Puls. Ran-sc. Rat. Rhus.* Sil. Spig. Stann. Stront. Sulph.
Inflammation of gums, Amm-c. Creos. Hep. Iod. Kali-c. Ntr-m. Nitr. *Nux.* Sil.
— — —, left upper side, Creos.
Infuriating toothache, Ars.
Itching in teeth, Spong.
— — gums, Bell. Merc. Rhod.
Knocking pain, Ars. Carb-an. Kali-c.
Lascinating, (compare Rending, tearing.)
Looseness of teeth, *Amm-c.* Arn. Ars. Aur. Bar-c. Bry. Calc. Camph. Carb-an. *Carb-veg.* Caust. Cham. Chelid. Chin. Cocc. Hep. Hyosc. Igt. Kali-c. Lach. Lyc. Mgn-c. Mgn-s. *Merc.* Merc-cor. Ntr-s. *Nitr-ac.* Nux-m. *Nux.* Op. Phosp. Plb. Psor. Puls. Rhod. Rhus. Sang. *Sec-c.* Sep. Spong. Stann. Staph. Sulph. Verat. Zinc.
— — — painful, Puls.
— — —, sensation, Bry. Hyosc. Lachn. Merc. Nicc. Nux-m. Oleand. Spong. Sulph.
Mucus on teeth, Hyosc. Iod. Mgn-c. Plb. Selen. Sulph.
— — — in morning, Iod.
— — — black, Chin.
— — — brown, Sulph.
— — — yellow, Iod. Plb.
— — — offensive, Mez.
Nerves as if extended, Coloc. Puls.
— — — — and let suddenly loose, Puls.
Nodosities on gums, Berb. Ntr-s. Phosp-ac. Plb. Staph.
Notching of teeth, Lach. Plb.
Numbness, sensation of, *Chin.* Ntr-m. Petr.
To the œsophagus, pain extending, Ntr-m.
Pain in paroxysms, first in upper front teeth to all the bones of face and eye worse from taking cold water in the mouth, Rumex.
— right side of face from root of tooth which had been sawn off extending to temples, next day same pain in left side from throat to left ear, causing earache, Lith.
Painfulness of gums, Agar. Ambr. Calc. Caust. Dolich. Hep. Phosp. Ruta. Staph.
— — — in spots, Ox-ac.
Pale gums, Nitr-ac. Nux. Phosp. Plb. Staph.
Periodical pain, Ars. Diad.
In pregnant women, toothache, Alum. Bell. Bry. Calc. Cham. Hyosc. *Mgn-c.* Merc. Nux-m. Puls. Rhus. *Sep.* Staph.
Pressing in teeth, Bism. Bov. Chin. Euph. Guaj. Iod. Ntr-c. Nux-m. Oleand. Staph. Tar. Verat.
— — roots, Staph.
— — gums, Ars. Staph.
Pressing asunder, expansive toothache, Kalm. Mur-ac. Ran-b. *Sabin.* Spig. Thuj.
Pricking toothache, Ant. Bar-m. Hell. Mgn-s. Nux-m. Phosp. Prun.
— in gums, Puls.
As if teeth were being pulled out, toothache,* Berb. Cocc. Cocc-c. Ip. Prun. Stront.
Pulsations in gums, Calc.
— — teeth, Bar-m. Cocc-c. Hyosc. Mgn-c. Merc. *Ntr-s.* Puls.
Purple colored thin border on gums nearest teeth, Plb.
Pustules on gums, Carb-an. Ntr-s. Petr.
Putrid gums, Amm-c. Cist. *Ntr-m.* Nux. (compare Scorbutic).
Rapid, quick pain, Lact.
Rasping pain, Mang.
Redness of gums, Aur. Berb. Carb-an. Cham. Creos. Iod. Merc. Ntr-s. Nux. Phell. Ran-sc.
— —, dirty, Berb.
— —, pale, Bar-c. Kali-chl.
Rending, tearing, in teeth, *Agar.* Alum. Ambr. *Amm-c.* Amm-m. Anac. Ang. Arn. Ars. Bar-m. Bell. Berb. Bruc. Bry. *Carb-veg.* Cast. Caust. Cham. Chenop: Chin. *Cocc-c.* Coff. *Colch.* Cupr. Daph. Graph. Grat. Hell. *Hyosc.* Hyper. Iod. Kali-c. Lach. Lyc. Mgn-c. Mang. *Merc.* Meph. Ntr-m. Ntr-s. *Nitr. Nux-m. Nux.* Oleand. Ol-an. Phell. *Phosp.* Phosp-ac. Plb. *Puls.* Ran-b. *Rat. Rhod. Rhus. Samb.* Sass. Sep. *Sil.* Spig. *Staph. Sulph.* Sulph-ac. Tabac. *Tong.* Verb. Viol-od. Zinc.
— on left side, Bel. Iod. Samb. Sulph. Sulph-ac.
— in molars, Amm-c.
— — — —, lower, Agar.
— — roots, Camph. Lach. Meph. *Merc.* Ol-an. Staph. Stront. *Teucr.*
— — gums, Ars. Bruc. Chin-sulph. Colch. Hyosc. Lyc. Sass. Staph. Teucr.
Rheumatic toothache, Nux. Staph.

9. TEETH AND GUMS.

Roots of teeth, pain in, Amm-c.
Scabs, gangrenous, on gums, Chin. Sulph.
Scorbutic gums, Amm-c. Amm-m. Cist. *Creos. Mur-ac.* Nitr. Sacch.
Screwing toothache, Euph.
Semi-lateral pains, Cham. Coloc. Nux. Puls.
Sensitiveness, (compare Tenderness.)
Separation of gums, Ant. Arg. Arg-n. Carb-veg. Cist. Dulc. Iod. Merc. Phosp. Phosp-ac. Sulph. Tereb.
Shocks, jerks, Anac. *Bar-c.* Cham. *Cocc-c.* *Lyc.* Meph. Merc. Nux-m. Plat. Sep. Sulph.
— in gums, Lyc.
Shooting, (compare Rending).
Sounds, painful reverberation of in teeth, Therid.
Shrivelled gums, Carb-veg. Merc. Par.
Softening of gums, Arg. *Iod.* Phosp-ac. *Tereb.*
Soreness of gums, Carb-an. Carb-veg. Dig. Nitr-ac. Sep. Sil.
—, sensation of, in teeth, Calc. Caust. Cina. Croton. Graph. Nux. Psor. Rhod. Rhus. *Zinc.*
— —, in gums, Alum. Bism. Bry. Carb-veg. Graph. *Merc.* Ntr-m. Puls. Rhus. Ruta. Sass. Tereb. Thuj. *Zinc.*
— — between gums, and cheek, Rhod.
Spasmodic pains, Anac. Borax. Lyc. *Nux-m.* *Plat.*
Splintered, pain as if teeth were, Sabin.
Spongy gums, Bry. Creos. Dulc. Merc.
Stinging stitches in gums, Amm-m. Ars. Bell. Calc. Kali-c. Kali-jod. Lyc. Petr. *Puls.* Sabad. Sep. Staph.
— — teeth, Acon. Ambr. *Amm-c.* Bar-c. Bell. Borax. Bry. *Calc. Caust.* Cham. Chin. *Clem.* Colch. Con. Cycl. Dros. *Euph.* Euphr. Gles. *Graph.* Guaj. Hœmatox. Hell. *Kali-c.* Kali-chl. Lach. Laur. Mgn-c. *Merc. Mez.* Ntr-c. Nitr-ac. *Nitr.* Nux-m. Nux. Phell. *Phosp.* Psor. Puls. *Ran-sc.* Raph. Rhus. *Sabad.* Sabin. *Samb.* Scill. *Sep. Sil.* Spong. *Sulph.* Tabac. Valer. Zinc.
— — lower teeth, Euphr.
Suppuration of gums, Amm-c. Canth. Carb-veg. Caust.
Suppurating pustules on gums, *Carb-an.* Ntr-s. Petr.
Swelling of gums, Agar. Alum. Ambr. *Amm-c.* Amm-m. Anac. Arg-n. Ars. Aur. *Bar-c.* Bell. Bism. *Borax.* Calc. Caps. Carb-an. Caust. Cham. Chin. Cist. Cocc. Cocc-c. Con. Croton. Dolich. *Graph.* Hep. Iod. Kali-c. Kali-jod. Lac-can. Lach. Lyc. Mgn-c. Mgn-m. *Merc.* Merc-cor. Mur-ac. Nicc. Nitr-ac. *Nitr.* Nux-jug. *Nux.* Petr. Phell. *Phosp.* Phosp-ac.

Plb. Rhod. Sass. Sep. Spong. Staph. Stront. *Sulph.* Sulph-ac. Thuj. Zinc.
— under gums, Rhod.
— around a decayed tooth, Sabin.
— painful, Carb-an. Croton. Kali-c. Kali-jod. Mgn-m. Nux. Phell. Ran-sc. Rhod. Sabin. Sass. Sil. Staph. *Sulph.* Thuj. Zinc.
— — when chewing, Spong.
— — to touch, Hep. Stront.
— sensation of, Puls.
— over upper incisors, with swelling of upper lip, Lyc.
—, convulsions from, over teeth which are not quite through, Creos. Stann.
— pale red, Bar-c.
— white, Nux. Sabin.
— at night, Cast. Merc.
— with headache, Cast.
— — toothache, Bar-c. Borax. Ntr-c.
Taste, acrid, foul, from roots of teeth, Fluor-ac.
Tenderness of gums, Agar. Ambr. Brom. Calc. Caust. Lach. Ntr-m. Nux. Phosp. Ruta. Staph.
— — to cold and warmth, Ntr-m.
— — teeth, Ferr-m. Gymnoc. Mang. Ntr-c. *Ntr-m.* Sass. Seneg. Sulph.
— — — to air, Berb.
— — — — and touch, Ntr-m.
— — — — cold water, Bry. Cina. Gymnoc. Hell. Merc. Sep.
— of points of teeth, Sulph.
To the temples, pain extending, Ant. Ars. Bar-c. Chin. Cupr. Hyosc. Merc. Mez. Nux-m. Nux. Sulph.
Tension in teeth, Anac. Coloc. Puls.
Throbbing in teeth, Acon. Aloe. Ang. Ars. Bar-c. Calc. Caust. Cham. Chin. Cocc-c. Coff. Coloc. Daph. Hyosc. Kali-c. Lyc. Mgn-c. Mgn-s. Merc. Mur-ac. Ntr-c. Ntr-m. *Ntr-s. Nitr-ac.* Nitr. Par. Phosp. Plat. Puls. Rat. Sabad. Sabin. Spig. Staph. Stram. Sulph. Verat.
— — roots of teeth, Ol-an.
— — gums, Bell. Calc. Daph. Nux. Puls. *Sulph.*
—, drawing, Hyosc. Sep.
— as from inflammation of periosteum, Hyosc.
— when breathing, Carb-veg.
— with headache, Glon.
To the throat, pain extending, Ntr-m.
Tingling in teeth, Mur-ac. *Rhus.*
— gums, Arn.
Topor, sense of, Chin. Petr.
Twisted, feeling as if teeth were, Lact.
Turbercle, painful on gums, Phosp-ac. Plb.
Ulcers on gums, Agn. Aur. Berb. Borax. Carb-veg. Creos. Iod. Kali-c. Lyc. Merc. Merc-cor. Millef. Mur-ac. Ntr-m. Nux. Ox-ac. Phosp. Psor. Sabin. Sep. Stann. Staph. Sulph-ac.

9. TEETH AND GUMS.

Ulcers on gums, with swollen cheeks, Aur. Iod. Stann
— — — with base like lard, Hep.
— — tooth, Agn.
Ulcerous pain in gums, Bell. Kali-jod.
— — — teeth, Amm-c. Bell. Kali-jod. Mgn-c. Phosp.
Ulceration of roots, Alum.
Vesicles on gums, Ntr-m.
— —, bleeding, Mgn-c.
— — burning, Bell. Mgn-c. Mez.
Wandering, shifting pain in all the teeth, Mang. Puls. Tilia.
Warm, teeth feel, left side upper jaw, Fluor-ac.
Water, sour, fetid, coming from teeth, Nicc.
White gums, Merc. Nitr-ac. Nux. Plb. Staph. Zinc.
— ulcerous fringes on gums, Merc.
Wrenching pain, Prun.
Yellow teeth, *Iod.* Lyc. Nitr-ac. *Phosp-ac.* Thuj.
Day and night toothache, Ambr.
In morning toothache, Creos. Hyosc. Lach. Nux. Phosp. Sulph. Tart.
— — in bed, Creos. Kali-c. Lach. Nux. Ran-b. Staph.
— — pain in gums, Par. Tereb.
— afternoon, after dinner, toothache, Berb. Lach. Nux. Puls.
— evening, toothache, Alum. Amm-c. Anac. Apis. Bar-c. Bell. Bov. Cham. Graph. Kali-c. *Mgn-s.* Mang. *Merc.* Mez. Nicc. Nitr-ac. *Phosp.* Puls. Rat. Sabin. *Sulph. Sulph-ac.*
— — in bed, Alum. Amm-c. Ant. Bar-c. Bov. Carb-an. Cham. Diad. Graph. Kali-c. Led. Mgn-c. Mgn-m. *Merc.* Nitr-ac. Phosp. Puls. *Sulph-ac.*
— — chilliness of teeth, Mez.
At night, toothache, Ambr. Amm-c. Anac. *Ars.* Bar-c. Bell. Berb. Bov. Bry. Calc. Cham. Chenop. Chin. Clem. Coff. *Cycl. Graph.* Grat. Hell. Hep. Kali-jod. Lyc. Mgn-c. Mgn-m. *Merc.* Ntr-c. Ntr-m. *Ntr-s.* Nitr-ac. Nitr. Nux-m. Nux. Oleand. Petr. *Phosp.* Phosp-ac. Puls. Rhod. *Rhus.* Sabin. Sep. Sil. *Spig.* Staph. *Sulph.*
— — only, Lyc.
— — out of bed, Ntr-s.
— — relieved, Oleand.
— — pain in gums, *Merc.* Rhus.
— — with restlessness, *Mgn-c.*
From air drawn in, toothache, Alum. Bell. Caust. Chin. Cic. *Ntr-m.* Nux-m. Nux. Petr. Rhus. Sabin. Selen. Sil. Spig. *Staph.* Sulph.
When biting the teeth together, pain, Amm-c. Colch. Graph. Guaj. Hep. Ip. Petr. Sep. Tabac. Zinc-ox.
From eating bread, toothache, Carb-an.
— chamomile, toothache, Alum.
— coffee, toothache, Cham. Lachn. Nux.
After coition, toothache, Daph.
From a cold toothache, Acon. Bar-c. Bell. *Cham.* Kali-c. *Hyosc.* Igt. Merc. Nux-m. *Nux.* Puls. Rhus.
— — — in spring, Puls.
— coldness, toothache, *Agar. Calc.* Hell. Mgn-c. Sulph-ac. *Therid.*
— cold air, toothache, Agar. Bell. Bry. Cina. Hyosc. Merc. Nux-m. Nux. Puls. Rhus. Sass. Seneg. Sep. Sil. *Staph.* Thuj.
— — — relieved, Ntr-s. *Puls.*
— cold drink, toothache, Ant. Arg-n. Borax. Bruc. Bry. Calc. Carb-an. Cham. Cina. Clem. Graph. Kali-c. Lac-can. Lach. Mang. Merc. *Mur-ac.* Nux-m. *Nux.* Rhus. Rumex. Sass. Spig. *Staph.* Sulph. Tilia. Thuj.
— — — relieved, Coff. Puls.
— food, toothache, Con.
— anything cold, toothache, Ant. *Calc.* Carb-veg. Cast. Hell. Kali-c. Kali-jod. Mgn-s. Mang. *Merc.* Par. Phosp-ac. Plb. Sil. *Spig.* Sulph. Thuj.
— a draft of air, toothache, Bell. *Calc. Chin.* Sass Sep. Sulph.
— drinking, toothache, *Cham.* Sabin.
— hot drinks, toothache, Ang. Cham. Dros.
— — — relieved, Lyc.
— eating, toothache, Ant. *Bell.* Bry. Canth. Cast. Cocc. Hep. Mgn-m. Mgn-s. Merc. Puls. Thuj. (compare Meals.)
— — — relieved, Rhod. Sil. Spig.
After fruits, toothache, Ntr-s.
When lying on unaffected side worse, Bry.
— — affected side, Ars. Nux.
— — — relieved, Bry.
— — in a horizontal position, Benz-ac. Clem.
From masticating, toothache, *Alum.* Amm-c. Bell. Bry. Chin. Ferr-m. Graph. Hyosc. Lach. Merc. Oleand. Phosp. Rhus. Sabin. Staph. Thuj. Verat. Zinc.
During meals, toothache, Bry. Carb-an. Cast. Cocc. Croton. Euph. Graph. Hep. Igt. *Kali-c. Lyc.* Mgn-m. Mgn-s. Merc. Ntr-c. Puls. Sabin. Sulph. Thuj.
— — pain in gums, Merc.
After meals, toothache, Ant. *Bell.* Borax. Bry. *Cham.* Chin. Coff. Graph. Igt. *Lach.* Mgn-c. Ntr-c. Ntr-m. Nux. *Sabin.* Spig. Stann. *Staph.*
From mental exertion, toothache, Bell. *Nux.*
— damp, moist air, Borax. Nux-m. Rhod. Seneg.
— movement, Mez.
By noise, pain increased, Calc.
From open air, toothache, Ambr. Ant. Bell. Bov. Cham. Chin. Con. *Nux.* Petr. *Phosp.* Rhus. Spig. Staph. Sulph.
— — — relieved, Ant. Bov.

9. TEETH AND GUMS. 73

By picking the teeth, pain excited, Puls. Sang.
Perspiration relieves, Chenop.
By pressure, pain increases, Ntr-m. Tong.
— — — relieved, Amm-c. Ars. Chin. Cocc. Euph. Grat. Mgn-m. Mur-ac. Ntr-c. Rhus. Tabac.
When at rest, intolerable pain, *Mgn-c.*
— riding in a carriage, toothache, Mgn-c.
After rising from bed, pain relieved, Oleand. Sabin.
In the room worse, Cham. Mgn-c. Nicc. Nux. Puls. Rhod. Sep. Sulph.
On entering into a room, worse, Mgn-s.
From salt food, toothache, Carb-veg.
When sitting, worse, Amm-m. Graph. Puls.
— sleep commences the pain abates, Merc.
— sucking the teeth, pain, Nux-m.
From sweet things, toothache, Sep.
— talking, toothache, Sep.
During a thunderstorm, toothache, Rhod.
From tobacco smoking, worse, Bry. Chin. Clem. Sabin. Spig. Thuj.
— — — relieved, Borax. Ntr-s.
When touched, toothache, Bell. Borax. Cast. Chelid. Chin. Cocc-c. Mgn-m. Mgn-s. Mez. Ntr-m. Nitr. Sep.
— — pain in gums, Arg. Arg-n. Hep. Merc. Petr. Stront.
By touch, pain increased, Amm-c. Bell. Calc. Cast. Clem. Euph. Hep. Graph. Igt. Lyc. Merc. Ntr-m. Nux-m. Nux. Phosp. Puls. Rhod. Sabin. Sep. Staph. Sulph.
— — with food, Kali-c. Mgn-m. Mgn-s. Sang.
— vinegar, pain relieved, Puls. Tong.
When walking in open air, toothache, Agn. Cham. Con. Dros. Mgn-s. Nux.
— — — — — relieved, Bov. Bry. Hep. Lyc. Mgn-m. Puls. Sep.
From warm food, toothache, Agn. Phosp. Sil.
— anything warm, toothache, Ambr. Amm-c. Anac. Agn. *Bar-c.* Bry. *Calc.* Carb-veg. Cham. Kali-c. Lachn. Mgn-s. Merc. Phosp. Phosp-ac. Puls. Sil. Sulph.
— — — — relieved, Kali-jod. Nux-m.
By external warmth, pain increased, Graph. Hell. Hep. Nux-m. Puls.
— — — — relieved, Amm-c. *Ars.* Bov. *Cast.* Kali-c. Lach. Lyc. Mgn-m. Merc. Mur-ac. Ntr-c. Nux-m. Nux. *Rhus.* Sabad. Staph. Sulph-ac.
— warmth of bed, pain increased, Cham. *Merc.* Phosp. Phosp-ac. *Puls.* Sabin.
— — — — relieved, Lyc. Mgn-s.
— — — room, pain increased, Cham. Hep. Iris. Mgn-s. Nux. *Puls.*
After washing, toothache, Nux-m. Phosp.
— — with cold water, Calc. Merc. Sulph.

In wet weather, toothache, *Borax.* Nux-m. *Rhod.* Seneg.
By wine, toothache excited, *Nux.*
Ailments from cutting wisdom teeth, Mgn-c. With anxiety, Clem. *Coff.* Oleand.
— pains in limbs as if bruised, Verat.
— cheeks swollen, *Arn.* Ars. Aur. Bar-c. Bell. Borax. Bry. Carb-veg. Caust. Cham. Graph. Iod. Kali-c. Lach. Lyc. Merc. Ntr-m. Nux. Petr. Puls. Samb. Sep. Staph. Sulph.
— — red, Cham. Nux.
— chilliness, Daph. Euph. Lach. Merc. Puls. Sulph.
— coldness of whole body, Verat.
— cough, Sep.
— discouragement, despair, Ars. Cham. Nux.
— dyspnœa, Ntr-m. Puls. Sep.
— ears, coldness of, Lach.
— — pain in, Bell. Borax. Nicc. *Puls.* Rhod.
— — stitches in, Bell. Cham. Creos. Lach. Merc. Ntr-m. Phosp. Sulph. Thuj.
— erections, Daph.
— excitability, irritability, Alum. Cham. Sep.
— eyes surrounded by a yellow mark, Spig.
— face bloated, Spig.
— — heat in, Cham. Graph. Stann.
— — pain in, Ars. Creos. Euph. *Kali-c.* Sil. Spig.
— — paleness, Puls. Spig.
— — redness and swelling, Cham. Verat.
— — swelling, Arn. Ars. Bell. Bry. Cham. Merc. Ntr-m. Nux. Puls. Staph. Verat.
— fainting, Verat.
— glands, submaxillary, swelling of, Amm-c. Bar-c. Camph. Carb-veg. Cham. Dulc. Merc. Nux. Sep. Staph.
— head, congestion to, Acon. Aur. Bell. Calc. Cham. Chin. Hyosc. Lach. Mez. Puls. Sep. Sulph.
— — heat, *Aur.*
— — pain in, Borax. Euph. Lach. Nitr. Puls. Thuj. Verat.
— heat, nocturnal, Sil.
— — universal, Lach. Verat.
— jaw, lameness of, Nux-m.
— — pain in, Nux. Thuj.
— — swelling of periosteum of, Sil.
— knees, tearing pain in, Chenop.
— lassitude, Clem.
— legs, heaviness of, Lach.
— lips, swollen, Bov. Ntr-c.
— nausea, Oleand. Verat.
— neck, pain in, Nux-m.
— — rigidity of, Lach.
— perspiration, Daph. Chin.
— — cold on forehead, Verat.
— pulsation in body, Sep.
— relaxation, Mang.

with restlessness, *Coff*. Mgn-c. Mang. Ntr-s.
— to run about, compelled, *Mgn-c*. Spig.
— saliva, collection of, Cham. Daph. Merc. Ntr-m. Phosp. Stront.
— sleep desire to, Sulph.
— sleeplessness, Sil.
— thirst, Verat.
— tossing about, Clem.
— twitching of feet and fingers, Mgn-c.
— urination frequent, Oleand.
— vomiting, Verat.
— weakness, Clem. Verat.
— weeping, Bell. Coff.

10. Mouth, Palate and Tongue.

Apthœ in mouth, Aeth. Arg. *Ars*. Aur. Bapt. *Borax*. Bry. Canth. Carb-veg. Cham. Chin. Cic. Corn-c. Dulc. Gum-gut. Hell. Hip-m. Iod. *Merc*. Nitr-ac. Nux-m. *Nux*. Plb. Staph. *Sulph*. *Sulph-ac*. Thuj. Vinca.
— on palate, Sass.
— — tongue, Agar. *Borax*. Sass.
— easily bleeding, Borax.
— in children, Borax. *Merc*. Nux. Sacch. Sulph. Sulph-ac.
Atrophy of tongue, Mur-ac.
Biting sensation in mouth, Ambr. Asar.
— — on palate, Carb-veg. Mez. Ran-sc.
— — — tongue, Arn. Asar. Ol-an. Teucr.
— tongue, Thuj.
— — at night in sleep, Phosp-ac.
— — when chewing or talking, Caust. Igt. Petr.
Black tongue, Aeth. *Ars*. Bufo. Chin. Cupr. Lach. Lyc. Op. Phosp. Sec-c.
— posterior part, *Verat*.
— coated tongue, Chin. Elaps. Merc. Phosp.
Blood, clotted in mouth, Canth.

Blueness of tongue, Ars. *Dig*. Mur-ac. Sabad. Spig.
— — mouth, Merc.
Bluish white coating on tongue, Gymnoc.
Boring, sense on palate, Aur.
— — tongue, Clem.
Brown tongue, Ars. Chin. Carb-veg. Lac-can. Lach. Merc. Nux. Phosp. Plb. Rhus. Sec-c. Spong. Sulph.
— coated tongue, Ars. *Bell*. Bry. Carb-veg. Cocc-c. Hyosc. Kali-b. Merc-jod. Phosp. Plb. Rumex. Sabin. Spong. Sulph. Verb.
— — in morning, Verb.
Burning in mouth, Ars. Arum-trif. Asar. Asa-f. Calc. *Cham*. Coloc. Cupr. Gels. Gymnoc. Hipp-m. Hyper. Iris. Jatr. Kali-chl. Mgn-m. Merc-sulph. Mercurial. Mez. *Ntr-s*. Nux. Plat. Scill. Seneg. Sulph. *Verat*.
— on palate, *Camph*. *Carb-veg*. Cinnab. Dulc. Hipp-m. Igt. Mgn-c. Merc-cor. Ntr-s. *Ran-b*. *Scill*. Seneg.
— from mouth to stomach, Brom. Camph. Merc-cor.
— on tongue, Acon. Apis. Asar. Bar-c.

10. MOUTH, PALATE AND TONGUE.

Bell. Bov. Calc. Carb-veg. Caust. Cocc-c. Colch. Hipp-m. Hyosc. Ind. Iod. Jac-c. Kali-chl. Mgn-m. Mercurial. Ntr-s. Ol-an. Ox-ac. Phell. Phosp. Phosp-ac. Plat. Plb. Prun. Ran-sc. Rat. Rhod. Seneg. Sulph. Verat.
Burning on tip, Coloc. Cycl. Gum-gut. Hydroc-ac. Kali-c. Kali-jod. Merc. Ntr-c. Ntr-m.
— — — as from pepper, Teucr.
— — — with ptyalism, Chin.
— — anterior half, Gum-gut.
Burnt as if, sensation in mouth, Hyosc. Jac-cor. Mgn-m. Plat. Psor. Sabad. Sep.
— — on palate, Cimex. Sep.
— — tongue, Cimex. Coloc. Daph. Hyosc. Laur. Merc. Plat. Prun. Puls. Psor. Sabad. Sang. Sep.
— — middle, Hyosc. Plat. Psor. Puls. Sabad. Sep.
— — tip, Lact. Merc-sulph.
Caries of palate, *Aur.* Merc.
Chapped tongue, (compare Cracked.)
Chewing motion, Bell. Mosch.
Clean tongue, Dig. Hyosc. Phosp.
Coldness, sensation of, in mouth, Tart-ac. Verat.
— — on tongue, Bell. Carb-veg. Cist. Hydroc-ac. Kali-chl. Laur. Verat.
— — tip, Cupr.
Contracting sensation in mouth, Asar.
— — on palate, Arn. Cinnab. Glon.
— — root of tongue, Hydroc-ac.
Contraction, spasmodic, of mouth, Calc.
Convulsions of tongue, *Cham. Lyc.* Ruta.
Cracked tongue, chapped, *Ars.* Bar-c. Bell. Benz-ac. Bry. *Cham.* Chin. Cic. Kali-b. Lach. Lyc. Mgn-m. Nux. Phosp. Phosp-ac. Plb. Puls. Ran-sc. Rhus. Sacch. Spig. Sulph. *Verat.*
— — in middle, Kobalt.
— — on tip, Lach.
Cramp-like sensation on tongue, Borax.
Like a cuticle on tongue, sensation, Rhus.
Cutting on palate, Hell.
— — tongue, Bov.
Dark red tongue, Bry.
Discoloured tongue, Sec-c.
Distortion of mouth and tongue when talking, Caust.
Drawing and jerking in tongue, Cast.
Dryness in mouth, *Acon.* Aeth. Aloe. Alum. Amm-c. Ang. Apis. Arg. Arn. Ars. *Bar-c.* Bar-m. *Bell.* Berb. *Bry.* Calc. Cannab. Carb-an. *Carb-veg.* Caust. Cham. Chelid. Chenop. *Chin.* Cina. Cinnab. Cist. Cocc. Con. Cor-r. Cupr. Euph. Graph. Gum-gut. Hipp. *Hyosc.* Hyper. *Igt.* Jatr. Kali-b. Kali-c. Kali-jod. Lac-can. *Lach.* Lact. *Laur.* Led. *Lyc.* Mgn-c. Mgn-m. Mgn-s. *Merc.* Merc-jod. Mercurial. Mosch. *Mur-ac.* Ntr-m. *Ntr-s.* Nitr-ac. Nux-m. *Nux.*

Oleand. Ol-an. Par. Petr. Phell. Phosp. Phosp-ac. *Plb.* Puls. Ran-sc. *Rhus.* Rumex. Ruta. Sass. Samb. Scill. Sec-c. *Seneg.* Sep. *Sil.* Stram. *Sulph.* Tabac. Tellur. Thea. Therid. *Verat.* Zinc.
— — in morning, Ambr. Arg-n. Berb. Cannab. Caps. Carb-an. Jac-cor. Lyc. Mgn-c. Mur-ac. Ntr-s. Nitr-ac. Nux. Ol-an. Op. Par. Petr. Pod. Puls. Sang. Seneg. Spig. Sulph. Thuj.
— — on awaking, Alum. Calc. Clem. Graph. Kali-c. Kobalt. Sep. Tar.
— — forenoon, Seneg.
— — evening, Cycl. Par.
— — at night, Amm-c. Arum-trif. Calc. Caust. Cinnab. Cocc. Mgn-c. Mgn-m. Nux-m. Nux. Phell.
— — with moist mouth, Acon. Sulph.
— — with thirst, Acon. Aloe. Arg-n. Arn. Berb. Bry. Canth. Cham. Chelid. Cinnab. Creos. Cycl. Laur. Merc-cor. Ntr-c. Ntr-s. Nitr-ac. Op. Petr. Rhus. Sec-c. *Sulph.* Tabac.
— — — only relieved for a short time by cold water, Kali-b.
— — with thirstlessness, Acon. Ang. *Bell.* Bry. Cannab. Carb-veg. Cocc. Euph. Euphr. Jatr. Kali-c. Lac-can. *Lyc.* Nux-m. Nux. Phosp-ac. Puls. Sabad. Samb.
— only of posterior part of mouth, Mez.
— of palate, Carb-an. Cist. Cycl. Glon. Hell. Mang. Mgn-c. Meny. Staph. Verat.
— — soft palate, like leather, Stict.
— — tongue, Acon. Aloe. Apis. Arg. Arg-n. Arn. *Ars.* Bapt. Bar-c. Bar-m. *Bell.* Bry. Calc. Carb-an. Caust. Cham. Chenop. Cist. Cocc-c. Con. Creos. Cupr. Daph. *Dulc.* Gels. Hell. Hipp-m. Hyosc. Iod. Kali-b. Kalm. Lach. Laur. Lyc. Merc. Merc-cor. Merc-sulph. Mercurial. Ntr-m. Nitr-ac. Nux. Nux-m. Ox-ac. Par. Phosp. Phosp-ac. Plb. Pod. Psor. Rhus. Rumex. Sec-c. Sep. Spong. Sulph. Sulph-ac. Tabac. Verat.
— — — and lips, Ars. Cham. Lach. Lyc. Phosp.
— — red and cracked at tip, Kali-b. Lach. Rhus. Sulph.
— — without thirst, Bry. Puls.
— — in the morning, Calc. Clem. Cist. Graph. Kali-c. Nitr-ac. Sep. Sulph. Tar.
— — at night, Calc. Nux.
— sensation of in mouth, Acon. Asa-f. Bell. Colch. Dros. Kali-c. Lyc. *Nux-m.* Sulph-ac. Viol-od.
— — mouth moist and coated with mucus, Acon. Bell. Kali-c.
— — on tongue, Arg. *Ars.* Bell. Calc. Colch. *Nux-m.* Puls.

10. MOUTH, PALATE AND TONGUE.

Dryness, sensation of, in the morning, Stront.
Enlarge.ment, sensation of on tongue, Par. Petr
Excrescences painful in mouth, Staph.
Exudations, lymphatic, [extending to tonsils, Merc-cor.
Filthy tongue, Bry. Hydroc-ac. Lyc. Oleand.
Flabby tongue, Creos.
Fissures deep in tongue, Raph.
Foam, froth from mouth, Aeth. Agar. *Bell.* Brom. *Camph.* Canth. *Cham. Cicc. Cocc.* Colch. *Cupr. Hyosc.* Igt. Lach. Lact. *Laur.* Par. Plb. *Sec-c. Stann. Stram.* Tart-ac. Verat.
— — bloody, Sec-c. Stram.
— — milky, Aeth.
— — reddish, Bell. Canth. Hyosc. Sec-c. Stram.
— — white, Mgn-m.
— — yellowish, greenish, Sec-c.
— — with odor of rotten eggs, Bell.
Furred tongue, Bar-c. Bar-m. Graph. Iod. Lyc. Ntr-c. (compare the different colors.)
— — semi-lateral, Daph. Lob.
— — evening, Bism.
— — morning, Ran-sc. Selen. Tart. Verat.
Gangrene of tongue, Ars. Sec-c.
Glandular swelling in mouth, Iod.
— — under tongue, Nux-m. Staph. Tabac.
Glued up, as if mouth were, Mur-ac.
Grayish coated tongue, *Ambr.* Puls. Tart.
— yellow coated tongue, *Ambr.*
— on roof of mouth, Lac-can. Rhus.
Greasy, tongue feels, Iris.
— mouth and palate feel, Ol-an.
Greenish coated tongue, Nitr-ac. Plb.
Hæmoptisis, *Acon. Arn.* Bell. Brom. *Chin. Cop.* Creos. Elaps. *Ferr.* Ham. Hipp. Ip. Lach. *Led. Millef.* Mur-ac. Ntr-m. Op. *Phosp. Plb. Sabin. Sec-c.* Stram. Sulph-ac.
Hœmmorrhage from mouth, Arn. *Bell.* Chin. Cina. *Creos. Dros.* Hipp-m. Ip. *Led.* Lyc. Nux. Phosp. (compare Section 7.)
Hair, sensation of on tongue, Kali-b. Ntr-m. Sil.
Hairy sensation of in interior of mouth, Therid.
Hard tongue, Cupr. Gum-gut. Merc.
Heat in mouth, Bad. Borax. Brom. Carb-veg. Cham. Cinnab. Clem. Colch. Croc. Jatr. Ntr-m.
— — — at night, Cinnab.
— on palate, Camph. Dulc.
— tongue, Bell. Caps. Caust. Plb. Stram.
Heaviness of tongue, Anac. Bell. Colch. Mercurial. Mur-ac. Ntr-c. Ntr-m. Nux. Plb.
— —, difficulty of moving, Calc. Carb-veg. Lach. Lyc. Merc.
Indented with marks of teeth, tongue, Merc.
Inflammation of mouth, *Acon.* Amm-c.

Bell. Canth. Igt. Lach. *Merc.* Nux. Sacch. Verat.
— palate, Calc. Cham. Merc. *Nux. Ran-b.*
— of velum paltati, *Acon. Bell. Coff.*
— tongue, Acon. Ang. Apis. Arn. Ars. Bell. Canth. Lach. *Merc.* Plb. Ran-sc.
— — papillæ, Bell.
— — in the middle, Gels.
— — glands, Kalm.
Insular deep patches on tongue, Gins. Kali-c. Mancin.
Itching on tongue, Alum. Sulph.
— — tip, Dulc.
— — palate, Ferr-m.
Lead colored tongue, Ars.
Lumbrici discharged by mouth, Sabad.
Lumps in mouth, Mgn-c.
— on tongue, Mang.
— under tongue, Ambr.
— bleeding and burning when touched, Mgn-c.
Mucus, collection of, in mouth, Alum. Ang. Arn. Asar. Bell. Brom. Bruc. Bry. Calc. Caps. *Caust.* Chenop. *Chin.* Cupr. Graph. Hep. Igt. Iod. Lach. Laur. Mgn-c. Merc. Ntr-m. *Nux-m.* Nux. Ox-ac. Petr. Phosp. *Phosp-ac.* Plb. Puls. Rhus. Scill. Selen. Sil. Spig. Stram. Sulph. Therid. Teucr.
— frothy, Brom. Chenop. Phosp-ac.
— — in corners of mouth, Par.
— viscid, Mur-ac. Phosp-ac. Puls. Scill.
— in morning, Bell. Cupr. Fluor-ac. Graph. Igt. Mgn-c. Merc. Nicc. Plb. Puls. Rheum. Sil. Spig. Stront. Tilia.
— evening, with thirst, Ang.
— sense of, Cycl.
— on tongue, Bell. Cupr. Dulc. Grat. Lach. Lact. Merc. Merc-cor. Ntr-s. Nitr. Nux-jug. Nux-m. Phosp. *Phosp-ac. Puls.* Sec-c. Sulph. Verb. Viol-tr.
— — tough, Bell. Cupr. Dulc. Lach. Merc. Nux. Phosp-ac. Puls. Sulph.
— — yellow, Kali-b.
— — in morning, and after meals, Verb.
Numbness, sense of in mouth, Ambr. Bov. Ind. Jatr. Mgn-s. Ntr-s.
— on palate, Verat.
— — tongue, Ambr. Ars. Bell. Borax. *Colch.* Hell. Hyosc. Laur. Lyc. Merc. Mercurial. Ntr-m. Nux. Poth. Puls. Rheum.
— one sided, Ntr-m.
Odor from mouth, cadaverous, Nitr-ac.
— cheese like, Aur.
— earthy in the morning, Mang.
— like garlic, Petr. Tellur.
— — horse-radish, Agar.
— as from mercury, Bar-m.
— offensive, Acon. *Agar.* Alum. *Ambr.* Amm-c. *Anac.* Apis Arg-n.

10. MOUTH, PALATE AND TONGUE.

Arn. Ars. Aur. Bar-c. Bar-m.
Bell. Bry. Caps. Carb-an. Cast.
Cist. Croc. Dros. Gels. Hyosc.
Iod. Kali-c. Led. *Lyc.* Merc.
Merc-cor. Nicc. *Nitr-ac.* Nitr.
Nux-m. Nux. *Petr.* Phosp-ac. Pod.
Rhus. *Sep.* Sil. Spig. Stann. Staph.
Sulph. Thea. Verb.
Odor from mouth, offensive, in the morning, Arn. Bell. Camph. Grat. Nux. Puls. Sil Thea.
— — — after meals, Arn. Aur. Carb-veg. Cham. Merc. Nux. *Sulph.* Zinc.
— — like onions, Kali-jod. Petr.
— — — pitch, Canth.
— — putrid, Alum. Arn. *Aur.* Bov. Bry. Cham. Graph. Iod. *Lyc.* Merc. *Nitr-ac.* Nux. Petr. Puls. Rhus. Sabin. Sec-c.
— — — in morning and at night, Puls.
— — — after meals, Cham. Nux.
— — sour, Sulph.
— — like urine, Graph.
To open the mouth, difficulty, Caust. Colch. Lach. Nux.
Painfulness of mouth, Ip. Par.
— — tongue, Bell. Nitr-ac.
— — — on moving it, Berb.
— — — — touch, Bell. Berb.
— — — tip, Croton. Hep.
— — under tongue, Selen.
Paleness of mucus membrane, Eupat.
Palate soft dry, like leather, Sticta.
— wrinkled, Borax. Phosp.
Papillæ erect, Arg-n. Arum-trif. Croc. Kali-b. Merc-cor. Merc-sulph. Oleand. Poth.
Paralysis of organs of speech, Canth. Caust. Graph.
— — tongue, Acon. Bell. *Caust. Dulc.* Euph. Gels. Hydroc-ac. Hyosc. Ip. Mur-ac. *Nux-m. Op.* Stram.
— — — in damp cold weather, Dulc.
Paralytic sensation on palate, Meny.
— — tongue, Cocc. Ip.
Pimples in mouth, Dulc.
— on palate and tongue, Nux.
Pinching pain in tongue, Nux.
Pressing on palate, Thuj.
— — velum palate, Ruta.
Pustules on tongue, Mur-ac.
— — palate, Phosp.
— sharp pointed on soft palate, pock shaped, Ambr.
Protruded tongue, Hydroc-ac.
Purple blotches in mouth, Plb.
— colored tongue, Raph.
Putting the fingers into the mouth, children, Cham.
Ranula, Ambr. Calc. Lac-can. Merc. Ntr-m. Nitr-ac. Sacch. *Staph. Thuj.*
— gelatinous, Mez. Nitr-ac. Staph.
— — bluish red, Thuj.

Rasping, smarting pain in mouth, Ambr. Asar.
— — — when eating solid food, Phosp-ac.
— — on palate, Carb-veg. Chenop. Mez. Mur-ac. Ran-sc.
Raw tongue, Gels. Kali-b.
— — pain on left side, Jac-cor.
Redness of cavity of mouth, Amm-c. Ars. Bell. Cycl. Igt. Kali-b. Merc-jod.
— — velum palati, Bell. Cham. Chenop. Kali-b. Merc.
— — tongue, Aloe. Apis. *Ars.* Arum-trif. Bell. Bry. Cham. Coloc. Elaps. Gels. Hyosc. Kali-b. *Lach.* Merc-cor. Nux. Ox-ac. Pallad. Poth. Ran-sc. Rhus. Stann. Sulph. Verat.
— — tip, Hipp. Merc-jod. Phyt. Poth. Rhus. Sulph.
— — painful, Arg-n. Cycl.
— — edges, Bell. Merc-jod. Nux. Sulph.
Red, glistening tongue, Glon. Kali-b. Lach.
— spots on tongue, Hipp-m. Raph.
Reddish blue color, Ars.
Roughness in mouth, Berb. Carb-veg. Cina. Cycl. Dig. Ntr-s. Phosp.
— on palate, Mgn-c. Mez.
— — tongue, Ang. Bell. Bry. Carb-veg. Casc. Coloc. Grat. Laur. Oleand. Par. Phyt. Sulph.
— — from erection of papillæ, Croc. Oleand.
Saliva, collection of, Alum. Amm-c. Anac. Ant. Arg. Arg-n. *Asar.* Bar-c. Bell. Bism. Bov. Brom. Bry. Calc-ph. Camph. *Carb-veg.* Chelid. Chenop. Croc. Croton. Creos. Cupr. Dig. Eugen. Ferr-m. Grat. Hell. *Hep.* Hydroc-ac. *Igt.* Ip. Kali-b. Kali-c. Kalm. Lach. Lact. Lob. Mgn-m. Mur-ac. Ntr-m. Ntr-s. Nicc. *Nux-m.* Nux. *Ol-an.* Ox-ac. Par. Phell. *Phosp. Plb.* Ran-b. Rat. Rhod. *Rhus.* Sabad. Sang. Seneg. Spig. Staph. Sulph. Tar. Tart. Thea. Thuj. *Tong.* Verb. Viol-tr. Zinc.
— diminished, Acon.
— with sense of dryness, Colch. Kali-c. Plb. Rhod.
— — headache, or sore throat, Hipp.
— acrid, Arum-trif. Igt. Kalm. Lact. Verat.
— astringent, Par.
— bitter, Ars. Kali-b. Kalm. Sulph. Thuj.
— bloody, Arg. Ars. Bad. Canth. Clem. Dros. Hyosc. Ind. Kali-jod. Mgn-c. Merc. Nux. Phosp. Rhus. Staph. Stram. Sulph. Thuj.
— mixed with blood, Acon. Kali-jod. Sulph.
— brownish, Bism.
— burning, Hipp-m.
— clammy, Arg. Bell. Berb. Camph. Cannab. Eugen. Lob.
— cool, Asar. Cist.
— like cotton, Nux-m. Puls.

10. MOUTH, PALATE AND TONGUE.

Saliva, frothy, Apis. Berb. Brom. Bry. Canth. Cham. Cinnab. Cocc. Cupr. Eugen. Kali-b. Phell. Plb. Ran-sc. Sabin. Spig, Stram. Sulph.
— gluey, Bad.
— hot, Daph.
— insipid, Mur-ac.
— metallic tasting, Phyt. Ran-b. Zinc.
— musty, Kali-b. Led.
— offensive, Ars. Bry. Dig. Hipp-m. *Merc.* Petr.
— oily, Cub.
— reddish, Sabin.
— saltish, Ant. Euph. Hyosc. Kali-b. Kali-jod. Lyc. Merc. Merc-cor. Mez. Sep. Stram. Sulph. Verat. Verb.
— slimy, Camph. Lach.
— soapy, Berb. Bry. Dulc.
— sour, Alum. Calc. Calc-ph. *Igt.* Lact. Merc. Ntr-s. Pod. Sulph. Stann. Tar.
— sweet, Alum. *Dig.* Nicc. Phosp. *Plb. Puls. Sabad.*
— thick, Bell. Bism. *Nux-m.*
— tough, Apis. Arg. Ars. Camph. Cinnab. Dulc. Eugen. Hydroph. Lachn. Merc.
— viscid, Cannab. Cycl. Kali-b. Kali-jod.
— watery, Asar. Creos. Jatr. Lob. Mgn-m. Puls. Thea.
— white, *Ol-an. Ran-b.* Sabin. Spig.
—, — of egg like, Calad.
— yellow, Gels. Hipp-m. Phyt. Rhus.
Salivation, Acon. Amm-c. Ant. Arum-trif. Asar. *Bell.* Brom. Bry. Calad. Calc. Camph. *Canth.* Carb-veg. Cham. Chin. *Cinnab.* Clem. *Colch.* Con. Croton. Cupr. Cycl. Daph. *Dig.* Dulc. *Euph.* Graph. Grat. Hell. *Hep.* Hipp-m. Hydroc-ac. Hydroph. *Hyosc.* Igt. *Iod.* Ip. Iris. Jatr. Kali-b. Kobalt. Lach. Lob. *Merc. Merc-cor.* Mez. Ntr-m. *Nitr-ac.* Nux. Op. Phosp. Phyt. Plb. Puls. Ran-b. Ran-sc. Rhus. Sabad. Sang. Seneg. *Sep. Spong.* Stann. Staph. Stram. *Sulph. Sulph-ac.* Tart. Tong. Verat. *Zinc.*
— at night, Nux. *Rhus.*
— in febrile paroxysms, Hell. Hep. Nitr-ac. Sulph.
— from mercury, Bell. Chin. Dig. Dulc. Hep. *Iod.* Lach. Nitr-ac. *Sulph.*
— with nausea, Chin. Euph. Puls. Verat.
— — — and vomiting, Sulph.
— — — retching, Euph. Puls.
— — shuddering, Arg. *Euph.*
— — sneezing, Fluor-ac.
— — continuous spitting, Hydroph.
— — pain in stomach, Euph.
— — thirst, *Dulc.* Ntr-m.
— — without thirst, Cinnab. Merc.
Salivary glands painful, Acon.
— — swollen, Bar-m. Thuj.
— — inflammation of, Sacch.
— — ulcerated, Merc.
Shining tongue, Apis. Glon. Lach.

Skin peeling of on interior of cheek, Sulph.
— — — — palate, Par.
— — — — tongue, Ran-sc. Tar.
Slimy coated tongue, Bell. Chelid. Cupr. Lact. Merc. Nux-m. Petr. *Phosp-ac. Puls.* Verb. Viol-tr.
Smooth tongue, Kali-b. Lach.
Soft tongue, Merc. Rhus. Stram.
Soreness of mouth, Arum-trif. Dig. Igt. Kali-c. Lach. Mgn-s. Merc. Ntr-m. Nux. Phosp.
— — palate, Lach. Mez. Nitr-ac. Nux.
— — velum palati, Phosp-ac.
— — tongue, *Agar.* Aloe. Ars. Canth. Carb-veg. Cic. Cist. Dig. Gels. Kali-c. Lyc. Merc. Ntr-m. Nitr-ac. Nux. *Sep.* Sil.
— sensation of in mouth, Agar. Alum. Amm-c. Asa-f. Bell. Bism. Caust. Dig. Glon. Hyosc. Ip. Lachn. Sabad. Stram.
— — on palate, Agar. Alum. Caust. Cinnab. Mur-ac. Par. Thuj.
— — velum palati, Ruta.
— — of on tongue, Alum. Ant. Arn. Bar-c. Calc. Caust. Cist. Glon. Graph. Ip. Ox-ac. Poth. Sabad. Sang. Thuj.
— — — tip, Arum-trif. Kali-c. Poth. Sep.
— — — middle, Samb.
— — — frenum, Kali-c.
Speech difficult, Acon. Amm-c. Anac. Aur. *Bell.* Calc. Cannab. *Caust.* Cic. Chin. Cocc. Con. Cupr. Cycl. Dulc. Euphr. Graph. Hep. Hyosc. Lach. Laur. Lyc. *Mez.* Mosch. Mur-ac. Ntr-m. Nicc. Nux. Op. Phosp-ac. Plb. Ruta. Seneg. Sil. Stann. *Stram.* Sulph.
— — for certain words, Lach.
— — from elongation of tonsils, Aur.
— — — jerks in head and arms, Cic.
— — — pain in back, Cinnab.
— — — spasm of throat, Cupr.
— — — spasm of tongue, Ruta.
— — — swelling of tongue, Dulc.
— — — weakness, Hipp-m.
— — — — of chest, Stann.
— crying, hoarse like a child, Cupr.
— drawling in reading, Tabac.
— hasty, Ars. Bell. Hep. Lach. Merc.
— high, Lach.
— utters, inarticulate sounds, Hyosc.
— indistinct, Bry. Calc. Caust. Lyc. Sec-c.
— — from dryness in throat, Bry. Seneg.
— murmuring, whispering, Stram.
— nasal, Bell. Lach. Lyc. Phosp-ac. Staph.
— slow, Thuj.
— stammering, Acon. Bell. *Bov.* Bufo. Caust. *Euphr.* Hyosc. Lach. Merc. Ntr-c. Nux. Op. Sec-c. *Stram.* Sulph. Verat.
— quick and stammering, Merc.
— — subdued, Tabac.

10. MOUTH, PALATE AND TONGUE.

Speech swallows his words, Staph.
— trembling, Acon. Igt.
— wanting, Alum. *Bell. Caust.* Chin. *Cic.* Con. Cupr. Hep. Hydroc-ac. *Hyosc. Laur. Merc.* Mosch. Oleand. Op. *Plb. Stram.* Tart. *Verat.*
— — after apoplexy, Laur.
— — with violent pain in stomach, Laur.
— weak, Bell. *Canth.* Chin. Igt. Op. Sec-c. Spong. *Stann.* Staph. Verat.
— — from debility of organs, Amm-c. Canth. Staph.
— whizzing, Bell. Caust.
Spongy tongue, Benz-ac.
Sticky, viscid mouth, Berb. Ruta. *Scill.* Verat.
— feverish feeling in mouth, Gels.
Stiffness of tongue, Berb. Borax. Carb-veg. *Colch.* Con. Euphr. Hell. Hydroc-ac. Lach. Lyc. Merc-cor. Mercurial. Ntr-m. Nicc.
Stinging, stitches in mouth, Aur. Calc. Kali-chl. Spig. Sulph.
— — on palate, Igt. Mez. Nitr-ac. Ran-sc. *Staph.*
— — roof of mouth, Kobalt.
— — tongue, *Acon.* Ang. Berb. Brom. Chin. Clem. Elaps. Kali-b. Kali-chl. Kalm. *Nitr-ac.* Phosp-ac. Prun. Sabad. Staph.
— — — tip, Ang. Brom. Cycl. Igt. Merc. Merc-sulph. Nux. Phosp Phosp-ac. Ran-b. Sabad. Sabin. Staph.
Stomacace, Ars. Borax. *Caps. Carb-veg.* Chin. Dulc. *Hell.* Hep. Iod. *Merc.* Millef. Ntr-m. Nitr-ac. *Nux.* Sep. Sil. Staph. Sulph. Sulph-ac.
— after a cold, Dulc.
Suppurating pustules on palate, Phosp.
Suppuration of tongue, Canth. *Merc.*
Swelling in interior of mouth, Acon. *Amm-c. Bell.* Canth. Caust. Glon. Igt. Lach. *Merc.* Nux. Par. Sep. Verat.
— tight, almost painless of roof of mouth, size of a pigeon's egg, Par.
— between gums and cheek, Rhod.
— palate, Bar-c. Bar-m. Bell. Calc. Chin. Coff. Croton. Merc. Ntr-s. *Nux.* Par. Seneg. Sil. Sulph.
— of velum palati, Bell. Calc. Carb-veg. Coff. (compare Uvula, section 11.)
— — tongue, Acon. Anac. Apis. Ars. *Bell.* Calad. Calc. Canth. Chin. Cic. Cocc-c. Con. Dig. Dulc. Elaps. Glon. *Hell.* Kali-c. Kali-jod. Lach. Lyc. Merc. Merc-cor. Millef. Ox-ac. Phosp-ac. Plb. Sec-c. Sil. Stram. Thuj.
— under the tongue, Ntr-m.
— tongue one sided, Calc. Sil.
— — painful to touch, Con. Phosp-ac. Thuj.
— — — when talking, Phosp-ac.
— — glands under, Nux-m. Staph. Tabac.
— sense of, Berb. Cimex.
— — of palate, Arg-n. Nux. Puls.

Thickening of tongue, sensation, Nux.
Tingling, crawling in mouth, Zinc.
— — on tongue, Acon. Ntr-m. Sec-c.
Trembling of tongue, Ars. Bell. Merc.
— — when extending it, Lach.
Tubercles on tongue, Lyc.
Ulcers in the mouth, *Agn.* Alum. Caust. Dulc. Hep. *Iod.* Jatr. Kali-jod. *Merc.* Merc-cor. Ntr-c. Ntr-m. *Nitr-ac.* Nux. Op. Petr. Phyt. Plb. Staph. Thuj. Zinc.
— on roof of mouth, Arum. Cinnab. Kali-b. Ntr-m. Sil.
— — palate, Aur. Lach. Merc. Nux. Sil.
— — velum palati, Dros. Phosp-ac.
— — reddish arola, yellow tenaceous pus, Kali-b. Lac-can.
— at orifice of salivary glands, Acon. Bell. Merc.
— on tongue, Agar. Benz-ac. Bov. Chin. Cic. Cinnab. Dig. Dros. Graph. Kali-b. Kali-jod. Lach. Lyc. Mercurial. Mur-ac. Ntr-m. Op. Phyt. Verat.
— — — blue, Ars.
— — — frenum, Agar.
— biting, Ntr-m.
— with black base, Mur-ac.
— bluish, Ars. Aur.
— burning, Caust. Chin. Cic. Merc. Ntr-c. Ntr-m. Phosp-ac.
— dirty looking, Plb.
— fetid, Nux. Plb.
— flat, Ntr-c. Ntr-m.
— itching, Chin.
— lardaceous base, Hep.
— mercurial, *Iod. Nitr-ac.*
— painful, Ars. Kali-b. Mur-ac. Ntr-m. Nitr-ac.
— — to touch, Cic. Ntr-c.
— — — food and liquids, Ntr-m.
— small, yellow, Zinc.
— sore smarting, Bov.
— stinging, stitches, Nitr-ac.
— syphilitic, *Merc.* Nitr-ac.
— white, Cic.
— yellow, Aloe. Zinc.
Vesicles in the mouth, Ambr. Bar-c. Calc. Caps. Carb-an. Cham. Hell. Kali-c. Mgn-c. Merc. Mez. Ntr-c. Ntr-m. Nux. Rhod. Spong. Staph. Sulph.
— on palate, Calc. Ntr-s. Nux. Spig.
— — tongue, Amm-c. *Amm-m.* Ant. *Arg.* Bar-c. Berb. Brom. Bry. Calc. Carb-an. Cham. Chenop. Graph. Hell. Hipp-m. Kali-c. Kali-jod. Mgn-c. Mgn-m. Mang. Mercurial. Mur-ac. *Ntr-m.* Ntr-s. Phell. Phyt. Puls. Scill. Sep. Spig. Spong. Staph. Zinc.
— — tip, Cycl. Ind. Kali-jod. Lyc. Nitr.
— biting, Ntr-m. Rhod.
— burning, Ambr. *Amm-m.* Apis. Arg. Bry. Caps. Carb-an. Cycl. Kali-c. Kali-jod. Mgn-c. Mang. Mercurial. Mez. Ntr-m. Ntr.s. Nitr. Phell. Spig. Spong.

10. MOUTH, PALATE AND TONGUE.

Vesicles cutting. Mgn-s.
— gangrenous blood vesicles, Sec-c.
— inflamed, Bar-c.
— painful, Berb. Kali-c. Nux.
— — when touched by food or liquids, Ntr-m.
— scalded and raw, Lyc.
— sore, smarting, Arg. Sulph.
— stinging, stitches, Apis. Cham. Hell. Spong.
— which soon become ulcers, Clem.
— whitish, Berb.
White coated tongue, Acon. Agar. Alum. Ambr. *Ant.* Apis. *Arn.* Ars. Bell. Berb. Bism. Bry. Calc. Cannab. Carb-veg. Cham. Chin. Chelid. Cimex. Cina. Cinnab. Colch. Coloc. Corn-c. Creos. Croc. Croton. Cupr. Cycl. Dig. Elaps. Eupat. Gels. Hell. Hipp. Hipp-m. Hydroc-ac. Hyper. Igt. Ip. Kali-jod. Kalm. Kobalt. Lach. Lact. Laur. Mgn-c. Mgn-m. Merc-cor. Merc-sulph. Mez. Ntr-m. Nitr-ac. Nitr. Nux-jug. Nux-m. Nux. Oleand. Ox-ac. Phosp.
Tar. Pod. Psor. Puls. Raph. Rumex. Sabin. Sang. Selen. Sep. Sulph. Verat. Verb. Viol-tr.
— — pale tongue, Acon. Ambr. Anac. Ang. Ars. Berb. Creos. Oleand. Phosp.
— — with clean red spots, Hipp-m.
— — shining, silvery white all over, Glon.
— — white stripes, Bell.
— — in middle, Bry. Phosp.
— — at root, Sep.
— — in morning, Mgn-m. Ran-sc. Selen.
— — — evening, Bism.
— — less after breakfast, Croc.
Withered tongue, Verat.
Yellowish coated tongue, Ars. Bell. *Bry.* Cannab. Carb-veg. Cham. Chin. Cocc. Coloc. Corn-c. Gels. Hyper. Ip. Lept. Merc. Merc-jod. Mez. Ntr-m. Nux. Plb. Pod. Psor. Puls. Rumex. Sabad. Sabin. Sec-c. Verat. Verb.
— thick at root, Kali-b.
— gray, Ambr.
Yellow spots in mouth and throat, Lac-can. Lach. Lyc.

11. Fauces, Pharynx and Oesophagus.

Abcesses on tonsils, small, painful, frequent, Plb.
Adhesion, sense of, Nitr-ac.
As of awns of barley in Pharynx, Berb. Mgn-c.
Ball rising up, sensation of, Asa-f. Con. Kalm. Lach. Lob. Lyc. Mgn-c. Plb.
Biting in throat, Carb-veg. Colch. Mez. Teucr. Zinc.
Boring, Arg.
Bruised, pain as if, Rhus.
— — — — when touched, Cic.
Burning in throat, *Acon*. Aloe. Alum.Apis. *Arn*. *Ars*. Arum-trif. Asa-f. Aur. Bar-c. Bell. Bism. Borax. *Bov*. Brom. Calc. *Camph*. Cannab. *Canth*. Caps. Carb-veg. Cast. Caust. Cham. Chelid. Chenop. Chin-sulph. Clem. Cocc. Cocc-c. Coloc. Con. Croton. Cupr.Cycl.*Euph*.Fluor-ac. Gels. Gymnoc. Hipp-m. Hyosc. Igt.Iod. Iris. Kali-b. Lach. Lact. *Laur*. Lob.Lyc. Mgn-c. *Merc*. Merc-cor. Merc-jod. Merc-sulph. Mercurial. *Mez*. Mur-ac. Ntr-c. Nitr-ac. Nux. Oleand. Ol-an. Ox-ac. Pæon. Par. *Phosp*. Plb. Psor. Puls. *Ran-b*. *Ran-sc*. *Rhod*. Rhus.*Sabad*. *Scill*. *Sec-c*. *Seneg*. Spong. Sulph. Sulph-ac. Tilia. Verat.
— in œsophagus, Nux.
— lessened by sugar, not by water, Bell.
Choking, Acon. Ambr. Bar-c. Bell. Dig. Canth. Chelid. Creos. Graph. Lach. Nicc. Ol-an. Ran-sc. Sabin. Verat.
Chronic affections of throat, Mang. Ntr-m. Sabad. *Sulph*.
Coldness, sense of, Carb-veg. Kali-chl. Verat.
Constriction, Aeth. *Alum*. Ars. Bell. Benz-ac. Cact. Calc. Carb-veg Chin-sulph. Coloc. Con. Croc. Croton. Cycl. Elaps. Ferr. Fluor-ac. Gels. Hell. Hydroph. *Hyosc*. Igt. *Iod*. Jac-cor. Jatr. Lach. Laur. Lob. Lyc. Mez. Ntr-s. Nitr. Ol-an. Phosp. *Plat*. Plb. Rhod. Sabad. *Sass*. Seneg. *Stram*. Thuj. *Verat*.
Contraction, Acon. Bar-c. *Calc*. Calc-ph. Caps.*Chelid*.Cinnab.Croton. Hœmatox. Laur. Mez. Nicc. Phosp-ac. Ran-sc. Rat. Rheum. *Verat*.
— sensation of, *Alum*. *Arum*. *Bell*. Bry. Calc. Caps. Carb-veg. Caust. Cic.

Cinnab. Dros. Elaps. Grat. Hœmatox. Hipp-m. Hyosc. Igt. Iod. Ip. Jac-cor. Lach. Lob. Lyc. Merc. Ntr-m. Nux. Plat. Puls. Rhus. Sabad. Sass. Stram. *Sulph*. Verat. Zinc.
Convulsions in throat, Lach.
Creeping in throat, Plb.
Crumbs of bread, as if in pharynx, Dros. Lach.
Cuticle like on uvula, Amm-c.
Cutting in throat, Mang. Nitr.
Denuded spots in pharynx, Brom.
Digging sensation, Arg.
Diphtheric patches on arches of palate and uvula, Apis.
— — over fauces, Caps.
— — on uvula, tonsils, and roof of mouth, Kali-b.
— — — left tonsil, Lach.
— — — right tonsil, Lyc.
— — from left to right and right to left, Lac-can.
— — on arches of palate, Merc-jod.
Distention of œsophagus, sensation of, Hyper. Op. Verat.
Drawing, Cupr. Laur. Plat. Plb. Stann. Sulph. Teucr. Zinc.
Dryness, *Acon*. Alum. Amm-c. Amm-m. Anac. Ant. Ars. *Asa-f*. *Bell*.*Berb*.Borax. Bruc. *Bry*. Bufo. Calad. Calc.Carb-veg. Caust. Cham. Chenop. Chin. Cist. *Cocc*. Cocc-c. Colch. Cor-r. Creos. Croton. Cupr. Cycl. Dros. Gels. Hep. Hipp. Hyosc. *Igt*. Ip. Jatr. Kali-chl. Kali-jod. Kalm. Kobalt. Lac-can.Lach.Laur.Lob. *Lyc*. Mgn-c. Mgn-m.Mgn-s.Mang.Meny. *Merc*. Merc-jod. Merc-sulph. Mur-ac. Ntr-c. Ntr-m. Nitr-ac. *Nux-m*. *Nux*. *Ol-an*. Op. Petr. Phell. *Phosp*. Phyt. Plb. Pod. Puls. Rhus. Sabad. Sabin. Samb. Sang. Sass. Scill. Sec-c. Selen. *Seneg*. Sep. Sil. Stann. Staph. Stram. Stront. *Sulph*. Tabac. Tar. Tellur.Verat. Verb. Zinc. Zing.
— not relieved by drinking, Sang.
— in posterior part of throat, Kali-c. Mez.
— extending to chest, ears and nose, Lach.
— painful, Lach. Merc.
— partial, Lach.
— after diarrhœa, Ox-ac.
— day and night, Phosp.

11. FAUCES, PHARYNX AND OESOPHAGUS.

Dryness in morning, Amm-c. Bov. Caust. Lachn. Lyc. Petr. Plb. Puls. Sass.
— at night, Cinnab. Phell.
— with difficulty in speaking, Bry. Merc. Seneg.
— — irritation to cough, Seneg.
— — thirst, Ars. Chenop. Cimex. Cinnab. Creos. Cupr.
— without thirst, Apis. *Calad.* Caust. Meny. Nux-m. Pallad. Phosp-ac. Psor. Samb.
— with water in the mouth, Merc.
— sensation of, Amm-m. Ars. *Bry.* Carb-veg. Chenop. Cist. Croton. Lyc. *Nux-m.* Phyt. Rhus. *Stann.*
Dust, sensation of, Cist. Merc.
Elongation of uvula, sensation of, Calc. Caps. Chelid. Croc. Croton. Hydroph. Hyosc. Iod. Kali-b. Lyc. Merc. Millef. Ntr-m. Sabad. Sep. Sil.
— — — with stiffness in nape of neck, Kali-c.
Empty, sensation in pharynx, Mur-ac.
Expectoration of mucus, Alum. Croton. Guaj. Mgn-s. *Ntr-m.* Rhus.
— by hawking, All-cep. Bism. Calc. Carb-an. Caust. Chenop. Con. Dros. *Kali-c.* Lach. Lam. Lyc. Ntr-m. Petr. *Phosp.* Phosp-ac. *Plat.* Rhus. Seneg. *Sep.* Stann. Tar. Teucr. Thuj.
— — in the morning, Ambr. Apis. Ntr-m. Petr. Phosp. Rhus. Sep.
— — with choking and vomiting, Ambr.
As of a soft piece of flesh hanging down in pharynx, Lach. Phosp. Thuj.
Food passes into the Choana, Petr. Sil.
Like a soft piece of fur in pharynx, Phosp.
As if grown together, sensation, Nitr-ac.
Gurgling in the throat, when drinking, Cina, Cupr. Laur. Thuj.
Hair, sensation of in throat, Sil. Sulph.
To hawk, irritation, All-cep. Bell. Berb. Chenop. Cocc-c. Colch. Cor-r. Croton. Dulc. Euphr. Fluor-ac. Gymnoc. Hep. Kali-b. Kali-c. Lach. Lob. Lyc. Nux-jug. Pæon. Par. Petr. Phosp. Phosp-ac. Plat. Plb. Psor. Sabad. Spig. Teucr.
Heat in throat, Aeth. Benz-ac. Brom. Camph. *Cham.* Cist. Clem. Ferr. Gels. Glon. Hydroc-ac. Laur. Merc. Merc-sulph Nitr-ac. Raph. Sang.
— — at night, Cinnab.
Herpes, bluish, after suppressed gonorrhœa, Zinc.
Inflammation, *Acon.* Alum. Arg. Arg-n. Ars. Bar-c. *Bell.* Berb. Bism. Brom. Bufo. Calc. Canth. Caps. Carb-veg. Caust. Cham. Cinnab. Cist. *Coff. Colch.* Con. Croton. Cupr. *Dulc.* Graph. Hep. Hydroc-ac. Igt. Iod. Kali-b. Lach. *Lyc.* Mang. *Merc.* Merc-jod. Mez. Ntr-c. Nicc. *Nitr-ac.* Nitr. Nux-m. Nux. Phosp-ac. Phyt. Plb. Puls. Ran-b. Sabad. Sang. *Seneg.* Sep. Stront. Sulph. Tellur.

Inflammation of oesophagus, Arn. Ars. Asa-f. Bell. Carb-veg. Cocc. Euph. Laur. Merc. Mez. Rhus. Sabad. Sec-c.
— — tonsils, Bar-c. Bell. Berb. Canth. Cham. Igt. Lach. Ntr-s. Plb. Puls. Sep.
— — uvula, Calc. Carb-veg. *Coff.* Colch. Kali-b. Merc. Ntr-s. Nitr. Nux. Puls. *Seneg.*
— gangrenous, Amm-c. Arn. Ars. Carb-veg. Con. Creos. Euph. Merc. Sec-c. Sulph.
— in children, *Cham.*
— erysipelatous, *Merc.*
— after a cold, *Cham. Dulc.*
— after mercury, *Arg. Nitr-ac.*
— with swelling of face, Nicc.
Irritability of œsoph., *Cocc.* Croton.
Itching in throat, Samb.
— periodical, Cist.
Liquids swallowed pass out through the nose, Aur. *Bell.* Lac-can. Lach. Merc. Petr.
Mucus, collection of, in throat, Alum. *Ambr.* Amm-m. Arg. Arn. Ars. Asar. Bell. Borax. Bry. Bufo. Carb-an. *Carb-veg. Caust.* Chenop. Colch. Dulc. Fluor-ac. Graph. Grat. Gymnoc. *Kali-c.* Kali-jod. Kalm. Lach. Lact. Lob. Mgn-c. Mgn-s. Merc. Merc-jod. Ntr-c. Nitr-ac. Nux-jug. Ol-an. Petr. Phosp-ac. Plat. Pod. *Puls. Ran-b.* Rhus. Rumex. Sabad. Samb. Sass. Seneg. Sep. Sil. Spig. *Stann. Tabac.* Tar. Thuj. Zinc.
— sensation of, Grat. Mez. Rhod.
— in the morning, Ambr. Amm-m. Caust. Hep. Kali-c. Lact. Ntr-m. Petr. Phosp. Plat. Puls. Rhus. Sep. Tar. Teucr.
— — in evening, Alum. Ang.
— — at night, Alum. Ntr-s. Puls.
— in posterior nares, Euph. Nitr-ac. Thuj. Zinc.
—, (compare Section 24.)
— albuminous, Merc-cor.
— bitter, Arn. Ars. Cist. Merc. Tar.
— bloody, Alum. Bism. Fluor-ac. Lyc. Mgn-c. Sep.
— easily discharged, Arg. *Carb-veg.*
— like a false membrane, Bell. Puls.
— frothy, Brom. Bry. Chenop. Par.
— gelatinous, Arg. Berb.
— gluey, bloody, mucus, from pharynx, Bad.
— grayish, *Ambr.* Arg. Ars.
— greenish, Ars. Colch. Dros.
— in small lumps, *Agar.* Seneg.
— lumpy, All-cep.
— lumps solid, Lith.
— mouldy tasting, Teucr.
— nauseates, Caust.
— putrid, Ang.
— red like blood, Thuj.
— saltish, Ars. Merc. Ntr-s. Phosp. Sulph. Therid.
— sour, Croton. Laur. Mgn-s. Phosp. Tar.

11. FAUCES, PHARYNX AND OESOPHAGUS.

Mucus tenacious, Alum. Amm-m. *Borax.* Cinnab. Cist. Cycl. Ferr-m. Grat. Kali-c. Lach. Lact. Mgn-c. Mgn-s. Merc. Merc-jod. Ol-an. Pæon. Puls. Raph. Sass. Seneg. Thuj.
— thick, Aloe. Alum. Arg-n. Berb. Bry. Cist. *Mgn-c.* Mgn-m. Merc. Nicc. Nux-m.
— tough, Aloe. Alum. Ambr. Ang. Ant. Asar. Borax. Bry. Caps. Cist. Hydroph. Lob. Lyc. *Mgn-c.* Mgn-m. Merc. *Ol-an.* Pallad. Phosp. *Phosp-ac.* Plb. Psor. *Puls. Ran-b.* Rhus. Sass. *Seneg. Tabac.*
— viscous, Alum. Ang. Ant. Arg-n. Asar. Borax. Bry. Caps. Chin-sulph. Lact. Lob. Mgn-c. Ol-an. Phosp. *Phosp-ac.* Plb. Puls. Ran-b. Raph. Rhus. Sass. Sep. Tabac.
— white, Bell. Mgn-c. Nux. Raph. Spig.
— yellow, Berb. Dros. Kali-b. Nux. Rumex. Sil. Spig.
Numbness sense of in throat, Mgn-s.
Paralysis of oesophagus, Bell. Caust.Gels. Lach. *Nux-m.* Op. *Plb.*
— — sense of, Ars. Cocc. Ip. Kali-c. Lach. Lact. Puls. Sil.
Partial pains which only affect a small spot, Lach.
Plug, as of a, in throat, All-cep. Ambr. Amm-c. Ant. Apis. Arn. *Bar-c.* Bell. Benz-ac. Berb. Calc. Caust. Cham. Chelid. Cocc-c. Croc. Croton. Gels. *Graph. Hep.* Hydroph. *Igt.* Kali-b. Kali-c. Lac-can. Lach. Led. Lob. Merc. Mez. *Ntr-n.* Nitr. *Nux.* Ol-an. Par. Phyt. *Plb.* Psor, Ruta. *Sabad.* Sabin. Sep. Sulph. Tabac. *Thuj.* Zing.
— — in pharynx, Lach.
Pressing pain in throat, Alum. Amm-m. Arum. Asa-f. Bar-c. Bry. Calc. Caust. Cinnab. Creos. Dulc. Ferr. Ferr-m. Grat. Hell. Hyosc. Iod. Kali-jod. Kalm. Lach. Merc. Mez. Nitr-c. Nitr. Nux. Par. Phell. Phosp. Plat. Rat. Rhus. Ruta. Sabad. Sabin. Seneg. Sep. Sulph. Tabac. Tar. Teucr. Thuj. Verat.Zinc-ox.
— as from anything hard, Arn. Bry. Ol-an.
— in oesophagus, Ferr-m. Lob. Merc.
— — as if pressed on by larynx, Chelid.
Pressing pain in tonsils. Bell. Nux.
Pricking pain, Acon. Aur-m.
Pulsation, Rhus.
Rasping, smarting, Bar-c. Merc. Mur-ac. Phosp. Phosp-ac.
Rawness, Mgn-m. Mur-ac.
Redness of throat, *Acon.* Arg-n. Berb. Calc. Carb-veg. Cycl. Igt. Lach. Lyc. Merc. Merc-cor. Merc-jod.
— — dark, Acon. Caps. Cham.
— erysipelatus, *Merc.*
— net like, Brom.
— dark red, glossy, puffed, veins enlarged, crack on left side, Kali-b.

Rending, tearing, *Aeth.* Ars. *Colch.* Staph. Teucr. Zinc.
Rigidity of throat, Chelid. Lach.
Risings in oesoph., *Asa-f.* Con. Euph. Lyc. Mgn-m. Plb. Ran-b. Spig.
— — cold, Caust.
— — hot, Merc. Phosp.
Roughness in throat, Aloe. Anac. Ant. Arg. Ars. Bar-c. Calc. Carb-veg. Caust. Chelid. Clem. Creos. Dig. Graph. Grat. Iris. Kobalt. Mgn-c. Mgn-m. Meny. Mez. Ntr-c. Nux. Phosp. Phyt. *Sabad.* Sass. Scill. Seneg. Spong. Stann. *Staph.* Stront. *Sulph-ac.* Tabac. Thuj. Tong. Verat. Verb. Zinc.
— — morning, Sass.
— — evening, Stann.
Sand in throat, sensation of, Cist.
Scraping in throat, Acon. Aloe. Alum. *Ambr.* Amm-c. Anac. Ant. Arg. Ars. Bell. Berb. Bov. Brom. Bry. Carb-an. *Carb-veg.* Caust. Chelid. Chenop. Chin-sulph. Cocc-c. Con. Creos. *Croc.* Croton. Cycl. Dig. Dros. Euphr. *Graph.* Grat. *Hep.* Hyosc. Iod. Kali-b. Kali-c. Kalm. Lob. Mgn-c. Mang. Meny. Mez. Ntr-c. Nitr-ac. Nux. *Ol-an.* Ox-ac. *Par.* Petr. *Phosp.* Phosp-ac. Plat.Pod.Ran-b. Ran-sc. *Sabad.* Sass. Scill. Seneg. Sep. Stann. Staph. Stront. Sulph. Tabac. *Teucr.* Thuj. Tong. Valer. Verat. Zinc.
— before and after, not during meals, Croc.
— in evening, Stann.
— morning, Chin-sulph. Sass.
Smarting-itching, Bar-c. Carb-veg. Cist. Kali-b. Merc. Mez. Mur-ac. Phosp. Phosp-ac. Puls. Teucr. Zinc.
Softness, sensation of, Cist.
Soreness, rawness, Alum. Ambr. Amm-c. *Arg.* Ars. Asa-f. Bell. *Bry.* Calc. Camph. Carb-an. Carb-veg. Caust. Cist. Cor-r. Creos. Dig. Gels. Gum-gut. Igt. Ip. Kali-c. Kobalt. Lach. Lith. Lob. Lyc. Mgn-c. Mgn-m. Mgn-s. Mang. Merc. Mez. Mur-ac. Ntr-m. *Nitr-ac.* Nux. Petr. Phosp. Phosp-ac. Plat. *Puls.* Ruta. Seneg. Sep. Sil. Stann. Staph. Sulph. *Thuj. Zinc.*
— — of oesophagus, Merc.
— — uvula, Lact.
— — with short cough, Lachn.
— — in scarlet fever, Hipp-m.
Spasm in oesoph., *Bell. Calc.* Coloc. *Con.* Graph. Hydroc-ac. Lach. Laur. Ntr-m. Nicc. Phosp. *Plat.* Ran-b. Sass. *Stram.* Sulph. Zinc.
— with eructation and palpitation of heart, Coloc.
Spasmodic pains, Alum.
As from splinters, pain, Arg-n. Dolich. Hep. Nitr-ac.
Stinging, stitches, in throat, *Acon.* Aeth. Alum. Amm-c. *Amm-m.* Apis. Arn.

11. FAUCES, PHARYNX AND OESOPHAGUS.

Asar. Aur. Bar-c. *Bell.* Berb. Bov. *Bry.*
Calc. Carb-an. Caust. *Chin.* Cist. Cupr.
Dig. Dros. Ferr-m. Graph. Gum-gut.
Gymnoc. Hep. Hipp-m. *Igt.* Ip. Kali-b.
Kali-c. Kali-jod. *Lach.* Laur. *Led.* Lyc.
Mgn-c. Mgn-s. Mang. Meny. *Merc.*
Merc-cor. Mez. Ntr-c. *Ntr-m.* Nicc.
Nitr-ac. Nitr. Nux-m. Nux. Par. *Petr.*
Phell. Phosp-ac. Pod. *Puls. Rhus.*
Sabin. Sass. *Sep.* Sil. Spig. Spong. Stann.
Staph. Stram. *Sulph.* Sulph-ac. Tar.
Teucr. Thuj.
Stinging in tonsils, *Bell. Merc. Ran-sc.* Raph.
— in left tonsil towards ear, relieved by swallowing, Kali-b.
— — side, Grat.
— to ears extending, Hep.
— between the acts of swallowing, Aeth. Igt.
Squeezing in oesoph., Alum.
Swallowing, difficult, Acon. Aeth. Alum.
Ambr. Amm-c. Apis. Arg. *Arum.* Bar-m.
Bell. Bry. Canth. Caust. Chelid. Cina.
Cocc. Croton. Dros. Elaps. Fluor-ac.
Gels. Grat. Hep. Hyosc. *Igt.* Iod. Ip.
Jac-c. Kali-c. Lyc. Meny. Merc. Nux-m.
Nux. Op. Phosp. Puls. Rhus. Sil.
Stram. Sulph.
— impeded, Ambr. Amm-c. Ang. Ant.
Arn. Ars. Bell. Bufo. Cact. *Canth.*
Carb-veg. Cic. *Cina.* Con. Cupr. Elaps.
Hep. Hipp-m. *Hyosc.* Iod. Kali-c. Lach.
Laur. Lob. Lyc. *Ntr-s. Op.* Plb. *Stram.*
Sulph.
— — of food, Dros. Rhus.
— — — when lying, Cham.
— — liquids, Bell. Canth. Cic. Cina.
Hyosc. Igt. Merc-cor.
— — by nausea, Arn. Merc-cor.
—, imagines he cannot, Hydroph.
— inability to, with hoarseness, Acon.
Bell. Phosp.
— incomplete, Bell. Merc. Petr. Sil.
— painless inability, Canth.
— with a rattling noise, Arn. Cina. Cupr.
Laur. Thuj.
— — cracking noise, Caust.
— food descends slowly and gets in lahrynx, Kali-c.
When swallowing, pain, Acon. *Alum.*
Amm-m. Arg. Ars. Arum-trif. Asa-f.
Bar-c. Bell. Bry. Calc. Camph. *Canth.*
Caps. Carb-an. Carb-veg. Casc. Caust.
Cham. Chin. Cinnab. Cor-r. Dros. Ferr.
Graph. Hœmatox. Hell. Hep. Igt. Ip.
Kali-c. Kali-jod. Laur. Led. Lyc. Mgn-s.
Mang. Meny. Merc. Mez. *Ntr-m.* Ntr-s.
Nicc. Nitr. Nux. Ol-an. Ox-ac. Petr.
Phosp-ac. Puls. Rhus. Ruta. Sabad.
Sabin. Sang. Sass. Sep. Sil. Staph.
Stront. *Sulph.* Sulph-ac. *Thuj.* Verat.
— — saliva, pain, Bry. Cinnab. Hep. *Lach.*
Merc. Merc-jod. Phell. Plat. Rat.

Rhus. Ruta. Thuj. Zinc.
— — food, Ambr. Dros. Lach. Phosp-ac.
— — stitches, Aeth. Alum. Amm-m. Bar-c.
Bell. Bov. Bry. Calc. Caust. Cham.
Graph. Hep. Lach. Merc. Ntr-m.
Rhus. Sulph.
— — cutting as of knives, Stann.
— — itching in a small spot—left side, Lachn.
— — pain shooting up, eustachian tube. Gels.
— — — at root of tongue, Phyt.
— not swallowing, pain, Arn. Cina. Grat.
Igt. Iod. Lac-can. Laur. Led. *Mang.*
Nux. Phell. Plat. Puls. Sabad. Sulph.
Thuj. Zinc.
On empty swallowing, cough, Ntr-m.
— — sensation as of swallowing a piece of meat, Sabad. Sulph.
To swallow, disposition to, Alum. Arum.
Bell. Cact. Caust. Cinnab. Cist. Cocc-c.
Con. Græt. Hœmatox. Hydroph. Ip.
Kobalt. Lach. *Merc.* Merc-jod. Ntr-s,
Nux-m. Phyt. Plb. Sabad. Seneg. Staph.
Tilia.
— — when speaking, Staph.
— — with danger of suffocation, Bell.
— — when walking in the wind, *Con.*
Swallowing involuntarily, Con.
Swelling in the throat, Amm-c. Amm-m.
Bell. Berb. Calc. Cinnab. Cocc-c. Lach.
Ntr-m. Nitr-ac. Nux. Op. Petr. Poth.
Seneg. Sep. Spig. Thuj. Verat.
— of uvula, Bar-m. Bell. Calc. Carb-veg.
Chin. Coff. Iod. Merc. Ntr-s. *Nux.* Par.
Phosp. Phosp-ac. *Seneg.* Sil. Sulph.
Tilia.
— sensation of, *Arg.* Ars. Bell. Benz-ac.
Bry. Calc. Carb-veg. Casc. Caust. Chin.
Coff. Colch. Gum-gut. Hep. Igt. Ip.
Kalm. Lac-can. Lach. Merc. Nitr-ac.
Nux. *Plb.* Puls. Rhus. Sabad. *Sabin.*
Sang. Stann. Sulph. Tar. Verat.
Tension, Asa-f. *Chelid.* Nitr. Nux. Puls.
Sep. Stann.
Tickling, Chin-sulph. Cist. Croton. Lach.
Nitr-ac. Nitr. Petr.
Tingling, creeping, Acon. Colch. Glon.
Grat. Lob. Pallad. Samb. *Sec-c.*
Tonsils indurated, Igt. Plb.
— inflamed, Bar-c. *Bell.* Berb. *Canth.* Cham.
Hipp-m. Igt. Lach. Ntr-s. Plb. Puls.
Sep.
— suppurating, Aur. Bar-c. *Bell. Canth.*
Hipp-m. Igt. Lyc. Merc. Merc-cor. Sep.
— swollen, Alum. Amm-c. Aur. *Bar-c.*
Bell. Berb. Calc. Canth. Cham. Croton.
Graph. *Hep.* Igt. Lach. Lyc. Merc.
Merc-cor. Ntr-s. Nicc. Nitr-ac. Nux.
Phosp. Phyt. Puls. Ran-sc. Raph. Sep.
Stann. Staph. Sulph. Thuj.
— swollen, right side, Bell. Lac-can. Lyc.
Phyt. Sabad. Spong.

11. FAUCES, PHARYNX AND OESOPHAGUS. 85

Tonsils, swollen left side, Apis. Bar-c. Lac-can. Lach. Sulph.
— ulcerated, Bar-c. Bell. Hep. Igt. Lyc. Merc. Merc-cor. Merc-jod. Sep.
Torn, as if, Caust.
Twisting sense in throat, Hyper. Op.
Ulcers in throat, Arg. Bell. Calc. Creos. Dros. Igt. *Iod.* Kali-b. Lach. Lyc. *Merc.* Millef. Ntr-m. *Nitr-ac.* Nux. Sacch. Sang. Thuj. Vinca.
— on velum palati, Croc.
— chancre-like, Creos. Lyc.
— mercurial, *Iod.* Lyc. *Nitr-ac.*
— shining, glistening, Lac-can.
— stinging painful, Kali-b. Lac-can. *Merc.* Nitr-ac.
— on tonsils, Aur. Igt. Lach. Lyc.
— irregular, gray-white, Lac-can. Merc-jod.
— when scarlet fever does not come out, Apis.
— white, yellowish, burning ulcers, Hipp-m.
Ulcerous pain in throat, Kali-jod.
Uvula redness, Calc. Puls.
Veins distended in throat, Puls.
Viscid throat, Sep.
To the ears, pain extending, Bell. Hep. Igt. Lach. Merc. Nux.
— glands of neck, Sep.
— — submaxillary, Merc,
To the gums, pain extending, Lach.
— larynx, Lach.
In the morning. pain in throat, Amm-c. Berb. Calc-ph. Chin-sulph. Cist. Nicc.
— — forenoon, pain relieved, Alum.
— — evening, pain, Alum. Lact. Mgn-m. Nicc. Puls. Sulph-ac. Viol-tr.
At night, Alum. Amm-m. Camph. Canth. Graph. Mgn-m. Mgn-s. Merc. Nitr.
When blowing the nose, pain, Carb-veg.
From brandy, pain, Rhus.
— eating bread, pain increased, Ran-sc.
When breathing, pain, Arg. Hep.
From a cold, pain in throat, Bar-c. Cham. Dulc.
— cold air inhaled, pain, Cist. *Merc.* Nux.
When coughing, Acon. Arg. Carb-veg. Hep.
From draft of air, Chin.
While eating, pain in throat, Aloe. Plb.

— — — relieved, Benz-ac. Lach.
— — warm food, Alum. Lach. Sil. Sulph.
After eating, pain, Ambr. Ars. Laur.
— — relieved, Cist.
From every emotion, pain, Cist.
When exerting one's self, pain, Caust.
— putting out the tongue, pain, Kali-b.
— speaking, Acon. Bell. Berb. Calc. Dros. Mgn-c. Merc. Nicc. Rhus. Staph.
— swallowing, Acon. Alum. Amm-m. Arg. Ars. Asa-f. Aur. Bar-c. Bell. Berb. Bry. Calc. Calc-ph. Camph. Canth. Caps. Carb-veg. Casc. Caust. Cham. Chin. Cocc. Coff. Cor-r. Creos. Croc. Dros. Ferr. Graph. Hell. Hep. Ip. Kali-c. Kali-jod. Lach. Laur. Led. Lyc. Mgn-c. Mgn-s. Mang. Merc. Mez. Ntr-m. Nicc. Nitr-ac. Nux. Ol-an. Petr. Phosp-ac. Plb. Puls. Rhus. Ruta. Sabad. Sabin. Sass. Sep. Sil. Staph. Stront. Sulph. Thuj. Verat.
— food, Ambr. Bar-c. Bry. Dros. *Hep.* Nitr-ac. Nux. Petr. Phosp. Phosp-ac. Rhus. Sep. *Sulph.*
— saliva only, Bry. *Cinnab.* Cocc. Hep. *Lach.* Phell. Plat. Puls. Rat. Rhus. Ruta. Zinc.
After swallowing, pain, Ambr. Bry. *Nux.* Phosp. Puls. Rhus. Sulph. *Zinc.*
— — relieved, Cist. Igt.
Empty swallowing, pain, Lach. Merc.
Between the acts of swallowing pain, Aeth. Caps. Grat. Igt. Mgn-s. Mang.
When swallowing pain between shoulders, Rhus.
— — — worse after sleeping, Lach.
— touched, pain in throat, Bell. Bry. Gum-gut. Lac-can. Lach. Mez. Nicc. Phyt. Spong. Teucr. Zinc.
— when turning the head, pain in throat, Bry. Hep.
From lifting, pain in throat, Calc.
With swelling of external glands, Sep.
— headache, Bell. Lac-can.
— deafness, Gels.
— dyspnœa, Lach. Merc.
— salivation, Lach. Merc.
— swelling of right side of face, Nicc.
— thirst at night, Lyc.
— yawning, Aloe. Nicc.

12. Appetite and Taste.

HUNGER AND THIRST.

After taste of food long, Ntr-m. *Phosp-ac.* Sil.
— — — beer, Sulph.
— — — bread, *Phosp-ac.*
— — — milk, Igt.
— — — acids, Ntr-m.
Appetite changing, Alum.
— increased, Alum. Amm-c. Ang. *Arg.* Berb. Bry. Coff. *Eugen.* Gels. Iod. Lact. Merc. Nux-m. Ox-ac. Par. *Sep.* Tart. Teucr.
— — excessively, Berb. *Ntr-m.* *Nux-m.* *Sulph.*
— — at noon, Lact. Mez. Ntr-m. Nux-m.
— — in evening, Arn. Mez. Ntr-m. *Nitr.*
— — while eating, Chin. Merc.
— — with sense of fulness in stomach, Arg.
— — — desire for coition, Cinnab.
— — feels better after eating a good deal, Iod.
— loss of, sudden while eating, Arg. Caust. Colch. Iod. *Lyc.* Mgn-s. Plat *Rheum.* Ruta. Tart. (compare Satiety.) .
— wanting, Acon. All-cep. Aloe. Alum. Ambr. Amm-m. Anac. *Ant.* Arn. Ars. Aur. *Bar-c.* Bar-m. Bell. Berb. Borax. *Bruc.* Bry. Calc. Canth. Carb-veg. Cham. Chelid. Chin. Cic. Cinnab. Cocc. Colch. Coloc. *Con.* Cop. Cor-r. Croton. *Cycl.* Dig. Fluor-ac. Guaj. Gum-gut. Hep. Hyosc. Igt. Iod. Iris. Kali-b. Lach. Lact. Laur. Led. Lith. *Lyc.* Mgn-c. Mgn-s. Merc. Murex. Nicc. *Ntr-m.* Nitr-ac. Nitr. Nux. Oleand. Ol-an. Petr. Phosp. Plat. *Plb.* Pod. Puls. Ran-sc. Rat. *Rhus.* Ruta. Sabad. Sang. Scill. Sec-c. *Seneg.* Senna. Sep. Sil. *Spig.* Spong. Stront. Stram. Sulph. Sulph-ac. Tabac. Tart. Tereb. Thromb. Thuj. Verat. Viol-tr. Zinc.
— — in the morning, Cycl. Lach. Selen. *Seneg.*
— — — evening, Cycl.
— — from fulness, sense of, *Chin.* Phosp. Rhus.
— — — sadness, Plat.
— wanting with clean tongue, Dig. Laur.

— — — dryness in mouth, Cic.
— — — hunger, Agar. Alum. Ars. Bar-c. Bry. Chin. Dulc. Hell. Mgn-m. Ntr-m. Op. Rhus. Sil. Sulph-ac.
— — — nausea, *Ant.* Con.
— — — thirst, Amm-c. Ars. Borax. *Calc.* Creos. *Nitr.* Nux. Phosp. Rhus. Sep. Sil. *Spig.* Sulph. Tart. Zinc-ox.
— — easily satisfied with little food, Gels. Prun.
Aversion to acids, Bell, *Cocc.* Ferr. Igt. Nux. Phosp-ac. Sabad. *Sulph.*
— — beer, Asa-f. Cham. Chin. Clem. Cocc. Croton. Ferr. Nux. Phosp. Rhus. Stann. Sulph.
— — brandy, Igt. Merc. Rhus.
— — bread, Agar. Con. Cycl. Hipp-m. Kali-c. Lach. Lact. Lyc. Mgn-c. Meny. *Ntr-m.* Nitr-ac. Nux. Phosp-ac. Puls. *Rhus.* *Sulph.*
— — — brown, Kali-c.
— — — white, Chenop.
— — — and butter, Cycl.
— — broth, Arn. Ars. Bell. Cham. Graph. Rhus.
— — butter, Ars. Carb-veg. Chin. Cycl. Meny. Petr. Puls.
— — cheese, Chelid. Oleand.
— — coffee, Bell. Bry. Calc. Cham. Chin. Coff. Fluor-ac. Lyc. Merc. Ntr-c. Ntr-m. Nitr. Nux. Phosp. Rheum. Rhus. Spig.
— — — without sugar, Rheum.
— — cold food, Cycl.
— — eggs, Ferr.
— — fish, Colch. Graph. Zinc.
— — — herrings, Phosp.
— — flour, Phosp-ac.
— — food in general, Acon. Ang. Ant. Arg. Ars. Aur. Bell. *Bry.* *Canth.* Cham. *Chin.* Cinnab. Cocc. Colch. Dulc. *Grat.* Guaj. *Hell.* *Igt. Ip.* Kali-b. Kali-c. Kali-jod. Lact. Laur. *Mgn-s.* Mang. *Merc.* Ntr-m. Ntr-s. *Nux.* Oleand. Ol-an. *Op. Plat.* Prun. *Puls.* Rat. *Rhus.* Sabad. Scill. Sep. Sil. Stront. Sulph. *Tart.* Thea.

12. APPETITE AND TASTE.

Aversion to fruit, Bar-c.
— — liquids, Agn. Arn. *Bell. Canth. Chin.* Cocc. Hyosc. Igt. Lach. Merc. Nux. Rat. *Samb. Stram.*
— — meal and flour and dishes made of it, Ars. Phosp.
— — meat, Aloe. Alum. Arn. Ars. Aur. Bell. *Calc. Carb-veg.* Chenop. Ferr. Graph. Hell. Hipp-m. Igt. Lact. Lyc. Mgn-c. Mgn-s. Merc. Mez. *Mur-ac.* Nicc. Nitr-ac. *Ol-an. Petr.* Plat. Puls. *Rhus. Sabad.* Sep. *Sil.* Sulph. Tereb. Zinc.
— — — boiled, Chelid. Nitr-ac.
— — milk, Aeth. Amm-c. Bell. Bry. Calc. Carb-veg. Cina. Guaj. *Igt.* Ntr-c. Nux. Puls. Sulph. Tart.
— — mother's milk, Cina. Lach. Merc. Sil. Stann.
— — pork, Ang. *Colch.* Dros. *Psor.*
— — potatoes, Thuj.
— — puddings, Ars. Phosp.
— — rich (fat) food, Ang. Bry. Carb-an. Carb-veg. Colch. Cycl. Hep. Ntr-m. Petr. Puls. Rheum. Sulph.
— — salt food, Carb-veg. Graph. Selen.
— — solid food, Ang. Bapt. Ferr. Merc. Staph.
— — sweetmeats, Ars. Caust. Graph. Hipp-m. Merc. Nitr-ac. Phosp. Sulph. Zinc.
— — tobacco, Arn. Brom. *Calc.* Camph. Canth. Carb-an. Cocc. *Igt.* Lach. Lyc. Meph. Ntr-m. Nux. Puls. Spig. Tar. Tart.
— — — snuffing, Spig.
— — veal, *Zinc.*
— — vegetables, Bell. Hell. Mgn-c.
— — warm, cooked food, Bell. Calc. Cupr. Graph. Igt. Lach. Lyc. Mgn-c. Merc. Petr. Sil. Verat. Zinc.
— — — —, cannot eat or drink anything hot, Ferr.
— — cold water, Bell. Bry. *Calad.* Canth. Caust. Chelid. Chin. Hydroph. Ntr-m. Nux. *Phell. Stram.* Tabac.
— — wine, Igt. Hipp-m. Lach. Merc. Nux-jug. Rhus. Sabad. Sulph.
Cold in stomach from ice-cream, fruits, water, etc., Ars. *Puls.*
Dainty, *Chin.* Mgn-m. Ntr-c. Rhus.
Desire for acids (compare Sour).
— almonds, Cub.
— apples, Aloe.
— beer, Acon. Aloe. Bry. Caust. Chin. *Cocc.* Kali-b. Lach. Merc. Ntr-c. Nux. Op. Petr. *Phell.* Phosp-ac. *Puls.* Sabad. Spig. Stram. Stront. Sulph.
— bitter drinks, Ntr-m.
— — food, *Dig.* Ntr-m.
— brandy, Ars. Cub. Hep. Lach. Nux. Op. Selen. Sep. Sulph.

— bread, Ars. Ntr-m. Plb. Puls. Stront.
— —, wheat, Aur.
— — and butter, Ferr. Mgn-c.
— butter, Merc.
— cakes, Plb.
— charcoal, Alum. *Cic.* Nitr-ac. Nux.
— cheese, Igt.
— cherries, Chin.
— chocolate, Hydroph.
— cloves, Alum.
— coffee, *Ang.* Arg. Ars. Aur. Bry. Caps. Carb-veg. Cham. Chin. Colch. Con. Selen.
— ground or burned, Alum.
— cold drinks, Amm-c. *Ang.* Ars. Aur. *Bov.* Bry. Calc. Caust. Cham. Chin. Clem. Cocc. Dulc. Euph. Led. *Merc.* Ntr-m. Ntr-s. Nitr. *Oleand.* Phosp. Phosp-ac. Plb. Psor. Rhus. Ruta. *Sabad.* Spig. Sulph. Tart. Thuj. *Verat.*
— — food, Cupr. Sil. Thuj. *Verat.*
— cucumbers, Ant. Verat.
— delicacies, Calc. Chin. Cub. Ip. Petr. Rhus. Sang.
— earth chalk, lime, Nitr-ac. Nux.
— eggs, soft boiled, Calc. Ol-an.
— farinaceous food, Sabad.
— fat, Nitr-ac. Nux.
— ham-fat, Mez.
— fried food, Plb.
— fruits, Aloe. Alum. Chin. Cub. Igt. Mgn-c. Phosp-ac. Sulph-ac. Tart. Verat.
— — acid, Chin.
— herrings, Nitr-ac. Verat.
— honey, Sabad. (compare Sweet).
— hot drinks, Chelid. Casc.
— indigestible things, Alum. Bry.
— indistinct, Bry. *Chin.* Igt. *Mgn-m.* Puls. Sang. Therid.
— juicy things, Aloe. Phosp-ac.
— lemonade, Bell. Sabin. Sec-c.
— liquid food, Ang. Ferr. Merc. Staph. Sulph. Verat.
— for many things, which become repugnant when little is eaten, Rheum.
— meal and flour, Lach. Sabad.
— meat, Hell. Mgn-c. Meny. Merc. Sulph.
— milk, Ars. Aur. Bapt. Bry. Calc. Chelid. Merc. Phell. Phosp-ac. Rhus. Sabad. Sil. Staph. Stront. Sulph.
— — cold, Phell. Phosp-ac. Rhus. Sabad. Staph.
— nuts, Cub.
— onions, Cub.
— oranges, Cub.
— oysters, Apis. Lach. Rhus.
— pastry, Plb.
— pickles, Hep. Staph.
— puddings, Sabad.

12. APPETITE AND TASTE.

Desire for raw potatoes and flour, Calc.
— rags, clean, Alum.
— refreshing things, Caust. Cocc. Phosp. Phosp-ac. Puls. Sang. Tilia. Verat.
— rice, dry, Alum.
— salt things, Calc. Carb-veg. Caust. Con. Cor-r. Meph. Merc-jod. Ntr-m. Nitr-ac. Thuj. Verat.
— seasoned highly, Fluor-ac, Hep.
— smoked things, Caust.
— sour-kraut, Carb-an. Cham.
— sour drinks, Ant. Borax. Bry. Cham. Dig. Hep. Phell. Plb. Scill. Verat.
— — food, Alum. Amm-c. Ant. Arn. Ars. Bell. Borax. Brom. Bry. Carb-veg. Cham. Chin. Cist. Con. Cor-r. Cub. Dig. Ferr. Hep. Hipp. Igt. Kali-b. Kali-c. Lach. Mgn-c. Merc-jod. Phell. Phosp. Pod. Puls. Sabin. Sacch. Scill. Sec-c. Sep. Stram. Sulph. *Tart.* Therid. *Verat.*
— spirituous liquors, Amm-c. Arn. Ars. Cupr. Puls. Staph. Sulph.
— starch, Alum. Nitr-ac.
— sweet things, Amm-c. Arg. Calc. Carb-veg. Chin. Ip. Kali-c. Lyc. Mgn-m. Merc. Ntr-c. Rheum. Rhus. Sabad. Sulph.
— — tea, Hep.
— — grounds, Alum.
— tobacco, Daph. Eugen. Staph. Therid.
— vegetables, Alum. Mgn-c.
— vinegar, Arn. (compare Sour).
— warm food, Ang. Chelid. Cupr. Cycl. Ferr.
— water, cold, Arn. Ars. Bell. Calc. Cop. Led. Mgn-c. Merc. Ntr-c. Oleand. Phosp. Plat. Plb. Rhus. Ruta. Sabad. Sass. Scill. Thuj.
— whiskey, Acon. Arn. *Ars.* Calc. Chin. Cub. Fluor-ac. Hep. *Lach.* Merc. Nux. Op. Puls. *Selen. Spig.* Staph. Sulph. Therid.
— wine, Acon. Arg. Bry. Calc. Chelid. Chin. Cic. Cub. Fluor-ac. Hep. Lach. Merc. Sep. Spig. Staph. *Sulph.* Therid.

Eat, constant desire to, Rat.
Hasty eating, Calad. Coff. Cupr. Plat. (compare Voracity).
Hunger increased, Amm-c. Ang. Ant. Arg. *Aur.* Bov. Calc. Chin. Chin-sulph. Cina. Coff. Dulc. Fluor-ac. Graph. Grat. *Hell. Iod.* Laur. Lyc. *Mgn-m.* Merc. Mez. *Ntr-c.* Nux-m. Nux. Oleand. Phosp. Phyt. Plb. Puls. Rheum. *Sabad.* Sec-c. Sep. *Spong.* Stann. Staph. Stront. Tabac. *Teucr.* Thea. Verat.
— constant, Bov. Merc. Rat. Tabac.

— excessive, Coff. *Graph.* Lyc. Merc-ac. Ntr-c. *Nux-m.* Verat.
— greedy, *Bell, Oleand.*
— insatiable, Ang. Ant. Arg. *Sec-c. Spong.* Stann. Staph. *Zinc.* (compare Voracity.)
— strong, Amm-c. Aur. Meny.
— tormenting, Arg. Bell. Seneg.
— in morning, Ant. Teucr.
— — forenoon. Hep. Ntr-c.
— at noon, Mez. Nux-m.
— in evening, Guaj. Mez. Nitr. Teucr.
— at night, Selen.
— after meals, Bov. Calc. Cic. Cina. Grat. Kali-chl. Merc. Par. Phosp. Plb. Staph. Stront.
— with aversion to food, Agar. Ang. Bry. Calc. Caust. Cham. Dulc. Grat. Hell. Lyc. Ntr-m. Ntr-nitr. Nicc. Nux. Op. Phosp. Rheum. Rhus. Sabad. Spig.
— — acidity of stomach, Graph.
— — colic, Cocc-c.
— — nausea, *Hell.* Mgn-m. Ntr-c. Oleand. Phosp. Tabac.
— — inability to swallow, Hyosc.
— — thirst and dryness of throat, Cycl.
— — — and flow of urine, Verat.
— — vomiting and diarrhoea, Verat.
— — water collected in mouth, Thea.
— as if stomach were empty, no appetite, Ntr-m.
— ravenous, *Agar.* Alum. Amm-c. Ang. Arn. Asa-f. Aur. Bell. Berb. Bry. Calc. Caps. Carb-veg. Casc. Caust. Chin. *Cina.* Cinnab. Cocc. Cocc-c. Coloc. Con. Croc. Dros. Elaps. Graph. Hell. Hep. *Hyosc.* Igt. *Iod.* Kali-c. Kali-chl. Lac-can. *Lyc.* Meny. Mgn-m. *Merc.* Mur. *Ntr-m.* Nitr-ac. Nitr. Nux-m. *Nux. Oleand.* Op. *Petr.* Phosp. Plat. Puls. Rhus. *Sabad. Scill.* Sec-c. Sep. *Sil. Spig.* Stann. Staph. Stront. *Sulph.* Sulph-ac. Valer. *Verat.* Zinc.
— — in morning, Ant. Calc. Sabad.
— — 10-11 A. M., Sulph.
— — forenoon, Ntr-c.
— — noon, Mez. Nux-m.
— — afternoon, Nux.
— — in evening, Agar. Aloe. Mez. Sabad. Teucr.
— — at night, Bry. *Chin.* Phosp. Selen. Sulph.
— — after meals, Bov. Calc. Chin-sulph. Cic. Cina. Lach. Merc. Phosp. Plb. Stront.
— — — beer drinking, Nux.
— — by cold water relieved, Kali-chl.
— — in open air relieved, Tart.
— — with abdomen, rumbling in, Sulph-ac.
— — with want of appetite, Bry. Ferr. Iod. Lach. Ntr-m. Oleand. Op. Sil.
— — — aversion to eat, Ang. Dulc. *Hell.* Nux. *Op.* Rheum. Sabad.
— — — alternating with, Caps.

12. APPETITE AND TASTE.

Hunger ravenous with colic, Cocc-c.
— — with dispising humor, Plat.
— — — disgust for life, Nitr-ac.
— — — emptiness, sense of in stomach, Arn. Igt. Sep.
— flushes of heat, Bry.
— — fulness of stomach, Asar. Staph.
— — headache, Sulph.
— — — if not satisfied, Lyc.
— — nausea, Hell. Lach. Mgn-m. Ntr-c. Oleand. Phosp. Spig. Tabac. Valer.
— — pain in stomach, Lach. Puls.
— — soon satisfied, Ntr-m.
— — taste disagreeable, Chin.
— — with thirst, Bry. Hyosc. Spig. Verat.
— — — trembling, from longing for food, Oleand.
— — vomiting, Chin. Hell.
— — weakness, Lach. Merc. Phosp. Sulph.
— — — — and fainting if hunger is not soon satisfied, Phosp.
— — yawning, Lach.
— — during an attack of gout, Ph.
— sense of in stomach, Ant. Asar. Aur. Ind. Millef. Nicc. Plat. Seneg. Stann.
— wanting, Amm-c. Ars. Caps. Cham Cic. Lach. Tabac. (compare Appetite wanting).
Indigestion, *Anac. Bar-c. Calc. Carb-an.* Carb-veg. Chin. *Graph.* Hep. Igt. Iod. Lach. Lyc. *Merc. Ntr-c. Nux-m.* Op. Par. Petr. Scill. Sep. Spong. Stann. *Sulph.* Valer. Zing.
Loathing during meals, Ars. Bell. Bry. Canth. Caust. Cham. Colch. Cycl. Ol-an. Sass. Tart.
Relish, of tobacco, Coff. Eugen.
— none until the first mouthful is taken, Sabad.
— of food too strong, Camph.
— — broth, Caps.
Satiety, sudden during meals, Amm-c. Ars. *Bar-c.* Bry. Cic. Colch. Con. Croc. Cycl. Igt. Led. Lyc. Merc. *Ntr-m.* Nux-m. Prun. *Rhod.* Spong. Thea. *Thuj.*
— sense of, Arn. Chin. Clem. Lyc. Mang. Prun. Rhus. Ruta.
Spoiled, stomach, *Ant.* Asa-f. Caust. Hep. *Nux. Puls.*
— by fat or rich food, Asa-f. *Puls.*
— by pastry or pork, *Puls.*
— readily, and often, Hep.
— with nausea and inclination to vomit, Ant.
Taste in mouth and pharynx, acrid, Aur. Berb. Hydroc-ac. Laur. Lob. Rhus.
— — acute, Chin. Coff.
— — like almonds, sweet, Coff. Croton. Dig.
— — — — after smoking, Dig.
— — astringent, Alum. Ars. Brom. Lach.

Mur-ac.
— — bad, Agar. Calc. Iod. Kali-c. Raph. *Sabad.* Selen. Zinc.
— — bitter, *Acon.* Aeth. Aloe. *Amm-c. Amm-m.* Anac. *Ang. Ant.* Arg-n. *Arn.* Ars. Asa-f. *Bar-c. Bell.* Berb. *Bry.* Calc. Calend. *Carb-an. Carb-veg.* Casc. Caust. *Cham.* Chelid. *Chin.* Colch. Coloc. Con. Corn-c. Creos. Croc. Diad. *Dig.* Dros. Dulc. Elat. Euph. Graph. *Grat.* Gum-gut. Hell. Hep. Hipp. Hipp-m. Igt. Iod. Iris. *Kali-c.* Kali-jod. *Lach.* Lact. Led. Lob. *Lyc.* Mgn-c. Mgn-m. Mgn-s. *Merc.* Mez. Ntr-c. *Ntr-m. Nitr-ac. Nux.* Op. Petr. Phosp. Phyt. Plb. Prun. *Puls.* Ran-b. *Rhus. Sabad. Sabin. Sass.* Sep. *Sil.* Spong. Stann. Stram. *Sulph.* Tabac. Tar. *Tart. Verat.*
— of everything, except water, Acon. Stann.
— — — even saliva, Borax.
— in morning, Amm-c. *Amm-m.* Arn. *Bar-c. Bry.* Calc. *Carb-an.* Carb-veg. Cham. Cinnab. Ip. *Lyc.* Mgn-s. Merc. Nicc. Nux. Puls. Rhus. Rumex. Sep. Sil. Sulph.
— — evening, *Amm-c,* Arn. Puls.
— after drinking, Ars. Chin. Puls.
— during meals and while chewing, Dros. *Puls.*
— — only when swallowing food, Creos.
— after meals, Amm-c. Ang. *Ars.* Bry. Creos. Hell. Lyc. Nitr-ac. Phosp. Ran-b. Teucr. Valer,
— especially after swallowing food, Puls. Sil. Sulph.
— — after smoking, Ang.
— — — relieved, Diad.
— — with expectoration of mucus and saliva, Nux.
— — relieved after breakfast, Kali-jod.
— bitterish, sour, Aloe. Petr. Ran-b. Rhus. Sulph.
— — sweet, Kali-jod. Mgn-s. Meny.
— — bloody, Alum. Amm-c. Bell. Berb. Bism. Bov. Ferr. Hipp-m. Ip. Jatr. Rhus. Sabin. Sil. Zinc.
— of blood in mouth before coughing, Elaps.
— chalky, Igt. Nux-m.
— cheese like, Phell. Phosp.
— clammy, Berb. Chin-sulph. Croton. Grat. Nux-m. Prun.
— — in morning, Nicc.
— clay like, Aloe. Chin.
— contracting, Alum.
— coppery, Ang. Cocc. Cupr. Kali-b. Meph. Nitr. Nux.
— as if stomach were deranged, Bar-c. Kali-c.
— earthy, Aloe. Cannab. Chin. *Hep. Nux-m.* Phosp. Puls. Stront.

12. APPETITE AND TASTE.

Taste empyrumatic, Bry. Calad. Cycl. Kali-chl. *Nux*. Phosp-ac. Puls. Ran-b. Sass. Scill. Sulph.
— — during meals, Scill.
— — after dry food, Ran-b.
— fatty, greasy, Alum. Asa-f. Caust. Cham. Cycl. Lyc. Mang. Mur-ac. Ol-an. Petr. Phosp. Puls. Rhus. Sabin. Sil. Thuj. Valer.
— like flour in the morning, Nicc.
— — hazel nuts, Coff.
— herby, Calad. Nux. Phosp-ac. Sass. Stann. Verat.
— like horse radish, Raph.
— like ink, Aloe.
— insipid, Acon. Agar. Ambr. Ant. Ars. Asa-f. Bell. Bruc. *Bry*. Caps. Chelid. Chin. Cor-r. Croton. Cycl. Dig. Dulc. Euph. Euphr. Guaj. Igt. Ip. Iris. Kali-c. Kobalt. Lyc. Mgn-m. Mang. Ntr-m. Nux-m. Oleand. Ol-an. Par. *Petr.* Phosp. Phosp-ac. *Puls*. Ran-b. *Rheum*. Rhus. Sabin. *Staph*. Sulph. Tabac. *Thuj*. Verb.
— — in morning, Rat. Valer.
— — evening, Thuj.
— — after beer, Chin.
— — meals, Thuj.
— like lead, Calc.
— — manure, Sep.
— metalic, Agn. Calc. Chelid. Cocc. Cocc-c. Cupr. Jatr. Hep. Lach. Meph. Merc. Merc-cor. Ran-b. Rhus. Sass. *Seneg*. Zinc.
— milky, Aur.
— like mint, *Verat*.
— mouldy, Led.
— — after hawking up mucus, Teucr.
— nauseous, Lach. Sabad. Selen.
— like nuts, Coff.
— offensive, Agar. Anac. Hydroc-ac. Spig. *Valer*.
— oily, Mang. Sil.
— pappy, Bruc. Graph. Nux-m.
— like pitch, Canth.
— pungent, Verat.
— purulent, Puls.
— putrid, Acon. *Arn*. Ars. Bar-m. Bell. Bov. *Bry*. Calc. Caps. Carb-veg. Caust. *Cham*. Cinnab. Con. Cupr. Cycl. Gels. Graph. Hydroc-ac. Iod. Iris. *Merc*. Mur-ac. *Ntr-m*. Nux. *Petr*. Phosp-ac. Pod. *Puls. Rhus. Sep.* Sil. Spig. *Sulph*. Sulph-ac. Valer. *Verat*. Zinc.
— — in morning, Chin. Nux. Rhus. Sulph.
— — after meals, Rhus.
— — from fauces, even when the food tastes naturally when eating and drinking, Bell.
— — low down in pharynx when hawking up mucus, Nux.
— — after first mouthful, Rhus.
— — like rotten eggs in morning, Amm-c.

Graph. Hep. Phosp. Phosp-ac. Thuj. Taste, rancid, Ambr. Asa-f. Euph. Kali-jod. Mur-ac.
— — after food or drink, Kali-jod.
— saltish, Ars. Bron. *Carb-veg.* Chin. Cupr. Iod. Lyc. *Merc*. Merc-cor. Ntr-c. Nux-m. Nux. Phosp. Puls. Rhus. Sep. Sulph. Therid. Verat. *Zinc*.
— — of water, Brom.
— slimy, mucus, Arn. Bell. Carb-an. Cham. Dig. Kali-c. Lyc. Merc. Ntr-s. Nux. Pallad. Par. *Petr*. Phell. Phosp. Plat. Prun. Puls. *Rheum*. Rhus. Sabin. Sass. Seneg. Sil. Tabac. Zing.
— — in morning, Lyc. Valer.
— — after drinking, Chin.
— soapy, Dulc. Iod.
— sour, Ars. *Bar-c*. Bell. *Calc. Caps*. Carb-an. Cham. *Chin. Cocc*. Con. Croc. Cupr. Graph. Hep. Igt. Iod. Kali-b. Kali-c. Kali-chl. Lach. *Lyc. Mgn-c*. Merc. *Ntr-m. Nitr-ac. Nitr. Nux*. Ol-an. Op. Ox-ac. Petr. *Phosp*. Phosp-ac. Puls. Rheum. Sass. *Sep*. Sil. Stann. *Sulph*. Tabac. Tar. Tart.
— — salt, Cupr.
— — sweet, Croton. Kali-jod. Mgn-s. Meny.
— — in morning, Berb. Lyc. *Nux*. Sulph.
— — with constipation, Lyc.
— — when coughing, Cocc.
— — after drinking, Nux. Sulph.
— — before meals, Bar-c.
— — after meals, Berb. *Carb-veg*. Cocc. Lye. Ntr-m. *Nux. Phosp*. Puls. Sabin. *Sep*. Sil.
— — milk, Ambr. Carb-veg. Lyc. Sulph.
— stale, Bry. Chin. Petr. Puls. Staph. Thuj.
— like sulphuric acid, Plb.
— sulphur, Cocc. Nux.
— sweetish, Acon. Aeth. Alum. Arg-m. Aur. Bry. Cocc-c. Coff. Croc. *Cupr*. Dig. Ferr. Hydroc-ac. Ip. Iod. Kali-b. Kali-jod. Laur. *Merc*. Mur-ac. Nitr-ac. Nux. Phosp. *Plat. Plb*. Puls. Ran-b. *Sabad*. Sass. *Scill*. Seneg. Spong. Stann. *Sulph*. Thuj. Zinc.
— — in morning, Aeth. Ran-sc. Sulph.
— — evening and after meals, Thuj.
— — gonorrhoea, Thuj.
— — after smoking, Selen.
— — drinking water, Phell.
— like tallow, Valer.
— like urine, Seneg.
— wine, Seneg.
— viscous, Calad. Plat.
— watery, Caps. Chin. *Staph*.
Taste, of food and drink,
— bitter, acrid, Rhus.
— —, beer, Ars. Chin. Igt. Merc. Mez. Phell. Puls. Stann.
— —, bread, Ars. *Asar*. Chin-sulph. Cina. Did. Dros. Ferr. Merc.

12. APPETITE AND TASTE.

Nux. Phosp-ac. Puls. Rhus. Sass. Sulph-ac. Thuj.
Taste bitter of butter Puls.
— — coffee and milk, Sabin.
— — liquids, Acon. Ars. *Chin.* Puls.
— — meals, Acon. Ang. Ars. Asar. Borax. *Bry. Camph.* Cham. *Chin.* Coloc. Dig. Dros. Ferr. Igt. Hell. Hep. Lyc. Nitr-ac. Nux. Phosp-ac. Puls. Ran-b. Rheum. *Rhus. Sabin.* Sass. Stann. Staph. Stram. Sulph. Teucr. Valer.
— — meat, Camph. Puls.
— — milk, Puls.
— — tobacco, (smoking), Asar. Camph.
— — wine, Puls.
— like clay, food, Chin.
— coarse, bread, Rhus.
— dry, bread, Phosp-ac. Rhus.
— — food in general, Ferr. Ruta.
— herby, beer, Nux.
— insipid, beer, Ip. Puls.
— — food, Amm-c. Calc. Chin. Cycl, Jac-cor. Oleand. Ruta. Stram.
— metallic, food, Amm-c.
— nauseous, food and meat, Chin-sulph, Scill.
— tobacco smoking, Ip. Poth. Selen.
— pungent, tobacco, Staph.
— putrid, beer, Igt.
— — food, Bar-m. Igt. Mosch.
— — meat, Puls.
— — water, Ntr-m.
— saltish, food, Ars. Bell. Carb-veg. Chin. Puls. Sep. Sulph. Tar.
— — water, Brom.
— sickly, beer, Ip.
— — food, Anac. Ars. Calc. Cycl. Ruta. Thuj.
— slimy, beer, Asa-f.
— smoky, bread, Nux.
— sour, beer, Merc. Puls.
— — bread, *Bell.* Cham. Chin. Cocc. Nitr-ac. Puls. Staph.
— — — wheat, Nux.
— — butter, Puls. Tar.
— — coffee, Chin.
— — food in general, Amm-c. Ars. Calc. Caps. Chin. Jac-cor. Lyc. Nux. Puls. Tabac. Tar.
— — liquids, Chin.
— — meat, Caps. Puls. Tar.
— of straw, Stram. Sulph.
— sweet, beer, Cor-r. Mur-ac. *Puls.*
— — bread, Merc. Puls.
— — butter, Puls.
— — food, Mur-ac. Puls. Scill.
— — meat, Puls. Scill.
— — milk, Puls.
— — tobacco, Selen.
— unsalted, food, Ars. Calc. Cocc. Thuj.
— watery, food, Cupr.
— of wine, water, Tabac.
— acuteness of, Bell. Camph. Coff.

— dulness of, *Rhod.* Sec-c. Seneg. Spong.
— loss of, Alum. Amm-m. *Anac.* Ars. *Bell.* Borax. Bry. Calc. Canth. Hep. Hyosc. Lyc. Mgn-c. Mgn-m. Mercurial. *Ntr-m.* Op. Ox-ac. Phosp. Puls. Rheum. Rhod. Sec-c. *Sil.* Stram. Sulph. *Verat.*
Tastelessness of food, Alum. Ars. Bell. Bry. *Colch. Cor-r.* Dros. Ferr-m. Igt. Kali-b. Kali-jod. Merc. Puls. Rhod. Ruta. Sass. Scill. Seneg. Sil. Staph. *Stram.* Tart. Viol-tr.
— — beer and butter, Puls.
— — coffee and milk, Nux.
— — meat, Alum. Nux. Puls.
Thirst, *Acon.* All-cep. Aloe. Amm-m. *Anac. Ang. Ant.* Arn. *Ars. Aur.* Bapt. Bar-m. *Bell.* Bov. *Bry. Calc.* Camph. Canth. *Cast.* Carb-veg. Caust. Cham. Chenop. *Chin.* Cic. Cina. Clem. *Cocc.* Colch. Coloc. Corn-c. Cor-r. Cupr. Dig. Dros. Dulc. Elaps. Eugen. Euph. Fluor-ac. Grat. Guaj. *Hep.* Hipp-m. Hydroc-ac. Hyosc. Hyper. *Iod.* Kali-b. Kali-jod. Lach. Lachn. Lact. Lam. *Laur.* Led. Lob. *Mgn-c. Mgn-m.* Mgn-s. *Merc.* Merc-cor. Mez. Mur-ac. Nit-c. *Ntr-m. Ntr-s.* Nicc. *Nitr-ac.* Nitr. Nux. Oleand. *Op.* Ox-ac. Petr. *Phell.* Phosp. Phosp-ac. *Plb.* Pod. *Puls.* Rhod. Rhus. *Sabad.* Samb. Sass. Scill. Sec-c. Senna. Sil. *Spig.* Stann. *Stram.* Stront. Sulph. Tart. Therid. Thuj. *Verat.* Verb. Zinc. Zing.
— constant, Aeth. Agar. Aloe. Amm-c. Ars. Bar-c. *Bell. Calc.* Lam. Merc. *Ntr-m.* Sulph.
— vehement, burning, *Acon. Anac.* Ars. *Aur. Bell. Bry. Calc.* Camph. Canth. *Carb-veg.* Caust. Cham. Chin. Colch. Cub. Cupr. *Cast.* Ferr. Graph. Hep. Hyosc. Iod. Jatr. *Laur.* Lyc. Mgn-m. *Merc.* Merc-cor. Merc-jod. Mur-ac. Ntr-c. Nicc. *Nitr. Op.* Phosp-ac. *Plb.* Puls. Raph. Rhus. Scill. *Sec-c. Sil.* Spong. Stann. *Stram.* Sulph. Thuj. Verat. Verb.
— — in ascites or diabites, Acet-ac.
— in morning, Borax. Calc. Carb-an. Dros. Graph. Grat. Mgn-s. *Nitr-ac.* Nux. Plb. Rhus. Sabad. Sass. Sep. Thuj.
— — 3 A.M. Mgn-m.
— afternoon, Berb. Bov. Ran-b. Ruta.
— evening, Amm-c. Bism. Bov. Croc. Mgn-c. Mgn-s. *Ntr-s.* Nicc. Rat. Sep. *Thuj.*
— night, Aloe. Arn. Ars. Bry. Calc. Cham. Cinnab. Coff. Cycl. Fluor-ac. *Mgn-c.* Mgn-m. Nicc. Nitr-ac. Rhus. Sulph. *Thuj.*
— by beer drinking increased, Bry.
— during meals, Aloe. Amm-c. *Cocc.*
— after meals, Aloe. Bell. *Bry.* Graph.
— in phthisis pulmon, Nitr-ac.

12. APPETITE AND TASTE.

Thirst, arrest of breathing when drinking, Anac.
— with loss of appetite, Amm-c. *Calc.* Coloc. *Nitr.* Ox-ac. Rhus. Seneg. Sil. Spig. Sulph. Tart.
— violent when drinking cold water, Jatr.
— with aversion to drink, Amm-c. Arn. *Bell. Canth.* Caust. *Hyosc.* Lach Merc. Ntr-m. Nux. Rhus. Samb. *Stram.*
— — choking sensation when drinking, Scill.
— for cold water, Arn. Bry. Calc. Dulc. Mgn-c.
— — — — without fever, Arn.
— without desire to drink, Ang. Mez.
— — drinking, Graph.
— drinking large quantities, Bad. Bry. Stram. *Verat.*
— — — — often, Bry. Lac-can. Ntr-m.
— — small quantities, *Ars.* Bell. Chin. Hell. Scill.
— — — — often, Acon. Ars. Bell. Chin. Hyosc. Lac-can. Puls.
— with dryness of tongue, Dulc.
— — — in back part of throat, accumulations of saliva in forepart, Mez.
— easily quenched, Caust.
— with heat in mouth, Hyper.
— — inability to swallow, Bell. Canth. Cic. Hyosc. Igt.
— — moist mouth, Stram.
— — nausea, Ntr-m.
— during spasms, Cic.
— with urging to urinate, Cast. Caust. Phosp-ac. Tart. Verat.
— after vomiting, Oleand.
Thirstlessness, Agn. Ambr. Amm-c. Apis. Arg-n. Ars. Bell. Bov. Calad. Camph. Canth. Caps. Chin. Cor-r. Croton. Cycl. Diosc. Dulc. Euph. Ferr. Gels. Hell. Hydroc-ac. Ip. Iris. Lyc. Mang. Meny. Merc. Nux-m. Oleand. Petr. Plat. Puls. Sabad. Samb. Sass. Sep. Spig. Staph. Tabac. Tart. Thuj.
— in dropsy, Apis.
— with inclination to drink, *Ars.* Calad. Cocc. Coloc. Nux-m.
— during meals, Nux-jug.
— with moist tongue, Calad. Hell. Meny. Nux-m. Puls. Sabad.
Voracity, voracious appetite, Chin. Cina. Cupr. Merc. *Mur-ac.* Petr. Scill. *Sep.* Staph. Verat. *Zinc.*
—, desire to eat often and much at a time, Cocc-c.
—, eats too much and too often and looses flesh, Iod.

13. Complaints During and After Meals.

During meals, abdomen distended, Con.
— — — movement and croaking in, Ferr-m.
— — — painful, Ars.
— — anxiety, Carb-veg. Sep.
— — chest, heaviness in, Mgn-m.
— — —, pain in, Led. Ol-an.
— — chilliness, Carb-an. Euph. Ran-sc.
— — cough, Calc.
— — dizziness, Amm-c. Mgn-c. Oleand.
— — eructation, Ntr-c. Nitr-ac. Oleand. Sass.
— — face, heat in, Amm-c.
— — — perspiration, *Ntr-m.*
— — fever, Staph. Tabac.
— — flatulency, Ferr-m.
— — giddiness, Amm-c. Arn. Mgn-c. Mgn-m.
— — head affected, Ntr-s.
— — headache, Graph. Ran-b.
— — — relieved, Phell.
— — hiccough, Mgn-m. Merc. Teucr.
— — hunger, Verat.
— — nausea, Aug. Arg. Bar-c. Bell. *Borax.* Caust. Cic. Cocc. Colch. Dig. Kali-c. Ferr. Mgn-c. Nux. Ruta. Verat.
— — — with retching to vomit, Cocc. Ferr.
— — nose, itching of, Jatr.
— — perspiration, *Carb-an. Carb-veg.* Igt. Ntr-c. Ntr-m. *Nitr-ac.* Ol-an.
— — — on face, Ntr-m. Sulph-ac.
— — — forehead, Nux.
— — feels as if food passed over raw places, Bar-c.
— — pressure in oesophagus, Ars.
— — reeling, Oleand.
— — regurgitation, Merc. Phosp. Sass.
— — risings up from stomach, Phosp.
— — sight obscuration of, Ntr-s.
— — sleepiness, Kali-c.
— — stomach distended, *Con.*
— — — pain in, Ang. Arn. Cic. Con. Sep. Tart. Verat.
— — — — when swallowing food, Bar-c. Nitr-ac. Sep.
— — syncope, Nux.
— — thirst, Aloe. Amm-c. Cocc. Ntr-c.
— — vomiting, Dig. Nitr.
— — —, sudden, Amm-c. Ars. Iod. Rhus. Sep. Sil. Stann. Verat.

After meals, complaints, Bry. Caps. Carb-an. Carb-veg.
— — dinner, Alum. Ars. Igt. Nux. Phosp. Valer. Zinc.
— — abdomen, colic, Coloc. Nux-m.
— — — aching in, Hell.
— — — cramps, hysteric, *Valer.*
— — — cutting, Kali-b. Petr.
— — — distention, Agar. Agn. *Ambr.* Anac. Ant. Arn. *Borax.* Bry. *Calc.* Carb-an. *Carb-veg.* Cast. Caust. Cham. Chin. Con. Croc. Dig. Dulc. *Graph.* Hep. Igt. Kali-c. Lach. Lact. Lyc. Mgn-s. Mang. Merc. Mur-ac. Ntr-c. Ntr-m. Nitr-ac. Nux. Petr. *Phosp.* Phosp-ac. Plat. Puls. Prun. Rhus. *Sep.* Sil. Spong. Sulph. Tabac. Tereb. Thuj. Zinc.
— — — fulness, Agar. Agn. Anac. *Ant.* Aur. *Cast.* Cham. *Chin.* Croc. Graph. Kobalt. Lach. *Lyc.* Mgn-c. Mur-ac. Ntr-m. *Nux.* Phosp-ac. Rhus. *Sil.* Spong. Sulph.
— — — — after eating but little, Bar-c. Cycl. Ntr-m. Rhod. Sulph.Thuj.
— — abdomen pain in, Alum. Ambr. Amm-m. Anac. Ant. Arg. Arn. Ars. Bar-c. Bell. Borax. Bov. Bruc. *Bry.* Calc. Carb-veg. *Cast.* Caust. *Chelid.* Chin. Cic. Coloc. Con. Croton. Dig. Ferr-m. Grat. Kali-c. Igt. *Iod.* Lach. Lob. Lyc. *Nux.* Ol-an. Ox-ac. Petr. Phosp. Plat. Puls. Rhus. Sil. Spong. Staph. *Sulph.* Sulph-ac. Valer. Zinc.
— — — pulsation, *Selen.*
— — — restlessness, Sulph-ac.
— — — rumbling, *Cycl.* Puls. Sep. Zinc.
— — after taste, long, of what has been eaten, Ntr-m. Phosp-ac. Sil.
— — anxiety, Ambr. Asa-f. Canth. Carb-an. Carb-veg. Caust. Chin. Ferr-m. Hyosc. Kali-c. Lach. Mgn-m. Ntr-m. Nitr-ac. Nux. Phosp. Phosp-ac. Sil. Thuj. Viol-tr.
— — anus, pain in, Lyc.
— — aversion to work, *Anac.* Bar-c.
— — bones, pain in, Hell.
— — chest fulness, *Lyc.*
— — — oppression, Asa-f. Cinnab. Lyc. Ntr-s. Nux. *Sulph.* Viol-tr.

13. COMPLAINTS DURING AND AFTER MEALS.

After meals, chest, pain in, Chin. Laur. Phosp. Thuj. Verat.
— — tightness, Carb-an. Puls.
— — chilliness, Asar. Calc. Carb-an. Caust. Kali-c. Nux. Rhus. Sil. Sulph. Tar. Teucr. Zinc.
— — — of feet, Cor-r.
— — coldness, Ran-b.
— — cough, Agar. Anac. Ars. Bell. Bry. Cham. Chin. Dig. Ferr. Kali-b. Kali-c. Laur. Mgn-c. Nux-m. Nux. Op. Puls. Ruta. Staph. Sulph. Tereb. Thuj. Zinc.
— — — spasmodic, Bay.
— — — with vomiting, Anac. Bry. Dig. Tart.
— — — dry, after dinner, Kali-b.
— — dejection, Nux-m. Phosp-ac.
— — disgust, Alum. Ip. Kali-c. Sass.
— — diarrhoea, Aloe. Ars. *Asar.* Brom. Bry. Calc. Carb-veg. Caust. *Chin.* Cist *Coloc.* Con. Corn-c. Croton. *Ferr.* Hep. Lach. Lyc. Mur-ac. Ntr-c. Nux-m. Raph. Rheum. Rhod. Sec-c. Sulph. Sulph-ac. Tabac. Thromb. *Verat.*
— — — (after breakfast,) Alum. Arg-n. Borax. Thuj.
— — — (after dinner,) Alum. Amm-m. Nitr-ac. Nux.
— — — relieved, Arg-n Brom. Diosc. Grat. Hep. Iod. Lith. Lyc. Ntr-c. Nicc. Sang.
— — eructations, Ang. Arg-n. Ars. Bar-c. *Bry.* Calc. Carb-veg. Cham. *Chin.* Con. *Cycl.* Dig. Ferr. Gymnoc. Kali-c. Lach. Merc. Nitr-c. Nitr-ac. Nux-m. Nux. Ox-ac. Petr. *Phosp.* Plat. Puls. Ran-sc. *Sass.* Sep. *Sil.* Spig. *Sulph.* Tar. *Thuj. Verat.* Zinc.
— — — bitter, *Bry. Chin.* Creos. *Sass.*
— — — empty, Ang. Calc. Ntr-c. *Ntr-m. Phosp. Ran-sc.* Rhus. *Sulph. Verat.*
— — — hiccoughing, *Cycl.*
— — — loud, Calc.
— — — scratching, Nux-m.
— — — sour, Bry. Carb-veg. Chin. Creos. Dig. Kali-c. Petr. Sass. Sil. Zinc.
— — — with taste of what has been eaten, Bry. Ran-sc. Sil. Sulph. Thuj.
— — evacuate, desire to, Anac. Ferr-m.
— — face, heat of, Amm-c. Amm-m. Anac. Asa-f. Caust. Cham. Cor-r. Lyc. Nux. Petr. Phyt. Sil. Sulph. Viol-tr.
— — — paleness, Kali-c.
— — — perspiration, Cham. Ntr-s. Viol-tr.
— — — redness, Arum. *Lyc.* Nux. Sil.
— — fever, Asar. Borax. Cham. Dig. Graph. Igt. Lach.
— — fingers, deadness of, Con.
— — flatulency, Aloe. Carb-veg. Con. Ferr-m. Kali-c. Lach. Ntr-s. Nitr-ac.

Nux. Puls. Sulph. Thuj. Zinc.
— — giddiness, vertigo, Cham. Chin. Cor-r. Lach. Mgn-s. Merc. Ntr-s. *Nux.* Petr. Phosp. Phosp-ac. Puls. Rhus. Sulph.
— — — relieved after breakfast, Alum. Cocc.
— — gnawing as from hunger, Grat.
— — hands, hot and burning, Lyc. Phosp. Sulph.
— — headache, Amm-c. Anac. Ant. Arn. Ars. Bruc. Bry. Calc. Carb-an. Carb-veg. Cham. Chin. Cinnab. Cocc. Croton. Graph. Hyosc. Kali-c. Lach. Lyc. Meny. Ntr-s. Nitr-ac. Nux-m. Nux. Pæon. Phosp. Puls. Rhus. Sep. Sil. Sulph. Zinc.
— — —(breakfast) after, Bufo. Lyc.Nux-m.
— — — head cloudiness of, Bell.Cocc. Meny. Ntr-m. Nux. Petr. Phosp-ac.
— — — confusion of, Bell. Lob. Ntr-c. Nux. Sulph.
— — — congestion to, Petr. Sil.
— — — heat of, Lyc. Nux.
— — — pulsation, Clem. Selen.
— — heartburn, *Amm-c. Calc.* Chin. Con. Croc. *Iod.* Lam. Ntr-m. Sep. Sil.
— —, heart, pressure at, Kali-b.
— —, heart, Asa-f. Bell. Calc. Cycl. Ferr-m. Nitr-ac. Phosp. Sep. Viol-tr.
— —, flushes of, Sil.
— — heaviness in body, Lach.
— —, hiccough, Alum. Borax. Bov. Carb-an. *Cycl.* Graph. *Hyosc* Igt. Kobalt. Lyc. Mgn-m. Merc. Ntr-c. Par. Phosp. Sep. Verat. Zinc.
— —hypochondres, pain in, Bry. Mgn-s. Zinc.
— — hypochondriac humor, Anac. Chin. *Ntr-c.* Nux. Zinc.
— — ill humor, Bov. Carb-veg. Cham. Iod. Kali-c. Merc-sulph. Ntr-c. Puls.
— — indolence, Asar. Bar-c. Chin. Lach. Phosp. Thuj.
— — irritability, Amm-m.'Carb-veg. Teucr.
— — laughter, involuntary, Puls.
— — leucorrhoea, Cham.
— — limbs, pain in, as if beaten, Lach. Meph.
— — lower, numbness of, Kali-c.
— — liver, pain in, Bry. Graph. Lyc.
— — loathing, Alum. *Ip.* Kali-c. Sass.
— — melancholy, Puls.
— — mind, fatigue of, Lach.
— — mouth, acidity, Carb-veg. Chin. Mgn-c. Sabin. Sep.
— — —, dryness of, Thea.
— — — odor offensive of, from, Cham. Sulph.
— — nausea, Agar. *Amm-c.* Amm-m. Anac. Ars. Bism. Bry. Calc. Carb-an. Carb-veg. Caust. Cham. Chin. Clem. Con. Cycl. Dig. Elaps.

13. COMPLAINTS DURING AND AFTER MEALS.

Euphr. Graph. Grat. Gymoc. Hell. Igt. Ip. Kali-c. Lach. Laur. Lyc. Mgn-c. Merc. *Ntr-m.* Nitr-rc. Nux. Ol-an. Ox-ac. Petr. Phosp. Plb. Puls. Rheum. *Rhus. Sep.* Sil. *Stann. Sulph.*
After meals, nausea with retching to vomit, Agar. Amm-c. Bism. *Bry. Cham.* Cycl. Graph. Kali-c. Ntr-s. Puls. *Rhus.*
— — palpitation of heart, Bruc. Calc. Camph. Lyc. Ntr-c. Ntr-m. Nitr-ac. Phosp. Sep. Thuj.
— — peevishness, Arn.
— — pulsation in head, Clem. Selen.
— — — rectum, Aloe.
— — pulse, quick or intermittent Ntr-m.
— — regurgitation, Asa-f. Bry. Ferr. Lach. Merc. Nux. Phosp. Puls. Sass. Thuj. Verat.
— — — bitter, Sass. Verat.
— — — sour, Con. Dig. Sass.
— — — into œsophagus, Asa-f.
— — — — of what has just been eaten, Phosp.
— — respiration obstructed, Cham. Viol-tr.
— — — short, Ars. Puls. Nux-m. Zinc.
— — — tight, Carb-an. Lach. Phosp. Puls.
— — sadness, Hyosc.
— — saliva, collected in mouth, Creos. Ntr-s.
— — scrobiculus (pit of stomach) pain in, Agar. Amm-c. Anac. *Bry. Caps. Cham.* Grat. Ntr-c. *Nux. Puls.* Sil. Tereb. Thuj.
— — — pulsation, Sep.
— — sexual irritation, Aloe.
— — shuddering, Rhus.
— — sleepiness, *Acon.* Agar. *Anac. Arum.* Asa-f. *Aur.* Berb. *Bov.* Bufo. Calc. *Chin.* Cic. Cinnab. Clem. Cocc-c. Croc. Cycl. Euph. Graph. Kali-c. Lach. Laur. Meph. Ntr-m. Nitr-ac. Nux-m. *Nux.* Ol-an. Petr. *Phosp.* Phosp-ac. Rat. Rhus. *Ruta.* Sil. *Sulph.* Tabac. *Verb.* Zinc.
— — sluggishness, Asar. Bar-c. Chin. Phosp. Thuj.
— — sourness in stomach, Sabin.
— — — mouth, Carb-veg. Ntr-m.
— — spleen, stitches in, Mgn-s.
— — stomach, cold feeling in, Cist.
— — — cramps. Bism. Bry. *Calc.* Chelid. Chin. Cic. *Cocc. Ferr.* Iod. Kali-c. Nux. Puls. *Sulph.* Tabac.
— — — cutting, Chelid.
— — — distention, Agar. Anac. Bar-c. Caust. Cham. Dig. Dulc. Nux. Sulph-ac.
— — — emptiness, Carb-veg. Oleand. Sass.
— — — fulness, Agar. Anac. Bar-c. Cham. Chin. Gymnoc. Lach. Mosch. Ntr-c. Ntr-m. Nicc. Nitr-ac. Phosp-ac. Rhus. Sil. Zinc.
— — — heaviness, Bar-c. Kali-b. Plb.

— — pain, Acon. Agar. Alum. *Amm-c. Anac.* Ars. Asa-f. *Bar-c.* Bell. Bism. *Bry. Calc.* Calc-ph. Caps. *Carb-veg.* Caust. Cham. *Chin.* Cic. Cist. Cocc. Coloc. Con. Daph. Dig. *Ferr.* Ferr-m. Graph. *Grat.* Gymnoc. Hep. *Iod. Kali-c.* Kobalt. Lach. *Led. Lyc.* Merc. Mosch. *Ntr-c. Nux.* Petr. *Phosp. Phosp-ac. Plat. Plb. Sep.* Sil. *Sulph.* Tabac. Tart. Verat. *Zinc.*
— — — —, especially after supper, Sep.
— — — pressure, Amm-c. Anac. Ars. Bar-c. Bell. Bism. Bruc. Bry. Calc. Carb-veg. Chin. Cocc. Ferr. Grat. Hyper. Iod. Kali-b. Kali-c. Lach. Led. Lyc. Merc. Ntr-c. Nux. Phosp. Plat. Plb. Puls. Rhus. Sep. Sil. Sulph. Zinc.
— — weakness, sinking, as if he would die, Dig.
— — sweat, Benz-ac. Con. Laur. *Nitr-ac.* Sep.
— —, cold, Sulph-ac.
— — swelling of body, sensation of, Cinnab.
— — syncope, Nux. Phosp-ac.
— — taciturnity, Ferr-m.
— — thirst, Aloe. Bell. Bry. Cocc-c. Graph. Ntr-c.
— — throat burning in, Laur.
— — — sensation of pressure, as from food, Amb. Ars.
— — throbbing through the body, Lyc.
— — — in coeliac artery, Cact.
— — tremulous sensation through whole body, *Lyc.*
— — uneasiness, · Bar-c. Chin. Cinnab. Lach. Nux-m. Nux. Phosp-ac. Rhod. Sulph.
— — vomiting, *Amm-c.* Anac. *Ars.* Bry. Calc. Cham. Coloc. Crotal. Cupr. Dig. Dros. Ferr. Graph. Hyosc. *Iod.* Ip. Iris. Lach. Lob. Mgn-c. Nitr-ac. Nux. Phosp. Puls. Ruta. Sec-c. *Sep. Sil. Stann.* Sulph. Tart. *Verat.*
— — — bitter, Mgn-c. Stann.
— — saltish, Mgn-c.
— — — of what has been eaten, *Ars. Calc.* Ferr. Hyosc. Lach. Nux. Phosp. *Puls.* Ruta.
— — — disposition to, Chin. Mgn-c.
— — water-brash, Amm-m. Calc. Chin. Con. Croc. Ind. Kali-c. Lam. Merc. Ntr-m. Nux. Sep. *Sil. Sulph.*
— — weakness, Alum. Anac. Ant. Asar. Calc. Cannab. Chin. Clem. Con. Ferr-m. Lach. Nux-m. Nux. Ox-ac. Phosp. Phosp-ac. Rhus. Sulph. Thuj.
— — weariness, Ferr-m. Lach. Meph.
— — weep, disposition to, Puls.
— — relieved in general, Anac. Bar-c. Carb-an.

13. COMPLAINTS DURING AND AFTER MEALS.

After meals, relieved, chill, Ambr.
— — —, clawing pain in stomach, Puls.
— — —, cough, Ferr.
— — —, cutting pain in abdomen, Bov. Kali-c. Nitr-ac. Nux. Ol-an. Rhod. Calc. Ntr-c.
— — —, emptiness and qualmishness of stomach, Mgn-c.
— — —, fulness, Ferr.
— — —, headache, Alum.
— — —, — (after supper), Colch.
— — — pressure in hypogastrium, Mgn-c.
— — — — and drawing pain, Mang.
— — — — below scrobiculus, Kali-c.
— — — — in stomach Chin. Petr. Stront.
— — — soreness in scrobiculus, Nux.
— — — tension across navel, Merc.
— — — twisting in scrobiculous, Sil.
— — — uneasiness in scrobiculus, Cham.
— — — vertigo, after breakfast, Alum. Cocc.
— drinking, complaints, Caps.
— — abdomen, coldness, Asa-f.
— — — colic, Bry. Chin. Ferr.
— — — distention, Ambr. Ntr-m.
— — — heaviness, Asa-f.
— — — pain in, Aloe. Ambr. Ars. Bry. Chin. Croc. Ferr. Ntr-m. Nitr-ac. Nux-m. Nux. Ol-an. Puls. Rhus. Staph. *Sulph.* Teucr.
— — — uneasiness, Croc.
— — bones, pain in, Hell.
— — breath obstructed, Anac. Nux.
— — chest cold feeling in, Elaps.
— — — pain in, Chin. *Thuj.* Verat.
— — — tightness of, Nux.
— — chilliness, Ars. Asar. Caps. Chin. Cocc-c. Nux. Tart. Verat.
— — cloudiness of head, Bell. Cocc.
— — convulsions, Hyosc.
— — cough, Acon. Arn. Ars. Carb-veg. Chin. Cina. Cocc. Dros. Ferr. Hep. Laur. Lyc. Ntr-m. Nux. Op. Phosp. Rhus.
— — — cold drinks, Amm-c. Carb-veg. Dig. Hep. Lyc. Rhus. Scill. Sil. Sulph-ac.
— — — spasmodic, Bry.
— — diarrhoea, Ars. Cina. Croton. Pod.
— drinking, cold drinks, diarrhoea, Ant. Ars. Bell. Bry. Carb-veg. Cocc. Dulc. Hep. Lept. Ntr-c. Nux-m. Puls. Rhus. Sulph-ac. Thromb.
— — eructations, Ars. Hyper. Mez. Rhus. Sulph. Tar.
— — flushes of heat in face, Cocc.
— — headache, Acon. Cocc. Merc.
— — heartburn, Lam.
— — hiccough, *Igt.* Lach. Puls.
— — hypochondres, pain in, Ntr-c.
— — nausea, Ars. Ntr-m. Nux.
— — — with retching, Nux. Puls. Rhus. Teucr.
— — scrobiculus, pain in, Nux. Ol-an.

— — stomach, cold in, Sulph-ac.
— — — cramp in, Ferr. Kali-c.
— — — pain in, Acon. Aloe Ferr. Iris. Kali-c. Nitr-ac. Nux. Ol-an. Rhod. Sil. Sulph-ac.
— — taste insipid, Coloc.
— — throat, sensation of erosion in, Nitr-ac.
— — vomiting, Arn. Ars. Bry. Bufo. Cina. Ferr. Mez. Nux. Puls. Sil. Verat.
— — — bitter, when drinking immediately after a meal, Bry.
From acids, complaints, Aloe. Ant. Ars. Bell. Dros. Ferr. Ip. Lach. Ntr-m. Nux. Phosp. Phosp-ac. Sep. Staph. Sulph. Thuj.
— — after taste, long, Ntr-m.
— — colic, Dros.
— — cough, Con. Lach. Nux. Sep.
— — — vinegar, Ant. Sep. Sulph.
— — diarrhoea, Aloe. Ant. Apis. Brom. Coloc. Lach. Phosp-ac. Sulph.
— — eructations, Phosp-ac.
— — — bitter, Staph.
— — heartburn, Nux.
— — vomiting, Ferr.
— — waterbrash, Phosp.
— bacon, relieved, Ran-b. Ran-sc.
— beer, Ars. Asa-f. Bell. Coloc. Euph. Ferr. Kali-b. Mez. Nux. Rhus. Sep. Stann. Sulph. Thuj.
— — after taste, long, Sulph.
— — agitation, congestion of blood, Sulph.
— — colic, Teucr.
— — congestion to head, Ferr.
— — cough, Mez. Rhus.
— — diarrhoea, Kali-b.
— — — relieved, Aloe.
— — heat and pain in head, Ferr. Rhus.
— — hunger, Nux.
— — loathing, Mur-ac.
— — uneasiness in stomach, Acon.
— — vomiting, Ferr. Mez.
— bread, Bry. Caust. Ntr-m. Nitr-ac. Nux. Phosp. Puls. Rhus. Sass. Sep. Sulph. Zinc.
— — relieved, Caust. Ntr-c.
— — after taste long. Phosp-ac.
— — colic, Bry.
— — cough, Kali-c.
— — black, cough, Phosp-ac.
— — and butter, Chin. Nitr-ac. Puls. Sep.
— — eructations, Bry.
— — headache, Zing.
— — hiccough after bread and butter, Ntr-s.
— — nausea, Zinc.
— — stomach, pain in, Acon. Bry. Caust. Kali-c. Merc. Puls. Rhus. Ruta. Sass. Sulph-ac. Zinc.
— — pressure in, Bry.
— — taste sour, Nitr-ac.
— — vomiting, Bry. Nitr-ac.
— cabbage, Bry. Chin. Lyc. Petr. Puls.

13. COMPLAINTS DURING AND AFTER MEALS.

— — diarrhoea, Bry. Petr.
— chocolate, diarrhoea, Borax. Lith.
— coffee, Calc-ph. Camph. Canth. Caps. Caust. *Cham.* Cist. *Igt.* Merc.*Nux.* Puls. Sulph.
— — abdomen, pain in as if diarrhoea would set in, Mgn-s.
— — asthma, Cham.
— — cough, Caps. Caust. Cham. Igt.
— — odor of, cough, Sulph-ac.
— — congestion to head, Millef.
— — diarrhoea, Brom. Canth. Cist. Coloc. Corn-c. Fluor-ac. Ox-ac. Phosp. Thuj.
— — giddiness, Cham.
— —, fulness, sense of extending into, chest and abdomen, Canth.
— — headache, Cham. Cocc. Igt. Nitr. *Nux*.
— — retching, Caps. Cham.
— — stomach, pain in, *Cham*. Igt. *Nux*.
— — toothache, Cham. Nux.
— — relief, Ambr. Anac. Bar-c. Bell. Bry. Carb-veg. Cham. Euph. Glon. Kali-c. Mez. Phosp. Phosp-ac. Puls.
— cold food, Ars. Carb-veg. Graph. Lyc. Mang. Nux-m. Nux. Puls. Rhod. Rhus. Spig. Sulph. Verat.
— — — cough, Carb-veg. Hep. Lyc. Mgn-c. Rhus. Sil. Verat.
— — — diarrhoea, Ant. Coloc. Lyc. Puls.
— — — relieved, Bry. Phosp. Puls.
— — —, nausea, Ip.
— dry meats, Calc. Lyc. Ntr-c. Puls.
— eggs, nausea, Colch.
— — vomiting, Ferr.
— farinaceous food. Sulph.
— — — diarrhoea, Ntr-s.
— fish, Carb-an. Kali-c. Plb.
— fish, stale, Carb-veg. Puls.
— fruits, Ars. Borax. Bry. Carb-veg. *Chin*. Mgn-m. Ntr-c. Puls. Selen. Sep. Verat.
— — relief, Lach.
— — cough, Mgn-m.
— — diarrhoea, Ars. Borax. *Chin*. Cist. Coloc. Lach. Lith. Puls. Rhod.
— — fermentation, Chin.
— — feel like ice in stomach, Elaps.
— — stomach pain in, Borax.
— — toothache, Ntr-c.
— herrings, Fluor-ac. Lyc.
— lemonade, headache, Selen.
— —, nausea relieved, Cycl.
— meat, *Colch*. Sil. Sulph.
— — cough, Staph.
— — diarrhoea, Caust. Ferr. Sep.
— — flatulency, Bry. Lyc. Petr.
— — pain in stomach, Calc. Ferr.
— — smell of, nausea and diarrhoea, Colch.
— — smoked, Calc. Sil.
— — — diarrhoea, Calc.
— — — relief, Caust. Verat.

— melons, Zing.
— milk, Ambr. Ang. Ars. Brom. Bry. Calc. Carb-veg. Cham. Chelid. Chin. Con. Cupr. Kali-c. Lach. Lyc. Ntr-c. Ntr-m. Nitr-ac. Nux. Phosp. Sep. Sulph.
— — relief, Chelid. Verat.
— — abdomen, distended, Carb-veg. Con.
— — — pain in, Ang. Bry. Bufo.
— — after taste, long, Igt.
— — cough, Amb. Brom. Kali-c. Sulph-ac. Tart. Zinc.
— — diarrhoea, Ars. Bry. Colc. Con. Kali-c. Lyc. Ntr-c. Nicc. Nux-m. Sep. Sulph.
— — eructation; nauseous, Ntr-m.
— — — sour, Calc. Carb-veg. Chin. Lyc. Sulph. Tart. Zinc.
— — flatulency, Sulph-ac.
— — headache, Brom.
— — heartburn, Ambr.
— — langor, Sulph-ac.
— — regurgitation, sour, Calc. Carb-veg. *Lyc*. Tart.
— — retching, *Calc*.
— — stomach distended, *Con*.
— — taste sour, Ambr. Carb-veg. Lyc. Sulph.
— — vomiting, Aeth. Samb. Spong.
— — water brash, Cupr.
— — weakness, Sulph-ac.
— — boiled, diarrhoea, Ntr-c. Nicc. Nitr-ac. Nux-m. Sep.
— — hot, relieves colic, Chelid. Croton.
— — with fruit, diarrhoea, Pod.
— mother's milk, vomiting, Sil.
— oil, Bry. Canth. Puls.
— onions, Lyc. Puls. Thuj.
— oysters, diarrhoea, Brom. Lyc.
— pancakes, Bry. Kali-c. Puls. Verat.
— pastry, rich, Ars. Carb-veg. Cycl. *Puls*.
— pears, Borax. Bry. Verat.
— pepper, cough, Cina.
— pork, Ant. Carb-veg. Colch. Cycl. Ip. Ntr-c. Ntr-m. *Puls*. Sep. Thuj.
— potatoes, Alum. Coloc. Sep. Verat.
— — colic, Alum. Coloc.
— — sudden evacuation, Coloc.
— pungent food, cough, Sulph.
— rich food, Ars. Asa-f. Carb-an. Carb-veg. Colch. Cycl. Dros. Ferr. Ip. Mgn-m. Ntr-m. Nitr-ac. Puls. Sep. Spong. Sulph. Tar. Thuj.
— — abdomen pain in, Ang. Bry.
— — eructations, *Carb-veg*. Ntr-m. Sep. Thuj.
— — — bitter, Ferr.
— — — nauseous, Ntr-m. Sep.
— — — rancid, Thuj.
— — — sour, Chin. Sulph. Zinc.
— — flatulency, Sulph-ac.
— — headache, Carb-veg. Colch. Cycl. Ip. Ntr-c. Ntr-m. Puls. Sep. Thuj.

13. COMPLAINTS DURING AND AFTER MEALS.

From rich food, heartburn, Ntr-c. Nux.
— — — nausea, Carb-an. Dros. Nitr-ac. Puls. Sep.
— — — regurgitation, sour, Calc. Carb-veg. Lyc. Tart.
— — — stomach spoiled, Asa-f. Chin. Puls.
— — — taste, acid, Ambr. Carb-veg. Lyc. Sulph.
— — — vomiting, Aeth. Samb. Spong. Sulph.
— salted food, Carb-veg. Dros. Ip. Selen.
— — — relief, Mgn-c.
— — — cough, Con.
— — — scraping in throat, Dros.
— solid food, Lyc.
— — cough, Cupr.
— — heartburn, Iod.
— sourkraut diarrhoea, Petr.
— spirituous liquors, Ant. *Ars.* Bell. Borax. Calc. Carb-an. Carb-veg. Con. Igt. Led. Ntr-m. *Nux.* Petr. Puls. Ran-b. Rhod. Rhus. Ruta. Selen. Sil. Stram. Stront. Zinc.
— strawberries, Sep. Ox-ac.
— sugar, Cham. Igt. Merc. Ntr-c. Ox-ac. Selen. Thuj.
— — cough, Zinc.
— — pain in stomach, Ox-ac.
— tea, Chin. Ferr. Selen. Thuj. Verat.
— — relief, Ferr. Kali-b.
— — cough, Ferr.
— — headache, Selen.
— — toothache, Thuj.
— tobacco, Ant. Calc. Clem. Cocc. Cycl. Euphr. Gels. *Igt.* Ip. Lach. Ntr-m. Nux. Par. Petr. Phosp. Puls. Ruta. Sass. Selen. Sep. Sil. Sol-m. *Spong. Staph.* Sulph. Sulph-ac. Tar. Thuj.
— — bitterness in mouth, Asar. Chin. Cocc. Euphr. Igt.
— — breath obstructed, Tar.
— — colic, Borax. Bufo. Igt.
— — cough, Acon. Brom. Carb-an. Cocc-c. Coloc. Dros. Euphr. Ferr. Hep. Igt. Iod. Mgn-c. Nux. Spong. Staph. Sulph-ac.
— — diarrhoea, Brom. Cham. Puls.
— — — relieved, Coloc.
— — eructations, Selen.
— — giddiness, Borax.
— — headache, Ant. Mgn-c.
— — — relieved, Diad.
— — heartburn, Staph. Tar.
— — heart palpitation of, Phosp.
— — hiccough, Ambr. Ant. Arg. Igt. Lach. Puls. Ruta. Selen.
— — nausea, Calc. Carb-an. Clem. Euphr. Igt. Ip. Lach. Nux. Phosp.
— — neuralgic pains in face, Sep.
— — perspiration, Igt.
— — toothache, Clem. Sabin. Spig.
— — vomiting, Ip.

— — weakness, Clem. Hep.
— — tobacco relief, Coloc. Hep. Merc. Ntr-c. Sep.
— — chewing, Ars.
— — undigested food, Caust. Iod. Lyc. Puls.
— — heartburn, Iod.
— turnips, Bry. Puls.
— uncooked, meats, Bry. Lyc. Puls. *Ruta.* Verat.
— veal, Ars. Calc. Caust. *Ip. Nitr.* Sep. Zinc.
— —, headache, and colic, Nitr.
— vegetables, Ars. Bry. Cist. Cupr. Hell. Ntr-c. Verat.
— vinegar, *Ant.* Ars. Bell. Borax. Caust. Dros. Ferr. Lach. Ntr-m. Nux. Phosp-ac. Sep. Staph. Sulph. Thuj.
— — colic, Aloe.
— — relief, Asar. Puls.
— warm food, Ambr. Anac. Bar-c. Bell. Bry. Carb-veg. Cham. Euph. Kali-c. Mez. Phosp. Phosp. Phyt. Puls. Stann.
— — — cough, Bar-c. Kali-c. Laur. Mez. Puls.
— — — diarrhoea, Phosp.
— — — — relieved, Acon.
— — — relieved, Ars. Bry. Con. Creos. Graph. Lyc. Mang. Nux-m. Nux. Rhus. Spig. Sulph. Verat.
— water, cold, Alum. Ars. Bell. Canth. Carb-an. Croc. Igt. Kali-b. Lyc. Mur-ac. *Nux.* Rhod. Rhus. Spig. Sulph. Tar.
— — — colic, Hipp-m. Tar.
— — — cough, Ars. Calc. Rhus. Stram. Sulph-ac. Verat.
— — — diarrhoea relieved, Cupr. Phosp.
— — — heaviness in stomach, Rhod.
— — — pain in stomach, Iris.
— — — — — and nausea, Rhus.
— — — relieves, Apis. Asar. Bry. Caust. Coff. Cupr. Lach. Phosp. Puls. Sep.
— wine, Ant. Arn. *Ars.* Bell. Bov. Calc. Camph. Carb-an. Coff. Con. Igt. Lach. *Lyc.* Ntr-c. Ntr-m. Nux-m. *Nux. Op.* Petr. Puls. *Ran-b.* Rhod. Sabad. Selen. *Sil* Stront. Thuj. Zinc.
— — congestion of blood, Sil.
— — cough, Arn. Borax. Ferr. Igt. Lach. Led. Stann. Stram. Zinc.
— — — sour wine, Ant.
— — diarrhoea, Lach.
— — — relieved, Chelid. Diosc.
— — eyes affection of, Zinc.
— — giddiness of, Ntr-c. Zinc.
— — headache, Calc. *Nux.* Ox-ac. *Rhod. Selen.* Zinc.
— — heat, excitement, Carb-veg.
— — intoxicated easily, Bov. Con. Cor-r. Kali-jod.
— — nausea, Ant.
— — stomach, cramp in, Lyc.

13. COMPLAINTS DURING AND AFTER MEALS.

From wine, toothache, Nux.
— — containing lead, Bell. Nux. Op. Plat. Sulph.
— — sour, Ant. Ars. Ferr. Sulph.
— — sulphurated, Ars. Merc. Puls. Sep.
— — relieves, Acon. Agar. Con. Lach. Op. Sulph-ac.
— — — vomiting, Kalm.

14. Eructations, Nausea and Vomiting.

HICCOUGH, HEARTBURN AND WATER BRASH.

Eructations, *Alum.* Ambr. Ant. Arn. Ars. Bar-c. Bell. Berb. Bry. Calc. Canth. Carb-an. Carb-veg. Caust. Chin. Cocc. Con. Cupr. Diosc. Dulc. Fluor-ac. *Graph.* Hœmatox. *Hep.* Igt. Ip. Iris. Kali-c. Laur. Lyc. Merc. *Mez.* Mosch. *Mur-ac.* Ntr-c. Ntr-m. Nux. Petr. Phell. *Phosp.* Puls. Ran-b. Rhus. Rumex. Sabad. Sass. Scill. *Sep.* Sil. Stann. *Staph.* Sulph. Sulph-ac. *Tabac.* Tart. Thuj. Tilia. Valer. Verat. Zing.
— relieve, Arg-n. Graph. Kali-c. Lach. Lyc. Ntr-m. Nux. Ol-an. Seneg. Tart.
— aggravate, Cham. Chin. Phosp. Stann.
— acrid, Alum. Asa-f. Cact. Lact. Merc. Pod.
— bitter, Aloe. Ambr. *Amm-m.* Ang. *Arn.* Ars. Bell. Berb. Bism. *Bry.* Calc. Carb-veg. Cast. *Chin.* Cocc. Dros. *Grat.* Hyosc. Laur. Lyc. Mgn-s. *Merc.* Mur-ac. Nicc. *Nux.* Petr. Phosp. Phosp-ac. Puls. Sass. Scill. Sep. Sil. Spong. Stann. Staph. *Sulph-ac.* Tar. Thuj. Tong. Verat. Verb.
— — almonds, Laur.
— burning, Bell. Canth. Hep. Iod. Lob. Lyc. Merc. Ol-an. Phosp-ac. Sulph. Tabac. Valer.
— constant, *Con.* Cupr. Sulph.
— cool, Cist.
— empty, of tasteless wind, Acon. Agar. Aloe. Amm-c. Amm-m. Ang. Arg-n. Arn. Ars. Bar-c. Bell. Bruc. Bry. Calad. Cannab. Carb-veg. *Caust.* Chelid. Chenop. Chin. Coce. Cocc-c. Colch. Coloc. *Con.* Cycl. Euph. Guaj. Gum-gut. Ind. Iod. Ip. Iris. Jac-cor. Kali-b. Kali-chl. Kali-jod. Kobalt. Lac-can. Lach. Lact. Laur. Lob. *Mgn-s.* Meny. Merc. *Mez.* *Ntr-m.* *Oleand.* Ol-an. Ox-ac. *Phosp.* Plat. Plb. Pod. Puls. Ran-sc. Rhus. Ruta. Sabad. *Sabin.* Seneg. Staph. *Sulph.* Tabac. Tar. *Tart.* Valer. *Verat.* *Verb.*
— — with asthma, Calad.
— fatty, Carb-veg. Lyc.
— like garlic, Asa-f. Mosch.
— hiccoughing, Cycl. Tart.
— impeded, with ineffectual efforts, Acon. Ambr. Amm-c. Ang. Bell. Carb-an.

Caust. Casc. Ferr. Graph. Nux. Phosp. Plat. Puls. Sulph.
— imperfect, Arn. Phosp-ac. Sabad.
— tasting like ink, Ind.
— interrupted, Arn.
— like juniper berries, tasting, Chelid.
— loud, Arg-n. Calc. Carb-veg. Con. Lact. Nux-jug. Petr. Plat. Sulph.
— of musk tasting, Caust. Mosch.
— obstructing breath, Grat.
— offensive smelling, Bism. Cocc. Kali-b. Phell. Sulph.
— — tasting, Senna.
— of onious tasting, Mgn-m.
— painful, Carb-an. Caust. Con. Ntr-c. Nux. Plb. Sabad. Sep.
— putrid, Arn. Asar. Bell. Cocc. Mgn-s. Merc. Mur-ac. Nux. Oleand. Psor. Puls. Sep. Sulph. Tabac. Thuj. Tilia.
— rancid, Asa-f. Merc. Ran-sc. Thuj. Valer.
— repugnant, disagreeable, Cina. Lact. Ntr-m. Sep.
— like rotten eggs, Arn. Bufo. Mgn-c. Psor. Sep. Stann. Sulph. *Tart.* *Valer.*
— saltish after eating meat, Staph.
— scratching, Ant. *Ntr-m.* Nux-m. Stann. Staph.
— sobbing, Cycl. Meph. Staph. Tart.
— sour, Acet-ac. All-cep. Aloe. *Alum.* *Ambr.* Amm-c. Ars. Asar. Bar-c. Bell. *Bry.* Cact. Calc. Carb-an. *Carb-veg.* Caust. Cham. Chin. Cimex. Cycl. Dig. Elaps. Ferr. Gels. Graph. Gymnoc. Hep. Igt. Iod. Kali-b. *Kali-c.* Kali-chl. Lach. Lact. Lith. Lob. *Lyc.* Mgn-c. Merc. *Ntr-m.* Nicc. Nitr-ac. Nitr. *Nux.* Ox-ac. *Petr.* *Phosp.* Phosp-ac. Pod. Puls. Ran-sc. Sacch. Sass. *Sep.* *Sil.* Spig. Stann. Stram. *Sulph.* *Sulph-ac.* Tabac. Tart. Verat. *Zinc.* Zing.
— — wat-r, Nicc.
— sour, with bitterness in mouth, Graph.
— spasmodic, Cocc-c. Nux. Phosp. Sang.
— suppressed, followed by pain in stomach, Con.
— tasting of what has been eaten, Agar. Agn. Aloe. Ambr. Amm-c. *Arn.* Bry. Calc. Carb-an. Carb-veg. Caust. Cham.

14. ERUCTATIONS, NAUSEA AND VOMITING,

Chelid. Chin. Cic. *Con.* Croc. Euphr. Lach. Laur. Ntr-m. Nux. Oleand. Phell. *Phosp.* Plb. *Puls. Ran-s·.* Rat. Rhus. Ruta. Sass. Sep. *Sil.* Spig. Sulph. *Thuj.* Verat.
Eructations tasting, after acid food, Staph.
— — — rich food, *Carb-veg.*
— sweetish, Grat. Plb. Zinc.
— like urine tasting, Ol-an.
— vehement, Arn. Bism. Lach. Merc. Plb. *Verat.*
— in morning, Arn. Croc. Valer.
— — afternoon, Lyc.
— — evening, Ran-sc.
— at night, Sulph. Tart.
— after drinking, Ars. Croton. Mez. Rhus. Tar.
— — — acids, Phosp-ac.
— — — water, Hyper.
— during meals, Ntr-c. Oleand. Sass.
— after meals, Ang. Arg-n. Ars. Bar-c. *Bry.* Calc. *Carb-veg.* Cham. Chin. Cic. *Con.* Daph. Dig. Ferr. Kali-c. Lach. Merc. Ntr-c. *Ntr-m.* Nitr-ac. Nux-m. Nux. Petr. Phosp. Plat. Puls. *Ran-sc.* Rhus. *Sass.* Sep. Sil. *Spig. Sulph.* Thuj. Verat. Zinc.
— meat, Ruta.
— milk, Chin. Ntr-m. Sulph. Zinc.
— rich food, *Carb-veg.* Ferr. Ntr-m. Staph. Thuj.
— when rising from lying, Rhus.
— after smoking tobacco, Selen.
— in hysterical women, Ruta.
— mitigated by omission of flatulence, Meph.
— with, chest pain in, Zinc.
— — colic, Cham.
— — diarrhoea, Zing.
— — loathing, Croton.
— — nausea, Chin-sulph. Croton.
— — obstructed breath, Grat.
— — retching, *Cocc.* Verb.
— — hot saliva in mouth, Mosch.
— — scrobiculus, pain in, Cocc.
— — stomach, pain in, Calad. Cham. Cocc. Merc. Phosp. Rhus. Spong.
— — throat choking, Caust.
— — — fulness, Con.
— — pain in, Nux.
— — water, flow of in mouth, Lob.
— alternating with yawning, Berb.
Heartburn, Alum. *Ambr. Amm-c.* Arg. Asar. Bar-c. Bell. *Calc. Canth. Caps.* Carb-an. Carb-veg. Caust. Chin. Cocc-c. Con. *Croc.* Daph. Guaj. *Iod.* Kali-c. Lach. Lob. Lyc. Mang. Merc. Mosch. *Ntr-m.* Nux. Ox-ac. Petr. Phosp. Puls. *Sabad.* Sep. Sil. Sulph. *Sulph-ac.* Tabac. Valer. Verat. *Zinc.*
— rising up in throat, Con. Lyc. Mang. Ntr-m. Tabac.
— scratching. *Carb-an.* Ntr-c.

— in evening, Ambr.
— continual, Lob.
— after drinking, Lam.
— — meals, Amm·c. Calc. Chin. Con. Croc. Iod. Lam. Lyc. Merc. Ntr-m. Sep. Sil.
— — — of solid food, Iod.
— — — with good appetite, Croc.
— — — of acid things, Nux.
— — — — fat food, Ntr-c. Nux.
— during meals, Merc.
— after sugar. Zinc.
— — tobacco, Staph. Tar.
— when walking in open air, Ambr.
— — with running of water from mouth, Lob.
Hiccough, Acon. Agar. Agn. Amm-m. Benz-ac. Bell. Bov. Bry. Carb-an. Chelid. Cic. Cina. Colch. Cupr. Cycl. Dros. Euph. Euphr. Graph. Grat. *Hyosc.* Igt. Iod, Kali-b. Kali-jod. Lach. Laur. *Mgn-m.* Merc-sulph. Ntr-s. *Nicc. Nux.* Phosp. Plb. Puls. Ran-b. Ruta. Selen. Sil. Spong. Stann. Stram. Stront. Tabac. Tar. Teucr. Verat. Verb. Zinc.
— painful, Mgn-m. Rat. Tabac. Teucr.
— spasmodic, Bell. Nux. *Kan-b.* Stram. Tabac.
— vehement, *Amm-m.* Cic. Lob. *Lyc. Nicc. Nux.* Rat. Stront. Teucr. Verat.
— — in evening, Kali-b. Ntr-s. Nicc. Sil.
— at night, Ars.
— in bed, Lachn.
— after breakfast, Zinc.
— — drinking, *Igt.* Lach. Puls.
— — exercise, Carb-veg.
— during meals, Mgn-m. Merc. Teucr.
— after meals, Alum. Bov. Carb-an. *Cycl.* Graph. Hyosc. *Igt.* Lyc. Mgn-m. Ntr-c. Par. Sep. Verat. Zinc.
— from smoking tobacco, Ambr. Ant. Arg. Igt. Lach. Puls. Ruta. Sang. Selen.
— precedes spasms, Cupr.
— with blows, in pit of stomach, Teucr.
— — chest, pain in, Amm-m.
— — choking, Puls.
— — convulsions, Bell.
— — irritability, Agn.
— — perspiration, Bell.
— — saliva, abundant flow of, Lob.
— — spasms, and rumbling in abdomen, Hyosc.
— — stomach pain in, Mgn-m. Rat.
Loathing, Ant. Arg-n. Arn. Asar. Bar-m. Bell. Cast. Croton. Cupr. *Grat.* Guaj. Hydroc-ac. Kali-jod. *Laur.* Mgn-c. Mgn-s. *Ol-an.* Phell. Plb. *Prun. Rat. Sec-c.* Seneg. Senna. Tart.
— at night, Rat.
— after beer, Mur-ac. Nux.
— — meals, Ip. Ol-an. Sass.
Nausea, Acon. Agar. Agn. *Alum.* Ambr. *Anac.* Ang. *Ant.* Apis. Arg-n. Arn. *Ars.*

14. ERUCTATIONS, NAUSEA AND VOMITING.

Asar. Bapt. Bar-c. *Bell.* Borax. *Bov.* Brom. *Bry.* Calad. *Calc.* Camph. Cannab. Caps. *Carb-an. Carb-veg.* Causť. *Cham.* Chin. Cic. Cist. *Cocc.* Cocc-c. Colch. Coloc. *Con.* Cop. Corn-c. Creos. Croc. Croton. Cub. *Cupr.* Cycl. *Dig.* Diosc. Dros. Dulc. Euphr. Ferr-m.*Graph.*Grat. Gum-gut. *Hell.* Hep. Hydroc-ac. Hyper. Hyosc *Igt. Iod. Ip.* Iris. Kali-b, *Kali-c. Lach.* Laur. Led. Lept. Lob. *Lyc. Merc. Mez. Mosch. Ntr-c. Ntr-m.* Nicc. Nitr-ac. *Nux.* Oleand. Ol-an. Op. Ox-ac. *Petr.* Phell. *Phosp. Phosp-ac.* Phyt. *Plat. Plb.* Pod. Prun. *Puls. Ran-b. Ran-sc.* Rat. Rheum. Rhod. *Rhus.* Rumex. Sabad. Sang. Sass. Scill. *Sec-c.* Seneg. *Sep. Sil.* Spong. Stann. Stram. Stront. *Sulph.* Sulph-ac. *Tabac. Tar. Tart.*Thea. *Therid.* Thuj. Valer. *Verat.* Viol-tr. Zinc. Zing.
— in abdomen, Agn. Bry. Croton. Cupr. Puls. *Rheum.*
— — upper part, Actea-r. Agn. Cupr. Puls.
— — chest, Acon. Bry. Croc. Merc. Ol-an. Rhus.
— on palate, Cupr. Cycl. Phosp-ac.
— in pit of stomach, Agn. Caps. Cupr. Lachn. Mosch. Ruta. Scill. Teucr.
— — stomach, Acon. Agn. Cycl. Eugen. Hell. Ip. Laur Lyc. Phosp. Puls. Seneg. Senna. Sulph. Sulph-ac. Tart. Thuj.
— — throat, Ars. Bell. Chin. Croc. Cupr. Cycl. Lyc. Mez. Oleand. Phosp-ac. Puls. Stann. Staph. Valer.
— chronic, Bar-c. Nux.
— constant, Arg. Ars. Carb-veg. Cast. Coloc. Dig.Graph. Ip. Lob. *Lyc.*Mgn-m. Ntr-c. Plat. Sass. Sil. *Tart.* Verat.
— faintish, Ang. Carb-an. Causť. Cham. Cocc. Kali-c. Mgn-m. *Tabac. Valer. Verat.*
— as after fat food, Acon. Cycl. Tar.
— with a disposition to vomit. Agar. Alum. Amm-c. *Ant.* Arn. Asar. Aur. Bar-m. Bell. Bism. *Borax.* Brom. *Bry.* Camph. Caps. Cast. *Cham. Cocc. Con.* Cop. Croton. Cupr. Cycl. *Dig.* Ferr. Graph. *Grat.* Hep. Iod. Ip. Iris. *Kali-c. Merc.* Ntr-s. Nitr-ac. Nitr. *Nux.* Oleand. *Ol-an.* Op. Petr. Phell. Phosp-ac. Plb. Pod. Puls. Ran-sc. Rhod. *Rhus. Sabad.* Sass. Scill. Seneg. Senna. Staph. Sulph. Tabac. *Tart. Valer. Verat.* Verb.
— as after sugar, Acon. Cycl. Merc. Tar.
— — if occasioned by a piece of thread in pharynx, Valer.
— with uneasiness, Carb-an. Causť. Cham. Cycl.Lyc. *Ntr-s.* Sulph. Thea. Thuj.
— as if all the viscera were turning inside out, Sep.
— in morning, Acon. Alum. Anac. *Arn.* Bar-c. Berb. Bry. Calad. Cact. *Calc.* Carb-veg. Causť. *Cham.* Cic. Dig. Graph. Hep. Kali-b. Lach. Lob. Lyc. Mgn-m. Ntr-m. Nicc. *Nux.* Petr. Phosp. Psor. Ran-sc. Rhus. Sacch. *Sep. Sil.* Spig. Staph. *Sulph.* Verat.
— — forenoon, Bov.
— — afternoon, Ran-b.
— — evening, Asar. Calc. Con. Cycl. Kali-b. Ntr-c. Nux. Petr. Phosp. Puls. Ran-b. Sep.
— at night, Alum. Amm-c. Calc. *Carb-an.* Carb-veg. Cham. Con. Kali-b. *Merc.* Nitr-ac. Nitr. Phosp. Puls. Rat. Rhus. Sulph. Therid.
— from midnight to morning, Dros.
— after midnight, Ran-sc.
— after breakfast, Bell. *Cham.* Kali-b.
— from draft of air, Hipp.
— when closing the eyes, Therid.
— after coffee, Caps. *Cham.*
— — a cold, Cocc.
— while drinking, Bry.
— after drinking, Ars. Croton. Cycl. Ntr-m. Nux. Puls. Rhus. Teucr.
— — water, relieved, Lob. Phosp.
— by eating relieved, Brom. Kali-b. Phosp. Sabad. Sep.
— from smell of eggs, *Colch.*
— on entering into a room, Alum.
— by eructation relieved, Cinnab. Rhod. Tart.
— after every exercise which raises the temperature of the body, Sil.
— from exercising, Aloe. Ars. Colch. Tabac. Therid.
— from flatulency discharged, relief, Tart.
— food, smell of, Sep.
— as from indigestion, Bar-c.
— in lying relieved, Rhus.
— before meals, Berb. Lyc. Ntr-s. Sabad. Sulph.
— during meals, Ang. Bell. *Borax.* Causť. Cic. Cocc. Colch. Dig. Ferr. Jac-cor. Kali-c. Mgn-c. Nux. Ol-an. Puls. Verat.
— after meals. Agar. Alum. *Amm-c.* Anac. Ars. Bism. *Bry.* Calc. Causť.*Cham.*Con. Cycl. Dig. Graph. Grat Kali-b. Kali-c. Lach. Lyc. Merc. Ntr-m. Ntr-s. Nitr-ac. *Nux.* Ol-an. Op. *Phosp.* Puls. *Rhus.* Sang. *Sep. Sil. Stann. Sulph.* Verat.
— with good appetite, Bry. Cannab.
— from meat, smell of, *Colch.*
— — fresh meat, Causť.
— when meditating. Borax.
— from mental troubles, Kali-c.
— — milk, Calc
— — a loud noise, Therid.
— in open air, Acon. Ang. Bell. Lyc.
— — relieved, Croc, Lyc. Tabac. Tar.
— — pregnant women, *Con.* Creos. *Ip.* Ntr-m. Nux-m. *Nux.* Petr. Puls. *Sep.*
— when pressing on pit of stomach, Hyosc.

14. ERUCTATIONS, NAUSEA AND VOMITING.

— from rich food, Carb-an. Cycl. Dros. Nitr-ac. Puls. Sep.
— — riding in a carriage, Borax. *Cocc.*Lyc. Nux-m. *Petr.* Sep. Sulph.
— when rising from lying, Bry. Cocc.
— in a room, caused or relieved, Lyc.
— when sitting, Bry.
— — — up in bed, Bry. Cocc. Cor-r.
— — smoking, Carb-an. Clem. Euphr. Igt. Kali-c. Lac-can Phosp. Tabac.
— from spitting, Led.
— when standing up, Colch.
— — when swallowing saliva, Colch.
— — talking, Alum. Borax.
— not relieved by vomiting, Dig. Sang.
— when walking in open air, Acon. Ang. Lachn.
— after walking in open air, Alum.
— from sour wine, Ant.
— with, abdomen, rumbling in, Arg-n. Puls.
— — agitation, Igt.
— — anxiety, Bry. Dig. Igt. *Kali-c.* Merc. Nitr-ac. Plat. Tar. *Tart.*
— — appetite, want of, Ant. *Bell.* Cocc. *Con.* Croton. Cupr. *Hell. Laur.* Mgn-s. Merc-jod. Ol-an. Prun.
— — — ravenous, Agar. Mosch. Rheum. Tabac.
— — asthmatic paroxysms, *Cham.* Petr,
— — backache, Psor. Puls.
— — — and tenesmus, Hipp-m.
— — bruised pain in intestines, Cocc.
— — buzzing in ears, Acon,
— — chest, fulness in, Cycl.
— — — pain in, Merc. Ol-an.
— — chills, Bov. Creos. Nitr-ac. Puls, Sulph-ac.
— — coldness, Croton. Hep. Kali-b. Valer.
— — colic, Agar. Cupr. Dig. Glon. Merc. Mosch. Puls. Rheum. Tabac.
— — drunkenness, Cupr.
— — ears, humming in, Acon.
— — — pain in, Puls.
— — eructations, Acon. Ars. Chin-sulph. Cocc. Con. Ip. Mosch. Petr. Sep. Spig. Sulph.
— — eyes aching in, Ntr-s. Sil.
— — — — when turned, Sil.
— — evacuations, loose, Scill.
— — face, earthy, Mgn-m.
— — — heat, Petr, Stront.
— —·— paleness, Gels. Glon. Hep. Tabac. Tart.
— — — redness. *Verat.*
— — feet, pain in, Ars.
— — flow of urine, *Verat.*
— — giddiness, Calad. Calc-ph. Camph. Cocc. Croton. Gels Graph. Kali-b. Mgn-c. Merc. Merc-jod. Millef. (compare Vertigo, Sect. 2.)
— — hawking, Hipp-m.
— — headache Asar. Chin-sulph. Cic. Cocc. Cor-r. Creos. Gels. Glon.

Hipp. Kalm. Lith. Merc. Mez. Ntr-s. Nux. Phyt. Sang. Sil. Tar. Tart.
— —heat, Fluor-ac. Kali-b. Merc.
— — — in stomach extending to throat, Nitr-ac.
— — heartburn, Cinnab. Gum-gut.
— — hunger, Cycl. *Hell.* Kali-b. Mgn-m. Ntr-c. Oleand. Phosp. Spig. Tabac.
— — itching and nettle rash before, Sang.
— — languor. Con. Ntr-s. Plat. Sulph.
— — lips pale, Valer.
— — lying down, need to, Ars. Asar, Cocc. Mosch. Phosp-ac.
— — mouth, bitterness in, Chin-sulph.
— — — burning in, Creos.
— — navel retracted, Mosch.
— — palpitation of heart, Sil.
— — perspiration, Glon.
— — — on forehead, Croton.
— — — on face, cold, Lob.
— — — profuse, Lob.
— — relieves Glon.
— — pressing down, as if intestines were, Agn.
— — restlessness, Igt.
— — rheumatic pains, Kalm.
— — saliva, collection of Asar. Cocc. Croton. Creos. Ip. Mgn-s. Mez. Oleand. Petr. Valer.
— — salivation, Bry. Colch. Croton. Cycl. Lob. Merc. Sang. Stram. Verat.
— — shivering of upper part of body, Lob.
— — shuddering, Ars. Asar. Calc. Euph. Mez. Sabad.
— — sleep, disposed to, Ars.
— — spitting, Sang.
— — stomach, coldness, Mgn-m. Grat. Tabac.
— — — emptiness, Meph. Merc-jod.
— — — fulness, Sabin.
— — — heat, Chelid.
— — — pain, Ars. Iod. Lact. Rhod.
— — — sour, Nitr-ac.
— — — pit of, pain, Amm-c. Calad. Caps. Dig. Puls. Tart.
— — syncope, fainting, Alum, Ang. Carb-an Caust. Cham. Cocc. Kali-c. Kalm. Lach. Mgh-m. Ntr-m. Nux. Petr. Tabac. Valer. Verat.
— — taste, bitter, *Bell.* Lyc. Sep.
— — putrid, Cupr.
— — sour, Spong.
— — sweet, *Merc.*
— — thirst, Bell, Phosp. Verat.
— — throat burning in, Puls.
— — — scraping in, Meph.
— — tongue dry, Cor-r.
— — — and white, Petr.
— — trembling, Ars. Nitr-ac. Plat. Sulph.
— — weakness, Con. Ntr-s. Plat Sulph.
— — sense of a worm in oesoph., Puls.
Regurgitation Asa-f. Con. Croton. Lyc.

14. ERUCTATIONS, NAUSEA AND VOMITING.

Mgn-m. Nux. Plb. Ran-b. *Sass.* Spig. Verb.
— acrid, Ars. Cannab. Dig. Tart.
— bitter, *Arn.* Ars. Cic. Croton. Graph. *Gra .* Igt. Kobalt. Nux. Petr. Puls. *Sars.* Teucr.
— — of what has been eaten, Teucr.
— bitterish sour, Amm-c. Cannab. Cast. Sulph-ac.
— of blood, Nux Sep.
— burning, Lob.
— of drink, Sulph-ac.
— — what has been eaten, Amm-n. Bell. Bry. Calc. Canth. Carb-veg. Ferr. Graph Igt. Kali-c. Lyc. Mgn-m. Merc. Ntr-m. Nitr-ac. Nux. Phosp. Pod. Puls. *Rhus.* Seneg. *Sulph.* Teucr.
— — by mouthfuls, Phosp.
— — a disagreeable fluid, Plat.
— — — greenish fluid, Ars. Graph.
— — milk, Lyc. Tart.
— rancid, Merc.
— saltish, Arn. Sulph-ac. Tart.
— scratching, *Cannab.*
— slimy, mucus, *Arn.* Mgn-s. Raph.
— sour, Ars. Calc. Carb-veg. Con. Dig. Graph. Gum-gut. Kali-c. Lob. Lyc. Mang. Ntr-c. Ntr-m. Nux. Petr. Phosp. Plb. Puls. Sass. Spong. Sulph. Tart. Thuj.
— — of food taken, Graph. Lyc. Ntr-m. Phosp. Sulph.
— — —milk taken, Lyc.
— sweetish, Ind. Merc. Plb. Sulph-ac.
— water, Acon.
— waterish, Ant. Arn. Grat. Kobalt. Mgn-s. Ntr-s. *Plb.* Senna. Tart.
— of a yellow fluid, Cic.
— at night, Canth.
— after drinking, Merc.
— during meals, Merc. Phosp. Sass.
— after meals, Asa-f. Bry. Con. Dig. Ferr. Lach. Merc. Nux. Phosp. Puls. Sass. Thuj. Verat.
— — cough, Sulph-ac.
— drinking milk, Calc. Carb-veg. Lyc. Tart.
— when stooping, Cic.
— walking, Mgn-m.
— with burning in throat, Cic.
— — pain in stomach, Bell.
— — trembling, Mgn-s.
Risings up in throat, Asa-f. Con. Lach. Lyc. Mgn-m. Merc. Phosp. Plb. Ran-b. Spig. Valer. Verat.
— — bitterish sweet, Plat.
— — nauseous fluid, Plat.
— — sour, Mang. Phosp.
— — sweet, Ind. Merc.
— — of sweetish fluid, *Acon.*
Vomiting. Ambr. Anac. *Ant.* Arg-n. *Ars.* Bell. Bry. *Calc. Camph.* Caust. Cham. Chin. Cic. Cina. *Cocc.* Con. *Cupr.* Dig.

Dros. Ferr. Grat. Igt. *Ip.* Iris. Lach. *Laur.* Lob. *Lyc.* Ntr-m. Nux-m. *Nux.* Op. Petr. *Phosp.* Plb. Puls. Sec-c. Sep. *Sil* *Sulph.* Sulph-ac. *Tart.* Therid. *Valer.* *Verat.* Zinc.
— relief after, Anac. Asar. Sang. Thuj.
— worse after Cupr. Oleand.
— acrid. Arg. Ferr. Hep. Ip. Iris.
— albuminous, Jatr. Merc-cor.
— bilious, Acon. Ant. Apis. Arn. Ars. Bell. Bism. *Bry.* Calc. Camph. *Cannab.* Canth. *Cham.* Chin. Cina. Cocc. *Colch.* Coloc. Con. *Cupr.* Dig. *Dros.* Dulc. Elaps. Eupat. *Grat.* Hep. Ign. Iod. *Ip.* Iris. Jatr. Kali-b. Lach. Lyc. Merc-cor. Mur-ac. Ntr-m. Nux. Petr. *Phosp.* Phyt. Plb. Pod. Puls. Raph. Sabad. *Sabin.* Samb. *Sec-c. Sep.* Stann. *Stram.* Sulph. Valer. *Verat.*
— — at night, Merc.
— — then ingesta, Bry.
— — — blood or mucus, Carb-veg. Verat.
— bitter, Acon. Ant. Apis. *Bry.* Calc. Cast. Colch. *Eupat.* Grat. Hipp-m. Kali-b. Mgn-c. Merc. Mez. Ntr-c. Nitr-ac. Oleand. Petr. Puls. Raph. Sang. Sil. Stann. Sulph. Thuj. Verat. Zinc.
— bitterish sour, Grat. Ip. Puls. Tart.
— black, Arg-n. *Ars.* Calc. Chin. Hell. Hydroc-ac. Ip. Laur. Lyc. Nux. Petr. Phosp. *Plb.* Puls. Sec-c. Sil. Sulph. Sulph-ac. *Verat.*
— of blood, Acon. Aeth. Aloe. Alum. Amm-c. Arg-n. *Arn.* Ars. Bell. Brom. Bry. Cact. Calc. Camph. *Canth.* Carb-veg. Caust. Chin. Cic. Creos. Cupr. Cycl. Dros. Ferr. Hamam. Hep. Hyosc. Igt. Ip. Kali-b. Lach. Lyc. Merc. Merc-cor. Mez. *Millef.* Nitr. *Nux.* Op. Petr. *Phosp.* Phyt. Puls. Sacch. Sep. Stann. Sulph. *Verat.* Zinc.
— — clotted, Arn. Caust. Lyc. Nux.
— of a brown substance, with violent pain in stomach, Ars.
— brownish, Ars. Bism.
— chronic, Ars. Borax. Graph. *Nux.* Osm. Puls. *Sil. Sulph.*
— like coffee grounds, Merc-cor.
— easy, Colch. *Igt.* Sec-c.
— of fat lumps, Hipp-m.
— — faces with constipation. Plb.
— — foetid matters, Ars. Cocc. Cupr. Ip Nux. Op. Pod. *Sep.* Stann. Sulph.
— foamy, frothy, Aeth. Croton. Cupr. Pod. Tart. *Verat.*
— of food, Aeth. Amm-c. Anac. Ant. *Ars.* Bell. Borax. *Bry. Calc.* Cauth. Carb-veg. Caust. Cham. Chin. Cina. Cocc. *Colch.* Coloc. Croton. Cupr. Diad. Dig. Dros. *Ferr.* Graph. Hipp-m. Hyosc. Igt. Ind. Iod. *Ip.* Iris. Jatr. Kali-b. Kali-c. Lach. Laur. Lob. Mgn-s. Merc. Millef. *Ntr-m.* Nitr-ac.

14. ERUCTATIONS, NAUSEA AND VOMITING,

Nux. Oleand. Phosp. Phosp-ac. Phyt. Plb. Pod. Puls. Raph. Rat. Rhus. Ruta. Sabin. Samb. Scill. Sep. Stann. *Sulph.* Sulph-ac. Tart. Tellur. Thuj. *Verat.* Zinc.
— — in evening, Carb-veg.
— — about midnight, Ferr.
— — some hours aftar eating, Meph.
— — when lying on back, Rhus.
— — hot, Lob.
— — sour, Calc. Hep. Kali-b. Pod. Sulph.
— food, then bile, Bell. Dig.
— — — blood, Nux.
— — — mucus, Dros. Nux. Puls. Sil.
— — — water, Puls.
— water then food, Nux.
— food undigested, Kali-b. Lyc. Ntr-m Phosp. Samb.
— gelatinous, Ind. *Ip.*
— glairy, *Jatr.* Kali-b.
— greasy, Ars. Hipp-m. Iod. Mez. Nux. Thuj.
— green, Acon. Aeth. Ars. Bry. *Cannab.* Coloc. Cupr. Dig. Elaps. Hell. Hipp-m. *Ip.* Jatr. Lach. Lyc. Merc-cor. Mez. Oleand. Op. Petr. Phosp. *Plb.* Puls. Raph. Stram. *Verat.*
— of liquids, Acon. Arn. Ars. Bism. Bry. Cham. Chin. Creos. Diad. Dulc. Ip. Nux. Phosp. Sil. Spong. Tart.
— — — as soon as warm in stomach, Phosp.
— — — cold water only, Sil.
— milky, Aeth. Arn. Sep.
— milk drank, *Aeth.* Arn. Calc. Samb. Spong. Sil. Sulph.
— mucus, Acon. Aeth. Ant. Ars. Bell. Borax. Carb-veg. Cham. Chin. Cina. Cocc-c. Colch. Con. Cor r. Cycl. Dig. Dros. Dulc. Elaps. Guaj. Dros. Hyosc. Igt. Ip. Iris. Kali-b. Lach. Mgn-s. Merc-cor. Mez. Ntr-s. Nitr-ac Nux. Oleand. Phyt. Puls. Raph. Sacch. Sec-c. Seneg. Stram. Sulph. Tabac. Tart. Thuj. Verat.
— — bloody, Acon. Brom. Hep. Hyosc. Lach. Nitr. Phosp.
— painless, without effort, Sec-c.
— periodical, Cupr. Nux. Sacch.
— of a substance like pitch, Ip.
— pus, Merc-cor.
— saltish, Iod. Mgn-c. Ntr-s.
— scanty, Asar.
— of solids only, Bry. Cupr. Verat.
— sour, Acet-ac. *Calc.* Ars. Bell. Borax. Borm. Cadm. Calc. Camph. *Caust.* Cham. Chin. Croton. Daph. Ferr. Gels. Graph. Hep. Ip. Iris. Kali-b. Kali-c. Lact-ac. Lyc. Mgn-c. Ntr-m. *Ntr-s.* Nitr-ac. Nux. Phosp-ac. Pod. Psor. Puls. Sacch. Sass. Stram. *Sulph.* Tabac. Thuj. Verat.
— — early in the morning. Kali-b. Nux.
— stercoraceous, Bell. Nux. *Op. Plb.*

— sweetish, Creos.
— — mucus, Calc. Iris. Psor.
— tenacious, Arg-n. Dulc.
— of urine, *Op.*
— vehement, *Ars. Cupr. Jatr. Iod.* Mez. *Plb.* Tart. *Verat.*
— violent, Bell. Bism. Lach. Lob. Merc. Mosch. Nux. Puls. Raph.
— watery, Acon. Aeth. Arg. Arn. Ars. Bar-c. Bell. Bism. Bry. Cannab. Caust. Chin. Con. Creos. Cupr. Grat. Hep. Hipp-m. •Ind. Iris. Ip. Jatr. Kali-b. Mgn-c. Mez. Ntr-s. Nux. Oleand. Puls. Raph. Rat. Sang. Sil. Stann. Stram. Sulph. Sulph-ac. Tabac. Verat.
— — frothy, Croton.
— — containing flakes and offensive, Cupr.
— of water then of food. Ip. Nux. Sep. Sil. Sulph. Sulph-ac.
— — worms, Acon. Cina. Ferr. Hyosc. Phyt. Sabad. Sang. Sec-c. Sil. Spig. Verat.
— — — lumbrici, Acon. Cina. Sabad.
— yellowish, Ars. Bry. Colch. Iod. Ip. Oleand. Plb. Verat.
— — green, Oleand. Verat.
— in the morning, Ars. Bar-c. Calc. Creos. Dig. Dros. Ferr. Guaj. Hep. Kali-c. Lyc. Mosch. Nux. Sep. Sil. Sulph.
— — in afternoon, Chin-sulph. Sulph.
— — evening, Anac. Bell. Bry. Croton. Phosp. Puls. Sulph.
— night, Ars. Bell. Bry. Calc. Dig. Dros. Ferr. Igt. Kali-c. Lyc. Merc. Mur-ac. Nux. Phosp. Puls. Rat. Sep. Sil. Sulph. Therid. Valer. Verat.
— at midnight, Ferr.
— after acids, Ferr.
— — beer, Ferr. Mez.
— — bread, Nitr-ac.
— — breakfast, Borax. Daph.
— — children, Calc. Hyosc.
— — a cold, Bell.
— when becoming cold, Cocc.
— after drinking, Am. Ars. Bry. Cocc. Dros. Eupat. Ip. Ntr-m. Nux. Puls. Sil. Verat.
— — relieved, Cupr.
— in drunkards, Nux. Op Sacch. Zinc.
— after exercise, Colch. Stram. Tabac. Therid. Verat. Zinc.
— when closing the eyes, Therid.
— after meals, Amm-c. Ant. *Ars.* Bry. *Calc.* Cham. Crotal. Cupr. Dig. Dros. *Ferr.* Graph. Hyosc. *Iod.* Ip. Iris. Lach. Lob. Mgn-c. Nitr-ac. *Nux.* Op. Phosp. *Puls.* Ruta. Sec-c. *Sep. Sil* Stann. Sulph. Tart. *Verat.*
— during meals, Dig. Puls. Rhus.
— as soon as he eats, Dig.
— — — — — relieved, Ferr.
— after milk, Aeth. Samb. Spong. Sulph.
— — nursing (in infants,) Sil.

14. ERUCTATIONS, NAUSEA AND VOMITING.

— in pregnancy, Con. Ip. Iris. Jatr. Ntr-m. Nux-m. Nux. Ox-ac. Petr. Sep.
— from riding in a carriage, Cocc. Petr.
— after smoking, Ip.
— — spitting, Dig.
— — stooping, Ip.
— in teething children, Calc. Bism. Hyosc.
— with abdominal cramps, *Cupr.* Op.
— — — pain, Ars. Asar. Bry. Cadm. Canth. Colch. Graph. Hell. Hyosc. Iod. Nux. Plb. Puls. Stram.
— — after taste, bitter, Croton. *Puls.*
— — — sour, Anac.
— — agitation congestion of blood, Verat.
— — alternating with tonic spasms of pectoral muscles and distortion of eyes, vomiting does not relieve, in tetanus, Cin.
— — anxiety, Ant. Arg-n. Ars. Asar. Bar-m. Bism. Nux. Sang. Seneg.
— — back pain in, Puls.
— with breath offensive, Ip.
— — chills, Puls. Tart. Valer.
— — choking, Hyosc.
— — colic, Dig.
— — — relieved, Hyosc.
— — congestion to chest, Nux.
— — convulsions, Ant. *Cupr.* Hyosc. Merc. Op.
— — cries, Ars.
— — diarrhoea, Aeth. Ant. Apis. Arg-n. Ars. Asar. Bell. Bism. Chin. Coloc. *Cupr.* Cycl. Dulc. Elaps. Eugen. Euph. Hipp. Ip. Jatr Lach. Merc. Merc-cor. Merc-sulph. Phosp. Plb. Puls. Sang. Seneg. Sep. Stann. Stram. Sulph. Tart. *Verat.*
— — — during pregnancy, Petr.
— — eructations, Caust. Mur-ac. Nitr-ac.
— — eyes convulsed, Cic.
— — face pale, Puls. Tart.
— — — sweat on, Camph. Sulph.
— — feet coldness and numbness, Creos. Phosp.
— — giddiness, Hyosc. Ntr-s Therid.
— — hand, coldness, of Creos. Phosp. Verat.
— — — heat, Ars. Bell. Ip. Verat.
— — headache, Asar. Chin. Cimex. Con. Creos. Lach. Nux. Sang. Sep.
— — heat, Acon. Ars. Bell. Ip. Lam. Verat.
— — hiccoughing, Bry.
— — hunger, Cina.
— — — craving to eat, Sang.
— — compelling one to lie down, Verat.
— — legs cold, Nux.
— — — cramps in, Hyosc.
— — nausea, Acon. Bar-m. Colch. Croton. Dig. Eupat. Graph. Lam. Lob. Mur-ac. Nux. Rhus. Sang. Sulph. Tart. *Verat.* Zinc.
— — nose, dryness in, Creos.

— — — obstructed, Grat.
— — perspiration, Acon. Bell. Ip. Sulph.
— — — cold, Cadm. Camph. Lob. Sulph.
— — salivation, Lob.
— — scratching and burning in throat, Arg.
— — shuddering, Verat.
— — sight, obscuration of, Lam. Lach.
— — green and yellow colors before the, Tabac.
— — sleepiness, Cycl. Tart.
— — stomach, pain in, Ars. Asar. Bar-m. Cupr. Hyosc. Ip. Lach. Mosch. Op. Phosp. Plb. Sulph. Tart.
— — — pit of, Dig. Verat.
— — stool, ineffectual urging to, Sang.
— — syncope, Elaps. Kali-c. Gum-gut.
— — the morning cough, Scill.
— — dejection, Dig.
— — taste, bitter, Puls.
— — — sour, after, Anac.
— — teeth, bluntness of, after, Puls.
— — thirst, Acon. Creos. Ip.
— — tongue clean, Cina.
— — trembling, Colch. Eupat. Nux. Tart.
— — — urination profuse, Acon. Lach. Verat.
— — weakness, Ars. Bism. Eupat. Ip. Kali-c. Lam. Phosp. Sec-c. Tart. Verat.
— followed by hunger and thirst, Oleand.
— — — thirst, Acon. Sulph-ac.
Vomiturition, retching, Acon. Arg. Arn. Ars. Bar-m. Bell. Brom. Bry. Cannab. Canth. Caps. Carb-veg. Cham. Chin. Cocc. Cupr. Dig. Dros. Dros. Graph. Hyosc. Iod. Ip. Kali-c. Lob. Mgn-c. Merc. Mez. Ntr-m. Nux. Puls. Rhus. Scill. *Sec-c.* Seneg. Sep. Sil. *Stann.* Sulph. *Tart.* Tereb. Verat. Viol-tr. Zinc.
— convulsive, Dig.
— empty, with ineffectual efforts, *Arn. Asar. Bell. Bry.* Chin. Creos. Croton. Grat. Ip. *Nux.* Op. Plb. Puls. Sulph. Verat.
— — relieving head, Asar.
— vehement, Ars. Asar. Asar. Dig. Sacch.
— in morning, Creos.
— evening, Kali-c.
— at night, Arn. Ran-sc. Rat.
— in drunkards, *Nux.*
— after, meals, Chin. Mgn-c.
— before meals, Berb.
— from cold liquids, Ip.
— when hawking up mucus, Ambr.
— after smoking, Ip.
— when making an effort to swallow, Merc-cor.
— with colic, Hyosc.
— perspiration on forehead, Tart.
— increase of all complaints, Asar. Oleand.
— langor, Tart.
— retching, and salivation, Hep. Tart.

14. ERUTATIONS, NAUSEA AND VOMITING.

— pain in pit of stomach, Arn.
Waterbrash, pyrosis, Acet-ac. Amm-m. Anac. Ars. Bar-c. Bry. Calc. *Carb-an.* Carb-veg. Con. Cycl. *Dros.* Graph. Kali-jod. Lach. *Led.* Lyc. Mez. *Ntr-m.* Ntr-s. Nux. *Petr.* Phosp. Puls. Rhod. Rhus. Sep. *Sil.* Staph. *Sulph.* Valer. Verat.
— in morning, Sulph.
— — evening, Anac. Cycl. Ntr-s.
— at night, Carb-veg. Graph.
— after acids, Phosp.
— chronic, *Sil.*
— after drinking, Nitr-ac. Sep.

— — — fast, Nitr-ac.
— — meals, Amm-c. Calc. Phosp. Sep. *Sil. Sulph.*
— — milk, Cupr. Phosp.
— every other day, Lyc.
— with acidity, Carb-an.
— — anxiety, heat, tremor, Euph.
— — colic, Led. Sulph.
— — nausea, Calc. *Cycl.*
— — shuddering, shivering, Sil.
— — stomach, pain in Ntr-m. *Sil.*
— — vomiting, Anac. Ntr-m. Sil.
— — — a bitter fluid, Lyc.

15. Stomach.

Aching, Amm-c. Ant. Ars. Bar-c. *Bell.* *Calc. Carb-veg.* Caust. *Cham. Chin. Cocc.* Con. Cupr. Dig. Graph. *Igt. Kali-c. Lach.* Lyc. Mgn-c. *Merc.* Ntr-c. Ntr-m. Nux-m. *Nux* Petr. Phosp. Puls. Sep. Sil. Stann. Staph. *Sulph.* Verat.
Acrid feeling in stomach, Hep.
Adhesion, sense of in pit of stomach, *Hep.*
Anxiety in stomach and pit of, *Ars. Caust* Cham. Cic. Cocc. Coff. Cupr. Guaj. *Jatr.* Lact. Laur. Nux. *Paeon.* Plb. *Sec-c. Stram.* Teucr. Thuj. Verat.
Atony of stomach, Bell.
Balanced up and down, as if stomach were, Phosp-ac.
Beaten, pain as if in stomach, Asa-f. Euph. Mgn-m. Ol-an.
— — — — pit of, Camph.
Biting sensation in stomach, Mosch. Stram.
Bitterness in stomach, Cupr.
Boring, Ars. Ntr-s Sep.
Bruised pain, Nux. Ol-an.
Burning in stomach, Acet-ac. Acon. Ambr. Amm-c. Amm-m. *Ars.* Asa-f. Bell. Berb. Bism. Brom. *Bry.* Cact. *Calad.* Calc. *Camph. Canth. Caps.* Carb-an. *Carb-veg.* Cham. Chelid. Chin. Cic. *Colch.* Croc. Crotal. Croton. Daph. Dig. Dulc. Elaps. Euph. Fluor-ac. Gels. Graph. Hell. Hep. Hipp. Hydroc-ac. Hyosc. Igt. Iod. *Jatr.* Kali-b. Kali-c. Kali-jod. Lach. Lact. *Laur.* Lob. *Mang.* Merc. Merc-cor. Merc-iod. Mez. *Millef.* Mosch. Ntr-s. Nicc. Nitr-ac. *Nitr.* Nux-m. *Nux.* Ol-an. Ox-ac. Par. Phell. *Phosp.* Plb. Ran-sc. Rhus. Ruta. *Sabad.* Sang. Sass. *Sec-c* Seneg. *Sep.* Sil. Sulph. Sulph-ac. Tabac. *Tereb.* Tilia. Verat.
— — — not relieved by drinking, Calad.
— — — causing hunger, Graph.
— — — ascending to chest, Arg.
— — — circumscribed of the size of a dollar, Gymnoc.
— — — with vomiting, Bar-m. Jatr.
— — pit of stomach, Acon. Ambr. Amm-m. Ant. Arg. Ars. Bell. Bry. *Caps.* Cham. Casc. Dig. Euph. Laur. Merc. Nux. *Phosp.* Phosp-ac. Plat. *Ran-b. Ran-sc. Sec-c.* Sep. Sil. Sulph. Verat.
— across pit of stomach, Cham.

Cancer of stomach, *Ars.* Bar-c. Con. Creos. *Lyc.* Nux. Phosp. Plat. Verat.
Chilliness of pit of stomach, Bell. Calc. Cist. Hipp.
Choking. Nux.
Clawing, Arn. Calc. *Carb-an.* Caust. *Cocc.* Euph. Graph. *Nux.* Puls. *Sulph-ac.* Tabac.
— in pit of stomach, Caust. Dros. Ntr-m.
Coldness, sense of, Acon. Bov. Caps. Chelid. Clem. *Colch.* Con. Grat. Hipp. Hydroc-ac. Igt. Kali-jod. Lach. Lact. Laur. Mgn-s. Nitr-ac. Nitr. Ol-an. Phosp. Phosp-ac. Rhus. Sabad. Sacch. Sep. Sulph. Sulph-ac. Tabac.
— — — in morning, Mgn-s.
— — — — pit of stomach, Ars. Bell. Laur. Phosp.
Colic with spasms in chest, Cupr. Sep. Verat.
Concussive pain when stepping, Casc.
— — — in pit of stomach, Anac. Mgn-m.
Constriction of pylorus, Bry. *Prosp.*
— — stomach, Amm-c. Euph. Ferr. Guaj. Lach. Nux. Sacch.
— — must press the stomach with the hand, Dros.
— pain, Acon. *Alum.* Arn. Ars. Asa-f. Bell. Borax. Brom. Calc. *Carb-an.* Carb-veg. Chelid. Cocc. Con. Croton. *Euph.* Guaj. Hydroc-ac. Jatr. Kali-b. Kali-c. Lact. Laur. Lob. Lyc. *Mgn-c.* Meny. Merc. Millef. Mur-ac. Ntr-c. Ntr-m. Nicc. Nitr-ac. *Nitr. Nux.* Ol-an. Op. Phosp. Phyt. Plat. *Plb.* Puls. Ran-c. *Rat.* Rheum. Rhod. Sass. Sep. Spong. *Sulph.* Sulph-ac. Tabac.
— sense in pit of stomach, Cact. Cast. Lob. Plat. Puls. Rhod. Sulph-ac.
— pain as if stomach were gathered up in a ball, Arn.
— — in upper part of stomach, Croton.
Corrosion sense of, Iod. Nux.
Cramp, Agar. Amm-c. *Ant.* Arn. Ars. Asa-f. Bar-m. Bell. *Bism.* Brom. *Bry. Calc.* Cannab. *Carb-an. Carb-veg. Caust. Cham.* Chelid. *Chin. Cocc. Coff.* Con. Cupr. Daph. Dig. Dulc. Euph. *Ferr. Graph.* Hydroc-ac. *Hyosc* Iod. Jatr. *Kali-c.* Lach. Lob. Lyc. Mgn-c. Merc.

15. STOMACH.

Millef. Ntr-c. *Ntr-m*. Nitr-ac. Nitr. Nux-m. *Nux*. Petr. Phosp. Plb. *Puls*. Sec-c. Seneg. Sep. *Stann*. Sulph. Tabac. Thuj. Verat.
Cramps in st., chronic, Bell. Chin. Stann.
— periodical, Hyosc.
— in morning, Puls.
— — — 2 A. M., Ars. Ntr-c.
— — evening increased, Thuj.
— at night, Calc. Kali-c. Seneg. Sulph.
— in coffee drinkers, *Cham. Nux*.
— after loss of animal fluids, Chin.
— by diseases of spleen, caused, Bry.
— by vomiting relieved, Hyosc.
— worse by drinking water, cold, Calc.
— from a cold, Nitr-ac.
— with weak digestion, Nux-m.
— — bitter eructations, Stann.
— — pale face, Cannab.
— — flatulency, Carb-veg.
— — nausea, Graph. *Ntr-m*. Nux Tabac.
— — perspiration, Cannab.
— — weak pulse, Cannab.
— — vomiting, Calc. Kali-c. *Puls*.
— in pit of stomach, Ang. Ant. Chelid. Zinc.
Cramping pain, Ant. Arn. Ars. Iod. (compare Spasmodic).
Crawling, Colch. Lact. Puls.
— in pit of stomach, Lact. Puls.
Cutting pain, Ang. Cannab. Chelid. Kali-chl. Ntr-c. Plb. Rat. Sep. Sulph-ac.
— — in pit of stomach, Ant. Bry. Calad. Calc. Cannab. Nicc. Rat.
— towards spine, Sep.
Digging, Graph. Kali-c. Staph. Sulph.
— pit of stomach, Arn. Phosp. Sabad. *Sulph*.
Distention, Ars. Calc. Caps. Con. Dulc. *Hell*. Ip. *Lyc*. Nux-m. Nux. Op. *Rat*. Sabin. Sacch.
— before eating, Croc.
— pit of stomach, Ars. *Bell*. Calc. Cic. Daph. Hell. *Hep*. Merc-cor. *Nux*. Op. Prun.
— sensation of, Mang.
Dragging downwards, sensation of, Merc.
Drawing, sensation, of Amn-m. Ars. Bry. Mang. Ntr-c.
Earth in stomach, sensation of, Millef.
Emptiness, sensation of, Amm-c. Ant. Bry. Bufo. Calad. Caust. Con. Croc. Croton. Dig. Gels. Glon. Grat. Gum-gut. Hell. Hipp. *Igt*. Ip. Kali-jod. Lac-can. Meph. Merc-jod. Mur-ac. Ntr-c. Ntr-m. *Nicc*. Phosp. Plb. Ruta. Sang. Seneg. Senna. Sep. Staph. Sulph. Tart. *Teucr*. Verb.
— with sense of fulness in abdomen, Oleand.
Extension, sense of in pit of stomach, Mang.
Faintish, pit of stomach, Alum. Brom.

Hep. Laur. Nitr.
Fermentation in pit of stomach, Croc.
Flabbiness, Euph. Ip. Merc. Spong. Tabac. Thea.
Fulness, sense of, Acon. Amm-c. Ant. *Arn*. Ars. Asar. Asa-f. *Bar-c*. Bell. *Bov*. Calc. Camph. Canth. Carb-an. Carb-veg. Casc. *Cast*. Cham. Chin. Chin-sulph. Cocc. Croton. *Cycl*. Daph. Dig. Fluor-ac. *Grat Hell*. Hyosc. Igt. Iod. Jac-cor. *Kali-c*. Lach. Lachn. Laur. Lith. Lob. *Lyc*. Mang. Merc. Mez. Millef. *Mosch*. Mur-ac. Ntr-c. *Ntr-s*. Nicc. Nux-jug. Nux-m. Nux. Ol-an. Op. Par. Petr. Phell. *Phosp*. Plat. Prun. Ran-sc. *Rheum*. Rhus. Sabin. Stann. Staph. Sulph. Sulph-ac. Tart.
— as if of undigested food, Kobalt.
— oppressing the breathing, Ntr-s. Nux-m. Prun.
— more in the morning, Ran-sc.
— in evening in bed, Ntr-s.
Gangrene of stomach, Sec-c.
Gnawing, Amm-m. Ars. Calad. Chelid. Colch. Cupr. Glon. Iod. Lith. Lyc. Millef. Ntr-c. Nitr. Nux. Ox-ac. *Ruta*. Sulph.
— left side, Arg-n.
Gurgling, Anac. Carb-an. Croc. Croton. Fluor-ac. Kali-jod. Lact. Laur. Lob. Meny. Sacch. Teucr. Thea. Verb.
— when drinking, Cina. Cupr. Laur. Thuj.
Hardness, sensation of in pylorus, Creos.
Heat, Bar-c. Chin-sulph. Cinnab. Hydroc-ac. Kali-chl. Mang. Mez. Ntr-m. Phosp. Pod. Sass.
— in pit of stomach, Apis. Phosp.
Hepatic eruption at pit of stomach, Ars.
Jerks at pit of stomach, Ntr-c. Ntr-m. Nux. Plat.
Induration. Ars. Bar-c. Con. Lyc. Mez. Nux. Phosp. Thuj. Verat.
Inflation, Ars. Calc. Caps. Con. Dulc. Hell. Ip. Lyc. Nux-m. Nux. Op. Rat. Sabin. Sacch.
Inflamation, *Acon*. Ant. Apis. Ars. Asa-f. Bar-c. Bell. Bism. Brom. *Bry*. *Camph*. *Canth*. Chelid. Euph. Hell. Hydroc-ac. Iod. Ip. Kali-jod. Lach. Laur. Mez. Nitr. *Nux*. Phosp. Plb. Puls. Ran-b. Ran-sc. Sabad. Sang. Scill. Sec-c. Stram. Tereb. *Verat*.
Jumping, sensation of, Croc.
Lime as if burned or slacked in stomach, Caust.
Living, as if something were in stomach. Croc.
Movements in stomach, Ntr-m. Nitr. Ol-an. Lyc. Nux. Phosp. Sulph.
Narrow, pylorus feels too, Calc. Chin. Lyc. Nux. Phosp. Sulph.
Numbness, sensation of, Cast.
Obstruction of pylorus, sensation of, Lach. Nux. Phosp.

15. STOMACH.

Open, as if stomach stood, sensation, Spong.
Oppression in pit of stomach, Bell. Bry. Cocc. Coff. Creos. *Mosch. Plat.* Prun. Sabad. Sec-c. Teucr.
Over-eating as from, pain, *Ant.* Cycl. Rheum. Tart.
Pain, Arn. Ars. Bell. Brom. Bry. Cist. Cocc. Corn-c. Creos. Cupr. Elat. Jatr. Iod. Lyc. Rumex. Zing.
— pain horrid and indescribable sick feeling, *Ip.*
— which compels one to eat, Graph.
— in pit of stomach after retrogression of small pox, Millef.
— — — — as if something were tearing off, Petr.
Painfulness when pressed upon, Apis. Bry. Calc. *Ntr-m.* Nux. Ol-an. *Sil.*
— when stepping, Bar-c.
— — talking, Ntr-m.
— — touched, Ant. Bry. *Colch.* Coloc. Hyosc. Lach. Lyc. Merc. Ntr-c. *Ntr-m.* Nux. Phosp. Spig. Sulph.
— — walking or coughing, Hell.
Pains violent, *Ars.* Aur. Cupr. *Hell.* Hydroc-ac. *Iod. Ip.* Lach. Merc. Phosp. *Plb.* Ran-b. Ran-sc. *Sec-c.* Stann. *Verat.*
— sudden, Elaps.
— when nursing, Carb-veg.
— at cardiac orifice on swallowing food, Alum. Bry. Nitr-ac. Phosp.
Periodical pain, Hyosc. Igt. Lyc.
Pinching, nipping, Arn. Asar. Calc. Cannab. Graph. Kali-c. Plat. Puls.
— — in pit of stomach, Calc. Cannab. *Cocc.* Ip.
Pregnant women, in, pain, Puls.
Pressing in pit of stomach, Coff.
Pressure, *Acon. Agar.* Alum. Ambr. *Anac.* Arg-n. *Ars.* Asaf. *Asa-f. Bar-c.* Bar-m. *Bell.* Berb. *Bism.* Brom. *Bry.* Calad. *Calc.* Cannab. Canth. *Carb-an. Carb-veg. Casc.* Caust. *Cic.* Chin. Coff. Coloc. Con. Dig. Dulc. Elat. *Ferr.* Fluor-ac. *Graph. Grat. Hep.* Hyper. *Iod.* Ip. Kali-b. Kali-jod. Lach. *Lact.* Laur. Led. Lob. *Lyc.* Mgn-c. Mgn-m. Meph. *Merc. Mez.* Mosch. *Ntr-c. Ntr-m.* Nicc. Nux-m. *Nux.* Ol-an. Op. Osm. Ox-ac. *Par. Petr.* Phosp. *Plat. Plb.* Puls. Rheum. *Rhod.* Rhus. Sabin. *Samb.* Scill. Sec-c. *Seneg.* Sep. *Sil.* Spong. *Stann.* Stram. Stront. Sulph. Sulph-ac. Tabac. *Tart.* Tereb. *Thea. Verat.* Verb. Zinc.
Pressure in pit of stomach, Acon. Agar. Amm-c. Anac. Arg. Arn. Asar. Aur. Bar-c. Bell. Berb. Bov. Calc. Cannab. Caust. Cham. Chin. Coloc. *Cupr. Cycl.* Dig. Grat. Hell. Hep. Hydroc-ac. Hyper. Igt. Jac-cor. Kali-c.

Kali-chl. Kalm. Lact. Lob. Lyc. Mang. Merc. *Ntr-m.* Ntr-nitr. *Nitr.* Nux. Ol-an. Pæon. Plat. Plb. Prun. Puls. Ran-b. *Ran-sc.* Rhod. Rhus. Sass. Sep. *Stann.* Staph. *Tart.* Teucr. Tereb. Thuj. *Valer. Verat.* Zinc.
— as if heart were being crushed, Ars. Carb-veg. Cham. Nux.
— after each meal with vomiting of ingesta, Bry. Caps. Cham. Nux. Puls.
— as from a weight, *Acon.* Arn. Ars. Brom. Bry. Calc. Carb-an. *Cham.* Elaps. Fluor-ac. Hep. Kali-b. Merc. Nux. Par. *Phosp-ac.* Rhus. Scill. Sec-c. Sep. Sil. Spig. Staph. Zing.
— of a cold stone, Acon. Colch.
— — from a weight in pit of stomach, Ars. Cact. Fluor-ac. Grat. Lob. Spig. Spong.
— from the clothes, Amm-c. Bry. Calc. Carb-veg. Caust. Chin. Coff. Creos. Kali-b. Lach. Lith. Lyc. Nux. Spong. Sulph.
Pulsation in pit of stomach, Ars. Asa-f. Bell. Chin. Dros. Graph. Iod. Jac-cor. Kali-c. Lach. Lam. Mgn-m. Ntr-m. Nitr-ac. Plat. Puls. Rhus. Sep. Sulph. Tart. Thuj. (compare Throbbing.)
Red spots on pit of stomach, Ntr-m.
Relaxed, stomach feels, Ip. Lob. Raph. Staph. Sulph-ac.
Rending, tearing, in pit of stomach, Aeth. Colch. Dig. Rhus. Ruta. Sep. Zinc.
Restlessness, *Canth.*
Retraction sense of, Dig. Hell. Mur-ac.
— pit of stomach, Calad. Dulc. Lach.
Rolling, rumbling, Carb-an. Caust. Chin. Croc. Croton. Hell. Kali-jod. Laur. Lyc. Meny. Nux. Phosp. Phosp-ac. Puls. Sulph. Teucr. Thea. Verb.
Scraping, Hell.
Sensitiveness, Amm-c. Amm-m. Ars. Bar-c. Canth. Carb-veg. Caust. Cocc-c. Colch. Creos. Croton. Elat. Fluor-ac. Glon. Hep. Hipp-m. Lach. Lyc. Mgn-c. Merc. Nux. Ol-an. Phyt. Sulph-ac. Tereb. *Verat.*
— to pressure, Bry. Calc. Lach. *Ntr-m.* Nux. Ol-an. Sil.
— — talking, Ntr-c.
— — touch, Acon. Ant. Ars. Bry. Camph. Cannab. Canth. Cham. *Colch.* Coloc. Creos. Croton. Hyosc. Lach. Lyc. Merc. Ntr-c. *Ntr-m.* Nux. Phosp. Puls. Sacch. Sulph. Tereb. Tilia. Verat.
— when walking, Calc. Phosp.
Shocks, blows in pit of stomach, Ntr-c. Nux. Plat.
Shuddering in pit of stomach, Bell. Caust.
Sickly feeling, Croc. Croton. Diad. Kali-jod. Lact. Lyc. Mgn-c. Mosch. Sabad. Sil. Sulph. Tart. Teucr. *Thea.* Verat.

15. STOMACH.

Sinking in pit of stomach, Igt. Jatr.
— — before meals, Sulph.
— — after meals, Dig.
Soreness, *Ang. Bar-c.* Bry. Chin. Cinnab. Colch. Con. Daph. Mosch. Nux. *Sabad*. Zinc.
— inside, Eupion.
— pit of stomach, Alum. Con. Mang. Merc-jod. Ran-b. Ran-sc.
Spasmodic pain, Bar-m. Calc. Cocc. Con. Dulc. Ferr. Igt.
— — pit of stomach, *Ang.* Chelid. Zinc.
Stinging, stitches, Bell. Berb. Bry. Chelid. Coff. Con. Hydroc-ac. Igt. Kali-c. Nitr. Nitr-ac. Ol-an. Sep. Sulph.
— — pit of stomach, Ambr. Amm-c. Anac. *Arn.* Aur. Bar-c. Bell. Berb. Borax. Bov. Bry. Calad. Calc. Canth. Caps. Carb-an. Caust. Chelid. Chin. Coff. Creos. Croc. Croton. Cupr. Cycl. Dros. Euph. Graph. Igt. Iod. Ip. Jac-cor. *Kali-c.* Lach. Lyc. Nicc. *Nitr-ac.* Nitr. Pod. Puls Ran-sc. Rheum. Rhod. Ruta. Sabin. Samb. Sep. Staph. Sulph, *Tabac.* Tart. Zinc.
Strain, pain as of a strain, Borax. Nitr. Ol-an.
Swelling in pit of stomach, Acon. Amm-c. Aur. *Calc.* Cham. Cic. Cocc c. Coff. Hep. Hipp-m. Igt. Kali-b. *Lyc Ntr-m.* Nux. Petr. Sulph. Thuj.
Tension, Acon. Asa-f. Bry. Carb-veg. Clem. Croton. Kali-c. Mgn-m. Merc. Staph.
— in pit of stomach, Acon. Ang. Ant. Cham. Croton. Nux. Ran-sc. Stann. Tar.
Throbbing in pit of stomach, Acon. Asa-f. Calad. Cact. Chelid. Chin. Cic. Croc. Dros. Hydroc-ac. Iod. Ip. Kali-c. Lachn. Mgn-m. Oleand. Plat. Rheum. Rhus. *Sep.* Sulph. Thuj.
— — — — — with nausea, Ntr-c.
Tingling, Colch. *Rhus.*
— pit of stomach, Ind. *Puls.*
Torn away as if something were, Poth. Rhus.
Turning sensation, Nitr. Ol-an.
Ulcerous pain, Cannab. *Mgn-m. Rat.* Rhus. Stann.
— — pit of stomach, Cast. Hell. Ntr-m. Rhus.
— — relieved by eating, Gum-gut.
Undulation sense of, after meals, Phosp-ac.
Uneasiness, Croton. Grat. Phosp. Sabad. Zinc.
— as after a severe disease, Mur-ac.
Warmth sense of, Casc. Nux-m. Seneg.
— — — rising to head and chest, Bar-m.
— — pit of stomach, Bry. Sabad,
Water as if full of, sensation, Millef. Ol-an. Phell.
Weakness sensation of, Bar-m. *Dig.* Igt. Lob. Merc-jod. Petr.

— — — pit of stomach, Croc. Lob. Nitr.
— like faintness, after congestion in head and nape of neck, Tellur.
Winding twisting sensation, Ntr-m.
Worm, sensation of, Lach.
In the morning pain, Anac. Chin. Lyc. Mgn-s. Ntr-m. Nux. Phosp. Puls. Ran-sc. Staph. Sulph.
— — evening, pain, Alum. Carb-an. Lob. Lyc. Phosp. Puls. Sep. *Sulph-ac.* Thuj.
— — — relieved, Lyc.
At night, Alum. Amm-c. Ars. Calc. Carb-veg. Cham. Con. Graph. Igt. Kali-c. Nitr-ac. Nux. Phosp. Puls. Rhod. Rhus. Seneg. Sep. Sil. Sulph.
— — in bed, Ntr-s.
Open air, Lyc. Nux.
Bed, warmth of, relieved, Graph. Lyc.
Bending double, Kalm.
— — relieved, Cham. Lact.
Brandy, Igt.
Bread, eating, relieved, Staph.
Breathing, pain in pit of stomach, Anac. Caps. Cocc-c.
Chill during a, Lob.
After a cold, Carb-veg. Caust. Lyc. Sulph-ac.
By cold drinks, relieved, Phosp.
— drinking, Arn. Iris.
— — quickly, Sil.
From contradiction, Carb-veg.
— disappointment, Carb-veg.
By eating, Arn. Cact.
After eating, Lob.
By eating, relieved, Cham. Chelid. Iris. Lith. Mez. Ntr-s. Ox-ac. Raph. Sacch. Staph.
— eructations, relieved, Nicc. Nux-jug. Pæon. Rat.
When exercising, Ang. Bry. Cannab. Caust. Cupr.
— — fasting, Lob.
From flatulent food, Carb-veg.
By emission of flatus, relieved, Lact.
From loss of animal fluids, Carb-veg. Chin.
— fright, Carb-veg.
By lying down, relieved, Amm-c. Bell. Caust. Chin. Graph. Stann.
When lying on the side, Bry. Cupr.
— pressed upon, Acon. Bry. Calc. Colch. Igt. *Lach. Ntr-m.* Ol-an. Ran-sc. Sabad. Samb. Sil.
From a misstep, Aloe. *Bry.* Puls. Rhus.
By rest relieved, Cham. (compare Lying down).
When sitting, Elaps. Hep. Puls. Sulph.
From speaking, pain pit of stomach, Caps. Ntr-c.
When stepping, Anac. Bry. Hell. Mgn-m.
— when stooping, Alum. Glon. Kalm. Rhus.

From a strain, Arn. Bry. Rhus.
When stretching, pain pit of stomach, Amm-c.
— swallowing food, Bar-c. Nitr-ac. Sep.
From touch, Ant. Arn. Ars. Aur. Bar-c. Bry. Calc. Canth. Coloc. Creos. Croton. Cupr. Hyosc. Lach. Lyc. Merc-cor. Ntr-c. *Ntr-m.* Ox-ac. Petr. Phosp. Phosp-ac. Spig. Stann. Sulph. Tereb. Thuj.
Vomiting, relieved by, Hyosc.
Walking, when, Bell. Calc. Phosp. Poth. Sep.
— after, pain in pit of stomach, Calad.
With anxiety, Bov. Cham. Croton. Op. Ran-sc. Sabad.
— apathy, Kali-chl.
— asthma, Alum. Cham. Chelid. Cocc. Dulc. Guaj. Hell. Lyc. Ntr-s. Nux-m. Phosp. Puls. Rhod. Rhus. Spig. Stram.
— chest, spasms in, Lyc. Nux. Sep.
— — oppression of, Nux.
— chilliness, Amm-c. Kali-chl. Lyc.
— constant desire to eat, Raph.
— deadness of hands, Lyc.
— despair, Ant.
— diarrhoea, Calc-ph. Staph.
— eructations, Kali-chl. Grat. Lach. Rhus.
— — bitter, Stann.
— — sour, Mgn-c.
— eructate, desire to, *Grat.*

— face, pale, Cannab. Mgn-c. Stann.
— fainting, Laur. Nitr.
— flatulency, Carb-veg.
— headache, Bov. Calc-ph. Sang.
— heat in head, Caust.
— hunger, Meny, Raph. Verat.
— loins, pain in, Borax.
— mouth, bitterness in, Lyc.
With nausea, *Amm-c.* Ars. Calad. Caps. Croc. Croton. Dig. Grat. Lact. Mgn-m. Mgn-s. Mang. Meph. Merc. *Ntr-m.* Puls. Sec-c. Stann. Sulph. Tabac. Tart.
— peevishness, Bry.
— perspiration, Cannab. Cham.
— — suppressed, Cham. Chelid. *Cocc.* Dulc. Guaj. Hell. Ntr-s. Nux-m. Phosp. *Rhod.* Rhus. Spig. Stram.
— rattling in throat, Cannab.
— retching, Lach. Nux.
— restlessness, Cham. Mang.
— shuddering, Caust.
— speechlessness, from violent pain in stomach, Laur.
— suicide, inclination to commit, Ant.
— taste bitter, Lyc.
— thirst, Verat.
— vomiting, Bry. Calc. Dig. Graph. Ip. Kali-c. Lach. Nux. Puls. Sulph.
— — billious, Iod.
— — of what has been eaten, Calc. Phosp. Puls.
— weakness, Calc-ph. Ntr-m. Sabad.

16. Hypochondres, Kidneys, Diaphragm, Liver and Spleen.

Abbreviations:—HYP., HYPOCHONDRES, KID., KIDNEYS, DIA., DIAPHRAGM, LIV., LIVER, SP., SPLEEN.

Abscess of liv., Lach. Sil.
Aching in hyp., Bell. Chin. Hyosc. Kali-c. Merc. Ntr-c. Puls. Sulph. Zinc.
Anxiety in hyp., Cham. Phosp-ac. Staph.
Bandage, as if a, around hyp., sensation, Con. Lyc.
Beaten, as if. hyp., *Carb-veg.* Cocc. Cupr. Lach. Ox-ac. Ran-b.
— — liv., Carb-veg. Clem. Lact.
— — sp., Sass.
Blood boils in region of liv., Nux-jug.
Boring, hyp., *Seneg.* Sep.
— liv., Amm-c.
Breath, pain, obstructing, Igt. Kali-c. Staph.
— — — sp., Amm-m. Arn.
Bruise, pain as of, in liv., Creos.
Burning, dia., Asa-f.
— hyp., Acon. Aeth. Bell. Cannab. Caust. *Chelid.* Grat. Graph. Plat. Seneg. Spig. Tabac. Tong.
— kid., Bell. Bufo. Canth. Hep. Kali-b. Tereb.
— — left, Benz-ac. Lachn.
— liv., *Acon.* Amm-c. *Bry.* Gum-gut. *Kali-c.* Lach. Merc. *Mur-ac.* Stann. *Staph. Tereb.*
— sp., Bell. Igt. Sec-c.
Colic, renal, Berb. Ind. Nux-m. Ocim. Sass. Zinc.
— — with vomiting, anguish, red urine, brick dust, or bloody sediment, Ocim.
Compression, dia., Op.
— liv,. Ars.
Constriction, Asar. *Nux.*
— hyp., Acon. Con. Dig. Dros.
Contraction, dia., Asar. Mez.
— hyp., Nux.
— kid., Clem.
— liv., Canth.
Cramps, dia., *Stann.* Zinc.
— kid., Ocim.
Cutting, hyp., Ang. Kali-b. Nicc. Tong.
— kid., Berb. Canth. Clem. Merc. Nux-m.
— liv., Ang. Carb-veg. Lach.
— sp., Crotal. Verb.
Digging, hyp., Asa-f. Seneg.
— liv., Lact. Sabad.

Diseases in, general of kid., Berb. Cocc. Colch. Lyc. *Nux-m.* Nux. Plb. Sass. Zinc.
— — — — sp., Plb.
Distention, hyp., Bell. *Igt.*
— liv., Sil.
— sp., Brom. Iod.
Drawing, hyp., Berb. Calc. Puls, Teucr.
— kid., Clem. Nux-m. Tereb.
— liv., Bry. Con. Lact. Ntr-m. Sabad. Sulph.
— sp., Berb. Cupr. Sulph.
Dull pain in liv., Chin-sulph. Hyosc.
Flatus, pain in spleen, as from, Meph.
Fulness sense of, hyp., Acon. Ant. Cham. *Igt.* Sulph.
— — liv., Creos. Pod.
Gangrene, liv., Sec-c.
Gnawing, liv., Ruta.
Gurgling in left hyp., Lyc.
— — sp., Verb.
Hardness, hyp., Borax. Bry. Chin-sulph.
— liv., Ars. Calc. Cannab. Chin. Graph. Lyc. Mgn-c. Mgn-m. Merc. Nux. Sil. Sulph.
— sp., *Agn.* Ars. Caps. Chin. Igt. Iod. Ran-b. Sulph.
Heat in liv., sensation of, Aloe. Sabad.
— from chest to liv., Sang.
Heaviness, sensation of, hyp., Acon. *Nux-m.* Sulph.
— — liv., Ars. Kali-c. Lact. Nux. Phosp-ac. Tabac.
— — sp., Sulph.
Induration, liv., Ars. Calc. Chin. Graph. Lact. Laur. Lyc. Mgn-m. *Nux.* Sacch. Sulph.
— — after abuse of quinine, *Nux.*
— sp., *Ang.* Brom. Chin.
Inflammation, dia., Acon. Bry. Cham. Cocc. Hyosc. Nux. Puls.
— kid., Acon. Bell. *Cannab. Canth.* Cocc. Colch. Hep. Merc. Sulph. Thuj.
— liv., *Acon.* Bell. *Bry. Canth. Cham.* Chin. Cocc. Igt. Kali-c. Lach. *Lyc. Mgn-m.* Merc. Ntr-c. Ntr-m. *Nux.* Puls. Sec-c. Sep. Sulph.
— — chronic, Lach. Lyc. Mgn-m. Ntr-c. Ntr-m. Nux. Ran-sc. Selen. Sulph.

16. HYPOCHONDRES, KIDNEYS, DIAPHRAGM, LIVER AND SPLEEN.

Inflamation, sp., Acon. Arn. Ars. *Chin.* Cupr. Igt. Nux. Sulph.
Jerks, hyp., Berb. Lact. Nux. Puls. Stann.
— kid., Canth. Ran-sc.
— liv., Croc. Valer.
Liver, affections of, Arn. Bell. Calc. Canth. Lach. Mgn-m. Merc. Ntr-c. Ntr-m. *Nux.* Puls. *Sulph.*
Lump, sensation of in liv., **Tabac.**
— — in sp., Sulph.
Miliary eruption in region of liv., Selen.
Obstruction in liv., Chin. Nux-m.
— — sp., Chin. Nux-m.
Oppression, hyp., Nux.
Pain across kid., Phyt.
— from kid., to hip, cannot straighten, Ox-ac.
Painfulness in general, hyp., Bell. Chin. Ntr-c. Sulph.
— hyp., right, during pregnancy, Phyt.
— — left, Merc-jod. Pallad. Sang.
— kid., All-cep. *Alum.* Berb. *Cannab.* Cocc. Colch. Nux. Ox-ac. Plb. Zing.
— liv., Acon. Aeth *Ambr.* Chin. Clem. Iod. Iris. Kalm. Lyc. Mgn-m. Millef. Pallad. Pod. Psor. Sulph.
— sp., Chin. Iod. Kobalt. Mez. Ntr-m. Pallad. Sacch.
Perspiration, hyp., Iris.
Pinching, hyp., Ip.
— liv., Lyc. Ntr-m.
— sp., 11 A. M. Fluor-ac.
Pressing, dia., Viol-tr.
— hyp., *Acon.* Ambr. Berb. *Borax.* Casc. Chin. Con. *Croton.* Mang. Mur-ac. Phosp-ac. Rhod. Spong. Sulph. Verat. Zinc.
— — expansive, Calc.
— kid., Canth. *Kali-c.* Ran-sc. Tereb. *Thuj.* Zinc.
— liv., Acon. Agn. Aloe. *Ambr.* Amm-c. Anac. Arn. Ars. *Asa-f.* Berb. Calc. Carb-an. Carb-veg. Chin. Cocc. Con. Creos. Dig. Graph. *Kali-c.* Lact. Laur. Lith. *Lyc. Mgn-m.* Merc. Nux-m. *Nux.* Ol-an. Phosp. Phosp-ac. Plb. Prun. Ran-sc. Raph. *Ruta.* Sabad. Sabin. Sep. Stann. Sulph. Tabac. Tereb. Thuj. Zinc.
— — with obstruction of breathing, Acon.
— sp., Borax. Creos. Igt. *Nitr-ac.* Ol-an. Stann. Sulph.
Pressure from clothes around hyp., Amm-m. Bry. Calc. Carb-veg. Caust. Chin. Coff. Creos. Hep. Nux. Spong. Sulph.
— — — sp., Fluor-ac. Kali-b. Ntr-m. Puls.
Pricking, sp., Ruta.
Pulsation, sp., Ran-b.
Rending, tearing, hyp., Teucr.
— kid., Berb. Canth.
— liv., Clem. *Con.* Creos.

— sp., Ambr. Con.
Rheumatic pain in region of liv., Meph.
Rumbling in sp., Verb.
Scraping liv., Sabad.
Sensation want of, in sp., Ars.
Smarting in sp., Asar.
Softening of liv., Lach.
Soreness, hyp., Alum. Bry. Phyt. Sulph.
— kid., Cinnab. Hipp-m. Zinc.
— — right, Phyt.
— — left, Benz-ac.
— liv., *Acon.* Amm-c. Carb-an. Dig. Eupat. Lyc. Ntr-s. Pallad. Raph.
— — beating, worse from motion, walking, lying on left side, breathing, Sil.
— sp., Asar. Ran-b.
Spasmodic pain, dia., Lyc. Ntr-m.
— hyp., *Mur-ac. Phosp-ac.* Rhod. *Stann.* Zinc.
— liv., Phosp-ac. Zinc.
— kid., Sulph.
— sp., Stann.
Spasms of dia., Stann.
Sprain, sensation of, in liv., Kali-c. Lyc.
Squeezing, liv., Lact.
Sticking in kid. and pain as if torn, Mez.
Stinging stitches, dia., Spig. Viol-tr.
— hyp., *Aeth.* Ars. Asa-f. Aur. Berb. Bry. *Carb-veg.* Graph. Kali-b. *Kali-c.* Lyc. Nitr-ac. Phosp. Pod. Puls. Rhod. Sabad. Sabin. *Sep.* Sil. Sulph. Sulph-ac.
— — right, Hyper.
— — left, Ntr-c. Sep.
— kid., Acon. Aeth. Bell. Berb. Canth. Chin. Croton. Cycl. Dig. Kali-c. Hep. Nitr. Phosp-ac. Ran-sc. Valer. Zinc.
— — right, Lob.
— — liv., *Acon.* Agar. Alum. Amm-m. Asar. Berb. Bry. *Calc.* Canth. *Carb-veg. Caust.* Chin. *Cocc. Con.* Creos. Cycl. Hep. *Kali-c.* Lact. Laur. Lyc. Mgn-c. Mgn-m. *Merc.* Merc-cor. Merc-jod. Mosch. *Ntr-c.* Ntr-m. *Ntr-s.* Ntr-ac. Nux-m. Nux. Ol-an. Ox-ac. Phosp. Phosp-ac. Plb. *Ran-b. Ran-sc.* Sabad. Selen. Sep. Sil. Stann. *Sulph.* Sulph-ac. *Tabac.* Zinc.
— — — to thighs, Kobalt.
— — sp., Agar. Amm-m. *Arn.* Bell. Carb-veg. Chin. Con. Hep. Kali-b. *Mgn-s. Ntr-c.* Ntr-m. Ntr-s. *Nitr.* Ol-an. Psor. Ran-sc. Rhod. Sass. Selen. Sep. Sil. Spig. Stann. Sulph. *Sulph-ac.* Tabac. Verat. Verb. Zinc. Zing.
Suppuration of kid., Canth.
Swelling, of hyp., Acon. Aur. Bry. Chin-sulph.

16. HYPOCHONDRES, KIDNEYS, DIAPHRAGM, LIVER AND SPLEEN.

Swelling liv., Ars. Bar-m. Ccal. Cannab. Chin. Dolich. Lach. Lact. Laur. Lyc. Merc. Nux-m. Nux. Sacch. Sulph.
— — after abuse of quinine, Nux.
— sp., Agn. Ars. Caps. Chin. Gymnoc. Igt. Iod. Ruta. Sacch.
— — after ague suppressed by quinine, Diad.
Tension, hyp., *Acon.* Bell. Calc. Casc. Cham. Chin-sulph. Con. Dig. Graph. Lyc. Mur-ac. Ntr-c. Nux. Puls. Sep. Staph. Sulph. Verat.
— liv., Aloe. Bry. Calc. Carb-veg. Caust. Cimex. Lact. *Lyc.* Mgn-m. Murex. Ntr-m. Ntr-s. Nux. Sulph.
— sp., Nitr-ac. Rhod. Sulph.
Throbbing, hyp., Acon. Graph. Puls.
— kid., Canth.
— liv., Ntr-s. Nux. Sep. Sil.
— sp., Grat. Ran-b. Ruta.
Torn off, as if something were in sp., Ambr.
Ulcerous pain, hyp., Chin-sulph. Puls.
— liv., Laur. Sil.
Uneasiness in liv., Aloe.
Warmth, sense of liv., Sabad.
Morning, in pain, hyp., Staph.
— — liv., Bry.
— sp., Amm-m.
Evening, pain, sp., Mgn-s.
Bending body, pain, kid., Chin.
— — — liv., Cocc.
Breakfast, after, pain, liv., Graph.
Breathing, when, pain, hyp., Asa-f. Kali-c. Ran-sc.
— — — liv., *Bry. Selen.*
— — sp., Agar.
— — deep, pain in hyp., Ran-sc.
— — — — in liv., Psor.
— — — — stitches in liv., Aloe.
— — — — — relieved, Ox-ac.
— — — — in sp., Bry. Chin. Mosch. Ntr-c. Ran-sc. Sabad. Sulph.

Coughing, when, pain, hyp., Dros. Sang.
— — — liv., Bry. Cocc. Psor.
Eructations relieved, by Pallad.
Exercising when, pain in hyp., Sep. Zinc.
— — — — liv., Ang. Iris. Merc. Nitr-ac. Nux.
— — — sp., Kali-b. Ran-b.
Lying on right side, when, pain in liv., Mgn-m. Psor.
Pregnancy, during, pain, hyp., Puls.
Pressed upon, when pain, hyp., Acon.
— — — relieved, left hyp., Sang.
— — liv., Berb. Bry. Clem. Psor. Sabad. Selen. Tabac.
— — — — relieved, Merc-jod.
— — — sp., Igt.
Riding in a carriage, pain, hyp., *Borax.*
— — — liv., Sep.
— — — sp., Borax. Lach.
Sitting down, when, pain, kid., Valer.
— when pain, hyp., Puls.
— — liv., Amm-c.
Stooping when, pain, dia., Lyc. Ntr-c.
— — — hyp., Alum.
— — — liv., Alum. Calc. Clem. Cocc. Kali-c. Lyc.
— — — sp., Rhod.
Touched when pain hyp., Aur. Cupr. Dros. Ran-b.
— — — liv., Aeth. Agar. Bry. Carb-an. Carb-veg. Chin. Clem. Lyc. Mgn-m. Merc. Ntr-s. Nux. Sep. Valer.
Walking, when, pain, hyp., Zinc.
— — — kid., Clem.
— — — liv., Hep. Mgn-m. Ntr-s. Psor. Sep.
— — sp., *Arn.* Hep. Igt. Lach. Rhod. Selen.
With giddiness, pain, hyp., Calc.
— necessity to lie down, pain, liv., Graph.
— obscuration of sight, pain, hyp., Calc.
— vomiting, pain, liv., Bry.

17. Abdomen, Groin, Flatulency.

Abbreviations:—ABD., ABDOMEN; INT., ABDOMINAL INTEGUMENT; NAV., NAVEL; EPIG., EPIGASTRIUM; HYPOG., HYPOGASTRUM; SID., SIDES OF ABDOMEN; ING., INGUINAL REGION OR GROIN.

Aching in abd., Ars. *Bell.* Calc. Caust Cham. Chin. Cocc. Coloc. Cupr. Hyosc. Igt. Lach. Lyc. Merc. *Nux.* Puls. Sulph. *Verat.*
Adhesion, sense of, hypog., Sep.
— as if intestines adhered to nav., Verb.
Arthritic pains which suddenly wander from extremities to abd., Daph.
Ascites, Acon. *Agn.* Apis. *Ars.* Bry. Cannab. Canth. Caust. *Chin.* Colch. Crotal. *Dig.* Dulc. Euph. Igt. *Kali-c.* Hell. Lact. *Led.* Lyc. *Merc.* Millef. Nux. Prun. Sabin. Sacch. Scill. Sep. Spong. *Sulph.*
— sacculated, Cannab. Chin. Sacch.
— from glandular affections, Merc.
— with a fold over pubic region, Colch.
— — induration of liver and asthma, Lact.
Bearing down, ing., Calc. Cham. Kali-jod. Mgn-s. Teucr.
— — sid., Phosp.
Beaten, as if, abd., Amm-c. Ang. Arg. Ars. Aur. Cannab. Carb-veg. Caust. Cham. Chin. *Cocc.* Coloc. Con. Ferr. Hep. Igt. Kali-jod. Lam. Led. Mgn-m. Merc-cor. *Ntr-s.* Ran-b. Ruta. Sabad. Samb. Sep. Staph. Stram. Sulph. Verat. Valer.
— — when lying on right side, Merc.
— — hypog., and ing., *Valer.*
— — int., Nux. Plb. Sabad. Sulph. Valer.
— — ing., left, Dolich.
— — nav., Ox-ac.
— — sid., Ang. Nux.
— — right, Ang. Camph.
Blood congestion of to abd., Chenop. Lact. Merc. Nux.
— stagnation in abd., Bell. Bry. Dig. *Nux.* Puls. Sulph.
— in abd., flowing backwards. sensation, Elaps.
Hard body, sensation of, moving in abd., Borax.

Boring in abd., Aloe. Arg. Ars. Calad. Cina. Coloc. Dig. Sabad. *Seneg.* Sep. Tar.
— — epig., Seneg.
— — hypog., Sabad.
— — sid., Par.
Brownish spots on abd., Ars. Carb-veg. Kali-c. Nitr-ac. Phosp. Sabad. Sep. Thuj.
Bruising pain, abd., Ntr-s.
— — epig., Stann.
— — integ., Sulph.
— — sid., Arn. Coloc. Ferr.
Bubbling in abd., Hell. Phosp-ac. Tar.
Burning in abd., Acon. Alum. Amm-c. Amm-m. Apis. *Ars.* Bell. Berb. Bov. Bry. Calc. *Camph.* *Canth.* Caps. Carb-an. Caust. Cham. Chelid. Cocc. Colch. Coloc. Cop. Crotal. Dulc.Eugen. Euph. Euphr. Graph. Grat. Hydroc-ac. Kali-c. Kali-jod. Lach. *Laur.* Lyc. Mgn-s. Merc. Merc-sulph. Mercurial. *Mez.* Ntr-c. Ntr-m. Ntr-s. Nux. Ol-an. Phell. Phosp. Phosp-ac. Plat. Plb. Raph. *Ran-b.* Rat. Rhus. Ruta. *Sabad.* Sass. Sec-c. *Sep.* Sil. Spig. Stann. Stront. Thuj. *Verat.*
— — left side of pelvis, Amm-c. Graph. Lac-can. Plat. Ruta. Sep.
— — epig., *Calad.* *Camph.* Canth. *Cham.* Raph.
— — hypog., *Camph.* Lac-can. Nitr. Phosp-ac. Stram.
— — int., Berb. Selen.
— — nav., Acon. Berb. Bov. Calc. Canth. Carb-veg. Cham. Crotal. Kali-c. Kali-jod. Lach. Mgn-s. Merc. Merc-jod. Ntr-c. Ol-an. Phosp-ac. Plat. Raph. Sabad. Sulph-ac. Tilia.
— — sid., Rat.
— — in small spots, Ox-ac.
Burst, as if it should, pain, abd., Anac. Coff. Sep. Valer.
— — — — when walking, Lac-can. Lach.

17. ABDOMEN, GROIN AND FLATULENCY.

Catamania, pain, abd., as if the, would appear, Cina. Croc. Kali-c. Lam. Mgn-c. Mosch. Mur-ac. Sep. Stann. Tilia.
Chilliness, abd., Ars. Kali-c. Par. Phosp. Plb. Sec-c. Sulph.
— — upper part, Ars. Camph. Kali-c. Mang. Oleand. Sec-c. Sulph.
— — disposition to suffer from, Caust. Nitr-ac.
Chill commences in abd., Calc.
Clawing in abd., Carb-an. Coloc. Hep. Ip. Mosch. Sep. Zinc.
— epig., Mosch.
— hypog., Bell. Lyc. Puls.
— nav., Acon. Stann.
— vig., Kali-jod.
Coldness, sense of in abd., Acon. *Aeth*. Alum. Ambr. Ars. Asa-f. Bell. Berb. Bov. Calc. Camph. Caust. Chin. Cist. Colch. Creos. Croton. Eugen. Grat. Hell. Hipp. Hydroc-ac. Kali-c. Laur. Meny. Merc-sulph. Mercurial. Oleand. Petr. Phell. Phosp. Plb. Pod. Rat. Ruta. Sabad. Sass. Sec-c. Seneg. Sep. Sulph. *Tereb*. Zinc.
— — — one side only, Ambr.
— int., Ambr. Tereb.
— nav., Rat.
Colic, Aloe. Alum. Arg-n. *Asar*. Bell. *Bov*. Calc. Cannab. Caps. Carb-veg. Canth. Chin. Coff. Colch. *Coloc*. Con. *Cop*. Croc. Croton. Cub. *Cupr*. Diosc. Elaps. *Euph*. Ferr. Hæmatox. Hipp. Hyosc. Iod. Ip. Kali-b. *Kali-c*. Lach. *Laur*. Led. Mgn-m. *Mez*. Mur-ac. Ntr-c. Ntr-m. Ntr-s. Nitr. Nux-m. *Nux*. Ox-ac. Pallad. Petr. Phosp. Plb. Pod. Puls. *Ran-b*. Rhus. Rumex. Sass. *Sec-c*. *Senna*. *Sil*. Spig. *Sulph*. *Verat*.
— dry, Coloc.
— alternates with affections of eyes, Euphr.
— anger, from, Cham.
— clutching with the nails, as if, Bell. Ip.
— cold, from a, as if diarrhœa would set in, Dulc.
— compelling to walk bent, Puls. Rhus.
— constipation, from, Sil.
— convulsions, with Sec-c.
— dysenteric, Led.
— every evening, Led.
— hemmorrhoids, from, Carb-veg. Coloc. Lach. Nux. Puls. *Sulph*. Valer.
— morning, in, 5 a. m., Kobalt.
— paralysis, of lower extremities, with, Plb.
— periodical, *Igt*. Lac-can. *Nux*. Sulph.
— — with diarrhoea, Gels.
— — daily, Arn. Diad. *Ntr-m*.
— restlessness, with, Ars. Bell.
— torpor of liver, with, Sang.
— weakness from, or loss of annimal fluids, Chin.

— worms, from, in children, Cic. Ruta. Sabad. Sil. Valer.
— yellow hands, with, and blue nails, Sil.
— relieved by lying down, Merc.
Colic, painter's, *Alum. Op. Plat*.
Collapsed, abd., Euph.
Compressing pain in abd., Ambr. Hyper. Puls.
— — nav., Acon.
— — ing., Igt. Thuj.
— — sid., left, Berb.
Congestion (portal system,) Aloe. Kali-chl.
Contracting pain in abd., Amm-c. Bell. Berb. Calc. Caust. Coloc. Creos. Dig. Gels. *Hep*. Kali-c. *Laur*. Lyc. Mgn-c. Mang. Merc. Mosch. Ntr-m. Ntr-s. Nux. Ol-an. Phosp. Rhus. Sabin. Sass. Sulph. Tar. Thuj.
— — — nav., Bell. Phosp.
— — — ing., Rat.
Contraction of abd., Dros. Hep. Ferr. Lach. *Plb*. Rhus.
— — — muscles, Arg. Ferr. Ntr-nitr. Sabad. Scill.
— — — — in walking, Arg.
— hypog., Con. Rhus.
— in ing., Rat.
— nav., Ntr-c. Phosp. Plb.
— — as of a hard twisted ball Creos.
— of intestines and pressure from above downwards, as if bowels would be pressed outwards, Sass.
Constriction, sensation in abd., Bell. Carb-an. Chin. *Coloc*. Dig. Euph. Kali-b. Mez. Mosch. *Plat*. *Plb*. Sabad. Thuj.
— — hypog, Bell. Clem. Evon. Verb.
— — nav., Bell. Plb. Puls. Verb.
Cramp in abd., Ambr. Amm-c. Ars. Aur. Bell. Berb. *Bry*. *Calc*. Camph. *Cham*. Chelid. Chin. *Cocc*. Coff. Con. Creos. Croton. *Cupr*. *Euph*. Ferr. Graph. Hep. *Hyosc*. *Igt*. Iod. *Ip*. *Kali-c*. Lach. Lyc. *Mgn-c*. Mgn-m. *Mosch*. *Mur-ac*. Nitr-ac. *Nux*. Ol-an. Petr. Phosp. Phosp-ac. Prun. *Puls*. *Rhus*. Seneg. *Sep*. Spong. Stann. *Stram*. Teucr. *Valer*. *Verat*.
— hypog., Stann.
— around nav., Stann.
— hysteric, Ars. Bell. Bry. *Cocc*. *Ip*. *Mgn-m*. Mosch. Nux. *Stann*. *Stram*. *Valer*.
— periodical, *Igt*.
— with chilliness, in suppressed menstruation, Puls.
— — menses irregular, *Cocc*.
— in parturient women, Cic.
— during pregnancy, Puls.
— with convulsions, *Cupr*. Sec-c.
— — leucorrhœa, discharge of, Mgn-c. *Mgn-m*.
— — shrieking, Cupr.
Crawling, sensation, abd., Camph. Croton. Mgn-m.
Creeping, sensation, abd., Dulc.

Cutting, in abd., Acon. Agar. Aloe. Alum. Ambr. Ant. Arg. Arn. Ars. Bar-c. Bell. Bov. Bry. Calc. Carb-an. Cham. Chelid. Chenop. Chin. Cic. Cina. Coloc. Con. Creos. Croton. Cub. Cycl. Dig. Dulc. Elat. Graph. Hep. Hyosc. Hyper. Igt. Iod. Ip. Kali-b. Kali-c. Lach. Lact. Laur. Led. Lept. Lob. Lyc. Mgn-c. Mgn-m. Merc. Mez. Murex. Mur-ac. Ntr-m. Nicc. Ntr-ac. Nitr. Nux-m. Nux. Ol-an Ox-ac. Petr. Phosp. Phosp-ac. Plb. Puls. Ran-sc. Rheum. Rhus. Sabad. Sass. Scill. Sec-c. Sep. Sil. Stann. Staph. Stront. Sulph. Sulph-ac. Tart. Valer. Verat. Verb. Viol-tr. Zinc.
— epig., Asar. Calc. Cham. Chin-sulph. Laur. Lyc. Mgn-m. Nux-m. Ol-an. Sulph. Tereb.
— hypog., Ang. Evon. Iris. Laur. Mgn-s. Nicc. Ol-an. Sep. Sil. Tereb.
— — relieved after stool, Pallad.
— ing., Calc. Carb-an. Gum-gut. Valer.
— nav, Aloe. Bov. Calad. Croton. Dulc. Glon. Hyper. Igt. Ip. Kali-b. Kali-jod. Mang. Merc-cor. Mur-ac. Nux. Ol-an. Puls. Raph. Sass. Spig. Verb.
— sid., Arn. Croton. Mur-ac. Par. Ruta.
— from worms, Cina.
— in left lower abdomen, with frequent burning urine, All-cep.
— with strangury, Arn.
— from both groins to sympheses pubis, Elaps.
— outwards, from within, Ang.
Cutting in abd., (as with a knife), Coloc. Lact. Merc. Murex. Sabad. Verat.
— — nav., Bov. Laur. Tart.
— — ing., Calc.
— from right to left across abd., Lyc.
Despair, to pain driving, Coff.
Diarrhœa, as if a would set in, pain in abd., Agar. Ang. Bar-c. Dig. Lach. Meph. Nux. Oleand. Sabin.
Digging in abd., Ars. Bell. Ntr-c. Rhus. Ruta. Sabad. Seneg. Spong. Stann. Sulph. Valer.
— epig. or hypog., Ol-an. Sep.
— nav., Con.
Distention of abd., Acon. Aloe. Anac. Apis. Arn. Ars. Bar-c. Bell. Borax. Bov. Calc. Carb-veg. Caust. Chin. Cic. Cimex. Cocc. Coff. Colch. Con. Cor-c. Creos. Croton. Cub. Cupr. Ferr. Graph. Hœmatox. Hell. Hipp-m. Hyosc. Jatr. Kali-b. Kali-c. Lach. Lyc. Mgn-c. Mgn-m. Mang. Merc. Merc-cor. Mez. Ntr-c. Ntr-s. Nux-m. Op. Petr. Phosp. Phosp-ac. Plb. Puls. Raph. Rheum. Rhus. Sacch. Sang. Scill. Sec-c. Sep. Sil. Spig. Spong. Stram. Stront. Sulph. Tilia. Verat. Zinc.
— on left side of colon, worse after eating, Aloe.

— relieved after stool, Hyper.
— sudden, painful, followed by diarrhœa, Kali-jod.
— with cold feet, Lyc.
— in children, Cina. Sil.
— painful, Acon. Bell. Hyosc. Ntr-c. Ntr-m. Nux. Rhus. Sulph. Verat.
— — of epig., and sensation as if contents were passing into the chest, Cham.
— sensation of in abd., Ntr-s. Sep. Valer.
Downwards pressure towards groin, Sass. Teucr.
Drawing in abd., Acon. Agn. Ars. Caps. Chin. Cocc. Creos. Dros. Lach. Led. Lob. Lyc. Mgn-c. Mgn-s. Ntr-m. Nux. Op. Staph. Verat.
— hypog., Chin. Valer.
— ing., Calc. Kali-c. Kali-jod. Ol-an. Plat. Thuj. Valer.
— int., Seneg. Valer.
— nav., Igt. Rat.
— sid., Lyc. Ntr-c. Par.
— right, Camph.
— of abdominal muscles towards back, Nitr.
Emptiness, sense of, abd., Ant. Arn. Arum. Cham. Cina. Cocc. Coloc. Dig. Dulc. Euph. Fluor-ac. Guaj. Gum-gut. Hep. Kali-c. Kobalt. Lach. Merc. Mez. Mur-ac. Oleand. Petr. Phosp. Puls. Sass. Scill. Seneg. Stann.
— at nav., better by bandaging and eating, Fluor-ac.
Enteritis, Acon. Ant. Arn. Ars. Bar-m. Bell. Bry. Canth. Cham. Chin-sulph. Croton. Cupr. Cupr-sulph. Graph. Hydroc-ac. Hyosc. Iod. Ip. Lach. Laur. Merc. Mez. Nux. Plb. Puls. Ran-flam. Rhus. Sabin. Scill. Sil. Tereb. Verat. Vipra-red.
Eruption on abd., Ntr-c.
— herpes zoster, Graph. Rhus. Thuj.
— rash, Hipp-m.
— ringworm, Tellur.
— yellow brown spots, Kobalt. Lyc.
— — scaby itching, moist when scratched, Kali-c.
Erysipelas on abd., Graph.
Exostosis, Aur.
Extension sense of, abd., Igt. Sep. Valer.
— — ing., Mgn-s.
Falling, sense of something in abd., Plb.
Fermentation/sense of, Ang. Croc. Gran. Lyc. Rhus. Seneg. Stram.
Flabbiness, sense of, abd., Phosp. Rhus. (compare Emptiness and weakness.)
Flatulency in general, Agn. Bell. Carb-veg. Cham. Chenop. Chin. Cinnab. Cocc. Coloc. Euph. Graph. Igt. Lach. Lyc. Merc. Ntr-c. Ntr-m. Nitr-ac. Nux-m. Nux. Phosp. Puls. Sacch. Sang. Sep. Sulph. Zinc.
— accumulation of, Ant. Bar-c. Borax.

17. ABDOMEN, GROIN AND FLATULENCY.

Calc-ph. Chin. Cic. *Graph.* Igt.Kali-jod. Lyc. Meny. Ntr-c. Ntr-s. *Nitr-ac. Nitr.* Nux. Ol-an. Phosp. Prun. Rhus. Senna. Sep. Tart. Zinc.
Flatulency, colic like, Acon.Ambr.Amm-c. Anac. Arn. *Asa-f. Aur. Bell.* Bry. *Caps.* Carb-veg. Casc. *Cham. Chin* Cocc. Colch. Con. Euph. Ferr. Graph. *Grat.* Hyosc. Igt. Ip. Iris. Kali-c. Lac-can. Laur. Lyc. Mang. *Mez.* Ntr-m. Ntr-nitr. Ntr-s, Nitr-ac. *Nux. Phosp.* Plb. Puls. Rhod. Rheum. Scill. Staph. Tart. Teucr.
— — hypog., Acon. Chin. Phosp.Sulph-ac.
— — with protrusion colon, relieved by pressure and leaning forward, Bell. Coloc.
— cutting, Con. Puls.
— drawing, Chin.
— griping, Anac. Asa-f. Aur. Graph. Lam. Ntr-s. Rhus. Tart. Teucr.
— obstructed, Aloe. Ambr. Ant.Arn.Asar. Aur. *Calc. Canth.* Carb-an. Carb-veg. Caust. Cham. Chin. Cocc. Coff. Coloc. Con. Graph. Guaj. Hep. Igt. *Iod.Kali-c.* Kalm. Lam. *Lyc.* Mosch. Ntr-c. *Ntr-m.* Ntr-s. *Nitr-ac. Nitr.* Nux. Ox-ac. Phell. *Phosp.* Phosp-ac. Plat. Plb. Prun. Puls. Rheum. Rhod. Scill. Sep. Sil. Stann. Staph. *Sulph.* Tart. Teucr. Tilia. Verat.
— — with a hard stool, Caust.
— painful, in general, Arn. Ntr-c. Ntr-s. *Puls.* Rhod.
— pressing, Casc. Chin. *Ntr-nitr.* Nux. Puls. Rheum. Sulph.
— rising up, Graph. Lyc Ntr-nitr. Rheum,
— squeezing, Carb-veg. Teucr.
— tightening, Chin. Graph. Rheum. Rhod.
— urging, Plb. Seneg.
— wandering about, Carb-veg. Ntr-c.Ntr-s. Ol-an. Phell. *Puls.* Rhus.
— in the morning, Hep. Nitr-ac. Nux.
— in afternoon, Nitr.
— in evening, *Nitr-ac. Puls.* Zinc.
— at night, Acon. Ambr. *Aur.* Carb-veg. Cocc. *Ferr.* Igt. Kali-c. Merc. Ntr-m. *Nux-m.* Puls.
— after acids, Phosp-ac.
— by bending forward, relieved, Bell. Coloc.
— in children, Cham.
— by cough, increased, Cocc.
— drinking, after, Nux.
— eructation by, or discharge of wind, relieved, Ntr-nitr.
— by exercise increased, Ntr-nitr.
— in gouty persons, Zing.
— — hysterical women, Colch. Igt. Puls.
— — lying, increased, Phosp.
— by pressure, external, relieved, Bell.
— with anxiety, Cic. Nux.
— — bowels contracted, Chin.
— — — protruded (transverse colon, Bell.) Pallad.

— — breath obstructed, *Mez.*
— — chilliness, *Mez.*
— — eructations, Grat. Rhod.
— — headache, Calc-ph.
— — nausea, Grat. Kalm.
— — peevishness, Cic.
— — spasms,Prun.
Flatus, no emission of, Kali-b. Lyc. Ntr-c. Raph. Sil.
— cold, Con.
— difficult, Calc-ph. Hep. Plat. Sil. Verat.
— frequent, *Agar.* Agn. Aloe. Aur. Bell. Borax. Bry. *Carb-veg.* Caust. Chenop. Chin. Chin-sulph. Croton. Dig. Gels. *Graph.* Gum-gut. Igt. Ind. *Kali-c.* Lact. Led. Lob. Mang. Millef. Ntr-c. Ntr-s. Nitr-ac. *Oleand.* Ol-an. Phosp. Phosp-ac. Plb. Ran-b. Rhod. Sass. Scill. Staph. Stram. Stront. Sulph. Tart-ac. Teucr. Zinc.
— hot, Acon. Aloe. Cham. Cocc. Phosp. Plb. Puls. Staph. Teucr. Zinc.
— — humid, Carb-veg.
— interrupted, small, Calad. Caust. Plb.
— painful, Con. Graph. Kali-c. Puls.
— noise of, croaking, Arg. Graph.
— — crying, as of something, Arg. Thuj.
— — fermenting, Ang. Gran. Rhus. Senna. Stram.
— — rumbling, Acon. *Anac. Ant.* Aur. Bism. Bry. Calc. Con. Cycl. Ferr-m. Guaj. Laur. Mur-ac. *Ntr-m.* Nitr-ac. *Oleand. Plb.* Raph. Rhod. Scill. Senna. *Sep. Sil.* Spig. Spong. Stront. *Sulph. Sulph-ac.* Tar. Tart.Tereb.Thuj.Verat. Zinc.
— grunting, Sil. Spong.
— — gurgling, Aloe. Cina. Gum-gut. Jatr.
— — — in epig., Puls.
— — rolling, Acon. Agar. Agn. Aloe. Ang. Ant. Arg. Arn. Aur. Berb. Bism. Boy. *Bry.* Calc. Canth. Carb-an. Carb-veg. Caust. Cham. Chenop. Chin. Coloc. Con. Corn-c. Cop. Cycl. Elaps. Ferr-m. Glon. Graph. Grat. Guaj. Gum-gut. Hell. Hipp-m. Igt. Jatr. Kali-jod. Lachn. Laur. *Lyc.* Mgn-c. Mgn-s. Meny. Merc. Mez. Ntr-c. Ntr-m. Ntr-s. Nicc. Nitr-ac. Nux. Oleand. Ol-an. Ox-ac. Par. Petr. Phosp. Phosp-ac. Plb. Puls. Rhod. Rhus. *Sass.* Scill. Sec-c. *Sep.* Sil. Spig. Staph. Stram. *Sulph. Sulph-ac.* Tabac. Tart. Terb. Teucr. Thuj. Verat. Zinc. Zing.
— — — in left side, feels it but does not hear it, Lachn.
— — — with drawing through legs down to toes, Ferr-m.
— in hypog., Aur. *Cycl.* Hydroc-ac. Sil. Sulph-ac.
— in epig., Caust. Chin. Lyc. Nux. Phosp. Phos-ac. Puls.

17. ABDOMEN, GROIN AND FLATULENCY,

Flatus, around nav., Caps.
— in evening, Puls. Spong.
— — — in bed, Bry.
— when taking a deep breath, Hell.
— on left side, Lyc.
— darting in urethra, on passing, Mgn-s.
— presses on bladder, Igt. Prun.
— in lying (morning), Spong.
— — sleep, Agn.
— scentless, Ambr. Lyc. Phosp. Teucr.
— smelling like rotten eggs, Arn. Coff. Ferr-m. Sulph. Tart. Teucr. Valer.
— — — garlic, Agar. Mosch. Phosp.
Flatulency smelling fetid, Agar. Aloe. Alum. Arn. Ars. Asa-f. Aur. Bar-c. Borax. *Bov.* Bry. Calc. Carb-an. *Carb-veg.* Caust.Cham.*Chin.*Chin-sulph. Cocc. Con. Croton. Dulc. Graph. Grat. Iod. Iris. Lact. Lith. Lob. *Mgn-c.* Millef. Ntr-c. Ntr-m. Ntr-s. Nicc. Nitr-ac. Nux. Oleand. Ol-an. Petr. Phosp. *Plb.* Psor. *Puls.* Ran-b. Rhod. *Rhus.* Ruta. Sang. Sass. Scill. Senna. *Sep. Sil.* Spig. *Staph.* Stront. Sulph. Teucr.Tilia.Valer.
— — of the medicine, Raph.
— — putrid, All-cep. Arn. Ars. Asa-f. Calad. Camph. Carb-veg. Cocc.Dulc. Igt. Ntr-c. Nitr-ac. Nux. Puls. Sass. Sil. Sulph. Valer. Zinc.
— — sour, Calc. Graph. Merc. Ntr-c. Rheum. Sulph.
Fulness in abd., Agar.Aloe.Alum.Amm-c. Anac. Ant. Ars. Asar. Aur.Bar-c.Calad. Calc.Camph.Carb-veg.Cast.Caust.Chin. Cocc. Cocc-c. Coff.Colch.Con.Croc.Dig. Graph. Hell. Lach. Lact. Laur. Led, Lyc. Mgn-m. Mgn-s. Mur-ac. Ntr-s. Nitr. Nux-jug. Nux-m. Nux. Ol-an. Phosp. Plb. Puls. Raph. Rhod. Sass. Spig. Stann. Sulph. Tart. Tereb. Verb. Zinc.
— — hypog., Aur. Diad.
— — in morning, Con.
Furuncles on abd., Phosp. Zinc.
Gangrene of abd., Plb.
Glands ing., drawing in, Dulc. Mez. Thuj.
— — hardness, Ars. Calc. Clem. Dulc.
— — inflammation, Dulc. *Merc.* Sil.
— — pain in, Ars. Berb. *Calc.* Graph. *Merc.* Tereb. Thuj.
— — — ulcerous, Amm-m. Bov. Creos. Dig. Hell. Mgn-c. Mang. Nitr-ac. Ran-b. Rhus.
— — pressure, pulsation and shooting, Berb.
— — suppurations, Ars. Hep. Merc. Nitr-ac. Phosp. Sulph.
— — swelling, Ars. Aur. Bad. Bell. *Calc.* Carb-veg. *Clem.* Dulc. Graph. Hep. *Iod. Merc.* Ntr-c. *Nitr-ac.* Ocim. Phosp. Phosp-ac. Rhus. Sil. Spong. *Staph.* Stram. Sulph. Tereb. *Thuj.*
— — — schirrous, Iod.

— — twitching, Clem.
— — mesenteric swelling, *Ars. Calc.* Con. Iod. Sacch.
— — induration, *Ars.Calc.*
Gnawing, abd., Ars. Calc. Cupr. Dulc. Oleand. Plat. Ruta.
— hypog., Gum-gut. Seneg.
— about nav., Ruta.
— — transverse colon, Gels.
Globus hystericus, Acon. Con. *Mgn-m.* Plb.
— — relieved by eructations, Mgn-m.
Grasping in abd., Carb-an. Coloc. Sep. Zinc.
— hypog., *Bell.* Lyc. Puls.
— ing., Kali-jod.
— nav., Stann.
Griping, pinching, abd., Agar. Aloe. Alum. *Amm-m.* Anac. *Asa-f.* Aur. Bar-c. Borax. Brom. Bruc. Bry. Calc. Carb-veg.Chenop.Chin.Cic. Cina. Cocc. Coloc.Con. Corn-c.Croc. Croton. Cycl. Dig.Dulc.*Euphr.*Graph.Grat.Guaj. *Hell.* Hyper. *Igt.* Iod. Ip. Lact. Lam. *Lyc.* Mgn-c. Mgn-m. Meny. *Merc.* Mez. *Ntr-m.* Ntr-s. Nitr-ac. Nux Ol-an. Petr. Phell. Phosp. Plat. Plb. Ran-b. Ran-sc. Rhus. Sabin. Samb. Scill. Sil. *Spig.* Stann. Sulph. *Sulph-ac.* Tabac. Tar. Tart. Tong. Valer. Verb. Zinc.
— — as with nails, Bell.
— — from worms, Cina.
— — epig., *Cocc.*
— — hypog., Aur. Ruta. *Sil.* Tart-ac.
— — ing., Rat.
— — int., Paeon. Sabin.
— — nav., Aloe. Croton. Dulc. Fluor-ac. Igt. Iod. Lact. Laur. Mur-ac. Nicc. Plat. Raph. Verb.
— — — as if grasped by hands, Ip.
— — side, Igt. *Lyc.* Mur-ac. Rat. Ruta.
— — — from left to right, Asar. Carb-veg.
Hardness of abd., Alum. Anac. Arn. *Ars.* Bar-c. Calc. Caps. Caust. Cham.Cholid. Chin. Con. Cupr. Ferr. Graph. Grat. Kali-c. Lac-can. Lach. Mgn-m. Mgn-s. Merc-jod. Mez. Ntr-c. Nux-jug. Nux. *Op.* Phosp. Plb. Puls. Sacch. Sec-c. *Sep. Sil.* Spig. Spong. Stram. Sulph. Valer.
— hypog., Clem. Graph. Sep.
— ing., Ant. Dulc.
— int., Ntr-c.
— nav., Bry. Plb. Rhus.
— sid., right, Mgn-m.
— children, Calc. Sacch. Sil.
As if hard pointed bodies were moving in confusion in abd., Borax.
Heat, abd., Aloe. Bell. Bry. *Camph.* Carb-an. Casc. Cic. Cina. Euph. Graph. Lach. Lachn. Lact. *Laur.* Mang. Meny. Mez. Plb. Pod. Raph. Ruta. Sabad. Sass. Sil. Spong.

17. ABDOMEN, GROIN AND FLATULENCY.

Heat, abd., flushes of, Cinnab.
— int., Croton.
— as if hot water from breast to abd., followed by diarrhœa, Sang.
Heaviness, abd., Aloe. *Ambr.* Ars. *Asa-f.* Calc. Carb-veg. Cop. Croc. Ferr. *Graph. Hell. Kali-c.* Lact. Lyc. Mgn-c. Mez. Ntr-nitr. Nux-jug. Nux. *Op.* Phosp. Rhus. *Sep.* Sulph. Tereb.
— epig., Croton. *Nux-m.*
— hypog., Diad. Croton. Ferr.
— ing., Calc. *Croc.*
— sense of, after drinking, Asa-f.
— — in walking, Ferr.
Hernia, femoral, *Nux.*
— inguinal, *Alum. Asar. Aur.* Berb. Carb-veg. *Cham.* Chin. Clem. *Cocc.* Guaj. Lach. *Lyc.* Mgn-c. *Nitr-ac. Nux.* Op. Petr. Phosp. Prun. Psor. Rhus. *Sil.* Spig. Staph. Sulph. *Sulph-ac.*Tereb. Thuj. *Verat. Zinc.*
— — strangulated, Acon. Alum. Ars. Bell. Lach. Millef. *Nux. Op.* Rhus. Sulph. Verat.
— — painful, *Sil.*
— — protruded, Alum. *Aur. Sulph-ac.*
— — in children, *Aur.* Nitr-ac.
Inflammation of hernial structure, Acon. Nux. Op. Sulph.
— — — — with vomiting of bile, Acon. Ars. Bell. Lach. Verat.
— right side, Lyc.
Hernia, pain in ing., as if would develop a, Berb. Cham. Chin. Clem. Coloc. Cupr. Guaj. Prun. Spong. Sulph-ac. Tereb.
Inactivity in abd., *Alum.* Ant. Arn. Camph. Chin. Croton. Igt. Kali-c. Nux-m. Nux. Sass.
Induration in abd., Ars. Calc. Chin. Lyc. Plb. (compare Hardness.)
Inflammation of intestines, (compare Enteritis.)
— of peritoneum, Acon. Bell. Bry. Cham. Cocc. Coff. Coloc. Hyosc. Nux. Puls. Rhus.
Inflation, distention, abd., Aeth. Aloe. Ambr. Amm-c. Anac. Ant. Arg. Arn. Ars. Asar. Asa-f. Aur. Bar-c. Bell. Bism. Bry. Calc. Calc-ph.Caps.Carb-an. Carb-veg. Cast. Caust. Cham. Chin. Chin-sulph. Cocc. Colch. Coloc. Creos. Croc. Croton. Dig. Ferr. Graph. Grat. Gum-gut. Hyosc. Hyper. Igt. Iod. Kali-c. Kali-jod. Lach. Lam. Lob. Lyc. Mgn-c. Mgn-m. Mang. Meny. Merc. Merc-cor. Mur-ac. Ntr-m. Nitr-ac. Nitr. Nux-m. Nux. Ol-an. Op. Ox-ac. Petr. Phosp. Phosp-ac. Plat. Plb. Poth. Puls. Raph. Rheum. Rhod. Rhus. Sabin.Scill. Sec-c. Sep. Spig. Stann. Stram. Stront. Sulph. Tabac. Thuj. Tilia. Valer. Verb.
— epig., Acon. Hell. Ruta.

— hyp., Bell.
— ing., Amm-c. Kali-c. Ntr-s.
— sid., *Caust. Ntr-m.* Zinc.
— painful, Bar-c. Bell. Cast. Caust. Cham. Kali-jod. Merc. Merc-cor.
— partial, Bell. Plb.
— puffy, Plb.
— in morning, Nitr-ac. Rhod.
— — evening, Rhod.
— with constipation, Mgn-m.
— — swelling of mesenteric glands, Ars. Calc. Con. Sacch.
Insensibility, abd., Ars.
Intussusception, of intestines, Thuj.
Inward pressure, ing., Igt. Thuj.
Itching on abd., Bell. Led. Merc. Ntr-c. Ol-an. Petr. Puls. Sass. Sep. Sulph. Zinc.
— in ing., not relieved by scratching, Mgn-s.
Jerks, Ars. Cannab. Murex. Ntr-m. Plat. Rhus.
— hyp., Arn. Sulph-ac.
— ing., Calc. Cannab.
— int., Ang. Guaj. Nux. Ran-sc. Sulph-ac.
Jumping sense, abd., *Croc.*
Labor-like pains, abd., Asa-f. Bry. Cham. Cina. Creos. Croc. Igt. Iod. Kali-c. Ntr-m. Nux. Pallad. Plat. Puls. Sec-c. Sep. Sulph-ac. Tilia.
Lead colic, *Alum. Op. Plat.*
Living, like something in abd., sensation, Cannab. Croc. Kali-jod. Merc. Nux. *Sabad.*
— — hypog., Sabad. Thuj.
— — ing., Kali-jod.
— sid., Rat.
Like a lump in abd., Plb. Rhus. *Sulph.* Tart.
— nav., *Spig.*
Movements in abd. Berb. Cannab. Carb-veg. Caps. Chin-sulph. Croc. Kali-jod. Lact. Mang. Merc. Ntr-c. Ntr-s. Ol-an. Phell. Puls. Rat. Rhus. Sabad. Sep. Sulph. Tar. Thuj.
— as from the fist of a foetus, Sulph.
— — — water, Casc. Hell, Phosp-ac.
Oppression, in abd., Arum. Euphr. Mgn-c. *Mosch.* Seneg.
— hypog., at night, Mgn-c.
Outpressing pain, abd., *Colch.*
— ing., Cannab. Clem. *Igt.* Kali-jod. Lyc. Rhus. *Tereb.*
Outward stinging, sid., Asa-f.
Pains running,upwards, forwards and hackwards, Gels.
Painfulness, abd., Acon. Aloe. Apis. Ars. Bell. Bov. Bry. Cannab. Canth. Carb-an. Cic. *Coff.* Coloc. Con. Creos. Croton. Cub. Dig. Ferr. Gymnoc. Hyosc. Jatr. Mang. *Merc.* Ntr-s. Nitr-ac. Nux. Ox-ac. Puls. Ran-b. Ran-sc. Scill. Sec-c. Sulph. Tilia. Valer.

17. ABDOMEN, GROIN AND FLATULENCY.

Painfulness, external, Acon. Bov. Canth. Nux. Puls. Tabac.
— to touch, *Acon.* Aeth. Aloe. Bell. Bism. Bry. Canth. Carb-veg. Caust. Cham. Con. Cycl. Hyosc. Jatr. Merc. Nux. Phosp. Puls. Stann. Stram. Tabac. Tereb. Tilia. *Verat.*
— when walking, Phosp. Ran-b. Sulph.
— epig., Stann.
— hypog., Arg-n. Caust. Cycl. Jac-cor. Merc. Psor. Stann. *Verb.*
— — right, Bapt. Merc. Ntr-s.
— ing., Graph. Therid.
— int., Acon. Bell. Bov. Canth. Hyosc. Nux. Puls. Tabac.
— nav., Aloe. Chin. Dulc. Kali-c. Stront. Verat.
— — deep behind, Jatr.
Pendulous, abd., Bell. Croc. Plat. Pod. Sep. Zinc.
—, of mothers, Iod. Ntr-c. *Sep.*
Perforation region of nav., sensation of, Aloe.
Perspiration on abd., Ambr. Anac. Ang. Cic. Dros. Plb.
Plug, as of a, behind nav., sensation, Ran-sc.
— — —, pressed in intestines, Anac.
Pressing in abd., Aloe. *Ambr. Arg.* Bell. *Bism. Calc. Caps. Casc. Caust. Chin.* Coff. Croton. *Cupr. Euph.* Euphr. *Grat.* Igt. Lach. Lyc. Mang. Meph. Merc. Mez. Ntr-m. *Ntr-nitr.* Nux. Op. *Par. Plat.* Plb. Prun. Puls. Rheum. Rhus. Sabin. Samb. *Sep.* Sil. Staph. *Sulph.* Tabac. Tar. Tart. *Tereb.* Verat. *Zinc.*
— outwards, Carb-an.
— epig., Ambr. Bry. *Caust.* Croton. Elat. *Nux.* Sulph. Teucr.
— hypog., Ambr. Arg. Aur. Bell. Carb-veg. Caust. Chin. Cocc. Colch. Diad. Elat. Kali-c. Ntr-m. Ruta. Scill. Sep. Thuj. Valer.
— ing., Bell. Berb. Kali-jod. Merc.
— nav., Anac. Chin-sulph. Cocc. Croton. Lach. Meny. *Ran-sc.* Raph. Rheum. *Spig.* Tabac. *Verb.*
— sid., Asar. Tar. Thuj. Zinc.
— — left, Sulph. Tar.
— — right, Prun.
— from left towards nav., Aloe.
— downwards, Agn.
Pressing asunder, sensation in abd., Colch. Euph. Igt.
— as from a weight, Bell. Cocc. Coloc. Diad. Lact. Merc. *Nux.* Sep. Spig. Tar. Tart. Verb.
— — epig., Nux. Tar.
— — hypog., Bell. Cocc. Diad. Sep.
— nav., Cocc. Lact. *Spig.* Verb.
Protrusion in various parts of abd., Igt.
— sensation of, abd., Igt.
Pulsation, abd., Acon. Aloe. Calad. Caps. Colch. Fluor-ac. Igt. Kali-c. Lach. Ntr-s. Plb. Sang. Sep. Stront. Sulph-ac. Tart.
— epig., Calad. Cannab.
— ing., Lyc. Sulph-ac.
— nav., Acon. Aloe.
Pustules in ing., Puls.
Rasping, abd., Hep.
— ing., Sulph-ac.
Red spots on abd., Bell. Sabad. Sep.
— points, Sabad.
Redness, scarlet, of abd., Rhus.
Rending, tearing, in abd., Aloe. Alum. Ars. Bry. *Cham.* Cocc. Colch. *Cop.* Croton. Cycl. Dig. Lyc. *Mgn-m.* Merc. Mez. Nux-m. Nux. *Phosp.* Puls. Rhus. Scill. Sec-c. Stram. Sulph. Tabac. Verb. Zinc.
— ing., Ars. Euph. Lyc. Sulph-ac.
— int., Berb. Stram.
— nav., Croton. Cycl. Nux. Stram. Verb.
— sid., Croton. Lyc.
Restlessness, abd., Agar. Kali-c.
Retraction, abd., Ang. Apis. Cupr. Ntr-nitr. Pod. Puls. Staph. Thuj. Verat.
— nav., Acon. Bar-c. Chelid. Ntr-c. Plb. Tabac. Tereb.
— abd., muscles, with colic, Pod.
Rhagades on int., Hep. Sep. Sil. Sulph.
Rigidity, on left side, Ntr-m.
Screwing pains at nav., as from worms, with sleepiness, Nux-m.
Shattering sensation, abd., Carb-an. Creos. Scill.
Shocks in abd., Calc. Ntr-m. Puls. Scill.
Shuddering on abd., Cannab. Coloc.
Softness on abd., Phosp. Rhus.
Soreness, abd., Acon. Arg-n. Ars. Bell. Calc. Cannab. Carb-an. Coloc. Con. Croton. Euph. Gels. Hell. Hep. Hipp-m. Hyosc. Ip. Kali-c. Mgn-m. Meny. Ntr-c. Nux. Pallad. Puls. Ran-b. Rhus. Sep. Stann. Sulph. Tilia. Trifol.
— — right side, Zinc.
— epig., Mang.
— int., Ambr. Bell. Meny.
— sid., Arn.
— — left, Colch.
— ing., Rhus.
— nav., Rhus. Thuj.
Spasms, hysterical in women, Cocc.
Spasmodic pain, abd., *Ang.* Carb-veg. Coloc. Dig. Graph. Igt. Kali-c. Ol-an. *Phosp-ac.* Ran-sc. Sass. Staph. Tart. Teucr. Thuj. Verb.
— — hypog., Amm-c. Bry. Camph. Carb-veg. Cham. Cocc. Con. Dig. Ferr. Hyosc. Igt. Ip. Iod. Mur-ac. Nux. Puls. Stann.
— ing., Dig. Igt.
— int., Ferr. Lyc. Sabin. Samb.
— nav., Bell. Calad. Phosp-ac. Verb. Zinc.

17. ABDOMEN, GROIN AND FLATULENCY.

Spamodic pain, sudden, in upper part, cries out, sense, of contraction, Gels.
Sprain, pain as from in ing., Euph.
Stinging, stitches, abd., Aloe. Alum. Ang. Arg-n. Ars. Bell. *Bry.* Calc. Carb-veg. Cham. Chin. Con. Croton. Cupr. Dig. Fluor-ac. *Grat.* Gymnoc. Jatr. Kali-b. *Kali-c.* Mgn-m. *Mgn-s.* Merc. Mez. Ntr-c. Ntr-nitr. Nitr-ac. Nitr. Nux. Pallad. Psor. Puls. Ruta. Sep. *Spig.* Stann. *Sulph. Tar. Verb.* Viol-tr. Zinc.
— — left side, Bell. Chin. Hep. Lach. Sass. Staph. Sulph. Tar.
— — sudden to pelvis, impeding breathing, Chelid. Chin. Kali-c. Ran-sc. Samb. Tilia.
— — — like electric shocks, left side, Arn-n.
— — epig., Croton. Kali-c.
— — hypog., Bell. Chelid. Chin. Kali-c. Nux. Samb. Sep.
— — ing., Ars. Bell. Calc. Carb-an. *Kali-c.* Lyc. Merc. Mur-ac. *Ntr-s.* Prun. Rat. Stront. Sep. Sulph-ac.
— — left, to axilla, Ntr-s.
— — int., Berb. Mgn-m. Ruta. Samb.
— — nav., Acon. Aloe. Anac. Asa-f. Dulc. Gymnoc. Hyosc. Mgn-s. Nux. Plat. Plb. Raph. Sep. Verb.
— — — left side, Jac-cor.
— — sid., Calc. Croton. Igt. Ntr-c. Nux. Plat. Sabad. *Sass.* Tar.
— — — left, Bell. Hep. Samb. *Sass.* Sep. *Sulph. Tar.*
Stones, like sharp, rubbing together, in abd., Coloc.
Strangulation in abd., sensation of, Spong.
Swelling of abd., Acon. Arg. Ars. Bry. Calc. *Caust.* Graph. *Iod.* Jatr. Kali-b. Kali-c. Lac-can. Mang. Ntr-c. Ntr-m. Sacch. Sep. *Staph.* Sulph. Verat.
— — blackish blue, *Aeth.*
— elastic, ing., Amm-c. Caps.
— hypog, Sil.
— nav., Bry. Caust. Prun. Puls.
— sid., left, Laur.
— in children, Calc. Caust. Sacch. Staph.
— — hard, after scarlet fever, Calc. Sacch.
— in mothers, Iod. Ntr-c. *Sep.*
— with danger of suffocation when in horizontal position, Iod.
— sense of, Amm-c. Ant. Kali-c.
Tension, in abd., Ambr. Ang. Arg. Bar-c. Bell. Bry. Calc. Carb-an. Carb-veg. Caust. Chin. Creos. Croton. Graph. Gum-gut. Hyosc. Kali-c. Lact. Laur. Lyc. Mgn-c. Mgn-m. Merc. Mez. Mosch. Ntr-m. Ntr-s. Nux. Par. Petr. Phosp. Phosp-ac. Plat. Plb. Poth. Puls. Rheum. Rhod. Sabin. Sec-c. Sep. Sil. Spong. *Staph.* Stram. Stront. Sulph. Thuj. Verat. Zinc.

— epig., Croton. Ntr-c.
— hypog., Aur. Chin.
— ing., Amm-c. Berb. Croton. Dig. Mgn-s. Merc. Spig.
— — nav., *Verat.*
— in sid., Croton. Merc. Zinc.
Throbbing, in abd., Igt. *Sang.* (compare Pulsations).
— epig., Calad. *Cannab.*
— ing , Sulph-ac.
— nav., Acon. Aloe.
Tickling in epig., Bar-c, Bry. Cham. Hep. Lach. Ntr-m. Nitr-ac. Phosp-ac.
Tingling, int., Mgn-m.
Torpor, abd., sensation of, Carb-veg.
Trembling, abd., Iod.
Tumors, as if intestines were distended by wind, here and there, Ntr-c.
Turburculosis abdominalis, Ntr-s.
Turning sensation, in abd., Caps. Igt. Lact. *Sabad.* Sep.
Twisting, abd., Dig. Diosc. Elaps. Pallad.
— nav., Cina. Ran-b.
Twitching, abd., Agar. Ars. Guaj. *Rhus.*
— hypog., Sulph-ac.
— int., Ang. Guaj. Ran-sc. Sulph-ac.
Tympanitis, Arn. Chin. *Coloc.* Hœmatox. Jatr. Kali-b. *Op.*
Ulcers in bowels, Cupr. Plb.
— about nav., Apis. Ars. Calc. Lach., Lyc. Sep. Sil. Sulph.
Ulcerous pain, abd., Cham. Cocc. Creos. Ran-b.
— hypog., Nitr-ac.
— — ing., Amm-m. Cic.
— — int., Rhus.
— — sid., left. Valer.
Uneasiness, abd., Asa-f. Aur. Cist. Cycl. Ferr-m. Ntr-c. Ntr-m. Tart.
— — after a grave disease, Mur-ac.
Varices in ing., Berb.
Violent pain, abd., Aloe. *Ars.* Bell. Cast. Cham. *Coloc. Cupr.* Nitr. *Plb.*
— sid., right, Nitr.
Veins distended, on abd., Sep.
Warmth, sensation of, on abd., Casc, Mang. Seneg.
— — — nav., Sulph-ac.
Water, as of sensation in abd., Casc. Hell. Phosp-ac.
— cold, as if running through abd., sensation, Cannab.
— tepid, as of, in abd., Croton.
Weakness, sensation of, in abd., Borax. Igt. Lil-tigr. Oleand. Phosp. Staph.
— — — extending to throat, relieved by eructations, Kalm.
Winding, wringing, whirling pain abd., Berb. Cap. Ran-b. Rhus. Sulph-ac.
— — — nav., Cina. Nux-m.
Yellow spots on abd., Ars. Canth. Carb-veg. Kali-c. Phosp. Sabad. Sep. Thuj.

17. ABDOMEN, GROIN AND FLATULENCY.

Morning, in the, pain, abd., Agar. Alum. Ambr. Amm-c. Borax. Bov. Calc. Caust. Cham. Creos. Hep. Ntr-m. Nitr-ac. Nux. Petr. *Phosp.* Ran-sc.
— in bed, Acon. Ambr. Ntr-c. Phosp. Sep.
— at sun-rise, *Cham.*
Afternoon, in the, pain, abd., Nitr.
Evening, in the, pain, abd., Ambr. Diad. Fluor-ac. Led. *Mgn-m.* Meph. Merc. Ntr-s. Nitr-ac. Par. Phosp. *Puls. Valer.* Verat. Zinc.
— — in bed, Par. *Valer.* Zinc.
— — — painfulness of int., Sabin.
— relieved, Nitr.
Night in the, pain, abd., Acon. Ambr. Amm-c. Ars. *Aur.* Borax. Calc. Carb-veg. Cocc. Creos. Dulc. *Ferr.* Graph. Ind. Kali-c. Lyc. Mgn-c. Mgn-s. Merc. Ntr-c. Ntr-m. Nitr-ac. *Nux-m.* Petr. Phosp. *Plb.* Prun. Puls. *Rhus. Sep.* Sulph. *Sulph-ac.* Tabac. Verat.
— pain, int., Lyc.
Midnight, after pain, abd., Ambr.
Acids from, pain, abd., Dros. Phosp-ac.
Air, open, Nux.
Anger, after, Cocc.
Bandaging, relieved, pain abd., Puls.
Bending the body by pain, abd., Acon. Brom.
— forward, relieved, *Bell.* Euph. Sulph. Verb.
— double, necessity for, Bell. Chelid. *Coloc.* Grat. Rheum. Rhus. Sabad.
Blowing the nose, when pain, abd., Canth.
Brandy, from pain, abd., Igt.
Breakfast, after pain abd., *Nux.* Phosp.
Breathing, when pain, abd., Anac. Arg. Berb. Creos. Dig. Hyosc. Mgn-c. Mosch. Seneg. Sulph.
— — hypog. of, Asa-f.
— — deep, Mang. Sulph.
— — out (expiring), Brom. Dig.
Children, in abd., complaints, Calc. *Caust.* Cham. Cic. *Jalap.* Nux-m. *Senna.* Sil. Staph.
Chinchona (bark) abuse of, pain abd., from, Verat.
Coffee, from, pain abd., Cham. Igt. Nux.
— — relieved, Coloc.
Cold, from a pain, abd., Alum. *Cham.* Chin. Coloc. *Dulc.* Merc. Nitr-ac. Nux. Verat.
Constipation from, pain, abd., Con. Sil.
Coughing, when, pain, abd., Anac. Ars. Bell. Canth. Cham. Cocc. Nux.
— — int., Ambr. Puls.
Crooked, when sitting, pain, abd., *Tart.*
— — relieved, Sulph.
Drawing in abd., pain, when, Valer.
Eating, after, pain, abd., Evon. Iod.
— — relieved, *Psor.*
Eructation, relieves pain, in abd., Bar-c.

Lach. Nitr.
Exercise, from, pain, abd., Aloe. Arn. Berb. Cocc. Creos. Cycl. Dig. Ip. Ntr-m. Nitr. Nux. Ol-an. Puls. Sep. Stram.
— — — int., Plb.
— — — relieved, Coloc.
Flatus discharged by, pain, abd., relieved. Aloe. Arn. Grat. Guaj. Iris. Ntr-m. Ntr-s. Nitr.
Hemmorrhoids, from, pain abd., *Sulph.* Valer.
Laughing, when pain, abd. Ars. Nux.
Lying, when, aggravation, Phosp.
— on side, pain, abd., Par. Phosp.
— — — relieved, Ntr-s.
— — — left side, relieved, Pallad.
Milk, from pain, abd., Ang. Bry. Carb-veg. Con. Sulph-ac.
Pregnancy, during pain, abd., Arn. Bry. Hyosc. Nux. *Puls.* Sep.
Pressed upon, when, pain, abd., Acon. Aloe. Anac. Bell. Carb-veg. Cina. Coff. Cycl. Eupat. Jac-cor. Kali-b. Lac-can. Nitr-ac. Nux. Puls. Ran-b. Samb. Sass. Sulph.
— — — colic, Bell. Mez. Plb-ac. Zinc.
— — relieved, Amm-c. Asa-f. *Bell.* Bov. Cina. *Coloc.* Dulc. Graph. Grat. Kali-c. Meny. Ntr-c. Ntr-m. Nitr. Plb.
Rest, by, pain, abd., Bov.
— — — relieved, Ip. Puls.
Riding in a carriage, pain, abd., Carb-veg.
Rising, when, from lying, relieved, Arg.
Room, in a, pain, abd., Kali-jod.
Singing, from, pain, int., Puls.
Sitting, in, pain, abd., Ruta.
Sitting down, when, pain, abd., Ruta.
Sneezing, when, pain, abd., Bell. Canth. Cham. Pallad.
Standing when, pain, abd, Aloe., Bell.
— — — ing., Thuj.
Stooping, when, pain, hyphog., Kali-c.
Strain in loins, from a, pain, abd., Arn. Carb-veg. Lach.
Stretching out, pain, ing., Mdgn-s.
— — in morning, pain, int., Rhus.
— — pains, compel, Tart.
Sugar, from, pain, abd., Igt. Sulph.
Tobacco, from, pain abd., Borax. Igt.
— — relieved, Chioc.
Touch, from, pain, abd., *Acon.* Aeth. Aloe. Apis. Bell. Berb. Canth. Cham. Cupr. Cycl. Hyosc. Merc. Merc-cor. Nitr-ac. Phosp. *Plb.* Puls. Sil. Stann. Stram. Tabac. Tereb. Tilia. *Verat.*
— — hypog., Cycl.
— — ing., Spig.
— — int., Plb.
— — nav., Carb-veg. Caust. Croton,
— — sid., left, Bell. Colch.
Turning the body, when, pain, int., Ambr.
Vexation, after, pain abd., *Coloc.*

17. ABDOMEN, GROIN AND FLATULENCY.

Walking, in pain, abd., Chin. Coloc. Ferr. Hyosc. Phosp. Ran-b. *Sulph.* Verat.
— — as if bowels were loose and shaking abcut, Mang.
— — pain, ing., Thuj.
— on stone pavements, Con.
— after, in open air, pain, abd., Kali-jod.
Warm food, from, pain, abd., Kali-c. Ol-an
Warmth, external, by, pain, relieved, Alum. Bar-c. Cast. Meph. Pallad. Sil.
Water, from drinking, pain, abd., Croc. Hipp-u. Teucr.
Worms, from, pain, abd., *Cic. Felix.* Nux-m. *Ruta.* Sabad. (compare Sect. 18.)
Colic, agitation, with, Igt.
— anus, contraction of, with, Verb.
— anxiety, with, in, abd., Cic. Cupr. Hep. Mosch. Nux. Plat. Sulph.
— bending double, compelling, Bell. Chelid. *Coloc.* Grat. *Rheum.* Rhus. Sabad
— bladder, pain in, Lach. Nux. Prun.
— chilliness, with, Coloc. Daph. Merc. Mez. Phosp. Spig. Stront. (compare Sect. 32.)
— coldness, general, Ars. Bov. Meph. (compare Sect. 32.)
— constipation, with, Bell.
— convulsions, with, *Cic. Cupr. Sec-c.*
— cough, with, Chin.
— cries, with, Cupr. Hyosc. Ip. Viol-tr.
— despair, Coff.
— diarrhœa, with, Ambr. Amm-c. Ars. Borax. Bry. Chelid. *Coloc. Jalap.* Lach. Ntr-c. Nicc. Ol-an. Petr. Phosp. Puls. Spig. *Stront.* Verat. Zinc.
— dislike to work, with, Tart.
— dyspnœa, with, Berb. Caps. Cham. Chin. *Cocc.* Creos. Lach. Lyc. Mez. Mosch. Rhod. Prun. Sulph.
— eructations, with, Grat. Kali-c. Kali-jod. Nux. Rhod.
— evacuation of hard fæces, Ant.
— — bloody fæces, Rhus.
— eyes, affections of, alternating with, Euphr.
— — surrounded with a livid circle, with, Cham.
— face, heat of, with, Hep. Merc. Nux.
— — pale, with, Cham. Phosp.
— — red, with, Cast. Merc. Nux.
— — shivering in, with, Coloc.

Colic, with fainting, Ran-sc.
— hands, yellowness of, with, Sil.
— headache, with, Hyosc. (compare Sect. 3.)
— heat in general, with, Ars. Carb-veg. (compare Sect. 32.)
— humor ill, with, Asa-f. Cic. Creos.
— leg cramps in, Coloc.
— — heaviness of, with, Diad.
— — lameness of, with, Carb-veg.
— — painfulness, with, Coloc. Cop. Sec-c.
— leucorrhœa, discharge of, with, Creos. Mgn-c. Mgn-m. (compare Sect. 21.)
— lying down, compelling, Nux. Tart.
— — — on abdomen, compelling, Aloe.
— — — unable to remain, Prun.
— mucus, discharge of, from, anus, with, Viol-tr.
— nails, blueness of with, Sil.
— nausea, with, Amm-c. Chelid. Cycl. Dig. Grat. Hep. Mang. Nux-m. Nux. Ol-an. Samb. Stann. Sulph. (compare Sect. 14.)
— peevishness, Asa-f. Cic.
— perspiration cold, with, Ars.
— restlessness, with, Aloe. Bell. Carb-veg. *Coloc.* Mosch. *Tart.*
— sacral region, pain, in, with, Kali-c. Ntr-c. Nux. Sec-c.
— shuddering, with, Chin. Diad. Ip.
— sighing, with, Igt.
— sleepiness, Nux. Tart.
— sleeplessness, Creos.
— stretch one's self out, compelling to, Tart.
— thirst with, Chin. Verat.
— trembling and chatering with the teeth, with, Bov. Meph.
— urging to stool, with, Aur. Bar-c. Bism. Petr. Phosp. Sep. Staph. Verb. Viol-tr.
— urine, copious, with, Bell. Lach. Spig. Verat.
— — suppressed, with, Arn. Graph.
— urinate, urgency to, with, Creos. Ferr-m. Meph.
— vomiting, *Asar.* Ars. Bell. Casc. Cupr-carb. Hyosc. Lach. Puls. Sec-c. (compare Sect. 14.)
— water, collection of in mouth, with, Amm-c.
— waterbrash, with, Bry. (compare Sect. 14.
— weakness, with, Nux.
— yawning, with, Cast.

18. Stool and Anus.

Beating, as of small hammer, in rectum, Lach.
Biting in anus and rectum, Dulc. Phosp-ac.
Black, rectum, Merc.
Blood, discharge of, from, anus, Aloe. Alum. *Amm-c.* Ant. Ars. Asar. Bar-m. *Borax.* Cact. Calc. Calc-ph. Carb-veg. Casc. Chin-sulph. Coloc. Cycl. Igt. Kali-jod. Lach. Lyc. *Merc. Merc-cor.* Millef. Mur-ac. Ntr-m. Nux. Phosp. Plat. Psor. Puls. Rat. Sabin. Sep. Stram. Sulph. Valer. Zinc.
— constant dripping, no blood with stool, Kobalt.
— and sanious matter, Ntr-m.
— bright red, Bufo. Casc. Hydroph. *Merc.* Zinc.
— black, Ant. Merc-cor.
— — liquid, Elaps.
— clotted, Merc-cor. Stram.
— dark, Alum. Asar. Caps. Lob. Verat.
— dark, bloody fluid oozes, Apis.
— fetid, Hipp-m.
— congestion of, to anus, Sep. Sulph-ac.
Boring in rectum, Valer.
Burning in anus, Aloe. Alum. Amm-c. Ang. Ant. Ars. Bar-c. Bry. Calc. Cupr. Carb-an. *Carb-veg.* Cast. Chenop. Cocc. Colch. Coloc. Cop. Croton. Cub. Euph. Graph. Hep. Hydroph. Iod. Kali-c. Lach. Lact. Laur. Lyc. Merc. Mur-ac. Ntr-c. Ntr-m. Nicc. Nitr-ac. Nitr. Nux. Oleand. Op. Phosp. Puls. Rat. Sass. *Sep.* Staph. Stront. *Sulph.* Tereb. Thuj. Verat. Zinc.
— as from pepper, Caps.
— after stool, relieved, Clem.
— between the nates, Thuj.
— in the rectum, All-cep. Aloe. *Ars.* Aur-fol. Calc. Canth. Caps. Carb-an. Cast. Con. Kali-c. Merc-cor. Merc-sulph. Mur-ac. Ntr-c. Ntr-m. Nitr-ac. Petr. Phosp. Puls. *Sep. Sulph.* Sulph-ac. Tereb. Verat.
Bruise, like pain in anus, Lact.
Chafed easily by riding on horseback, Carb-an.
Clawing, squeezing, as from a claw, in anus, Phell.
Closed, sensation as if anus were, Lach. Plb.

Condylomation on anus, *Nitr-ac.* Sabin. Staph. *Thuj.*
Constriction of anus, Cimex. Croton. Lach. Laur. Mez. Ntr-m. Nux. Plb. Therid.
Contraction of anus, Ang. Borax. Croton. Hipp-m. Igt. Mang. Plumb. Sec-c. Thuj.
— of perineum, Sep.
— — rectum, Alum. Borax. Cact. Calc. Cocc. Coloc. Ferr. Lach. Ntr-m. Nux. Plb. Plb-ac. Sep. Stront.
— — sense of, Ntr-m. Nux.
Contractive pain at anus, Lyc.
Cracks in anus, Agn. All-cep. Graph.
Cramp in anus, Colch.
— in rectum, Calc. Lyc. Phosp.
Cutting in anus, Caust. Jac-cor. Kali-c. Laur. Ntr-c. Staph.
— in rectum, Caust. Lyc. Mang. Ntr-c.
Darting from perineum to rectum and genitals, Bov.
Drawing in anus and perineum, Cycl. Lact.
— pain, from anus, through urethra, Hipp.
— in rectum, Chenop. Creos. Mang. Rhod.
Dropping from anus, sense as if cold water were, Cannab.
Eruption on anus, Calc. Kali-c. Lyc.
— burning and in groups, Calc.
— herpetic, Ntr-m.
— itching, Lyc. Petr.
— little pimples around anus, burning and itching, Cinnab.
— pustules, Amm-m.
— ulcerous, Kali-c.
— on perineum, furuncles, Ant.
— — vesicular, Carb-veg.
Excrescences at anus, Jac-cor.
— — sycotic, Nitr-ac. Sabin. Staph. Thuj.
Fissures at anus, Aesc-hipp. Ars. Caust. Grat. Igt. Lach. Mez. Ntr-m. Nitr-ac. Nux. Phosp. Plb. Sep. Sil. Sulph. Thuj.
Fistula in ano, (in rectum,) Aur. Berb. Caust. Creos. Petr. Sil. Sulph. Thuj.
Formication, as from a large worm, Cinnab.
Gnawing at anus, Ang. Spong.
Griping in rectum, Sabad.
Grumbling in rectum, Mang.
Hemorrhoidal tumors of the anus, Acon. Aesc-hipp. Aloe. Alum. Ambr. Amm-c. Amm-m. *Anac.* Ant. Apis. Arn. Ars. *Bar-c,* Bell. Berb. Borax. Calc. Calc-ph.

18. STOOL AND ANUS.

Caps. Carb-an. Carb-veg. Casc. Caust. Cham. Cimex. Collin. Coloc. Cupr. Ferr. Fluor-ac. Graph. Hipp-m. Kali-c. Lach. Lact. Lyc. Mur-ac. Ntr-m. Nitr-ac. Nux. Phosp. Puls. Sang. Sep. Sulph. Sulph-ac. Zing.
Hemmorrhoidal tumors of the rectum, Ars. *Calc.* Caust. *Coloc.* Hep. Lyc. *Phosp.* Phosp-ac. Sep. Stront.
— disposition to, Calc. Carb-veg. Caust. Graph. Lach. Nux. Petr. Sulph.
— bleeding, *Acon.* Aesc-hipp. Amm-c. Ant. Bell. Borax. Bufo. Calc. Caps. Carb-veg. Cham. Chin. Collin. Coloc. Cupr. Elat. *Ferr.* Ham. Hyosc. Kali-c. Lach. Lob. Meny. *Millef.* *Mur-ac.* Nitr-ac. Phosp. Puls. Sabin. Sacch. Sep. Sulph.
— blind, Ant. Caps. Ferr. Grat. *Nux.* Puls. Verat.
— bluish, livid, Aesc-hipp. Carb-veg. *Mur-ac.*
— burning, Acon. Aloe. Ant. Apis. *Ars.* Berb. Calc. Caps. Carb-an. Carb-veg. Caust. Cham. Chin. Lach. Mur-ac. Nitr-ac. Psor. Sulph-ac.
— — as from hot needles, Ars.
— congestion, Sacch.
— cracked, Cham. Caust.
— crawling, Ant. Chin.
— cutting, Kali-c. Lach.
— fulness of, Kali-b.
— inveterate, *Nitr-ac.*
— itching, Ars. Berb. Clem. Chin. Graph. Kali-c. Sulph-ac.
— large, Caust. Graph. Lach.
— like ground-nuts, blue, painful and burning, Aesc-hipp.
— oozing, Alum. Bar-c. Caust. Clem. Kali-c. Ntr-m. Sulph. Sulph-ac.
— painful, Aloe. Alum. Anac. Ars. Cact. Calc. Carb-veg. Caust. Coloc. *Graph.* *Kali-c.* *Mur-ac.* Ntr-m. Nux. Sabin. Sacch. Stront. Thuj.
— — in sitting and lying, Phosp.
— — when walking, Caust.
— painless, Ars.
— protruded, Aloe. Amm-c. Bar-c. Calc. Caust. Ferr. Gran. Ham. Hep. Kali-c. Lyc. Me c. Nitr. Nitr-ac. Phosp. Phosp-ac. Plat. Puls. Rat. Rhus. Sep. Sil. Sulph. Zinc.
— rasping, Puls.
— smarting, Amm-c. Puls.
— sore, smarting, Aloe. Apis. Graph. Kali-c. Mur-ac. Phosp. Puls. Rhus. Zinc.
— stinging, Apis. Ars. Bar-c. Carb-an. Caust. Kali-c. Ntr-m. Sulph-ac.
— suppressed, Ars. Calc. Carb-veg. Caps. Nux. Phosp. Sulph.
— swollen, Aloe. Ang. Cact. Calc. Carb-veg. Caust. Coloc. Kali-c. Mur-ac. Nitr-ac. Thuj.

— tingling, Ant.
— ulcerated, Cham.
— between them, burning rhagades at anus, Graph.
— with congestion at anus, Lach.
— at climacteric period, Lach.
— after suppression of leucorrhea, Amm-m.
Heat of rectum, Aloe. Con.
Heaviness at anus, Sep.
— in perineum, Therid.
Herpes on anus, Ntr-m.
— perineum, Petr.
Inactivity of rectum, Alum. Anac. Arn. Camph. Carb-veg. Chin. Cocc. Croton. Hep. Igt. Kali-c. Mur-ac. Ntr-c. Nux-m. Nux. Op. Petr. Phyt. Plb. Puls. Ruta. Staph. Sulph. Verat. Zinc.
Itching of anus, Agar. All-cep. Aloe. Alum. Ambr. Amm-c. Anac. Ant. Arg-n. Bar-c. Borax. Cact. Calc. *Carb-veg.* *Caust.* Cina. Cocc-c. Colch. *Croc.* Croton. Cub. Elaps. Ferr-m. Fluor-ac. Graph. Grat. *Igt.* Iod. Kali-c. Lith. *Lyc.* Merc. Mur-ac. Ntr-c. Ntr-s. Nitr-ac. Nux-jug. Nux. Petr. Phosp. Phosp-ac. Plat. Rhus. Rumex. Sass. Sep. *Sil.* Spig. Spong. *Sulph.* *Teucr.* Zinc. Zing.
— — when sitting, Jac-cor.
— — after stool, relieved, Clem.
— — perineum, Agn. Fluor-ac. Ntr-s. Nux. Petr. Tar.
— — rectum, Ambr. Borax. Bov. Calc. Chin-sulph. Cic. Ferr-m. Gran. Nitr-ac. Nux. Phosp. Phosp-ac. Rhus. Sep. Sil. Spig. Sulph.
Jerking pains from anus up rectum, Sep.
Meals, after, pain in anus, Lyc.
Moistness of anus, *Bar-c.* Carb-an. Carb-veg. Nitr-ac.
— between anus and coccyx, Led.
— of perineum, Carb-an. Carb-veg. Pæon.
— rectum, Anac. Carb-an. Carb-veg. Caust. Coloc. Sep.
Mucus, discharge of, Acon. *Alum.* *Ant.* Ars. *Borax.* Caps. Carb-veg. Coff. Colch. Coloc. Dulc. Hell. Lach. *Merc.* Merc-cor. Nux. *Phosp.* Pod. Rhus. Sep. *Spig.* Stann. Sulph.
— serous, Kali-jod.
Openness, constant of anus, Phosp.
Painfulness of rectum, Acon. Caust. Con. Kali-chl. Nux. Seneg.
Paralysis of anus, Acon. Coloc. Graph. Laur. Selen.
— of sphincter, Bell. Gels. Graph. Hyosc. Phosp. Selen.
— — intestinal canal, *Phosp.*
Perspiration of perinæum, Alum. Carb-veg. Hep. Thuj.
— at anus, offensive, Alum. Carb-an. Thuj.
Pinching in rectum, Sabad.
Plug was pressing out, sensation as if, Croton.

18. STOOL AND ANUS.

Plug in anus, sensation of, cannot sit down, Kali-b. Lach.
— — rectum, Anac.
Pressure in anus, Acon. Ang. Ant. Bar-c. Cact. Chelid. Chin. Collin. Cycl. Kali-b. Lach. Lact. Laur. Lob. Nitr. Nux. Ol-an. Phell. Phosp. Puls. Seneg. Spig. Staph. Tong. Verat. Verb. Zinc.
— — perineum, Alum. Berb. Cop. Cycl.
— — rectum, Aloe. Ant. Arg. Arn. Cannab. Chenop. Chin. Croton. Cycl. Hipp-m. Kali-c. Kobalt. Nitr-ac. Nux. Op. Ox-ac. Phosp. Seneg.
— outwards, perineum, Asa-f.
Pricking at anus, Lact.
Prolapsus, of rectum, Ant. Ars. Calc. Colch. Croton. *Dig.* Elaps. Gels. Graph. Gum-gut. *Igt. Lach. Lyc.* Mgn-m. *Merc.* Mez. Ntr-m. Nitr-ac. Nitr. Plb. *Pod. Sep. Sulph.* Therid. Valer. Zinc.
— while passing water, Mur-ac.
Rasping pain in anus, Ant. Grat. Verat.
— — rectum, Ntr-m.
Rending tearing in anus, *Colch.* Kali-c. Phosp-ac. Zinc.
— up rectum, Sep.
— in rectum, Chenop. Kali-c. Ntr-m. Phosp-ac. Ruta. Sabad. Sep. Thuj.
Retraction of anus, Kali-b. Plb.
Rumbling in rectum, Mang.
Scraping in anus. Croton.
Sitting, when pain in anus, Amm-c. Phosp. Therid.
Smarting in anus, Ant. Dulc. Grat. Mur-ac. Phosp-ac. Puls. Verat.
— — rectum, Igt. Mur-ac. Ntr-m. Phosp-ac. Puls.
Soreness, excoriation, of anus, Amm-c. Ars. *Bar-c.* Calc. Carb-an. Grat. Hep. Kali-c. Merc. Ntr-m. Nitr-ac. *Sulph.*
— between the nates, Calc. Ntr-m. Sep.
— — when walking, Ntr-m.
— of perineum, Carb-veg. Rhod.
— — rectum, when riding in a vehicle, Psor.
— sense of, in anus, Amm-m. Ars. Berb. Caust. Croton. Euph. Graph. Hep. Igt. Kali-b. Nux. Phell. Puls. Sass. Spong. Zinc.
— — followed by blisters, from horse-back riding, Carb-an.
— — with burning and tenderness in sitting, Berb.
— of rectum, Amm-m. Ars. Caust. Grat. Lyc. Nux. Puls.
Spasms in anus, Colch.
— — sphincter, Colch.
— — rectum, Calc. Lyc. Phosp.
Stinging stitches, at anus, Acon. Ambr. Ars. Borax. *Carb-an.* Carb-veg. Chin. Coloc. Con. Croc. Croton. Ferr-m. Grat. Hydroph. Igt. Jac-cor. Jatr. Kali-c. Lob. Lyc. Mgn-c. Merc. Mosch. Ntr-m. Nitr-ac. Nux-jug. Nux. Ol-an.
Phosp. *Sep.* Sil. Spong. *Sulph.* Sulph-ac. Teucr. Zinc.
Stinging, stitches from anus to sacral region and adomen, Aloe.
— in rectum, Bell. Borax. Carb-an. Igt. Kali-c. Lach. Lachn. Lyc. Mez. Sep. Sil. Sulph.
— — to left groin, Creos. Croc.
— from anus to rectum, Igt.
— — to urethra, Cocc. Thuj.
— in perineum, from above downwards, and from within outwards, Lith.
Stitches in rectum, All-cep.
Stoppage of anus, Nux.
Stricture of rectum, Bell. *Borax. Camph.* Igt. Phosp.
Swelling of anus, Apis. Graph. Nux. Sulph. Teucr.
Tenesmus, Acon. Aeth. Aloe. Ars. Bell. Calc. *Caps.* Cocc-c. Croton. Euph. Grat. *Hell.* Hep. Ip. Lach. Lact. Laur. Merc. Merc-cor. Ntr-c. Nicc. Nitr. Nux. Op. Ox-ac. Phosp. Phosp-ac. Plat. *Rheum.* Rhus. Selen. Senna. Sep. Spong. Sulph. Tabac.
— in morning, after rising, Aeth.
— at night, *Merc.*
— with nausea, and pain in abdomen, Rhus.
— succeeded by fluid, discharge, mixed with blood and mucus, Aloe.
Tension of anus, Lyc. Sep.
— — rectum, Sep.
Throbbing at anus, Aloe. Croton. Grat. Lach. Rhod.
— — rectum, Ntr-m.
— — as of a small hammer, Lach.
— at perineum, Caust.
Tingling, crawling, at anus, Agar. Ambr. Chin. Colch. *Croc. Igt.* Kali-c. Ntr-c. Nux. *Plat.* Rhus. Sabin. Sep. Spig. Tereb. *Teucr. Zinc.*
— at rectum, Calc. Rhus. *Sabad.* Sep. Spig. Spong. Tart.
Torn away, pain as if something were, in anus, Aur-m. Calc.
Ulcer in the anus, Cub. Kali-c. Pæon.
Ulcerous pain at anus, and perineum, Cycl.
— — when walking, Agn.
Weight in perineum, and feeling as if a plug was wedged between symphysis pubis and coccygis, Aloe. Caust. Hep. Thuj.
Worm-complaints, Acon. All-cep. Ars. Calc. Carb-veg. *Cic. Cina.* Dolich. Ferr. Felix. Graph. Igt. Merc. Ntr-m. *Nux-m.* Nux. Petr. Ruta. *Sabad.* Sacch. Scill. Sec-c. *Sil. Spig.* Spong. Stann. Sulph. Tereb. Teucr. Verat.
— solitary, Croton.
— — in scrofulous individuals, Sil.
— ascarides, Acon. Asar. Bar-c. *Calc.*

18. STOOL AND ANUS.

Chin. *Cina*. Croton. *Ferr.* Graph. Grat. *Ign*. Mgn-c. *Mgn-s.* Merc. Nux. Phosp. Plat. Scill. Sil. *Spig.* Spong. *Sulph.* *Teucr. Valer.* Yuba.

Worm complaints, lumbricoides, Acon. All-sat. Anac. Asar. Bar-c. Bell. Calc. *Cic.* Cham. *Cina.* Graph Hyosc. Kali-c. Lyc. Mgn-c. Merc. Ntr-m. Nux. Rhus. Ruta. Sabad. Sec-c. *Sil.* Spig. *Sulph.* Tereb. Yuba.

— tenia, *Calc.* Carb-an. Carb-veg. Chin. *Felix.* Frag-ves. Grat. *Graph.* Kali-c. Mgn-m. Merc. Ntr-c. Nux. Petr. Phosp. Plat. *Puls.* Sabad. Sep. *Sil.* Stann. Sulph. Tereb.

Stool, bubbling, Eugen.
— copious, Ang. Ant. *Aur.* Benz-ac. Berb. Cact. Colch. Cop. Cub. Diosc. Elat. Gum-gut. Jatr. Iod. Ip. Iris. Kali-b. Lept. Mgn-c. Nux-m. Pod. *Ran-b.* Raph. Rumex. Sec-c. Tart. Teucr. Thuj. Verat.
— difficult, Agn. *Alum.* Amm-c. Anac. Ant. Asa-f. Bar-c. Bov. Bry. Calc. Camph. *Carb-veg.* Cast. Caust. Chin. Clem. *Coco.* Colch. Creos. Euph. Gels. Grat. Hep. *Ign.* *Kali-c.* Kali-jod. Lact. Lyc. *Mgn-m.* Mang. *Merc.* Mez. Mur-ac. Murex. Ntr-m. Ntr-nitr. Nicc. Nitr. Nitr-ac. *Nux-jug.* Nux. Ol-an. Petr. Phosp. Phosp-ac. Plat. *Plumb.* Pod. Prun. Psor. Puls. *Rhod.* Ruta. Sabad. Sabin. Sacch. *Sass.* Sep. Sil. Staph. Stront. Tart. *Thuj.*
— — as if sphincter contracted, Gels.
— — the stool being soft, Alum. Anac. Carb-veg. *Chin.* Colch. Diad. Hep. Ign. Nicc. *Nux-m.* Phosp-ac. Psor. Puls. Rhod. Sep. Sil. Staph. Tart. Therid.
— — easier in a standing posture, Caust.
— easy, Berb.
— frequent, in day time, Acon. Amm-m. Ang. Ang-spur. Arn. Borax. Calc. Carb-an. Chin. Cic. Cinnab. Coff. Cycl. Dros. Lob. Mang. Mez. Ntr-ac. Nux. Ol-an. Par. Petr. Phosp-ac. Pod. Poth. *Ran-b. Ran-sc.* Senna. Sil. Tart.
— gushing, with flatulence, Croton. Grat. Gum-gut. Jatr. Lac-can. Ntr-c. Ntr-s. Pod. Rhod. Sulph. Tabac. Thuj.
— insufficient, Alum. *Arn.* Bar-c. Carb-veg. *Cham.* Colch. Euphr. Graph. Gum-gut. Hyosc. *Lach.* Lact. *Mgn-m. Ntr-c.* Nux. Par. Petr. Sabad. Scill. Sep. Staph. *Sulph.* Zinc.
— interrupted, *Ambr.* Ang-spur. Calc. Con. Kali-c. Ntr-m. Nitr-ac. Ol-an. Phosp. Ruta. Sabad. Sulph. Verb.
— — every other day, Ambr. Calc. Con. Kali-c. Ntr-m. Sulph.
— — for two or three days, Sulph.
— involuntary, Acon. Apis. Arg. Arn.

Ars. *Bell.* Bry. Calc. Camph. Carb-veg. *Chin.* Cina. Colch. Con. Cop. Cub. Dig. Grat. *Hyosc.* Kali-c. Lach. *Laur.* Merc. Mosch. Mur-ac. *Ntr-m.* Oleand. Op. Ox-ac. Phosp. *Phosp-ac.* Puls. Rhus. *Sec-c. Sulph.* Sulph-ac. Tart. Verat. Vipr-toro.

Stool involuntary during a meal, Ferr.
— — at night, Arn. Bry. Con. Hyosc. Mosch. Puls. Rhus.
— — during sleep, Arn. Bry. Con. Hyosc. Mosch. Puls. Rhus. Sulph. Verat.
— — when urinating, Aloe. Mur-ac. Scill. Sulph. Verat.
— — when passing wind, Acon. Aloe. Caust. Ferr-m. Jatr Kali-c Mur-ac. Ntr-m. Oleand. Phosp-ac. Pod. Staph. Sulph. Verat.
— quick, Ant. Bar-c. Cast. Croton. Cupr. Grat. Gum-gut. Iod. Jatr. Kali-c. Mgn-m. Merc-sulph. Mez. Ntr-c. Nicc. Tabac. Thuj. Verat. Viol-tr.
— scanty, Alum. Arg. Bell. Berb. Bry. *Calad.* Calc. Carb-veg. Chin. Cinnab. Colch. Daph. Eugen. *Grat.* Hep. Hyosc. Kali-b. Kali-jod. Kalm. Kobalt. Mgn-c. Mgn-m. *Merc.* *Merc-cor.* Merc-jod. Ntr-c. Ntr-m. Plat. Ruta. Sabad. Sass. *Seneg.* Sep. Stann. Staph. *Tereb.* Therid.
— seldom, Lact. Mang.
— but soft, Meph.
— slow, Lach. Rhus.
— small, Acon. Aloe. Arg. Arn. Ars. Asar. Bell. Canth. Caps. Caust. Cham. Colch. Coloc. Corn-c. Dulc. Eugen. Lach. Lyc. Merc. Merc-cor. Mez. Nux. Oleand. Phosp. Ruta. Sang. Sep. Sulph. Thromb.
— tardy, *Amni-c.* Asa-f. *Colch.* Hyosc. *Mgn-m.* Ntr-nitr. Nicc. *Nux-m.* Phosp. Ran-b. Ran-sc. *Rhod.* Sass. *Seneg.* Sep. *Sil.* Spong. *Stront.* Sulph-ac.
— unobserved, Aloe. Ars. Colch. Ferr-m. Grat. Phosp-ac. Staph. Verat.
— ash-colored, Asar. Dig.
— black, *Ars.* Brom. *Bry.* Cact. Camph. Caps. *Chin.* Cub. Elaps. Hep. Hipp-m. Ip. Kali-b. *Lept.* Merc. Nux. Op. Phosp. Scill. *Sulph-ac.* Tabac. Tart. Tellur. *Verat.*
— brown, Ambr. Arn. Ars. Asa-f. Camph. Canth. Casc. Chelid. Creos. Croton. Dulc. Fluor-ac. Graph. Gum-gut. Kali-b. Mgn-c. Mgn-m. Merc-cor. Mez. Psor. Rheum. Rumex. Sabad. Scill. Sulph. Tarant. Tereb. Verat.
— changeable, Colch. Puls. Sulph.
— clay-colored, Calc. Hep. Kali-b. Petr.
— dark, *Agar.* Iod.
— gray, Aloe. Asar. Aur. Cist. Dig. Kali-c. Merc. Phosp. Phosp-ac. Rheum.
— greasy, shining, Caust. Thuj.

18. STOOL AND ANUS.

Stool greenish, *Aeth*. Aloe. Amm-m. Arg-n. *Ars*. Bar-m. Bell. Borax. Canth. Carb-an. Cham. Chin. Coloc. Croton. Dulc. Elat. Grat. Gum-gut. Hep. Ip. Iris. Laur. Lob. Mgn-m. Merc. Merc-cor. Nux. Paullina. *Phosp*. Phosp-ac. Pod. *Puls*. Raph.! Rheum. *Sep*. Stann. *Sulph. Sulph-ac*. Tabac. Tereb. Valer. Verat.
— — scum, Mgn-c.
— — like flakes of spinach, Arg-n.
— — scraped eggs, Nux-m.
— light colored, Benz-ac. Carb-veg. Caust.
— liver, brown, Anac. Mgn-c.
— pale, Carb-veg. Lyc.
— red, Rhus. Sil.
— of sepia, Mosch.
— tea-colored, Gels.
— white, *Acon*. Ars. Asar. Aur. Bell. Benz-ac. Bufo. Calc. Cast. Caust. Cham. Chelid. Chin. Cimex. Cina. Colch. Cop. *Dig*. Dulc. Hell. *Hep. Igt*. Iod. Lach. Lob. Merc. Ntr-s. Nux. Pallad. Petr. Phosp-ac. Pod. *Puls. Rhus*. Spig. Spong. *Sulph*.
— — like chyle or milk, Arn. *B. ll.* Bufo. Dig. Dulc. Hell. Merc. Nux. Pod. Rheum. Stront.
— — clay, in chronic diarrhœa, Petr.
— white, flocky, Ip. Scill.
— — grains or particles, Cub. Phosp.
— — masses, like tallow, Mgn-c.
— — streaked, Rhus.
— yellow, Aeth. Aloe. Ambr. *Ars*. Asa-f. Borax. Brom. Calc. Cham. Chelid. Chin. Cist. Cocc. Coloc. Croton. Elaps. Fluor-ac. Gels. Gum-gut. Hyosc. *Igt*. Ip. Iris. Mgn-m. Mang. Merc. Merc-cor. Merc-sulph. Ntr-s. Nicc. Oleand. Petr. Phosp. Plb. Pod. Puls. Raph Sabad. Stront. Tabac. Tart. Tereb.
— — streaked, Rhus.
— — gray, Cist.
— — green, Apis. Croton. Grat.
— — granular, Mang.
— — watery, Apis. Ars. Borax. Canth. Chin. Croton. Dulc. Grat. Gum-gut. Hyosc. Merc-sulph. Stront. Thuj.
— — and copious during day, scanty, hard and black at night, Merc-jod.
— acrid, excoriating, Ant. *Ars*. Canth. Cham. *Chin*. Coloc. Dulc. Ferr. Graph. Gum-gut. Igt. Iris. Kali-c. Lach. *Merc*. Nux. Phosp. *Puls*. Sass. Staph *Sulph*. Verat.
— bilious, *Aeth*. Aloe. Ars. Cact. *Cham*. Chin. Cina. Coloc. Corn-c. Croton. Cub. Diosc. Dulc. Elaps. Ip. Lept. Merc. *Merc-cor*. Oleand. Phyt. Pod. *Puls*. Sacch. Sulph. Verat.
— — in albuminuria, Tereb.
— bloody, Acon. Aeth. Aloe. Alum. Apis. Arg-n. Arn. Ars. Asar. Bapt. Benz-ac. Bry. Cact. Calc. *Canth*. Caps. Carb-veg.

Caust. Chin. Cinnab. Colch. Coloc. Cop. Creos. Cupr. Daph. Dros. Dulc. Elaps. Ferr. Hipp-m. Hydroph. *Ip*. Iris. Jalap. Kali-b. Kali-c. Lach. Led. Lyc. Mgn-m. *Merc*. Merc-cor. Millef. *Ntr-c*. Ntr-m. Ntr-s. *Nitr-ac*. Nitr. Nux-m. Nux. Ox-ac. *Phosp*. Plb. *Puls*. Raph. *Rat. Rhus*. Sabin. Sass. Sep. Sil. *Sulph. Tart*. Tereb. Valer. Verat. Vipr-toro.
Stool, bloody, painless, Apis.
— — dark, stringy, Croc.
— blood-streaked, Cina. Led. Mgn-m. Ntr-s. Nux. Scill. Thuj.
— burning, Ars. Lach. Merc.
— as if burnt, Bry.
— chalk-like, Bell. Calc. Dig. Hep. Lach. Spong.
— clay-like, adhering, Plat.
— clotty, Nux.
— crumbling, Amm-c. Casc. Guaj. Mgn-m. Merc. Ntr-m. Phosp-ac. Ruta.
— curdled, Bar-m. *Cham*. Merc. Nux-m. Puls. Sulph. Sulph-ac. Viol-tr.
— dry, Arg. Arg-n. Creos. *Hep*. Kali-chl. Kobalt. Lact. Mang. Ntr-m. Nitr-ac. Phosp. Pod. Stann. Tereb. Zinc.
— fermented, Calc. Ip. Mez. Rhod. Sabad.
— with filaments like hair, Selen.
— flakey, Cupr. Phosp. Verat.
— flocky (white), Dulc. Ip. Scill.
— frothy, foamy, Arn. Benz-ac. Calc. Chin. Coloc. Croton. Elaps. Elat. Graph. Grat. Iod. Kali-b. Lach. *Mgn-c*. Mgn-m. *Merc*. Ntr-s. Op. Pod. Raph. Rhus. Ruta. Sil. Sulph. Sulph-ac.
— — with bubbles, Scill.
— gelatinous, Colch. Hell. Rhus. Sep.
— globular, Cimex. Hipp-m. Mez. *Plb*. Thuj.
— like glue, Euph.
— like grains of boiled rice in stool, Plb.
— granular, Mang.
— greasy, Caust. Thuj.
— hard, Acon. *Agar*. Alum. Amm-c. Amm-m. Ant. Asa-f. Aur. Bar-c. Bell. Berb. Bov. Bry. Cact. Calc. Cannab. Canth. Carb-an. *Casc*. Caust. Chelid. Cimex. Clem. *Cocc*. Con. Creos. Croton. Cycl. Euph. Euphr. Fluor-ac. Graph. *Grat*. Guaj. *Hep*. Hyper. Igt. Iod. Kali-b. Kali-c. Kali-chl. Kali-jod. Kobalt. Lach. Lact. Lam. *Laur*. Lyc. Mgn-c. *Mgn-m*. Meny. Ntr-c. Ntr-s. Nicc. *Nitr. Nux*. Ol-an. Op. Pallad. *Petr*. Phell. Phosp. Phosp-ac. Phyt. Plat. *Plb*. Pod. Prun. Puls. Ran-b. *Rat*. Rumex. Ruta. Sabad. Sabin. Sass. Scill. Selen. *Seneg*. Sep. *Sil*. Stann. Staph. *Stront. Sulph*. Sulph-ac. Tereb. Thuj. Verat. *Verb*. Viol-tr. Zinc.
— — with constipation, Agn. Asa-f. Bry. Calc. *Cocc. Con*. Dulc. Graph. *Kali-c. Lyc*. Mgn-c. Ntr-m. *Nitr-ac. Nux. Sil. Staph. Verat*.

18. STOOL AND ANUS.

Stool, hard, chronic, *Bry. Caust. Cocc. Graph. Lyc.* Ntr-m. *Nux. Sil. Sulph.* Verat. (compare, Constipation.)
— — with hardness of the liver, Graph.
— — — copious hemorrhage from bowels, Ant.
— — long, dry and narrow, Phosp.
— — hard, tough and greasy, Caust.
— — round hard, black balls, Op.
— — like hazel nuts, with dulness in head, Kobalt.
— hard first, then fluid, Aloe. Lact.
— — — diarrhoea, Agar.
— — lumps united by a mucus thread, Graph.
— — — covered with mucus, Caust. Mgn-m. Nux. Plb.
— — and soft alternately, Ars. Borax. Iod. Lach. Mgn-s. Nitr-ac. Phosp.
— — involuntary, Aloe.
— partly hard and partly liquid, Nux.
— hot, Aloe. Cham. Cist. Merc-sulph. Phosp. Pod.
— undigested, Aloe. Ant. *Arn. Ars.* Asar. Bry. Calc. Cham. *Chin.* Coloc. *Con.* Creos. *Ferr.* Graph. Hep. Iris. Lach. Meny. Merc. *Ntr-ac.* Nux-m. *Oleand.* Phosp. Phosp-ac. Plat. Pod. Raph. Rhod. Sang. Scill. Sulph. Sulph-ac.
— — of flood of day previous, Oleand.
— — at night or after meals, Amm-m. Borax. Bry. *Chin.* Coloc. Ferr. Verat.
— knotty, Amm-c. Aur. Bar-c. Berb. Carb-an. Caust. Chelid. Graph. Iod. Kali-b. Lact. Led. *Mgn-m.* Meny. *Merc.* Mez. Ntr-s. Nux. *Op.* Petr. *Plb.* Prun. Ruta. Sep. Sil. Stann. *Stront. Sulph.* Sulph-ac. Thuj. Verb. Viol-od.
— liquid, Aeth. Ang. *Arn. Ars.* Calc. Carb-veg. Chenop. Chin. *Cic.* Clem. Con. Croton. Diad. Gels. Ind. Kobalt. Lach. Mgn-s. Meph. Mur-ac. Ntr-c. Ntr-s. Nitr. *Oleand.* Phell. *Phosp.* Psor. Raph. Rat. Rheum. Sabad. *Sec-c.* Sil. Staph. *Tereb. Verat.*
— — black, Ars. Scill. Stram.
— — brown, Graph. Mgn-c. Nux. Phosp. Psor. Raph. Scill.
— — greenish, Aeth. Croton. Raph.
— — reddish yellow, Lyc.
— — yellow, Aeth. Calc. Croton. Iris. Ntr-s. Nux-m. Raph. Rhus.
— — yellow white, Nitr-ac.
— — with tinea capitis, Psor.
— lubricated, Ferr-m.
— lumpy, Con. Lyc.
— lumps like chalk, Bell. Calc. Dig. Hip. Lact. Spong.
— membranes, false, Canth. Colch.
— mucus, Acon. Agar. Aloe. Amm-m. Ang. Apis. Arn. Ars. *Asar.* Bar-m. Bell.

Borax. Brom. Cact. Canth. *Caps. Carb-veg.* Casc. Cast. Cham. *Chelid. Chin.* Cina. Cocc. *Colch.* Coloc. Corn-c. Dig. *Dulc.* Elaps. Ferr. *Graph.* Grat. Gum-gut. *Hell.* Hyosc. Hyper. Iod. Ip. Iris. Kali-c. Kali-chl. Lach. Laur. Lept. Mgn-c. Mgn-m. *Merc.* Merc-cor. Millef. Nicc. Nitr-ac. Nux-m. *Nux.* Ox-ac. Petr. *Phosp.* Phosp-ac. Phyt. Pod. Prun. *Puls.* Raph. *Rheum.* Rhod. *Rhus.* Ruta. *Scill. Sec-c. Sep.* Spig. Sil. *Stann. Sulph.* Sulph-ac. Tabac. Tart. Thromb. Viol-tr.
Stool, mucus, adhesive, Caps.
— — with blood, Acon. Aeth. Aloe. Ang-spur. Apis. Arg-n. Arn. Bapt. Bell. Canth. Caps. Carb-veg. Cast. Chenop. Colch. Coloc. Creos. Cub. Dros. Elaps. Elat. Graph. Gum-gut. Hep. Hydroph. Igt. Iod. Ip. Iris. Lach. Led. Mgn-m. *Merc. Merc-cor.* Nitr-ac. *Nux.* Ox-ac. *Petr.* Pod. Psor. *Puls.* Raph. Sabad. Sabin. Sacch. Sep. Sil. Staph. Sulph. Sulph-ac.
— — brown, Ars. Grat. Nux. Zing.
— — dark, Arg-n.
— — draws out like a rope, Zanthox.
— — frothy, Iod. Pod. Sil. Sûlph-ac.
— — gelatinous, Aloe. Colch. Cub. Hell. Kali-b. Pod. Rhus. Sep.
— — glazed, Kalm.
— — granular, Bell. Borax.
— — green, Aeth. Amm-m. Apis. Arg-n. Bell. Borax. Canth. Cast. Cham. Cina. Colch. Corn-c. Dulc. Elat. Gum-gut. Ip. Laur. Mgn-c. Merc. Nitr-ac. Nux. Phosp. Phosp-ac. Psor. Sep. Sulph.
— — liquid, Laur.
— — in masses, Aloe.
— — like mush, Kalm.
— — red, Canth. Graph. Rhus. Sulph.
— — stringy, Asar. Sulph-ac.
— — tenacious, Asar. Caps. Croton. Hell.
— — white, Bell. Canth. Caust. Cham. Cina. Cocc. Colch. Dulc. Elat. Graph. Hell. Iod. Ip. Phosp-ac. Pod. Puls. Sulph.
— — yellow, Agar. Apis. Asar. Bell. Borax. Brom. Cham. Chin. Cub. Mgn-c. Nicc. Pod. Puls. Rhus. Sulph-ac.
— pappy, papescent, *Agar.* Aloe. Ant. *Arn.* Asa-f. *Calad.* Chenop. Chin. Cina. Creos. Croton. Cycl. Eugen. *Euph.* Fluor-ac. Kali-b. Kalm. Lach. Lact. Lam. Lob. Mang. Merc. Mez. Ol-an. Paeon. Par. Phosp. *Phosp-ac.* Plat. *Rheum.* Rhod. Selen. Seneg. *Sil. Sulph.* Sulph-ac. Tabac. *Tart.* Teucr. Therid. Valer. Zinc.
— in small pieces, Amm-c. Casc. Guaj. Mgn-m. Merc. Phosp-ac. Ruta.
— pitch like, *Merc.* Mez. Nux.

18. STOOL AND ANUS.

Stool purulent, *Arn.* Ars. Canth. Iod. Lach. Lyc. *Merc. Sil.* Puls. Sulph.
— sandy, Arg.
— with scraping of the intestines, Canth. Colch.
— with sediment like meal, Pod.
— like sheep's dung, Aur-sulph. Berb. Kali-c. *Mgn-m.* Merc. Ntr-m. Nitr-ac. Op. *Plumb.* Ruta. Sep. Verb.
— soft, Acon. Aeth. *Agn.* Aloe. Ambr. Amm-m. *Anac.* Arg. *Bar-c.* Berb. Borax. *Calc.* Carb-vég. Cocc. Coff. *Graph.* Ferr-m. Hipp-m. Hyper. Iod. Iris. Kobalt. Lach. Lact. Lob. Mang. Merc-sulph. Mez. Ntr-c. Ntr-m. *Nitr-ac.* Nitr. *Nux-m.* Ol-an. *Oleand.* Ox-ac. *Phosp.* Phosp-ac. Poth. *Puls. Ran-sc. Rat. Rhod.* Ruta. Sabin. *Sep.* Sulph. Tabac. Tilia. *Viol-tr.* Zinc.
— — twice a day, Cinnab.
— — difficult to pass, Agn.
— — after coffee, Fluor-ac.
— — with disposition to frequent evacutation, (looseness of the bowels), Calc.
— — chronic, *Calc. Graph.* Ntr-m. *Phosp. Sulph-ac.*
— soft first, then hard, Oleand. Sabin.
— soft and hard alternately, Mgn-s.
— — the whole evacuated with one effort, Gum-gut.
— stercoraceous, slimy, Cham. *Dig.* Led. Merc-cor. Nux. *Rheum.* Viol-tr.
— tenacious, Asar. Caust. *Merc. Plat.* Plb. Sass.
— large in size, *Bry.* Graph. Igt. *Kali-c.* Ntr-nitr. Nux. Puls. Sil. Sulph-ac. Thuj. Verat.
— small in size, Borax. Caust. Hyosc. *Merc.* Mur-ac. Phosp. Sep. Staph. Sulph.
— — soft, Graph.
— thin first, then knotty, Euph.
— tough, Mang. Merc-jod. Rumex.
— watery, Acon. Agar. *Ant. Arn.* Ars. Bell. Benz-ac. Berb. Bry. Cact. Calc. Camph. *Cham. Chin.* Cist. Cocc. Colch. Con. Cop. Creos. Croton. Cupr. Cycl. Dig. Diosc. Dulc. Elaps. *Ferr.* Fluor-ac. Grat. Gum-gut. Hell. Hipp-m. *Hyosc.* Iod. Ip. Iris. *Jatr.* Kali-b. Lach. Lept. Mgn-s. Merc. Merc-sulph. Mur-ac. Ntr-c. Ntr-m. Nitr. Nux-m. *Nux.* Oleand. Op. Ox-ac. Phosp. Phosp-ac. Plb. Pod. Puls. Ran-sc. *Rhus.* Sacch. Sang. *Sec-c.* Stront. Sulph. Sulph-ac. Tart. Tereb. Verat.
— — colorless, Apis.
— — dark, Nux.
— — with flakes, Cupr. Phosp. Verat.
— odorless, Hyosc. Rhus.
— smelling, like brown paper burning, Coloc

Stool, smelling like rotten cheese, Bry.
— cadaverous, Ars. Bism. Carb-veg. Creos. Lach. Phosp. Rhus. Sil. Stront.
— — like rotten eggs, Cham. Psor. Sulph-ac.
— — fetid, offensive, Apis. Arn. Arg-n. Ars. Asa-f. Aur. Bell. Benz-ac. Bry. Calc. Calc-ph. *Carb-veg.* Cham. Chin. Cocc. Coff. *Coloc.* Corn-c. Dulc. Eugen. Fluor-ac. Graph. Guaj. Gum-gut. Hipp-m. Iod. Lach. Lept. Lith. Lyc. Merc-cor. Mez. Mur-ac. Nitr-ac. Nux. Oleand. *Op. Par.* Phosp-ac. Plb. Pod. Psor. *Puls.* Ran-sc. Rheum. Rhus. Rumex. Scill. Sec-c. *Sil.* Staph. *Sulph. Sulph-ac.* Tabac. Teucr.
— — mouldy, Coloc.
— — musty, Coloc.
— — like onions, Nux-jug.
— — peculiar, Aloe.
— — putrid, Arn. *Ars* Asa-f. Aur. Benz-ac. Bry. Calc. Carb-veg. Cham. Chin. Cocc. Coloc. Creos. Dulc. Graph. Ip. Lach. Lyc. Merc. Nitr-ac. Nux-m. Nux. Oleand. Par. Plb. Pcd. Puls. Scill. Sec-c. Sep. Sil. Staph. Stram. Sulph. *Sulph-ac.*
— — sour, Arn. Bell. *Calc. Cham.* Coloc. Dulc. *Graph. Hep. Mgn-c.* Merc. Mez. *Ntr-c.* Phosp. *Rheum.* Sep. *Sulph.*
— — sweetish, Mosch.
Constipation, Agar. Aloe. Alum. Ambr. *Amm-c.* Amm-m. Apis. Arg-n. Arn. Ars. Aur. Bar-c. *Bell.* Bov. *Bry.* Cret. *Calc.* Camph. Cannab. Canth. *Carb-veg.* Caust. Cham. Cic. *Cocc.* Colch. Coloc. Con. Cor-r. Creos. Croton. Cupr. Daph. Dulc. Eugen. *Graph.* Grat. Guaj. Gymnoc. Hep. Hyosc. Jac-cor. Kali-b. *Kali-c.* Lach. Lact. *Laur.* Led. *Lyc.* Mgn-m. Mang. Meny. Mosch. Murex. *Ntr-m.* Nicc. Nitr-ac. Nux-m. *Nux.* Ol-an. *Op.* Ox-ac. Phosp. *Phyt. Plat.* Plb. Pcd. Puls. Rhus. *Sabad.* Scill. Selen. Sep. *Sil.* Stann. *Staph.* Stram. *Sulph.* Sulph-ac. Tabac. Tereb. Therid. Thuj. *Verat.* Verb. Viol-od. Zinc.
— chronic, *Bry. Caust.* Chin-sulph. *Graph.* Lach. *Lyc.* Ntr-m. *Nux.* Op. *Plb. Sulph.* Thuj. *Verat.*
— for several days, *Con. Sulph. Thuj.*
— — six days, followed by copious papescent stool, Cor-r.
— every other day, Ambr. Calc. Cocc. Con. Kali-c. Ntr-m. Sulph.
— every three months, Kali-b.
— with diarrhœa, alternately, Ant. Arg-n. Ars. Bry. *Iod.* Lach. Ntr-m. Nux. Rhus. Ruta. Sacch. Tart.
— — in elderly people, Ant. Op.
— painless, Op. Puls. Scill.

18. STOOL AND ANUS.

Constipation from taking cold by riding in a carriage, Igt.
— in nursing infants, Alum. Nux. Op. Sulph. Verat.
— after intermittent fever, suppressed by quinine, Puls.
— from lead-poisoning, *Alum. Op. Plat.*
— after pollutions, Thuj.
— in pregnant women, Alum. Coloc. Lyc. Nux. Sep.
— on a voyage, Plat.
— with bloated, swollen abdomen, Dolich.
— — distended abdomen, Bell. Mgn-m.
— — backache, Lach. Psor.
— — belching, Zing.
— — colic, Plb.
— — discharge of blood from rectum, Psor.
— — coldness of body and hot head, Bufo.
— — — extremities, Kali-b.
— — catarrh, Eupat.
— — debility, Kali-b.
— — want of desire, Alum. Graph. Lyc.
— — incarcerated flatulence, in left side, Aur. Iod. Lyc. Rhod. Sulph.
— — gastric derangement, Iod.
— — headache, Con. Kali-b. Nux. Pod. Verat.
— — heat of head, Bell.
— — — body, Cupr. Verat.
— — leucorrhœa, Pod.
— — induration of liver, *Graph.*
— — nausea and vomiting, Nux.
— — perspiration, Bell.
— — fruitless pressing to stool, Caust. Con. Igt. Merc. Ntr-m. Nux. Rhus. Sabad. Sep. Sulph. Verat.
— in pregnancy, Alum. Coloc.
— with spasmodic retention of faeces, especially in small intestine, Op.
— — painful retraction of anus, Kali-b.
— stool slips back, as if not power enough, Sil.
— with sour taste, Sep.
— — coated tongue, Kali-b.
— — clean patches on tongue, Kali-b. Ntr-m. Tar.
— — urging to stool, Cocc. Con. Op. Sec-c. Viol-od.
— — frequent desire to urinate, Sass.
— — vomiting, Plb.
— — vomiting of faeces, Plb.
Diarrhœa, Acon. Aeth. Agar. Aloe. Alum. Ambr. Amm-c. *Ant.* Apis. Arg-n. *Arn.* Asar. Asa-f Bar-c. Bell. Berb. Borax. Bov. *Bry.* Calad. *Calc.* Calc-ph. Cannab. Canth. Caps. Carb-veg. Cast. *Cham.* Chelid. *Chin.* Cina. Clem. Cocc. Colch. *Coloc.* Con. Cop. Creos. Croton. *Cupr.* Dig. Dulc. Eugen. Ferr. Graph. Hell. *Hep.* Hyosc. *Igt.* Ind. Iod. *Ip.* Jatr. *Kali-c.* Kali-jod. Lach. Lact. *Laur.* Led. Lob. *Mgn-c. Mgn-m.* Meph. *Merc. Merc-cor.* Mur-ac. Ntr-c. Ntr-m. Nicc.

Nitr-ac. Nitr. Nux-m. *Nux.* Op. *Paf.* Pæon. Petr. Phell. *Phosp. Phosp-ac.* Pod. Prun. *Puls.* Ran-sc. Raph. Rat. *Rheum. Rhus.* Ruta. Sabad. Sabin. Sass. Scill. Sec-c. Senna. Seneg. *Sep.* Sil. Spig. Spong. Staph. Stram. Stront. *Sulph.* Sulph-ac. Tabac. *Tart.* Tereb. Tong. Vater. *Verat.* Zinc.
Diarrhœa chronic, Agar. Bar-m. Bruc. Calc. Cinnab. Dulc. Ip. Mgn-c. *Mgn-m.* Ntr-s. Oleand. Petros. *Plb.* Pod. *Rhus.*
— colliquative, Ars. Chin. Ip. Tart. Verat.
— with constipation, alternately, Ant. Bry. *Iod.* Kali-b. Lach. Lact. Nux. Rhus. Ruta. Tart.
— in elderly persons, Ant. Op.
— debilitating, Ars. Bry. Calc. Chin. *Con.* Ferr. Merc. Nux-m. Oleand. Petr. Phosp. Rheum. Sacch. *Sec-c. Sep.* Sulph. Sulph-ac.
— painless, Chin. Clem. Ntr-s.
— not debilitating, Phosp-ac.
— dysenteric, Acon. Aloe. Ars. Bell. Canth. Caps. Carb-veg. Cinnab. *Colch.* Coloc. Creos. Dig. Euph. Gum-gut. *Hep.* Iod. *Ip.* Merc. Merc-cor. Millef. Nitr-ac. Nux. Plb. Rhus. Sang. Staph. *Sulph.* Urt-ur.
— feculent, Cina. Hep. Led. Mosch. Mur-ac. Plb. Prun. Spig.
— alternating with headache, Pod.
— after exciting news, Gels.
— painful, Ars. Bry. Caps. Carb-veg. Cham. Colch. Croton. Dulc. Fluor-ac. Jalap. Kali-chl. Mgn-c. Merc. Nux. Petr. Plumb. Pod. Puls. *Rheum.* Rhus. Sec-c. Sulph. *Verat.*
— painless, Apis. Arg-n. Ars. Bar-m. Bell. Camph. Carb-an. Cham. Chelid. *Chin.* Cinnab. Clem. Colch. Coloc. Croton. Ferr. Hep. *Hyosc.* Kali-c. Lyc. Merc. Ntr-s. Nitr. Nux-m. Nux. Op. Phosp. Phosp-ac. Plat. *Pod.* Rhus. Rumex. Scill. Sil. Stram. *Sulph.* Sulph-ac.
— relieving the pains with the evacuation, Ang-spur.
— vehement, Cist. Croton. Cupr. Grat. Gum-gut. Iod. *Jatr.* Kali-b. Mgn-m. *Mez.* Ntr-c. Nicc. Phosp. Pod. Raph. Rhod. Sep. Sulph. *Tabac.* Thuj. *Verat.*
— in morning, Aeth. All-cep. Aloe. Alum. Amm-m. Ant. Apis. Arg-n. Bov. Bry. Caps. Cist. Cop. Corn-c. Eupat. Fluor-ac. Formica. Hipp. Iod. Kali-b. Lac-can. Lach. Lith. Lyc. Merc. Mur-ac. Ntr-s. Nicc. Nitr. Nitr-ac. Nux-m. Nux. Oleand. Op. Ox-ac. Petr. Phosp. Pod. Rumex. Sabad. Scill. Sulph. Thromb. Thuj. Zing.
— as soon as he rises from bed, Lyc. Nuphar. Sulph.
— in forenoon, Cact. Gum-gut.
— afternoon, Aloe. Bell. Borax. Chin. Dulc. Laur.

18. STOOL AND ANUS.

Diarrhœa in the evening, Aloe. Borax. Bov. Canth. Caust. Colch. Gels. Kali-c. Lach. Merc. Mez. Mur-ac.
— — 4 to 6, Carb-veg.
— — 4 to 8, Lyc.
— — 5 to 6, Dig.
— at night, Aloe. Ant. Arg-n. Ars. Aur. Bov. Brom. Bry. Canth. Caps. Caust. Cham. Chelid. Chin. Cinnab. Cist. Colch. Cub. Dulc. Graph. Grat. Hep. Ip. Iris. Kali-brom. Kali-c. Lach. Lith. Merc. Mosch. Nux-m. Phosp Pod. *Puls.* Rhus. Selen. Sulph. Tabac. Verat.
— at midnight, Hipp-m.
— after midnight, All-cep. Arg-n. Ars. Hipp-m. Lyc.
— — to morning, Ars. Cist.
— in day, not at night, Amm-m. Canth. Cina. Glon. Gum-gut. Hep. Mgn-c. Ntr-s. Nitr. Petr. Scill.
— day and night, Kali-c. Merc-sulph. Sil. Sulph. Tarant.
— periodically, at same hour, Apis. Sabad. Selen. Thuj.
— every three weeks, Mgn-c.
— every year, in early part of summer, Kali-b.
— from acute diseases, Carb-veg. Chin. Psor.
— from anger and chagrin, Acon. Cham.
— mucus, in apyrexia of intermittent fever, Puls.
— in autumn, Bapt. Colch.
— after breakfast, Arg-n. Borax. Thuj.
— — — not, Thromb.
— in children, Aeth. Benz-ac. Calc. Carb-veg. *Cham.* Cina. Hell. *Hep.* Ip. *Jalap.* Mgn-c. Merc. *Nux-m.* Oleand. *Rheum.* Sep. Sil. Sulph. Sulph-ac.
— after cholera, Sec-c.
— — a cold, Acon. Aloe. Ars. Bar-c. Bell. Bry. Caust. Cham. Chin. Coff. Dulc. Elat. Graph. Ip. Kali-c. Merc. Ntr-c. *Nux-m.* Nux. Op. Puls. Sep. Sulph. Verat. Zing.
— in damp weather, Lach. *Rhod.*
— during dentition, Aeth. Arg-n. Ars. Benz-ac. Borax. Calc. Canth. Cham. Chin. *Coff.* Coloc. Dulc. Hell. Ip. Mgn-c. Merc. Nux. Pod. Psor. Rheum. Sep. Sil. Sulph. Sulph-ac.
— after drinking, (compare Sect. 13.)
— from evening air, cold, Colch. Merc.
— — eruption, suppressed, Bry. Hep. Mez. Sulph.
— during exanthanata, Ars. Chin. Scill. Tart.
— from fruits, Ars. Chin. Lach. Puls. Rhod.
— — ice-cream or ice-water, Puls.
— after and when lying on abdomen, relieved, Amm-m. Bov. Dros. Ntr-c. Nux. Puls. Rheum. Rhus. Seneg. Sulph. Verat.

Diarrhœa in lying in women, Ant. Dulc. Hyosc. *Rheum.*
— after measels, Chin. Merc. Puls. Scill.
— from opium, Mur-ac. Nux.
— during pneumonia, Tart.
— in pregnant women, Dulc. Hyosc. Lyc. Nux-m. Petr. Phosp. Sep. Sulph.
— during rheumatism, Kali-b.
— in scrofulous persons, Calc.
— during small-pox, Ars. Chin. Tart.
— in spring, Lach.
— — summer, Acon. Aeth. Bry. Creos. Dulc. Kali-b. Nux-m.
— — typhus fever, Nux-m.
— — warm weather, Lach.
— from impure water, Zing.
— as soon as he hears water run, Hydroph.
— from weaknesss, Asar. Chin. Nux-m. Phosp-ac.
— in young persons of rapid growth, Phosp-ac.
— with abdomen, distention of, Sulph. Verat.
— — pain in, *Agar.* Alum. Amm-c. Amm-m. *Ang. Ant. Asa-f.* Bar-c. Borax. *Bov. Bry.* Cannab. *Canth.* Caps. Cast. *Cham. Coloc.* Con. Cop. Croton. Dig. Euph. Gels. Hell. Hep. Hipp-m. Ind. Iris. *Jalap.* Kali-b. Kali-c. Kali-chl. Kali-jod. Lach. *Merc. Merc-cor.* Mez. Mosch. Ntr-c. Ntr-m. Nicc. *Nux. Ol-an. Petr.* Plb. Prun. Pod. *Puls. Rat.* Rheum. *Rhus.* Sass. Sil. Spig. Staph. Stann. *Stront. Sulph.* Tart. Tereb. Tong. *Verat.*
— — colicky, Cannab. *Cham. Coloc.* Dulc. Ip. Merc.
— — cramping, Ferr.
— anorexia, Nux-m.
— anus, with burning in, Hipp-m.
— —, — smarting at, Kali-c.
— —, — soreness of, Cham. Ferr. Merc. Sass.
— —, anxiety, Ant. Lach. Merc.
— back, with pain in, Ferr. Kali-jod.
— with chilling, Cast. Cop. Dig.
— — coldness, Spig.
— after coryza, Sang.
— with dispnoea, Sulph.
— — eructations, Con. Dulc. Merc.
— — flatulence, discharge of, Arg-n. Asa-f. Ferr-m. Glon. Hipp-m. Kali-chl.
— — faintness Dulc. Nux-m,
— — fainting, Nux-m.
— — headache, Merc.
— — heat, Merc.
— — feeling as of hot water poured from chest to abdomen, Sang.
— limbs, with painfulness of, Amm-m. Rhus.

18. STOOL AND ANUS.

Diarrhœa, with micturition and perspiration, Bell.
— — nausea, Ars. Bell. Bism. Hell. Ip. Lach. Merc. Prun. Rhus.
— — cold perspiration on head, Merc.
— — rumbling in stomach, Pæon.
— sacral region, with pain in, Colch. Kali-jod. Nux. Puls.
— with shuddering, Merc. Puls.
— — — and shivering, Ang. Cast. Cop. Dig. Sulph.
— — shreiking and whining, (in children,) Carb-veg. *Cham. Jalap. Senna.* Sulph.
— — sleepiness, Hipp-m. Nux-m.
— — tenesmus, Ars. Lach. Merc. Nux.
— — thirst, Ars. Dulc. Mgn-s. Pod.
— — trembling, Merc.
— — urine, profuse, Acon.
— — vomiting, Aeth. Ant. Ars. Asar. Bell. Coloc. Cupr. Dulc. Eugen. Jatr. Ip. Lach. Phosp. Rheum. Seneg. Stram. Tart. Verat.
— — weakness, Ars. Bry. Chin. Con. Kali-c. Merc. Phosp. Rheum. Sec-c. Sep. Sulph.
— — yawning, Cast.
Evacuate, desire to, urgent, Ant. Arg. Arn. Ars. *Bar-c.* Berb. Con. Elaps. Ferr-m. Mgn-c. Mgn-m.*Merc.* Merc-cor. Mez. *Ntr-c. Ntr-m.* Ntr-s. Nitr-ac. Nitr. Phosp. Puls. *Rheum.* Rhod. *Rhus.* Sabad. Sass. Sec-c. Staph. Stram.
— — frequent, Aloe. *Arg.* Caust. Chenop. Hyosc. *Igt.* Lachn. Mgn-c. Mgn-m. *Ntr-c.* Ntr-m. Ntr-s. Nux. Plat.Puls. Ran-sc. *Rheum.*Ruta. Sil. Spig.Stann. *Sulph.* Tabac. Tilia.
— — small stools with tenesmus, Acon. Aeth. Ars. Bell. Caps. Gum-gut. Laur. Merc-cor.
— ineffectual, Ambr. *Anac.* Arn. Asa-f. Bell. Bism. Bov. *Carb-an. Caust.* Chenop. Cocc. Colch. Con. Corn-c. Grat. Gymnoc. *Igt.* Kali-c. Lac-can. Lach. Lachn. Laur. Lyc. Mgn-c. Mgn-m. *Merc.* Merc-cor. *Ntr-c. Ntr-m.* Ntr-s. Nicc. Nitr-ac. Nux. Oleand. Plumb. Rat. Rheum. Rhus. *Sep.* Sil. Spig. *Stann.* Staph. *Sulph. Sulph-ac.* Tabac. Tereb. Thuj. Tong. Verat. Viol-od.
— — with vomiting, Sang.
— felt mostly in upper intestines, Igt.
— pressing, Nitr-ac.
— strong, Ferr. Merc-jod.
— — voiding wind only, Ferr. *Mgn-c.* Sang.
— sudden, Aloe. Anac. Ant. *Bar-c.* Carb-an. Ferr-m. Hipp-m. Merc-sulph. Ntr-c. Viol-tr.
— in evening, Bism.
— at night, *Merc.* Puls. Sulph.
— after meals, Aloe. Ferr-m.

Evacuate, desire to, when walking or exercising, Rheum.
— abdomen, with pain in, *Ars. Bar-c.* Meny. Puls. Rhus.
— anus, with pain in, Ars. Caust. Mgn-c. Sulph.
— — followed by painful constriction of, Lyc.
— with anxiety, Ambr. Caust.
— back, with pain in, Rat.
— bladder, with pain in, Sulph.
— efections, with, Thuj.
— eructations, with Ferr-m.
— exertion from, Thuj.
— face, with redness of, Caust.
— flatulency, with discharge of, Carb-an. Lach. Mgn-c. Mgn-m. *Sep.*
— lumbar region, with pain in, *Bar-c. Rat.*
— with nausea, Rhus.
— — prolapsus, recti, Ruta.
— rectum, with itching in, Euph.
— sacral region, with pain in, Rat.
— scrotum, with contraction of, Ferr-m.
— with sweat on back, Kali-b.
Evacuation, before,
— — abdomen pain in, Agar. Aloe. Alum. Amm-c. *Amm-m.* Arg-n. Ars. Bapt. *Bar-c.* Bell. Borax. *Bry.* Cact. Cannab. Canth. Caps. Carb-veg. Cast. Cham. Chenop. Chin. Cinnab. Colch. Coloc. Dig. Dros. Dulc. *Eugen.* Gels. Glon. Graph. Gum-gut. Hell. Hipp-m. Ip. Jatr. Kali-c. Kobalt. Lept. Lyc. Mgn-c. Merc. Mez. Mur-ac. Ntr-s. Nicc. Nitr-ac. Nitr. Ol-an. Ox-ac. Petr. Phosp. Pod. Puls. *Rat.* Rheum. Rumex. Sang. Stann. Staph. Sulph. Tabac. Tart. Thromb. *Thuj. Verat.* Viol-tr.
— — colicky, Alum. Kobalt. Sulph.
— — in traverse colon, Croton.
— — contractive, to chest, with shortness of breath, Ntr-s.
— — cutting, Acon. Aeth. Agar. Ant. Ars. Bar-c. Bry. Caps. Carb-veg. Cast. Chelid. Coloc. Con. Dig. Gels. Grat. Iris. Laur. Mgn-c. Merc. Merc-cor. Ntr-c. Nicc. Nitr-ac. Nux-m. Nux. Petr. Puls. Rhus. Sang. Sep. Sulph. Tart. Thuj. Verat.
— — drawing, Nitr-ac.
— — feeling of distension in, Fluor-ac.
— — fulness in, Phyt.
— — griping in, Bell.
— — heat in, Bell.
— — pain in left side of, Thromb.
— — pinching of, Aeth. Agar. Bell. Canth. Cast. Cina. Chenop. Cinnab. Fluor-ac. Gum-gut. Kali-c. Mgn-c. Merc. Ntr-s. Nicc. Petr. Verat. Zing.
— — tearing in, Dig. Rhus.

18. STOOL AND ANUS.

Evacuations before twisting in, Caust. Ox-ac. Stram,
— — anus, pain in, Carb-an. Carb-veg. Lach. Merc. Nux. Oleand. Phosp. Puls. Rat. Spong.
— — burning in, Aloe. Berb. Fluor-ac. Iris. Oleand. Rat.
— — creeping in, Mez.
— — itching in, Euph.
— — pressing in, Sulph-ac.
— — stinging in, Berb. Spong.
— anxiety, Ant. Ars. Bar-c. Caust. Cham. Croton. Kali-c. Merc. Poth.
— sudden, with dyspnoea and perspiration, relieved, after stool, Poth.
— backache, Nux. Puls.
— chill, Aloe. Ars. Bar-c. Benz-ac. Cast. Dig. Mez.
— — in rectum, Lyc.
— colic, Alum. Ars. Bry. Merc. Petr. Puls. Sulph. Verat.
— — only in daytime, Petr.
— creeping in rectum, Mez.
— discharge of blood, Lob.
— — of black blood, Merc.
— erections, Thuj.
— fainting, Dig.
— flatulency, Aloe. Ars. Cact. Caps. Carb-an. Carb-veg. Cast. Chelid. Chenop. Cocc. Formica. Gels. Grat. Iris. Kali-c. Kobalt. Lac-can. Lach. Lept. Mgn-s. Merc. Mez. Mur-ac. Ntr-s. Oleand. Phosp-ac. Puls. Rat. Sec-c. Spong. Sulph. Thuj. Tilia.
— — hot, Cocc.
— fulness and weight, in pelvis, Aloe.
— gaping, Cast.
— groins, pain in, Ntr-s.
— — pressing, in, Cast. Thromb.
— headache, Ox-ac.
— heat, Croton. Mgn-c. Merc. Phosp.
— intestines, burning in, Aloe.
— — gurgling, Pod.
— — pricking in, Aloe.
— — sore pain in, Thromb.
— mucus, white, Kali-c.
— muscles, involuntary jerking of,
— naval, pain about, Aloe. Amm-m. Caps. Fluor-ac. Grat. Nux. Ox-ac.
— nausea, Acon. Bry. Calc. Chelid. Dulc. Grat. Hell. Ip. Merc. Rhus. Rumex. Sep. Tart.
— perspiration, Acon. Bell. Dulc. Merc. Thromb.
— ptyalism, Fluor-ac.
— rectum, pain in, Nux.
— restlessness, Ars.
— sacrum, pains in, Berb. Carb-veg. Ntr-c. Nitr.
— sensitiveness, irritability, Borax. Calc.
— shuddering, Bar-c. Cast. Dig. Mez.
— tenesmus, Merc. Merc-cor.

Evacuations before thirst, Ars.
— tremor, Merc.
— urging, Aloe. Amm-m. Apis. Borax. Bov. Canth. Cist. Coloc. Corn-c. Gum-gut. Kali-b. Lept. Merc. Merc-cor. Ntr-c. Nicc. Nitr. Nux. Phosp. Rhus. Rheum. Sang. Sulph.
— — sudden, Bar-c. Cist. Hipp-m. Kali-c. Phosp. Pod. Sulph.
— vomiting, Ars. Ip. Ox-ac. Tart.
Between the stools, chilliness, Merc.
Evacuation, during,
— abdomen, pain in, Aeth. Agar. Aloe. Ang. Ars. Borax. Bov. Bry. Cannab. Carb-veg. Cham. Con. Cop. Croton. Cub. Cupr. Diad. Dros. Dulc. Eugen. Euph. Gum-gut. Hell. Ind. Lach. Mgn-c. Merc. Merc-cor. Mllef. Nitr. Nux. Ol-an. Ox-ac. Rheum. Sass. Selen. Sep. Sulph. Tereb. Verat. Zinc.
— — colic, in, Aloe. Alum. Apis. Arg-n. Canth. Caps. Cham. Coloc. Cop. Corn-c. Croton. Dulc. Gels. Hipp. Ind. Ip. Iris. Kali-c. Kobalt. Lyc. Mgn-c. Merc. Mez. Mur-ac. Ntr-m. Nitr. Nitr-ac. Ox-ac. Petr. Plb. Rheum. Rhus. Sil. Tabac. Tart.
— — cutting in, Acon. Agar. Aloe. Ars. Caps. Cham. Chelid. Coloc. Iris. Merc. Merc-cor. Nitr. Rhus. Sec-c. Staph.
— — distention of, Carb-an. Lyc.
— — fermentation in, Agar.
— — gnawing pains in, Kali-b.
— — griping in, Apis. Thromb.
— — left side, pain, in, Thromb.
— — pinching in, Agar. Canth. Merc. Verat.
— — retraction of, Agar.
— — rumbling in, Chelid. Corn-c. Iris. Elaps. Kali-b.
— — soreness, in, Euph.
— — tearing, Aloe. Cop.
— — twisting in, Bov. Elaps.
— anus, congestion of blood to, Puls.
— — contracted, Staph. Thuj.
— — constricted, Igt. Lach.
— — pain in, Mur-ac. Ox-ac. Sass. Stront.
— — — biting, Dulc. Lyc.
— — — burning, Aloe. Ang. Ars. Bar-c. Berb. Bov. Bry. Canth. Caps. Carb-veg. Cast. Chenop. Clem. Cocc. Colch. Croton. Euph. Ferr. Hipp-m. Iris. Kali-b. Lach. Lact. Laur. Lyc. Merc-sulph. Mur-ac. Ntr-c. Ntr-m. Nicc. Op. Puls. Staph. Stront. Sulph. Tereb. Verat.
— — — constringing, Mang. Staph.
— — — cutting, Caust. Laur. Ntr-c. Staph.
— — — grasping, Phell.

18. STOOL AND ANUS.

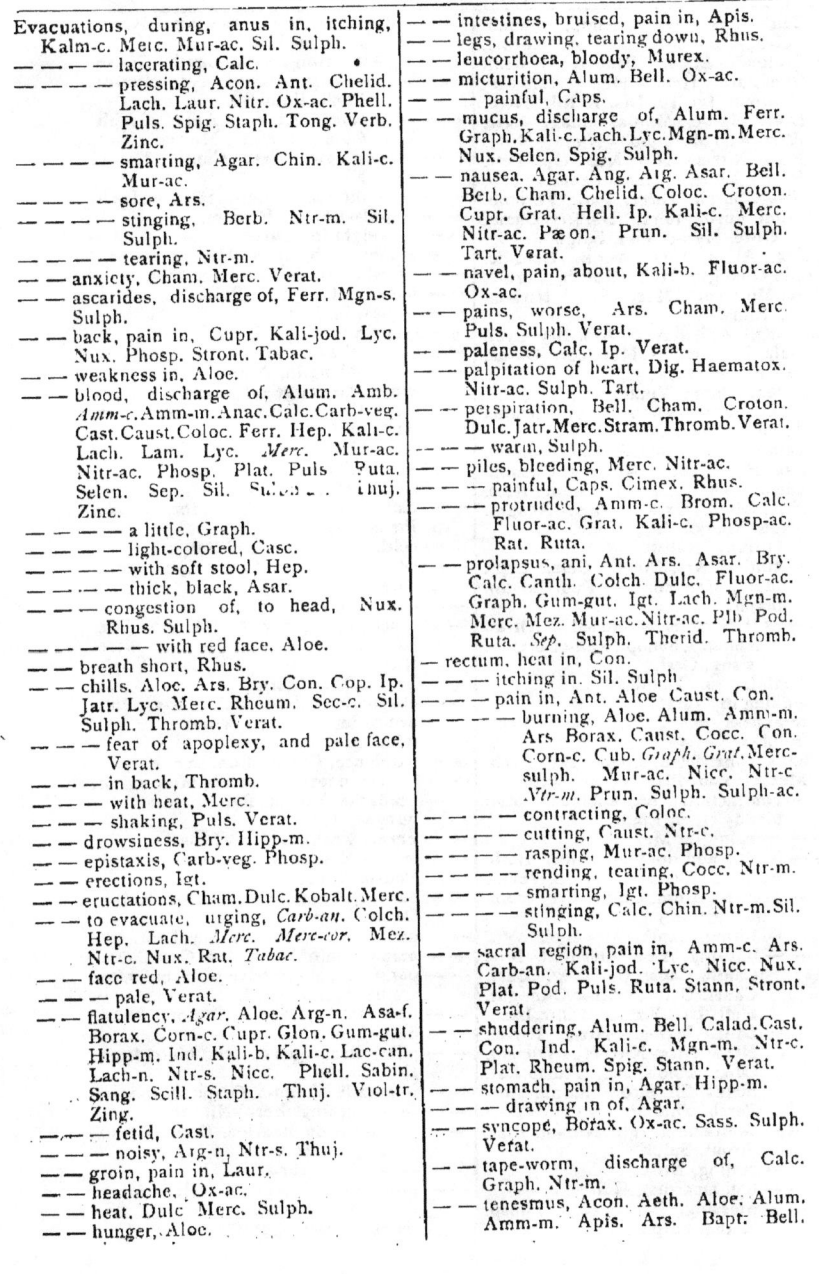

Evacuations, during, anus in, itching, Kalm-c. Merc. Mur-ac. Sil. Sulph.
— — — — lacerating, Calc.
— — — — pressing, Acon. Ant. Chelid. Lach. Laur. Nitr. Ox-ac. Phell. Puls. Spig. Staph. Tong. Verb. Zinc.
— — — — smarting, Agar. Chin. Kali-c. Mur-ac.
— — — — sore, Ars.
— — — — stinging, Berb. Ntr-m. Sil. Sulph.
— — — — tearing, Ntr-m.
— — anxiety, Cham. Merc. Verat.
— — ascarides, discharge of, Ferr. Mgn-s. Sulph.
— — back, pain in, Cupr. Kali-jod. Lyc. Nux. Phosp. Stront. Tabac.
— — weakness in, Aloe.
— — blood, discharge of, Alum. Amb. Amm-c. Amm-m. Anac. Calc. Carb-veg. Cast. Caust. Coloc. Ferr. Hep. Kali-c. Lach. Lam. Lyc. *Merc.* Mur-ac. Nitr-ac. Phosp. Plat. Puls Puta. Selen. Sep. Sil. Su... ... Thuj. Zinc.
— — — — a little, Graph.
— — — — light-colored, Casc.
— — — — with soft stool, Hep.
— — — — thick, black, Asar.
— — — — congestion of, to head, Nux. Rhus. Sulph.
— — — — with red face, Aloe.
— — breath short, Rhus.
— — chills, Aloe. Ars. Bry. Con. Cop. Ip. Jatr. Lyc. Merc. Rheum. Sec-c. Sil. Sulph. Thromb. Verat.
— — — — fear of apoplexy, and pale face, Verat.
— — — — in back, Thromb.
— — — — with heat, Merc.
— — — — shaking, Puls. Verat.
— — drowsiness, Bry. Hipp-m.
— — epistaxis, Carb-veg. Phosp.
— — erections, Igt.
— — eructations, Cham. Dulc. Kobalt. Merc.
— — to evacuate, urging, *Carb-an.* Colch. Hep. Lach. *Merc.* Merc-cor. Mez. Ntr-c. Nux. Rat. *Tabac.*
— — face red, Aloe.
— — — pale, Verat.
— — flatulency, *Agar.* Aloe. Arg-n. Asa-f. Borax. Corn-c. Cupr. Glon. Gum-gut. Hipp-m. Ind. Kali-b. Kali-c. Lac-can. Lach-n. Ntr-s. Nicc. Phell. Sabin. Sang. Scill. Staph. Thuj. Viol-tr. Zing.
— — — fetid, Cast.
— — — noisy, Arg-n. Ntr-s. Thuj.
— — groin, pain in, Laur.
— — headache, Ox-ac.
— — heat, Dulc. Merc. Sulph.
— — hunger, Aloe.

— — intestines, bruised, pain in, Apis.
— — legs, drawing, tearing down, Rhus.
— — leucorrhoea, bloody, Murex.
— — micturition, Alum. Bell. Ox-ac.
— — painful, Caps.
— — mucus, discharge of, Alum. Ferr. Graph. Kali-c. Lach. Lyc. Mgn-m. Merc. Nux. Selen. Spig. Sulph.
— — nausea. Agar. Ang. Arg. Asar. Bell. Berb. Cham. Chelid. Coloc. Croton. Cupr. Grat. Hell. Ip. Kali-c. Merc. Nitr-ac. Pæon. Prun. Sil. Sulph. Tart. Verat.
— — navel, pain, about, Kali-b. Fluor-ac. Ox-ac.
— — pains, worse, Ars. Cham. Merc. Puls. Sulph. Verat.
— — paleness, Calc. Ip. Verat.
— — palpitation of heart, Dig. Haematox. Nitr-ac. Sulph. Tart.
— — perspiration, Bell. Cham. Croton. Dulc. Jatr. Merc. Stram. Thromb. Verat.
— — — warm, Sulph.
— — piles, bleeding, Merc. Nitr-ac.
— — — painful, Caps. Cimex. Rhus.
— — — protruded, Amm-c. Brom. Calc. Fluor-ac. Grat. Kali-c. Phosp-ac. Rat. Ruta.
— — prolapsus, ani, Ant. Ars. Asar. Bry. Calc. Canth. Colch. Dulc. Fluor-ac. Graph. Gum-gut. Igt. Lach. Mgn-m. Merc. Mez. Mur-ac. Nitr-ac. Plb. Pod. Ruta. *Sep.* Sulph. Therid. Thromb.
— rectum, heat in, Con.
— — — itching in, Sil. Sulph.
— — — pain in, Ant. Aloe Caust. Con.
— — — burning, Aloe. Alum. Amm-m. Ars. Borax. Caust. Cocc. Con. Corn-c. Cub. *Graph. Grat.* Merc-sulph. Mur-ac. Nicc. Ntr-c. Ntr-m. Prun. Sulph. Sulph-ac.
— — — contracting, Coloc.
— — — cutting, Caust. Ntr-c.
— — — rasping, Mur-ac. Phosp.
— — — rending, tearing, Cocc. Ntr-m.
— — — smarting, Igt. Phosp.
— — — stinging, Calc. Chin. Ntr-m. Sil. Sulph.
— — sacral region, pain in, Amm-c. Ars. Carb-an. Kali-jod. Lyc. Nicc. Nux. Plat. Pod. Puls. Ruta. Stann. Stront. Verat.
— — shuddering, Alum. Bell. Calad. Cast. Con. Ind. Kali-c. Mgn-m. Ntr-c. Plat. Rheum. Spig. Stann. Verat.
— — stomach, pain in, Agar. Hipp-m.
— — — drawing in of, Agar.
— — syncope, Borax. Ox-ac. Sass. Sulph. Verat.
— — tape-worm, discharge of, Calc. Graph. Ntr-m.
— — tenesmus, Acon. Aeth. Aloe. Alum. Amm-m. Apis. Ars. Bapt. Bell.

18. STOOL AND ANUS.

Calc. Caps. *Caust.* Chenop. Cinnab. Colch. Coloc. Con. Cop. Corn-c. Croton. *Euph.* Fluor-ac. Grat. Gum-gut. Hell. Hep. Hipp-m. Hydroph. Igt. Ip. Iris. Kali-b. Lach. Laur. Mgn-c. Mgn-s. Mang. *Merc.* Merc-cor. Merc-jod. Nicc. Ntr-c. Ntr-s. Nitr-ac. Nitr. Nux. Op. Petr. Phyt. Rhus. Selen. Senna. Sep. *Spong.* Sulph. *Tabac.* Tart. Thromb.
Evacuation, during thirst, Ars. Bry. Cham. Chin. Dulc. Mgn-c. Pod. Sulph.
— urging, Alum. Apis. Arg-n. Benz-ac. Canth. Gum-gut. Hell. Kali-b. Mgn-c. Merc. Merc-cor. Mez. Nicc. Nux-m. Ox-ac. Rhus.
— vomiting, Apis. Arg. Ars. Bry. Cycl. Dulc. Hipp-m. Ip. Merc-cor. Ox-ac. Plb. Seneg. Verat.
— weakness, Borax. Verat.
Evacuation after abdomen, empty feeling in, Sulph-ac. Verat.
— — pain in, Agar. Ambr. Amm-c. Amm-m. Arg. Bov. Canth. Carb-veg. Chenop. Cimex. Diosc. Dros. Glon. Nicc. Nux. Ol-an. Ox-ac. Puls. Rheum. Staph. Tongo. Verat. Zinc.
— — burning, Kali-b.
— — cutting, Ars. Coloc. Gels. Lept. Merc. Merc-cor. Nitr. Pod. Rheum. Staph.
— — as if diarrhœa would set in, Ntr-m.
— — pinching, Chenop. Kali-c. Merc.
— — pressing, Grat.
— — rumbling in, Chelid.
— — sinking in, Verat.
— — weakness of, Chin. Diosc. Lept. Sulph-ac.
— — anus, constricted, Elaps. Igt. Lach. Mez. Nux-m. Plat. Stront. Sulph.
— — — contraction of sphincter after bloody stool, Elaps.
— — — creeping in, Mez.
— — — itching and tingling, Aloe. Berb. Euph. Kali-c. Nicc. Tereb. Teucr.
— — — pain in, Alum. Coloc. Lyc. (compare Rectum.)
— — — — biting, Canth.
— — — — burning, Aloe. Ars. Berb. Bov. Canth. Caps. Carb-veg. Cast. Caust. Coloc. Corn-c. Gum-gut. Hell. Iris. Kali-b. Kali-c. Lach. Laur. Mgn-c. Ntr-c. Ntr-m. Ntr-s. Nicc. Nitr. Nux. Oleand. Ol-an. Pæon. Petr. Phosp. Rat. Senna. Sil. Stront. Sulph. Tart. Tereb. Thromb.
— — — — contracting, Igt. Nux-m. Plat. Stront. Sulph.
— — — — cutting, Ntr-c.
— — — — hot, smarting, Hell.
— — — — pressing, Berb. *Lach.* Phosp. Senna. Sulph-ac.

Evacuation, after, anus, pricking, Iris.
— — — rending, Kali-c.
— — — smarting, Agar. Canth. Graph. Gum-gut. Hep. *Igt.* Nux-m. Phell. Puls. Sil.
— — — sore, Alum. Apis. Graph. Gum-gut. Merc. Mur-ac. Nux.
— — — stinging, Berb. Canth. Kali-c. Nicc. Nitr.
— — — throbbing, Berb. Hipp-m. Lach.
— — pulsation in, Hipp-m.
— — weight in, Aloe.
— — anxiety with, Caust. Nitr-ac.
— — aversion to open cold air, Mez.
— — back, chilliness in, Puls.
— — heat in, Pod.
— — pain in, Caps. Dros.
— — — relieved, Ox-ac.
— — throbbing in, Alum.
— — blood, discharge of, Alum. Amm-c. Apis. Canth. Caps. Casc. Lyc. Merc. *Sabin.* Scill. Sep.
— — — black, Lob.
— — — thin, red, Calad.
— — calves, tension in, Ox-ac.
— — chills, Canth. Grat. Mez. Ox-ac. Pæon. Plat.
— — cold, surface and feet, Sulph.
— — desire continues, Lach. Lyc. (compare Urgency to.)
— — — drowsiness, Bry.
— — evacuate, urgency, Aeth. Croton. Dig. Lach. Lyc. Merc-cor. Ntr-nitr. Nicc. Nitr-ac. Nux-m. Rheum. Staph. Tabac. Tar. Therid.
— — exhaustion, Merc-sulph. Nitr-ac. Pod. Sec-c. Sep. Thromb. Verat.
— — fainting, Croton.
— — flatulence, Cimex. Con. Lyc. Ntr-s.
— — fulness in feet, feel numb, Merc-sulph.
— — headache, Kobalt. Rat.
— — hunger, Petr.
— — knees, weakness in, Thromb.
— — mucus, discharge of, Asar. Calad. Phosp. Selen.
— — nausea, Acon. Caust. Croton. Kali-b. Ox-ac. Zing.
— — navel, pain about, Croton. Lept.
— — palpitation of heart, Ars. Con. Caust.
— — perineum, contractive pain in, after scanty, hard stool, Lyc.
— — perspiration, Acon. Croton. Merc. Sulph.
— — piles, discharges of fetid blood from, Hipp-m.
— — — pain in, Amm-c. Graph. Nitr-ac.
— — — — burning, Berb. Nitr-ac.
— — — protrusion of, Aloe. Brom. Diosc. Graph. Rat.
— — — blue, Mur-ac.
— — prolapsus ani, Ars. *Igt.* Hipp. Merc. Pod. Sep. Thromb.
— — rectum closes tight, Cimex.

18. STOOL AND ANUS.

Evacuation, after rectum creeping in, Mez. Teucr.
— — — pain in, Asar. Grat. Kali-c. Ntr-c. Ntr-m. Nux. Petr. Phosp. Puls. Seneg.
— — — aching, with fulness, Gymnoc. Lyc.
— — — burning, Amm-m. Ars. Bry. Corn-c. Grat. Kali-c. Ntr-m. Ntr-s. Petr. Phosp. Tereb.
— — — cutting, Ntr-c.
— — — pressing. Caust. Kalm. Nux. Phosp. Seneg.
— — — stitches, Cham.
— — — tearing, stinging, Kali-c.
— — — tingling, Chin.
— — — pressure, straining. and discharge of viscid white mucus, Asar.
— — — prolapsus of, Croton. Iris. Mez.
— — — soreness of, with ichor, Hep.
— — relaxation, Calc. Nitr-ac. Phosp.
— — relief of colic, tenesmus and urging, Acon. Alum. Ars. Canth. Cham. Colch. Coloc. Corn-c. Gum-gut. Nux. Rhus. Tart.
Evacuation, after, relief of head-symptoms, Corn-c.
— — sacral region, pain in, Tabac.
— — sensitiveness, Nitr-ac.
— — shuddering, Canth. Mez. Plat.
— — soreness, general, Calc.
— — tenesmus, Amm-m. Apis. Asar. Bapt. Bell. Bov. Canth. Caps. Cocc. Colch. Cub. Hipp-m. Hydroph. Ip. Kali-b. Kobalt. Lach. Mgn-c. *Merc.* Nicc. Nitr. Phell. Phosp. Phosp-ac. Rheum. Rhus. Senna. Staph. Sulph. *Tabac.* Tart. Thromb.
— — — to perineum and urethra, Mez.
— — thirst, Caps. Dulc. Ox-ac. Thromb.
— — trembling, Con.
— — vertigo, Petr.
— — vomiting, Eugen. Kali-b. Merc-cor.
— — weakness, Ars. Bov. Calc. Carb-veg. Chin. Coloc. Con. Ip. Lach. Mez. Nitr-ac. Petr. Pod. Sep. Thromb. Thuj. Verat.

19. Urine and Urinary Organs.

Agglutination of orifice of urethra by mucus, Petros.
As if a ball were rolling in bladder, Lach.
Biting in urethra, Prun. Teucr. Thuj.
Blood, discharge of from urethra, Amm-c. Ant. Arg-n. Arn. Ars. Cact. Calc. Camph. Cannab. *Canth Caps.* Caust. Chin. Con. *Euph.* Hep. Ip. *Lyc.* Merc. Mez. Millef. Murex. Nux. Phosp. Plb. Puls. *Sec-c.* Scill. Sep. Sulph. Tart. Tereb. Zinc.
— — with burning, Ambr. Chenop. Chin. Graph. Kali-c. Puls. Seneg.
— — — constipation, Lyc.
— — — dyspnœa, Con.
— — — pains in kidneys and bladder, Ip. Puls.
— — — — stomach and vomiting, Ip.
— — painless, Lyc.
— — with paralysis of legs, Lyc.
— — in urine, from a cut, hæmorrhagic diathesis, Tereb.
Burning in bladder, Acon. Ars. Berb. Canth. Cham. Chelid. Colch. Ind. Lach. Nux. Petr. Prun. Puls. Rheum. Rhus. Sabin. Sep. Staph. Tereb.
— — urethra, All-cep. Ambr. Amm-c. *Ant.* Apis. Arg-n. Ars. Asar. Aspar. Berb. Bov. Bruc. Bry. *Calc.* Cann. Canth. Carb-veg. Caust. Chenop. Chin. Clem. *Colch.* Coloc. Con. Croton. Cupr. Hipp-m. Igt. Ip. *Kali-c.* Kobalt. Lact. Lith. Lyc. Merc. Ntr-c. Nitr-ac. Nitr. Ol-an. Ox-ac. Par. Petr. Phosp-ac. Prun. Puls. Sep. *Staph.* Sulph. Tereb. Thuj.
— — smarting and stinging, as if scalded, Apis.
— — at neck of bladder, Acon. Cham. Nux. Petr. Puls. Staph.
— — — orifice, Ambr. Bry. Cannab. Chenop. Chin. Cochlear. Graph. Kali-c. Lact. Nitr-ac. Seneg. Sep. Sulph. Thuj.
— — when not urinating, Bry.
Calculi in bladder and kidneys, *Sass. Zinc.*
Catarrh of bladder, Dulc.
Constricting, sensation of, in bladder, Alum. Cact. Caps. Cocc. Phosp-ac. Puls. Sass.

Contracting, sensation of, in urethra, Carb-veg. Clem. Cop. Dig.
— in bladder, Berb.
Crawling in urethra, Petros.
Cutting pain in bladder, Berb. Canth. Caps. Kali-c. Lach. Lyc. Mang. Tereb.
— — — urethra, Ang-spur. Berb. Canth. Caps. Chelid. Colch. Con. Dig. Ip. Lach. Lyc. Merc. Sep. Zinc.
Diabetes, Bar-m. Bov. *Carb-veg,* Chin. Creos. Led. Mgn-c. Ntr-m. Phosp. *Phosp-ac.* Sacch. Scill. Tart. Thuj.
— with great pain, Con.
Dilation of orifice of urethra, Cop.
Drawing pain in bladder, Berb. Chenop. Rhod.
— from perineum to urethra, Kali-b.
— in urethra, Colch. *Petros.* Puls. Zinc.
— in fossa navic, Petros.
Dribbling, sensation of, Lact. Thuj.
Drop, sensation remained at upper part of urethra, Kali-b.
— — in fossa navic, All-cep. Thuj.
Dysuria, Arn. Ars. Cannab. Canth. Caps. Colch. Dig. Euph. Mgn-m. Merc. Nux. Plb. Puls. Ran-b. Sass. Sec-c. Sil.
Enuresis, Bar-c. Bry. *Nitr-ac.* Puls. *Rhus.* Spong.
Fulness, sense of, in bladder, Calad.
— — — — without desire to urinate, Calad. Pallad. Stann. Verat.
— — — after urinating, Calc. Con. Lac-can. Ruta.
Glued up, urethra feels, Bov.
Gonorrhoea, *Agn.* Arg-n. *Cannab. Canth.* Caps. Cinnab. *Cop.* Cub. Led. *Merc. Merc-cor.* Mez. Ntr-s. *Nitr-ac. Petros.* Psor. Puls. Rhod. Sabad. Sabin. Tereb. Thuj.
— with great congestion to parts, Merc-sulph.
— — chorde, Agave-amsric. Canth.
— — penis turned up, Berb. Selen.
— urethra feels as if glued up, Bov.
— with tenesmus and strangury, Tereb.
— first thin then thicker discharge, Merc-cor.
— secundaria, (chronic.) *Agn.* Bar-c. Bar-m. Canth. Caps. Cinnab. Dulc.

19. URINE AND URINARY ORGANS.

Ferr. Gels. Hep. Hydrast. Kobalt. Lyc. Merc. Mur-ac. Ntr-m. Ntr-s. Nitr-ac. Petr. Phosp-ac. Psor. Selen. Sep.Sulph. Tellur. Thuj. Zinc.
Gonorrhoea, chronic with green discharge, Kobalt.
— — — white discharge, Caps. Cinnab. Ferr. Kobalt. Merc. Ntr-m. Nitr-ac. Sep. Sulph. Thuj. Zinc.
— — with impotence, Agn. Calad. Kobalt.
— — — and fetid urine, Calad.
— — suppressed, Berb.Canth.Clem. Daph. Puls. Sass. Tussil.
From gonorrhoea suppressed, affections, testicles of, *Agn.* Aur. Bell. Canth.Clem. Merc. Ntr-c. Ntr-m. Nitr-ac. *Puls.* Rhus. Selen.
— — — — right testicle, Brom. Mez. Ocim. Rhod.
— — — — left testicle, Arg. Clem.
— — rheumatism, Cop. Daph. Sass.
Griping in bladder and urethra, Lyc.
Haematuria, Ambr. *Arn.* Ars. *Calc. Camph. Cannab. Canth.* Chin. Con. Cop. *Hep.* Ip. *Mez. Millef. Nux.* Op. *Phosp.* Plb. *Puls.* Sass. *Scill.* Sulph. *Tart.* Tereb. Thuj. Uva-ursi. Zinc.
Hæmorrhoids of bladder, Ant. Borax. Nux. Puls. Sulph.
Inflammation, of bladder, Apis. *Canth. Dig.*
— — urethra, Arg-n. Bov. Cannab. *Canth. Cop.* Hep. Sabin. Sulph. Tabac.
— — — burning, or shooting pain and increased gonorrhoea, Arg-n. Cannab.
Induration, cartilaginous, bladder, Pareira.
Insensibility in urethra, Mgn-s.
Irritation of urinary passages, Arg-n. Chenop.
Ischuria, Acon. *Arn. Aur. Camph. Canth.* Cic. *Dig.* Dulc. Hyosc. Merc-cor. Nux. Op. *Plb. Puls.* Rhus. Sabin. Stann. Sulph. Verat. (compare Urine, discharge of, suppressed).
— painful, Acon. *Arn. Aur. Canth.* Puls.
— after parturition, Arn. Ars. Bell. Canth. Caust. Hyosc. Lyc. Nux. Puls. Stann.
Itching, in urethra, Alum. Ambr. Anac. Arn. Berb. Bov. Canth. Caust. Cocc-c. Cop. Igt. Ind. Kali-chl. Laur. Lyc. Merc-cor. Mez. Ntr-m. Nux. Ol-an. Sep. Tabac. Thuj. Zinc.
— — with desire to urinate, Coloc.
— — fossa navic. Petros.
Jerking in urethra, Ntr-c. Phosp.
Mucus, discharge of, Agar. Agn. Ant. Calc. Cannab. Canth. Con. Dulc.Elaps. Ferr. Hep. Kali-jod. *Merc.* Mez. Ntr-m. Nitr-ac. Nux. Petr. Rhod. Sabin. Sabin. Sass. Sulph. Thuj.
— albuminous, Petros.
— bloody, Canth. Nitr-ac.
— dark-reddish color, Cub.

— green, Kobalt Merc.
— painless discharge of, Cannab. Psor.
— purulent, Cannab. Canth. Caps. Clem. Cop. Merc. Merc-cor. Nitr-ac. Nux. Sass. Thuj.
— a drop of pus before urinating,Tussilago.
— slimy, Cannab. Caps. Dulc. Hep. Merc. Ntr-m. Nitr ac. Puls. Sulph.
— thick, Cannab. Caps. Clem. Ferr. Merc. Merc-cor. Nux. Puls.
— — milky, Cannab. Caps. Ferr. Nux.
— viscid, Agar. Bov. Dig. Nitr-ac. Nux. Phosp. Tart.
— watery, Cannab. Merc. Merc-cor.
— — copious, Thuj.
— yellow, Agar. Cannab. Cop. *Merc.* Ntr-m. Petros. Thuj.
Narrowness of urethra, sense of, Bry. Dig. Graph.
Numbness of urethra, Mgn-mur.
— sense of, want of power, Thuj.
Paralysis of bladder, Acon. Ars. Bell. Canth. Caust. Cic. Dulc. Hyosc. Lach. Laur. Op.
— — after parturition, no desire, Ars. Caust.
Pinching in urethra and bladder, Lyc.
Polypus of bladder. Calc. Con. Graph. Lyc. Thuj.
Pressing pain or sensation, in bladder, Acon. All-cep. Alum. Amm-c. Arn. Aur. Berb. Canth. Carb-veg. Chenop. Chin. Colch. Con. Creos. Cycl. Dig. Hyosc. Lach. Lact. Ntr-m. Ol-an. Pallad. Puls. Rhus. Ruta. Sass. Scill. Sep Tart. Zinc.
— in urethra, Colch. Petros. Puls. Teucr.
— — relieved by pressing on glands, Canth.
Pulsation in bladder, Canth.
— — penis, Cop.
— — urethra, Canth. Merc.
Purulent, discharge from urethra, Cannab. *Canth.* Caps. Clem. Con. Ip. Nitr-ac, Nux. Sabad. Sabin. Sass.
Redness of orifice of urethra, Gels. *Hep.* Sulph. (compare Inflamation.)
Relaxation of bladder, Mur-ac.
Smarting in urethra, Berb. Borax. Ntr-c. Phosp. Sep. Teucr.
Soreness, sensation of in urethra, Berb. Caps. Clem. Cop. Lach. Mez. Prun. Teucr.
— of bladder when touched, Canth. Puls.
Spasm of bladder, Asa-f. Berb. Canth. Caps. Op. Phosp-ac. Prun. Sass. Sep. Tereb.
— at neck of bladder, tenesmus from, Arn.
Spasmodic pains at bladder, Berb.
— — — at night, Prun.
Stinging in bladder, Berb. Canth. Lyc. Pallad. Sulph. Tart.
— — urethra, Apis. Arg. Arg-n. Berb. Bor. Bruc. Bry. Calc. Cannab. Caps.

19. URINE AND URINARY ORGANS.

Chin. Cocc. Con. Cupr. Hep. Igt. Lach. Lyc. Mang. Merc. Merc-cor. Ntr-m. Nux. Pallad. Par. Petr. Scill. Sep. *Sulph.* Tart. Thuj. Tilia. Viol-tr.
Stone in bladder, Nux-m. Sass. *Zinc.*
Strangury, Apis. Arn. Ars. Camph. *Cannab. Canth.* Caps. Chin. Clem. Cocc-c. Colch. Coloc. Con. Cop. Dig. Dros. Dulc. Elaps. *Euph.* Graph. Hell. Led. Mgn-s. Merc. Merc-cor. Nux-m. Nux. Pareira. Petr. Phosp-ac. Plb. Prun. *Puls.* Ruta. Sabin. Sec-c. Sil. *Staph.* Stram. Sulph. Tart. Zinc.
— from 3 to 6 a. m., Pareira.
— can only urinate by getting on knees and pressing head against floor, Pareira.
Stricture of urethra, Arg-n. Bell. *Clem.* Dulc. *Petr.* Puls.
— sensation of, Bry. Dig. Graph.
Sugar in urine, Chin. Phosp-ac. Thuj. (compare Diabetes.)
Suppuration of bladder and urethra, Canth.
Swelling of interior of urethra, Led. Nitr-ac. Rhus.
— — orifice of urethra, *Cop.*
— in region of neck of bladder, Puls.
Tearing in urethra, Colch. Ntr-c. Ruta. Sulph.
— in bladder, Chenop.
Tenesmus vesicae, Acon. Arn. Calc. Canth. Caps. Colch. Lach. Merc. Mur-ac. Nitr-ac Nux. Ol-an Plb. Prun. Puls. Rhus. Sabad. Sass. Sil. Viol-tr.
— amelioration on walking in afternoon, Lith.
Tension of bladder, Tart.
— — urethra, Phosp.
Thickening of bladder, Dulc.
Tingling of urethra, Petros.
Tumor (small,) in urethra, Lach.
Twitching in urethra, Alum. Cannab. Canth. Kali-chl. Ntr-c. Nux. Phosp.
Ulcers in bladder, Ran-b.
— — urethra, Nitr-ac.
Weakness of bladder, All-cep. Alum. Mgn-m. Mur-ac. Pallad. Rheum.
Worm in bladder, like a, Bell.
Urine, discharge of copious, Acet-ac. Acon. Aeth. *Alum.* Ambr. Amm-c. Ang. Ant. Apis. Arg. *Arg-n.* Aur. *Bar-c.* Bism. Calc-ph. Canth. Carb-an. Carb-veg. Caust. Cham. Chelid. Cina. Cinnab. Coff. Colch. Coloc. Creos. Cycl. Daph. Eupat. *Euphr.* Ferr-m. Glon. Guaj. Hell. Hep. Hydroc-ac. Hyosc. Igt. Iod. Kali jod. Lac-can. Led. *Merc.* Merc-jod. Mosch. *Mur-ac. Ntr-c. Ntr-m.* Ntr-s. Nitr. Ol-an. Ox-ac. *Phosp-ac.* Psor. Raph. Rat. *Rhus.* Ruta. Sabin. Sacch. *Samb.* Sang. *Sass. Scill.* Seneg. *Spig. Sulph.* Tart. *Valer. Verb.* Viol-tr.
— — at midnight, Coff.

— — difficult, Ant. Apis. Arn. Ars. Bell Camph. Cannab. Canth. Clem. Cochlear. Con. *Dig.* Dros. Dulc. Euph. Hep. Mgn-m. Pareira. Petr. Plb. Puls. Ran-b. Sec-c. Staph. Sulph. Tart. Thuj.
— — diminished, Alum. Ambr. Amm-m. Apis. Bell. *Bry.* Carb-veg. Chin-sulph. Clem. *Colch. Coloc.* Dig. Dulc. Graph. Grat. Hæmatox. Hyper. Ind. Ip. Led. Lob. Merc-sulph. Mez. Op. Osm. Par. Phell. Pod. Puls. Rhus. Sacch. Scill. Selen. *Seneg.* Stann. Sraph. Stront. Sulph. *Sulph-ac.* Tereb. Tong. Verat.
— — — with burning, Colch.
— — — although he drinks much, Creos. Rhus.
— — by drops, Agar. Ang. Ant. Arn. Ars. Aur. Bell. Cact. Camph. *Cannab. Canth.* Caps. Caust. Clem. Con. Cop. Dig. Dros. Dulc. *Euph.* Graph. Gum-gut. Ka'i-c. Lyc. Mgn-m. Mgn-s. Merc. Merc-cor. Nux-m. Nux. Pareira. Petr. Phosp-ac. Plb. Prun. *Puls.* Rhus. Sabin. Sec-c. Sil. Spig. Staph. Stram. *Sulph.* Tart. Tereb. Thuj. Zinc.
— drops out perpendicularly, Hep.
— frequent, Actae-r. Agar. Amm-c. Anac. *Ant.* Apis. Arg. Arg-n. Arn. Aur. *Bar-c. Bar-m.* Bell. Benz-ac. Bism. Borax. Bov. Bry. Bufo. *Calc.* Cannab. *Canth.* Carb-an. Casc. *Cast.* Caust. Chelid. Chin. Cic. Cinnab. Clem. Cocc. Cocc-c. Cochlear. Colch. Coloc. Con. Creos. Cupr. Cycl. Daph. Dig. Dros. *Euphr.* Ferr-phosp. Gels. Glon. Graph. Hipp. Hyosc. Igt. Ind. Iod. Jatr. Kali-b. Kali-c. Kalm. Lac-can. Lach. Lact. *Led. Lyc.* Meph. *Merc.* Mur-ac. Nitr-c. Ntr-s. Ntr-ac. Nux. Ox-ac. Pallad. Par. Petr. Phosp. Phosp-ac. Plat. Plb. Psor. Rat. *Rhus.* Ruta. Sang. Sass. Scill. Selen. Sep. Sil. Spig. Staph. *Sulph.* Thuj. *Valer.* Zinc.
— — from acidity in urethra, Chenop.
— — at night, Alum. Ambr. Amm-c. Calc. Carb-veg. Cinnab. Creos. Graph. Lach. Lyc. Merc. Sep. Sulph.
— — towards morning, Amm-m. Mez.
— — too frequent, *Lach. Merc.*
— — incontinent, Bell. Bar-c. Bry. Caust. Cic. Dulc. Led. Lyc. Merc. Ntr-m. *Nitr-ac.* Petr. Pod. *Puls. Rhus.* Ruta. Sep. Sil. Spig. Spong. *Sulph.*
— increased, Agn. *Alum. Ambr. Amm-m.* Arg. Arn. Berb. Canth. Carb-an. Caust. Cinnab. *Clem.* Colch. Creos. Croton. Dig. Ind. Kali-jod. Kobalt. Lact. Lob. *Mgn-c. Mgn-s.* Merc-cor. Merc-sulph. Nicc. Oleand. *Ol-an. Phosp.* Plb. Puls. Rat. Rheum. *Rhod.* Sabad. Sec-c. Seneg.

19. URINE AND URINARY ORGANS.

Spong. Stront. Tabac. Tereb. *Teucr. Tcurid.* Zing.

Urine, discharge of, increased with coryza, A l-cep.
— — at night, Aloe. Ant.
— interrupted, Agar. Caust. *Clem.* Con. Dulc. Gum-gut. Led. Phosp-ac. Puls. Sulph. Thuj. Zinc.
— involuntary, *Acon.* Ant. Apis. Arn. Ars. Bar-m. *Bell.* Bry. Cainca. Calc. Camph. Canth. Carb-an. Carb-veg. *Caust.* Cham. Chin. Cic. Cina. Colch. Con. Creos. Dig. *Dulc.* Ferr. Graph. Hep. Hydroc-ac. *Hyosc.* Igt. Iod. *Laur.* Lyc. Mgn-c. Millef. Mosch. Mur-ac. *Ntr-m.* Nitr-ac. Petr. Phosp. Phosp-ac. Psor. Puls. Rhus. Ruta. Scill Seneg. Sep. Sil. Spig. Spong. Staph. Stram. Sulph. *Verat.Zinc.*
— — in daytime, Fluor-ac.
— — day and night, Caust.
— — when coughing, *Ant.* Caust. Creos. Ntr-m. Phosp. Puls. *Sep.* Staph. Sulph. Thuj. *Verat.* Zinc.
— — dribbling, Arn. Bell. Petr. Puls. Spig.
— — — after micturition and stool, Selen.
— — — when sitting, or standing, urine passing freely, Sass.
— — expelling flatus, Puls. Sulph.
— — at rest, Rhus.
— — running, Arn.
— — sitting, Puls. Rhus.
— — standing, Bell. Caust. Lyc. Ntr-m. Puls. Rhus.
— — with thirst, Acon.
— — when walking, Arn. Bry. Caust. *Mgn-c.* Mgn-m. Ntr-m. Puls. Ruta. Selen. Zinc.
— nocturnal, *Alum. Amm-c. Amm-m.* Arac. Arn. Ars. Bell. Bov. Borax. Bry. Calc. Carb-an. Carb-veg. Casc. Caust. Coff. Con. Creos. *Cupr.* Daph. Dig Dros. Dulc. Glon. Graph. *Hep.* Hyper. *Iod.* Kali-b. Lach. Lact. Lob. Mgn-m. Mgn-s. Merc. Ntr-c. Ntr-m. Nicc. Nitr-ac. Ox-ac. Petr. Phosp. Phosp-ac. Phyt. Pod. Puls. Rat. Rhus. Ruta. Sabin. Sang. *Sass.* Scill. Seneg. Sep. Sil. Spig. *Sulph.* Sulph-ac. Tart. Thuj.
— — conscious, Creos. Plantago-maj.
— — unconscious, Caust.
— involuntary wetting the bed, Acon. *Amm-c.* Arn. Ars. Bar-c. Bell. Bry. Calc. *Carb-veg. Caust.* Chin. *Cina.* Con. Creos. Dulc. Graph. Hep. Hyosc. Igt. Kali-c. Lyc. Mgn-s. Merc. Ntr-c. Ntr-m. Nux. Petr. Pod. *Puls.* Rhus. Ruta. *Seneg. Sep. Sil.* Stram. Staph. *Sulph.* Verat. Zinc.
— — — early morning, Amm-c.
— — — in sleep, Graph.
— — — — the first sleep, Sep.

— — during pregnancy, Pod.
— painful, Ars. Bar-m. Colch. Con. Ind. Nitr-ac. Nux-m. Nux. Ran-b. Stann. Sulph. Uva-ursi. Zinc.
— retarded, Coc-c. Hep. Hydroc-ac. Ip. Op.
— retention, *Acon. Arn. Ars.* Aur. Bell. *Canth.* Caps. Caust. Chin. Cic. Colch. Con. Cupr. Dig. Graph. Hep. Hyosc. Laur. *Lyc.* Nux. Op. Plb. *Puls. Ruta.* Sec-c. *Stram.* Sulph. Verat.
— — in new-born infants, Acon. Benz-ac. Hyosc.
— — painful, Acon. Arn. Aur. Canth. Crotal. Puls.
— — with pressure on bladder, Aur. Hyosc.
— — after typhus, Zing.
— scanty, smell, *Acon.* Agar. Aloe. Amm-c. Anac. Ang. Ant. Apis. Arg-n. Arn. Ars. Arum-trif. Aur. Bell. *Bry. Cannab. Canth.* Caust. Chelid. Chin. Clem. Cocc. Colch. Creos. Cupr. *Dig.* Dros. Dulc. Eupat. Euph. *Graph.* Grat. *Hell.* Hep. Hyosc. Kali-b. Kali-c. Kobalt. Lac-can. Lach. Lam. Laur. Led. Mgn-m. Meny. Merc. Merc-cor. Ntr-c. Nitr. Nitr-ac. Nux. Oleand. Ol-an. Op. Pallad. Petr. Phosp. Phosp-ac. Plb. Prun. Puls. *Rat.* Rhus. *Ruta.* Sabad. *Sabin.* Sacch. Sass. Sil. Spong. *Staph.* Sulph. Tar. *Tart.* Tereb. Verat. Zinc.
— — in daytime, Lyc.
— seldom, Acon. Agar. Aloe. Arn. Ars. Aur. Bell. Bry. Camph. *Canth.* Cupr. Hep. Hyosc. Laur. Nux. Op. Plb. Prun. Puls. Ruta. Sec-c. Stann. Stram. Stront.
— slow, Amm-m. Camph. Chin. Hep. Kali-c. Mur-ac. *Merc-acet.* Plat. Raph.
— stream divided, Cannab. Canth. Rhus.
— — feeble, Cham. Hell. Merc.
— — forcible, Agn.
— — intermittent, *Clem.* Con. Caust. Dulc. Op. Phosp-ac. Puls. Sulph. Thuj. Zinc.
— — thin, Agar. Camph. Canth. Chin. Clem. Graph. Gymnoc. Hell. Hipp. Merc. Ntr-ac. Ol-an. Petr. Prun. Puls. Samb. Sass. Spong. Staph. Sulph. Zinc.
— suppressed, *Acon. Ars. Aur. Bell.* Bism. Calend. Camph. Canth. Cupr. Diad. Dulc. Elaps. Hep. Hyosc. Iod. Lac-can. Laur. Merc-cor. Nux. Op. Osm. Plb. Pod. Puls. *Sec-c. Stram.* Sulph. Tereb. Vipr-r.
— violent, Cic. Cycl. Sulph.
— flow of, *Acon.* Bar-m. Bell. Cannab. Dig. Hyosc. *Merc.* Scill. Stram. *Verat.*
— with diarrhoea, Bell. Puls.
— — and perspiration, Acon.
— — emaciation, Merc.

19. URINE AND URINARY ORGANS.

Urine, flow of, with fatigue, Calc.-ph.
— — headache, Verat.
— — hunger, Bell. Verat.
— — nausea, headache, coryza and constipation, Verat.
— — pain in abdomen, Acon. Verat.
— — — — lo.ns, Phosp-ac.
— — perspiration, Acon. Bell
— — thirst, Bell. Cast. Verat.
Urinate, desire to, urging, *Acon.* Alum. Amm-c. Arn. Bar-c. Berb. *Cannab.* Carb-an. Colch. Coloc. Con. Euph. Hipp-m. *Hyosc. Lyc. Merc. Ntr-c. Ntr-m.* Pareira. Par. Phosp-ac. Sabad. Scill. Sec-c. *Sep.* Staph. Viol-tr.
— anxious, *Acon. Carb-veg.* Cham. *Dig.* Graph. Phosp-ac. Phyt.
— frequent, Acon. Ant. Apis. Arg. Asar. Bar-c. Bell. Benz-ac. *Bov.* Bry. Calc. Caps Carb-veg. *Caust.* Cic. Chin. Cina. Cocc-c. *Cop.* Diad. Dros. Guaj. Gymnoc. *Hell.* Hyosc. *Kali-c. Led. Lyc.* Mgn-m. *Mang.* Meny. *Merc.* Merc-sulph. Murex. *Mur-ac.* Ntr-m. Nitr-ac. Nux-jug. Nux. Ol-an. Petr. *Petros.* Phosp. Prun. Psor. *Puls.* Rat. *Rhus.* Rumex. *Sabad.* Sabin. *Samb.* Sass. Scill. *Sep.* Sil. *Spig. Stann.* Staph. Stram. *Sulph.* Tar. *Tart. Thuj.* Verb.
— — — — in evening, Creos. Lyc. Sabad. Sep. Zinc.
— — — small discharge, Amm-c. Ang. Ant. Camph. Caust. Chelid. Cupr. *Dig.* Dros. Euph. Hell. Hyosc. Kali-c. Kobalt. Lach. Laur. *Led.* Mgn-m. Meny. Merc. Nitr-ac. Nux. Ol-an. Op. Pareira. Petr. Phosp. Phosp-ac. Raph. Rat. Ruta. Sabad. Sabin. Sass. Sil. Spong. *Staph. Tart.*
— the urine only reaches the glans, and causes pains and spasms and tenesmus of rectum, pain in bladder relieved momentarily when urine passes, Prun.
— can only pass urine in a sitting posture, Zinc.
— — — — on standing, Sass.
— urine can be passed only during stool, Aloe. Alum.
— — more abundant during stool, Amm-m. Ox-ac.
— desire, urging, ineffectual, *Acon.* Alum. Arn. Borax. Camph. *Canth.* Caps. Caust. Cham. Chin. Coloc. *Cop. Dig.* Guaj. Hell. Hyosc. Ip. Kali-c. Nux. *Petros.* Phosp. Phosp-ac. Plb. Puls. *Sass.* Sep. Stram. Sulph. Verat.
— painful, Acon. Bov. Cannab. Graph. Hell. Kali-jod. Tart. Verat.
— sudden, Ambr. *Bar-c.* Bry. Igt. *Merc. Nitr-ac.* Phosp-ac. Puls. Rhus. *Ruta.* Spong. Sulph.
— no urging, only a sensation of fulness indicates the necessity for urinating. Calad. Stann. Verat.
— in morning, Ambr. Berb.
— — afternoon, Bell.
— — evening, Amm-c. Bell. *Sabad.*
— — at night, Ars Calc. Creos. Hyper. Lach. Mgn-m. Meph. Nux. Rhus. Sabin. Samb. Spig. Tart. Thuj.
— day and night, Cact. *Carb-veg.* Cast. Kali-c. Kali-jod. Mgn-m. Merc. Ntr-c. *Ntr-m.* Sass.
— in pregnant women, *Puls.*
— with burning in abdomen, **Lach.**
— — heat, Phosp-ac.
— — when lifting a load, Bry.
— with pain in abdomen, Lach. Puls.
— — — back and loins, Lach.
— — — bladder, Hell. Nux. Puls. Rhod. Ruta. Sulph-ac.
— — — groin, Rhod.
— — — perineum, Tart.
— — pale face, Phosp-ac.
— — tearing in urethra, Hyper.
— — thirst, Phosp-ac.
— — vertigo, Hyper.
Before micturition:
— — abdomen, cutting in, Sulph.
— — pain in back, Lyc.
— — bladder, pain in, Lith.
— — — pressing, Ang. Chin. Con. Nux.
— — — — neck of, Nux.
— — —, flushes of pain in, more to right side, Lith.
— — burning, Berb. Calc. Cannab. Chelid. Ntr-c. Rhod. Seneg. Zinc.
— — on rising to urinate, pressing at heart, relieved after urination, Lith.
— — hips, burning in, Dulc.
— — mucus, Calc. Merc.
— — nausea, Dig.
— — a drop of pus, Tussilago.
— — urethra, biting and itching, Cop.
— — — burning, Berb. Bry. Calc. Cannab. Canth. Chelid. Cop. Dig. Merc-cor. Ntr-c. Rhod. Seneg. Zinc.
— — — cutting, Bry. Canth. Dig.
— — — itching, Cop. Nux.
— — weakness, Nux.
During micturition:
— — bladder, burning, Aloe. Nux. Rheum.
— — — cutting, Canth.
— — — discharge of viscid purulent mucus from, Nux.
— — — pain in general, Ind. *Tart.*
— — — pressing, Asar. Berb. Hep Lachn. Verat.
— — — spasm, *Asa-f.*
— — — stinging. Ntr-m.
— — blood, emission of, Crotal. Murex.
— — os coccygis, pain in, Graph.
— — colic, Acon. Verat.
— — genitals, female, pain in, Thuj.
— — — burning, between labia, Creos.

19. URINE AND URINARY ORGANS.　　145

During micturition, genitals, soreness in vagina, Creos.
— — — and smarting in vulvae, Ntr-m.
— — glans, penis, pain in, Acon. Anac Casc. Ox-ac.
— — kidneys, pain in, Berb. Rheum.
— — seminal chord, pain in, Bell. Clem.
— — — drawing in, Bell. Canth. Caps. Clem.
— — stomach, pain in, Laur.
— — stool, involuntary, Mur-ac.
— — thighs, pain in, Berb.
— — urethra, itching in, Lyc.
— — — pain in, Berb. Colch. Diad. Zing.
— — — — biting, Canth. Carb-veg. Clem. Igt. Lyc. Mgn-c. Merc. Merc-cor. Nitr-ac. Phosp. Sep.
— — — — burning, Aloe. Alum. Ambr. Anac. Ang. Ars. Bar-c. Benz-ac. Berb. Cact. Calc. Camph. *Cannab.* Canth. Caps. Carb-an. Carb-veg. Cast. *Caust.* Cham. Chenop. Clem. Cocc-c. Cochlear. *Colch.* Con. Cop. Croton. Cupr. Dig. Dulc. Eugen. Ferr. Grat Gum-gut. Hep. Igt. Ip. Kali-b. *Kali-c.* Lach. Laur. Lyc. Mgn-c. Mang. Merc. Mez. *Ntr-c.* Ntr-m. *Ntr-s.* Nicc. Nitr. Nitr-ac. Nux-m. *Nux. Ol-an. Par.* Petr. Petros. Phosp. Phosp-ac. Plb. Prun. Psor. Puls. Raph. Rat Rheum. Rhod. Rhus. *Sabad.* Sabin. *Sass.* Sec-c. Seneg. Sil. Spig. Stann. *Staph.* Sulph. Sulph-ac. Tereb. Teucr. *Thuj.* Uva-ursi. Viol-tr. Zinc.
— — — — in forepart, Ars Calc. Caps. Carb-veg. Cochlear. Merc. Ntr-c. Nux. Seneg. Sulph.
— — — — glandular portion and for long after, Kali-b.
— — — contracting, Bry. Dig. Ind.
— — — — cutting, Ant. Bry. Canth. Con. Graph. Guaj. Hell. Iris. Merc. Nux-m. Phosp-ac. Sass. Sulph. Thuj.
— — — — in middle of, urethra, between the acts, Mgn-s.
— — — — itching, Lyc. Nux.
— — — — rasping, Carb-veg. Lyc. Mgn-c. Nitr-ac. Phosp. Sep.
— — — — smarting, Cannab. Kobalt. Merc-cor. Ntr-c. Nitr-ac. Phosp. Sep. Sil. Thuj.
— — — — sore, Bov. Carb-an. Cinnab. Cochlear. Daph. Nux.
— — — — as of a sore, Nitr-ac.
— — — — stinging stitches, Cannab. Clem. Cupr. Cycl. Graph. Iris. Merc. Merc-cor. Seneg. Sulph. Thuj.
— — — — itching stitch in external portion, between the acts, Euph.

— — — tearing, Nux. Sulph.
— — — the contact of urine causes tearing pains which are felt in the whole organism, Jac-cor.
— — tenesmus, Ang. Arn. *Colch.* Rhus.
— — varicies, protrusion of, oozing first blood, then mucus, Kali-c.
After micturition, abdomen, spasmodic contraction of, Ntr-m.
— — bladder, pressing pain in, Asar. Berb. Canth. Chin. Lac-can. Lith. Ntr-m. Ruta.
— — pressure in as if too full, Dig.
— — — spasm in, *Asa-f.* Puls.
— — os coccygis, pain in, Kali-b.
— — blood, discharge of, Hep. Zinc.
— — desire continues, Bov. Cact. Calc. Con. Guaj. Lac-can. Laur. Ruta.
— — thin gelatinous fluid, discharge of, Ntr-m.
— — glands, pain in, Anac.
— — loathing, and inclination to vomit, Cast.
— — mucus, discharge of, Murex. Phosp-ac.
— — — viscid, purulent, from bladder, Nux.
— — nausea, Cast. Dig.
— — residuary urination, Bry. Clem. *Hep.* Kali-c. Lac-can. *Lach.* Lyc. Ntr-c. Petr. *Selen.* Sil. Thuj.
— — bloody, Hep.
— — dribbling, Thuj.
— — shuddering, Eugen. Plat.
— — sight, great distinctness of, Eugen.
— — spermatic chord, pain in, Lith.
— — urethra, itching in, Clem. Cop. Lyc. Nux.
— — — prepuce, Mez.
— — — pain in, Bov.
— — — — biting, Borax. Chin-sulph. Cop.
— — — — burning, Berb. Can.iab. Canth. Clem. Coloc. Con. Grat. Kali-b. Kali-c. Led. Mgn-m. *Merc. Ntr-c.* Ntr-m. Ntr-s. Seneg. Teucr. *Thuj.* Zinc.
— — — — the last drops cause violent burning, Clem.
— — — — cutting, Berb. Canth. Dig. Ntr-m.
— — — — sensation, as if a drop remained, Kali-b.
— — — — in fossa navice, All-cep. Thuj.
— — — stinging, Berb. Con. Kali-b. Merc.
— — tenesmus, Ang. Scill.
— — weakness, Nux.
Urine acrid, Borax. Calc. Cannab. Canth. Caust. Clem. Creos. Graph. *Hep.* Iod. Kali-c. Laur. *Merc.* Ntr-m. Par. Prun. Rhus. Tart. Tellur Thuj. Verat.
— albuminous, Glon. Kalm. Tereb. Phyt.
— black, Colch. Lach. Ntr-m.

19. URINE AND URINARY ORGANS.

Urine bloody, Actea-r. Ambr. *Arn.* Ars. Bell. Berb. *Calc. Camph. Cannab. Canth.* Caps. Carb-veg. Chin. *Con. Hep.* Ip. Lyc. Merc. Merc-cor. *Mez. Millef. Nux.* Ocim-c. *Op. Phosp. Puls.* Rhus. Sass. *Scill.* Sec-c. Sep. Sulph. *Tart.* Tereb. Thuj. Uva-ursi. Zinc.
— — like water mixed with blood, Pallad.
— brown, Acon. *Ambr.* Ant. *Arn.* Asa-f. Bell. *Bry.* Bufo. Calc. Canth. Chenop. Cimex. Colch. Dig. Dros. Graph. Lact. Lach. Merc. Merc-cor. Nitr-ac. Oleand. Petr. Phosp. Prun. *Puls.* Stram. Sulph. Sulph-ac. *Tart.*
— burning, Acon. Aloe. Ang. Apis. Ars. Benz-ac. Borax. Bry. Camph. Cannab. *Canth.* Caps. Carb-an. Cham. Cochlear. Colch. Cor-r. Creos. Dig. Dulc. Haematox. *Hep.* Lach. Lyc. Merc. Oleand. Phosp. Prun. Rhus. Scill Sec-c. Sil.
— chestnut colored, Creos.
— clay colored, Anac. Berb. Cor-r. Sabad. Sass. Sulph-ac. Zinc.
— cloudy, Carb-an. Croton. Lob.
— like coffee, Ntr-m.
— cold, Agar. Nitr-ac.
— a cuticle forming on surface, Alum. Calc. Croton. Hep. Iod. Lyc. Par. Phosp. Psor. Sep. Sulph. Thuj.
— — greasy, Alum. Calc. Hep. Iod. Kobalt. Lyc. Par. Petr. Phosp. Puls. Sulph.
— — variegated, Iod. Phosp.
— dark, Acon. Ant. Apis. Arn. Ars. *Bell.* Benz-ac. Berb. Bry. Calc. Canth. *Carb-veg.* Chin Clem. *Colch.* Croton. Cupr. Cycl. Dig. Dros. *Eugen.* Graph. Hell. *Hep.* Igt. Iod. Ip. Lach. Lyc. *Merc.* Merc-sulph. Mez. Ntr-c. Nitr-ac. Nitr. Nux-m. Op. Pallad. Par. Phosp-ac. Poth. Puls. Rhus. Scill. Selen. *Sep.* Staph. Stront. Sulph. *Tart.* Tellur. *Verat.*
— — dark brown, Calc. Caust. Colch. Dig. Eupat. Nitr-ac. Op. Petr. Puls. *Tart.*
— — red, Ant. *Hep.* Ip. *Merc.* Merc-jod. Sulph-ac. *Tart.*
— fetid, Agar. Ambr. Ars. *Aur. Benz-ar.* Borax. Bufo. Calad. *Calc.* Carb-an. Carb-veg. Coloc. Creos. Cupr. Daph. *Dulc.* Guaj. *Merc.* Murex. Ntr-c. Ntr-m. *Nitr-ac.* Petr. Phosp-ac. Puls. *Rhod.* Sep. Sulph. *Viol-tr.*
— — acrid, Asa-f. Borax. Calc.
— — like ammonia, *Asa-f.* Chin-sulph. Ferr. Mosch. Nitr-ac. Pareira. Phosp. Stront.
— — cat's urine, Viol-tr.
— — horse's urine, Nitr-ac.
— — rotten eggs, Daph.
— — onions, Gum-gut.
— — pungent, Kobalt.

— sourish, Ambr. Graph. Merc. Ntr-c.
— — strong smelling, Benz-ac. Chin-sulph. Dros. Kali-b.
— fiery, Bell. *Colch.* Croton. *Kali-c.* Merc. Par. Plb. Sass. Tart.
— flakey, Cannab. Canth. Cham. Cycl. Mez. Nitr-ac. Sass. Zinc.
— flakes of mucus, Clem.
— frothy, Chenop. Chin. Chin-sulph. Clem. Cop. Croton. Iris. Jatr. Kali-c. Lach. Laur. *Lyc.* Seneg. Spong. Thuj.
— gelatinous, lumpy, Coloc. Phosp-ac.
— gravelly, Lyc. Nitr-ac. *Sass.* Sil *Zinc.*
— greenish, Ars. Berb. *Camph.* Chin. Cop. Iod. Kali-c. *Mgn-c.* Mgn-s. Ol-an. Rheum. Ruta. Verat.
— hot, Ars. *Bry.* Calc-ph. Cham. Cor-r. *Hep.* Lact. Merc-cor. Prun. Rhus. Scill. Sec-c. Sil. (compare Burning.)
— light colored, Ant. Arum. Colch. Coloc. Cycl. Dulc. *Euphr.* Fluor-ac. Igt. Lach. Mgn-s. Ntr-m. *Nitr.*
— light yellow, Agar. Aloe. Ambr *Ang.* Apis. Aur. Bell. Berb. Cact. Camph. Carb-an. Carb-veg. Cham. Chenop. Chin. Colch. Croton. Daph. Hydroc-ac. Hyosc. Iod. Jatr. Kalm. Kali-b. Lach. Lact. Laur. Led. Mgn-m. Ntr-c. Nitr. Ocim-c. Plb. Prun. Raph. Samb. Tong. Verat. Zinc.
— milky, Apis. Arn. Chin-sulph. Cina. Clem. Dulc. Merc. Mur-ac.
— mucus, Ant. Berb. Calc. Canth. Caust. Chin-sulph. Coloc. Con. Dulc. Ind. Merc. *Ntr-m.* Pareira. Puls. Seneg. Tilia. Uva-ursi. Valer.
— muddy, Hyper. Pallad.
— like musk, smelling, Ocim.
— pale, Aeth. Agar. Alum. Amm-c. Anac. Ang. Arg-n. Arn. Bell. Bufo. Canth. Cham. *Chelid.* Cocc. Colch. Coloc. Con. Creos. Eupat. Glon. Hell. Hep. Igt. Kali-jod. Kobalt. Lam. *Mgn-c. Mez.* Ntr-m. Nitr. *Nitr-ac. Ol-an.* Phell. Phosp. Phosp-ac. Puls. Rhus. *Sass.* Scill. Sec-c. Staph. Stram. *Stront.* Teucr.
— purulent, Benz-ac. Cannab. Canth. *Clem.* Con. Lyc. Merc. Nitr-ac. Ocim-c. Puls. *Sabin.* Sep. Sil. *Uva-ursi.* Sulph.
— red, *Acon.* Agar. All-cep. Aloe. Alum. Amm-m. Ant. *Bell.* Benz-ac. Berb. *Bry.* Calc. Camph. Cannab. Canth. Caps. Carb-veg. Chelid. Chenop. Colch. Creos. Cupr. Cycl. Daph. *Dig.* Dulc. Elaps. Ferr-m. Grat. Haemotox. *Hep.* Iod. Ipec. Kali-b. Kali-jod. Lach. Led. Lob. *Merc.* Nitr. Nux. Op. Par. Petr. Phosp. Plat. Plb. *Puls.* Rheum. Sass. *Scill.* Sep. *Sil.* Staph. Sulph-ac. Tabac. *Tart.* Thuj. Tong. Verat. Zinc.
— — like blood, Bell. Berb. Calc. Carb-veg. Croton. Merc. Rhus. Sep.

19. URINE AND URINARY ORGANS. 147

Urine deep red, Ant. Carb-veg. Cupr-acet. Hep. Lob. Merc. Phyt. Sulph-ac. Tart
— fiery red, Ars. Bell. Camph. Chinin. Haematox. Selen.
— leaves a stain of a mahogany color, Phyt.
— like pieces of half burnt straw, Lach.
— sugar in, Chin. Phosp. Thuj. (compare Diabetes.)
— thick, Camph. Carb-veg. *Con.* Daph. Dulc. Elaps. Nux. Ocim-c. Pareira. Plb. Psor. Sabad. Sulph-ac.
— — as oil, Stram.
— becoming thick, Berb. Coloc. Meph. Seneg.
— turbid, Alum.*Ambr.*Anac. Ars Aur.*Bell.* Berb. Bry. Calc. Camph. *Cannab.* Canth. Carb-veg. Cham. Chin. Chin-sulph. *Cina.* Clem. *Con.* Cop. Creos. Croton. Cupr. Cycl. Daph. Dig. Dulc. Hep. Igt. Ind. Iod. Ip. Kali-b. Kali-c. Kali-chl. Lach. Lith. *Merc.* Mez. Ntr-c. Ocim. Phosp. Phosp-ac. Plb. Psor. Puls. Raph. Rhus. *Sabad.* Sass. Sep. Sulph. Tart. Verat. Viol-tr. Zing.
— becoming turbid, Acet-ac. Ang. Aur. *Bry.* Caust. *Cham.* Chin-sulph. Cina. Cocc-c. Dulc. Ferr-m. Graph. Grat. Lob. Lyc. Meph. Merc. Merc-sulph. Ol-an. Phosp-ac. Plat. Rat. Rhus. Sang. Seneg. Sulph-ac. Valer. Zinc.
— like valerian, smelling, Mosch.
— — violets, smelling, Cop. Lact. Nux-m. Tereb.
— viscid, Arg-n. Canth. *Coloc.* Creos. Cupr. Dulc. Phosp-ac.
— watery, Acet-ac. *Alum.* Anac. Ant. Arn. Arum. Aur. Bell. Berb. Bism. Bry. Caust. Cham. Cocc. Creos. Dig. Euphr. Hell. Hipp. Hydroc-ac. Hyosc. Igt. Kali-b. Kali-jod. Lam. Mgn-c. Meph. Mez. Mosch. Murex. Mur-ac. Ntr-m. Nux. *Phosp. Phosp-ac.* Plb. Puls. Rhus. Sang. *Scill. Sec-c.* Stann. Sulph. Sulph-ac. *Teucr.* Thuj.
— — inodorous, with fetid stool of white mucus, Dros.
— whitish, Alum. Amm-c. Berb. Bry. Carb-veg. Cina. Cycl. Dulc. Merc. Ntr-m. Phosp. Rhus. Sec-c.
— white, like milk, Aur. Iod. Phosp. Phosp-ac.
— — turbid, Bry. Cannab. Chin. Con. Cycl. Dulc. Psor. Rhus.
— yellow, deep, like rotten eggs, Daph.
Urine, sediment of, Acon. Ambr.Arn. Ars. Calc. Cimex. Coloc. Con. Lyc. Tart. Tereb. Thuj. Zinc.
— abundant, Bell.
— adherent, Daph. Coloc.
— albuminous, Ocim-c.
— bloody, Acon. Cannab. *Canth.* Dulc. Hell. Lyc. Phosp. *Phosp-ac. Puls. Sep.*

Sulph. Sulph-ac. Tereb. Uva-ursi.
— bluish, Prun.
— bran like, Berb.
— brown, Ambr. Lach. Thuj.
— — white, Coloc.
— burnt, as if, Sep.
— calculi, *Sass. Zinc.*
— like chalk, Phyt.
— clay colored, Berb. Chin-sulph. Cor-r. Ol-an. Tong. Zinc.
— cloudy, Ambr. Arum. Bry. Carb-veg. Cham. Elaps. Grat. Hydroc-ac. Merc. Nitr. Ol-an. Par. Phosp-ac. Plat. Rat. Seneg. Thuj.
— — in middle, Par.
— like coffee grounds, Hell. Tereb.
— crusty, hard, Sep.
— earthy, Mang.
— farinaceous, Berb.
— flakey, Berb. Cannab. Canth. Cham. Croton. Kobalt. Merc. Mez.Sass.Seneg. Zinc.
— like flour, Calc. Graph. Merc. Ntr-m.
— gelatinous, Berb. Cocc-c. Phosp-ac. Puls.
— gravelly, Ambr. Amm-c. Ant. Arn. *Calc.* Chin. *Lyc.* Meny. Ntr-m. Nitr-ac. Nux-m. Nux. *Phosp.* Puls. *Ruta. Sass.* Selen. *Sil.* Thuj. *Zinc.*
— gray, Berb. Phosp-ac. Spong.
— jelly like lumps. Phosp-ac.
— purple, Fluor-ac.
— purulent, Calc. *Canth.* Cham. Con. Kali-c. *Lyc.* Merc. Nitr-ac. *Puls.* Sep. Sil.
— red, reddish, Acon. Ambr. Amm-c.Ant. Apis. *Arn.* Bell. Berb. Camph. *Canth.* Chin. Chin-sulph. Cocc-c. Creos. Daph. Elaps. Graph. Hydroc-ac. Ip. Lach. Laur. Lith. Lob. Lyc. Merc-cor. *Mez.* Ntr-m. Ntr-s. Nitr-ac. Ocim-c. Op. Pallad. Par. Phosp. Piat. Psor. *Puls.* Scill. Selen. *Sep.* Sulph. *Valer.*
— — blood color, Amm-c.
— — bodies, Ant. Coloc.
— — cloudy, Ambr. Nitr.
— — grainy, Selen.
— — filaments, fibres, Tart.
— — sandy, All-cep. Alum. Amm-c. Bapt. Cact. Chin-sulph. Lach. Lyc. Ntr-m. Nitr-s. Ntr-ac. *Phosp.* Petr. Sep. Sil.
— pale sandy, Sass.
— slimy, (mucus,) Ant. Ars. Aur. Benz-ac. Berb. Bry. Calc. Caust. Coloc. Con. Dulc. Kali-b. Lyc. Merc. Ntr-c. Ntr-m. Phosp-ac Sass. Seneg. Sulph-ac. Tereb. Tong. Thuj. Tilia. Valer.
— slimy filaments, Croton. Seneg.
— thick, Alum. Bell. Camph. Chenop. Hydroc-ac. Laur. Lob. Merc. Phosp-ac. Spong. Sulph. Tereb.
-- turbid, Con. Croton. Rhus. Zinc.
— violet coloured, Mang. Puls.

19. URINE AND URINARY ORGANS.

Urine, sediment white, Alum. Bar-m. Bell. Berb. Calc. Carb-veg. Colch. Coloc. Con. Creos. Eupat. Euph. Fluor-ac. Graph. Hep. Kali-b. Mgn-c. Murex. Ocim-c. Oleand. Petr. *Phosp.* Phosp-ac. Prun. *Rhus.* Sep Spig. Spong. Sulph. Tereb. Tong. Valer. Zinc.

— whitish, cloudy, Phosp-ac. Plat.
— — turbid, Con. Rhus.
— — yellow, Chin-sulph. Tereb.
— yeast like, Raph.
— yellow, Cham. Chenop. Chin-sulph. Cupr. Ntr-s. Phosp. Sil. Spong. Sulph-ac. Tereb. Zinc.

20. Male Sexual Organs.

Abcess in penis, Bov.
Amorous fits, Acon. Ant. Hyosc. Op. Stram. Verat.
Aversion to the other sex, Amm-c.
Bearing down to the genitals, Asa-f. Coloc.
Biting, in glans, Nux.
— — prepuce, Nux. Puls.
— — scrotum, Ran-sc.
Blennorrhoea of the glans, Alum. Caust. *Cinnab.* Cor-r. Dig. Jac-cor. Lach. *Lyc.* *Merc.* Mez. Ntr-c. *Ntr-m.* *Nitr-ac.* *Nux.* *Sep.* *Sulph.* Thuj.
— — yellowish white fluid from prepuce, Jac-cor.
Bloatedness of genitals, Calad.
Bruising pain in genitals, Arn.
— in scrotum, Acon. Kali-c.
— of testicles, Acon. Arg. Clem. Cocc. *Dig.* Hep. Ntr-c. Ox-ac. Pallad. *Rhod.*
Burning in genitals, Anac. Arn. Bov. Cannab. Canth. Creos. Jac-cor. Mgn-m. Puls.
— — glans, Ars. Berb. Croton. Nux. Pareira. Tart. Viol-tr.
— — prepuce, Ars. Berb. Calc. Merc. Nux. Puls Sil. Sulph.
— — penis, Merc-acet.
— — prostate gland, Cop.
— — scrotum, Euph. Lachn. Sil.
— — spermatic chord, Berb. Mang.
— — — vesicles, Ambr.
— — testicles, Berb. Plat. Staph.
— — — without swelling, Puls.
Chafed glans, Ntr-c.
— prepuce, Alum. *Calad.* *Igt.* Mur-ac. Ntr-c. Nux. *Sil.* Verat.
— scrotum, Arn. Ntr-c. *Petr.* Plb. *Sulph.* Zinc.
— between the thighs, *Bar-c.* Caust. *Cinnab.* Hep. Lyc. Merc. Nitr-ac. *Petr.* Rhod. Sulph.
Chancre, Arg-n. Hep. Jac-cor. Lac-can. *Merc.*
Choking, pains in relaxed testes, Amm-c.
Coition, aversion to, Agn. Cannab. Clem. Kali-c. Lyc. Rhod.
Crab-lice, *Sabad.*
Cramping pain in seminal chord, Arg. Nux.
— in testicles, Amm-c. Igt. Nux. Plb. Spong.
During coition, burning when semen is discharged, Creos.
— — and stinging when semen is discharged, Calc.
— — flatulent colic, Graph.
— — cramp in calves, Graph.
— — enjoyment, want of, Anac. Calad. Ntr-m. Plat.
— — sleepiness and sleep, Bar-c. Lyc.
— — stinging, Calc.
After coition, anxiety, Sep.
— — burning in back, Mgn-m.
— — coldness of legs, Graph.
— — — with heat of body, Graph.
— — erections, Rhod. Sep.
— — eyes, weakness of, Kali-c.
— — fatigue, mental and bodily, Sep.
— — head, affection of, Bov. Calc.
— — knees, weakness of, Sep.
— — limbs, soreness of, Sil.
— — nervous irritation, Petr.
— — night sweats, *Agar.*
— — peevishness, Selen.
— — perspiration, Eugen. Graph. Ntr-c.
— — pollutions, Ntr-m. Rhod.
— — prepuce retracted behind glans, Calad.
— — reeling, Bov.
— — roaring in head, Carb-veg.
— — late sleep, Bov.
— — tightness of chest, Staph.
— — thirst, Eugen.
— — toothache, Daph
— — tremor of legs, Calc.
— — weakness, Agar. Berb. Calc. Con. Graph. Kali-c. *Lyc.* Nitr-ac. Petr. Selen. Sep. Sil.
Coldness of the genitals, *Agn.* Aloe. Brom. Calad. Cannab. Caps. Gels. Iris. Lyc. Merc. Sulph.
— scrotum, Aloe. Caps. Merc.
— testes, Agn-c. Aloe. Brom. Caps. Merc.
— — left, Brom.
Coldness, sensation of, on prepuce and glands, Berb. Sulph. Zinc.
Condylomata, *Cinnab.* Euphr. Lyc. Millef. *Nitr-ac.* Phosp-ac. Sabin. Staph. *Thuj.*
— on glands, Nitr-ac. Phosp-ac. Staph.
— — prepuce, Nitr-ac. Sabin.
— — edge of prepuce, itching and burning, Psor.
— with heat and burning, Phosp-ac.
— oozing, Nitr-ac. Thuj.

20. MALE SEXUAL ORGANS.

Condylomata, soreness in, Euphr. Sabin.
Constriction of prepuce, Merc. Nitr-ac. Rhus. Sabin. *Sulph.* (compare Phimosis.)
— behind the glans, Coloc.
— — after coition, Calad.
Constructive pain at root of penis, in morning on waking, Kali-b.
Constringing sensation in spermatic cord, Nux.
— in testes, Bufo. Nux. Plb. Sulph.
— — penis, Arn. Kali-c. Mosch.
— — scrotum, Arn.
Contraction of spermatic chord, Alum. Berb. Nux.
— in testes, Alum. Camph. Merc-acet. Nux. Plb.
Cracks in the glands, Ars. Kali-c. Mosch.
— — prepuce, Merc. Sulph.
Cutting pain in glans, Lyc.
— — penis, Ol-an.
— — testicles, Berb. Phosp-ac. Sep. Tereb.
Drawing in glans, Iod. Kali-c. Lact. Lyc.
— — penis, Kali-c. Lact. Ol-an. Ran-sc. Rhod.
— — spermatic chord, Agn. Berb. Clem. Croton. Lact. *Mang.* Merc. Nitr-ac. Ox-ac. Puls. Tereb. Zinc.
— — testes, Agar. Amm-c. Berb. Chin. Clem. Cocc. Hipp. Merc. Ntr-c. Nitr-ac. Ox-ac. Psor. *Puls.* Rhod. Staph. Tereb. *Thuj.* Verat. *Zinc.*
Drawn up of testes, Bell. Berb. Croton. Euphr. Meny. Nux. Ol-an. Plb. Rhod. Thuj. Zinc.
— — right, Clem. Puls. Thuj. Zinc.
— — left, Calc. Croton. Pareira. Zinc.
Dryness of glans, Calad.
— — prostate glans, Cop.
Erections in general, Amm-m. Anac. Arn. *Canth.* Creos. Dig. *Euph.* Ferr. Igt. *Kali-c.* Led. *Merc.* Mgn-m. *Ntr-c. Ntr-m.* Nux. *Op.* Phosp-ac. Plat. *Plb. Puls.* Ran-b. Seneg. Sep. Sil. Staph. Tabac. Tar. Viol-tr.
— without desire, Calad. Euph. Mgn-s. Nitr-ac.
— too easily excited, Lyc. Nux. Phosp. Sabin.
— with gonorrhoea, Canth.
— insufficient, Con.
— painful, Cannab. *Canth.* Hep. Igt. *Kali-c.* Merc. Ntr-c. Nitr-ac. Nux. *Puls.* Sabad. Seneg. *Thuj.* Zing.
— too short, Calc. Con. Nux.
— — strong, *Canth.* Creos. Fluor-ac. Graph. Mez. *Phosp.* Puls. Sabin. Tar.
— caused by swelling of prepuce, Jac-cor.
— without any voluptuous irritation, Ambr. Eugen. *Phosp-ac.* Sabad. Spig.
— want of, Agn. Caust. *Con.* Graph. Kali-c. Lyc. *Mgn-c. Nitr-ac.* Nux-m. Rhod. Spong. Teucr.
— — in morning, Graph. Lact.

— too weak, Agar. Bar-c. Calad. Calc. Hep. Lyc. Selen. Sulph.
— in the morning, *Ambr.* Caps. Mgn-m. Mtr-s. Nux. Petr. Phosp. Puls. *Thuj.*
— — before rising, Bar-c.
— — day-time, Anac.
— — evening, Cinnab. Phosp.
— at night, Alum. *Aur.* Caps. *Merc.* Merc-cor. Ntr-c. Ntr-m. Nitr-ac. Ol-an. Par. Plat. Plb. Rhus. Sep. Staph. *Thuj.* Zinc.
— after midnight, Osm.
— — dinner, Nicc.
— with urging to stool, Thuj.
— during stool, Igt.
— with desire to urinate, Mosch.
— after urinating, Aloe.
— at night relieved, Lith.
Eruption on the genitals, Ant. Carb-veg. Iod. Merc. Nitr-ac. Rhus. Sep. Sil. Tart.
— — glans, Bry. Calad. Cinnab. Lach. Lyc. Nitr-ac. Rhus. Sep.
— — hairy part, Lach.
— — penis, Graph. Phosp-ac.
— — prepuce, Graph. Nitr-ac. Phosp-ac. Sass. Sep. Sil.
— — scrotum, Croton. Petr. Phosp-ac. Rhus.
— between the thighs, Hep. Petr.
— biting, Lyc.
— closing urethra by swelling, Rhus.
— elevations, Lyc.
— erysipelas of scrotum, Arn. Canth. Graph. Merc. Ntr-m. Puls. Rhus.
— granulated, Cinnab.
— herpetic, Croton. Dulc. Petr. Sass.
— itching, Arn. Bry. Nitr-ac. Petr. Sep. Sil.
— miliary, Bry.
— moist, Carb-veg. Hep. Phosp-ac. Rhus. Sil.
— pimples, Graph. Lach. Sil.
— points, Calad.
— small pustules, size of pin's head, Kali-b.
— red, Nitr-ac.
— specks, Arn. Carb-veg. Sil.
— vesicular, Carb-veg. Merc. Nitr-ac. Phosp-ac. Rhus. Tart.
Excitement of the genitals, Aur. Carb-veg. Cocc. Coff. Graph. Lyc. Ntr-m *Phosp.* Plat. Sil. Sulph.
Flaccidity of the genitals, *Agar.* Calad. Hell.
— of penis, Merc. Prun.
Fretting sensation, (corrosion,) in the testes, Phosp-ac. Plat.
Fullness sensation of in spermatic cords, Fluor-ac.
Gangrene of genitals, Ars. *Canth.* Laur.
Gnawing in testes, Phosp-ac. Plat.
From gonorrhoea suppressed, affections of the testes, *Agn.* Aur. Bell. Canth. Clem. Ntr-c. Nitr-ac. *Puls.* Rhus. Selen.

20. MALE SEXUAL ORGANS. 151

Hair falling off from the genitals, Bell. Ntr-c. Ntr-m. Rhus. Sass. Selen. Zinc.
Hanging down of testes, Amm-c. Bell. Camph. Chin. Gels. Iod. Lyc. Mgn-m. Nitr-ac. Puls. Sil. Sulph. Sulph-ac.
Hardness of testes, *Agn. Arn.* Bell. Nux. Spong. (compare Induration.)
Heat, sensation of in genitals, Sulph-ac.
Heaviness in testes, Amm-c. Elaps. Lob. Ntr-c. Ox-ac.
Hernia scrotalis, Mgn-m. Nux.
— — symptoms of, Lach.
Herpetic eruptions of genitals, Dulc. Nitr-ac. Sil.
— — — prepuce, Sass.
— — — scrotum, Croton. Petr.
— — between thighs, Petr. Ntr-m.
Hydrocele, *Arn. Graph.* Hydroph. Iod. *Nux.* Psor. *Puls.* Rhod. *Sil. Sulph.*
— like a bladder filled with water, Dig.
Impotence, *Agn. Calad. Calc. Camph. Cannab. Caps.* Caust. Chin. Coff. *Coloc. Con.* Creos. Elaps. Eugen. Ferr. Hyosc. Iod. Kobalt. Lach. *Lyc. Mosch. Mur-ac* Ntr-m. *Nitr-ac. Nux-m.* Nux. Op. Phosp. Phosp-ac. Plb. Psor. *Selen.* Sep. Stram. *Sulph.* Tussil.
— chronic, Lyc.
— from a cold, Mosch.
— after gonorrhoea, Cub. Kobalt. Thuj.
— with gloomy thoughts, Calad.
— penis relaxed when excited, Calad.
Induration of the testes, Agn. *Aur. Clem.* Cop. *Iod.* Merc. Nux. *Rhod.* Spong. Sulph.
— — — left, Brom.. Mez. Ocim-c. Rhod.
— — — right, Clem. Nitr-ac. Ox-ac,
— prepuce, Lach. Sulph.
— prostate, Cop. Iod. Thuj.
Inflammation of the genitals, Acon. Ars. Calc. Cannab. Canth. Con. Merc. Merc-acet. Mur-ac. Ntr-c. Ntr-m. Nitr-ac. Nux. Phosp-ac. Plb. Puls. Rhus. Sep. Spong. Staph. Thuj.
— — glans, Arn. Ars. Cannab. Cupr. Led. Merc. Ntr-c. Rnus. Sass. Thuj.
— — penis, Cannab. Canth. Cub. Led. Plb. Sep.
— — lymphatic glands, Merc.
— — prepuce, Ars. Calc. *Cannab.* Merc. Ntr-c. Nitr-ac. Sulph.
— — prostate, Hipp. Puls. Thuj. (compare Prostate gland.)
— — scrotum, Ars. Mur-ac. Ntr-m. Phosp-ac. Plb.
— — erysipelatous, *Ars.* Phosp-ac. Plb. *Puls.* Rhus.
— — spermatic cord, Nux. Puls.
·— — testes, Aur. Bell. *Clem.* Con. Lyc. Merc. *Nitr-ac. Nux.* Pod. *Puls.* Spong. Staph. Zinc.
Itching of genitals, Agar. *Ambr. Ang.* Benz-ac. Berb. Calc. Carb-veg. Caust.

Clem. Con. Euphr. Igt. Kali-c. Lyc. Mgn-m. Merc. Ntr-m. Ntr-s. Nitr-ac. Poth. Selen. Sep. Sil. Sulph.
— — — painful, Poth.
— — glans, Ang. Ars. Benz-ac. Cannab. Cinnab. Colch. Euphr. Ferr-m. Gymnoc. Hep. Ind. Kali-b. Mang. Merc. Ntr-m. Ntr-s. Nux. Poth. Sil.
— — hairy parts, skin inflamed, with small pustules, Kali-b.
— — prepuce, Cannab. Cham. Colch. Euph. Euphr. Gymnoc. Igt. Jac-cor. Lyc. Nitr-ac. Nux. Puls. Rhus. Sep. Sil. Viol-tr. Zing.
— — scrotum, Amm-c. Aur. Caust. Cist. Cocc. Ferr-m. Hipp-m. Ind. Kali c. Lachn. Mgn-m. Meph. Ntr-m. Ntr-s. Nitr-ac. Nux. *Petr.* Prun. Puls. Rhod. Rhus. Selen. Sil. Staph.
— — — in a small part, Nicc.
— — spermatic cord, Mang.
— between the thighs, Carb-veg. Ntr-m. *Petr.*
— voluptuous, Euph. Euphr. Staph.
— in morning, Puls.
— — evening, Igt. Puls.
Jerking in penis, Mez.
— — spermatic cord, Mang. Plb. Ox-ac.
Laxity of genitals, *Agn.* Calad. Hell.
Lustfulness, *Calc. Carb-veg. Chin.* Graph.
Moisture on scrotum, Ntr-c. *Petr. Sil.* Sulph. Zinc.
— between the thighs, Bar-c. Carb-veg. *Hep.* Lyc. Merc. Ntr-c. Petr. Rhod.
— frenum, Phosp-ac.
Numbness, Ambr.
— of glands and prepuce, Berb.
Painfulness of prepuce, Cor-r. Cycl. Osm. Sabin.
— — — as if small bundle of fibres were seized, Jac-cor.
— — penis, Jac-cor. Osm.
— — spermatic chord, Meny.
— of testes, Arn. Asa-f. Aur. Cannab. Caust. Clem. Cocc. Igt. Ol-an. Phosp-ac. Sep. Tar. Zinc.
— — left, Jac-cor.
— — right, ameliorated, after urinating, Kobalt.
Pains, aggravation of from movement, Berb.
Paraphimosis, Merc-cor.
Perspiration on genitals, Aur. Calad. Canth. Cor-r. Lachn. Merc. Sep. Sulph. Thuj.
— — at night, Bell.
— — scrotum, Daph. Igt. Lachn. Ntr-s. Rhod. Sep. Sil. Thuj.
— between the thighs, Cinnab.
Phimosis, Cannab. Dig. Jac-cor. Merc. Nitr-ac. Rhus. Sabin. Sep. *Sulph.* Thuj. (compare Swelling.)
— penis becoming smaller, Prun.

20. MALE SEXUAL ORGANS.

Pimple itching at glands chancre like, red point when dry, Jac-cor.
Pinching in glaus, Acon. Brom.
Pollutions, seminal emissions, Aloe. *Alum.* Amm-c. Anac. Ant. *Arg. Aur. Bell.* Bism. *Calc.* Canth. Carb-an. Caust. *Chin. Con.* Cor-r. Dig. Ferr. Kali-c. Kobalt. Lach. *Lact.* Lyc. Merc. Mosch. Ntr-c. Ntr-m. Nitr-ac. *Nux.* Ol-an. Op. Par. Petr. Petros. Phosp. *Phosp-ac. Puls.* Ran-b. Ran-sc. Ruta. Saccn. *Sep.* Sil. Stann. *Sulph.* Tabac. Tar. Thuj. Verb. Viol-od. Viol-tr.
— bloody, Caust. Led. Merc.
— easily, excited in daytime, Canth. Graph.
— — without erections, Graph.
— frequent, *Amm-c.* Bar-m. Bov. Calc. Carb-an. Carb-veg. Caust. *Con.* Dig. Ferr. *Kali-c.* Kobalt. Lyc. Ntr-c. Ntr-m. Nitr-ac. Nux. Op. Petr. Phosp. *Phosp ac. Plb. Puls.* Sacch. Sass. *Sep.* Stann. *Staph.* Sulph.
— too frequent, Carb-veg. Con. Kali-c. Lyc. Nitr-ac. *Phosp.*
— painful, Calc. Clem. Mosch. Sass. Thuj.
— after onanism, Chin. Sep.
— with backache, Kobalt.
— — amorous dreams, Kali-c. Kobalt. Led. Merc-jod. Par.
— without amorous dreams, Bism. Cor-r. Guaj. Merc-jod.
— without erections, Bell. Calad. Con. Gels. Kobalt. Mosch. Sabad. Selen.
— during sleep in afternoon, Caust. Clem. Merc. Phosp. Sulph.
After pollutions, affection of the head, Bov. Calc.
— anxiousness, Carb-an.
— brain as if partially paralyzed, Sil.
— burning in urethra, Carb-veg. Merc. Sulph.
— coldness, general, Merc.
— constipation, Thuj.
— erections, Ars. Grat. Kali-c. Rhod.
— eyes, weakness of, Kali-c.
— fatigue, Sep. Viol-od.
— heat, anxious, Petr.
— hypochondria, tension in, Agar.
— increase of all complaints, Alum.
— loins, weakness in, Phosp.
— micturition, stool and restless sleep, Aloe.
— peevishness, Ntr-c.
— sexual passion excited, Aloe. Mez.
— sluggishness, Ntr-c. Sep.
— vertigo, Caust.
Pressure, in penis, Viol-tr.
— — spermatic chord, Berb. Spong. Sulph.
— — testes, Aur. Berb. *Bism.* Calc. Cannab. Carb-veg. Caust Igt. Lach. Ntr-c. *Puls.* Sabad. Scill. Spong. Steph.
— — — right, *Bism.*

Priapism, Clem. *Coloc. Graph. Ntr-c. Ntr-m.* Phosp. *Plat. Puls.* Sil.
Prickling, in glans, Kali-b. Mez. Phosp-ac.
— — prepuce, Jac-cor.
Prostate glands, enlargement of, Benz-ac.
— induration of, Cop. Iod. Thuj.
— inflammation of, Agn. Alum. Apis. Caust. Cop. Cycl. Dig. Hep. Lyc. Puls. Sec-c. Selen. Sulph-ac. Thuj. Zinc.
— pressure in, Ol-an.
— swelling of, Cannab. Hipp. Iod. Thuj.
Prostatic fluid, emission of, *Anac.* Bell. Dig. Elaps. Euph. *Hep.* Lyc. Ntr-c. Nitr-ac. Nux-m. Petr. Phosp-ac. Puls. *Selen. Sep.* Sil. Spig. Staph. *Sulph.* Tabac. Thuj. Zinc.
— with the flatulence, Mgn-c.
— — stool, Anac. Ars. Carb-veg. Caust. Con. Selen. Sep. Sil. Sulph.
— — difficult, Agn. Alum. Amm-c. Anac. Con. Hep. Ntr-c. Nitr-ac. Sep. Staph.
— with the urine, Anac. *Hep.* Ntr-c. Sep. Sulph.
— after urinating, Daph. Hipp. Kali-c.
— without erection, Aur. Bell. Euph. Lyc.
Pulsation in penis, Cop.
Pustules on penis, Bov.
Redness of genitals, Cocc-c.
— — glans, Ars. Calad. Cannab. Croton. Merc. Sabin. Sass.
— — penis, Cannab.
— — prepuce, Calc. Cannab. *Cinnab.* Merc. Rhus. Sil. Sulph.
— — scrotum, *Arn.* Merc. Petr. Puls.
— between thighs, *Petr.*
— of urethra, Gels.
Relaxation of genitals, Gels.
— — testes. Nitr-ac. Sulph. (compare Hanging down).
Retraction of penis. Berb.
— — prepuce, Bell. Colch. Nux. Prun. Sulph. (compare Phimosis.)
— — after coition, Calad.
Scrabs, on corona glans, Kali-b.
— — prepuce, Caust. Nitr-ac.
Seminal emissions, (compare Pollutions).
Seminal discharge, bloody, Caust. Led. Merc.
— easily excited in daytime, Canth. Graph.
— — without erection, Graph.
— painful, Calc. Clem. Sass. Thuj.
— during coition, failing, Calad. Eugen. Graph. Lyc. Millef. Psor.
— — insufficient, Agar Berb. Plb.
— — larger and continues longer, Osm.
— — too late, Borax. Calc. Eugen. Lyc. Zinc.
— — powerless, Calc. *Con.* Ntr-m. Phosp. Sulph-ac.
— — too quick, too early, Berb. Borax. Calad. Carb-veg. Con. Lyc. Phosp. Plat. Selen. Sulph. *Zinc.*

20. MALE SEXUAL ORGANS.

Semen dribbling out, Canth.
— — in sleep, Sil.
— — during stool, Phosp-ac.
Sensitiveness of genitals, Cocc. Verat.
Sexual passion, diminished, Acon. Arg-n.
Bar-c. Bell. Carb-an. Hell. Hep. Ind.
Kali-c. Kali-jod. Lyc. Mgn-c. Op. Petr.
Phosp-ac. Sabad. Spong. Teucr.
— increased, *Agar.* Aloe. Alum. Amm-c.
Ant. Apis. Arn. Aur. Bell. Bov. *Calc.*
Cannab. *Canth.* Carb-veg. Caust. Cham.
Chin. Cinnab. Cocc. *Coff.* Croc. Dig.
Ferr. Graph. Hipp. *Hyosc. Igt. Iod.*
Lach. Laur. Led. Lyc. Mang. Meny.
Merc. Mez. *Mosch. Ntr-c. Ntr-m.*
Ntr-s. Nitr. Nitr-ac. *Nux. Op.* Ox-ac.
Par. *Phosp. Plat.* Plb. *Puls.* Rhus.
Ruta. *Sabin.* Sacch. Sass. Seneg. Sep.
Sil. Stann. Staph. Stram. Sulph-ac.
Verat. Zinc.
— — in old men, Fluor-ac,
— excitement of, easy, Kali-c. Lyc. Nux.
Phosp.
— excessive, *Alum.* Coloc. *Kali-c. Lyc.*
Ntr-c. Ntr-m. Plat. Plb. Psor. Sil.
Therid. Zinc.
— lustful, *Chin.* Con. *Merc.*
— — without erections, Agar. Aur. Calad.
Crotal. Ferr. Igt. Lach. Ntr-m. Puls.
Sabad. Sep. Sulph. Trifol.
— strong, Amm-c. *Canth.* Ferr-m. *Kali-c.*
Lach. Mosch. Nux. Plat. Plb.
— — with many erections, *Canth.* Dig.
Ferr. *Merc. Ntr-c. Ntr-m.* Nux. *Op.*
Plat. *Plb. Puls.* Sabin. Seneg. Sep.
Sil. Spig. Staph.
— — with pollutions, Dig. Ferr. Ntr-c. *Nux.*
Op. *Plb.* Sass.
— excitement of, strong, with discharge of
prostatic fluid, Nitr-ac.
— wanton, with inclination to co-habit, Ant.
Calc. Con. Igt. Kobalt. *Lach.* Ntr-m. Nitr-ac.
Phosp. Puls. Sass. Sil. Spig. Stram.
Zinc.
— with weakness, of faculty, Agar. Amm-c.
Graph. *Ignat.* Meny. Nux-m. Selen.
Sexual passion, wanting, suppressed,
Agn. Alum. Bell. Berb. Calc. *Camph.*
Carb-an. Cop. Ferr-m. *Graph.* Hell.
Hep. Igt. *Kali-c.* Lach. *Lyc.* Mur-ac.
Nitr-ac. Nux-m. Phosp-ac. Sil. Sulph.
— power weak, *Bar-c. Calad.* Calc. *Igt.*
Nux-m. *Sep.* Sil. *Sulph.*
Shivering in scrotum, Zinc.
Shrinking of penis, Aloe. Arg-n. Igt. Lyc.
— of scrotum, with coldness and pain in
testes, Berb.
— testes, Hydroph.
Shrivelling, of penis, Berb.
— — scrotum, Berb. Rhod. Therid. Zinc.
Smarting, in glans, Berb. Nux.
— in prepuce, Benz-ac. Nux. Puls.
— — scrotum, Ran-sc.

— — spermatic, cord, Berb.
— between thighs, Hep.
Sore pain, in penis, Arn. Cannab.
— — prepuce, Cham. Cor-r. Lob.
— — scrotum, Berb. Zinc.
— between thighs, Rhod.
Spasmodic pain in genitals, Graph.
— — — testicles, Spong.
Spots, on glans, itching, Arn.
— — moist, smooth, Carb-veg.
— — red, Arn. Carb-veg. Lach. Sil.
— — yellow-brown, Kobalt.
— — penis, Calc.
— — prepuce, Nitr-ac. Rhus.
Stench of the genitals, Ntr-m. Sass. Sulph.
Stinging, Stitches in glands, Acon. Ars. Berb.
Euph. Euphr. Ferr-m. Lyc. Merc. Mez.
Ntr-m. Phosp-ac. Ran-sc. Rhod. Sabin.
Sulph.
— — when pressing on it, Thuj.
— — penis, Berb. Lyc. Mgn-s. Merc.
Merc-jod. Mez. Mur-ac. Ntr-m.
Ol-an. Petr. Phosp. Puls. Spig. Thuj.
Viol-tr.
— — prepuce, Ars. Cham. Euphr. Mang.
— — Merc. Puls. Rhus. Sulph.
— — prostate gland, when walking, Kali-b.
— — scrotum, Ferr-m. Merc. Ntr-m.
Sulph. Thuj.
— — spermatic chord, Amm-m. Arn.
Berb. Grat. Nux. Sulph. Thuj.
— — testes, Arn. Bell. Berb. Bry. Caust.
Merc. Nux. Rhod. Staph. Sulph.
— — — left, Merc-cor.
Swelling of genitals, Ars. Canth. Cocc-c.
Kali-b. Lyc. Merc. Plb.
— glans, *Ars.* Cannab. Cinnab. Cor-r.
Merc. Ntr-c. Plb. *Rhus.* Sacch. Sulph.
Thuj.
— — one sided, Spig.
— penis, *Arn.* Cannab. Canth. Cinnab.
Creos. Cupr. Graph. Led. Mez. Millef.
Plb. Sabin.
— — lymphatic glands, Lact. *Merc.*
— — on the ridge, Sabin.
— prepuce, *Calad.* Cannab. *Cinnab.* Cor-r.
Graph. *Merc.* Ntr-c. Nitr-ac. *Rhus.* Sil.
Sulph. Thuj. Viol-tr.
— — on the frenulum, Sabin.
— of prostate gland, Cannab. Hipp. Iod.
— scrotum, *Arn.* Brom. Canth. Carb-veg.
Clem. Graph. Jac-cor. Phosp-ac. Plb.
Puls. Rhus. Sacch. Sep.
— — with chronic gonorrhoea, Brom.
— — painless, Mez.
— of spermatic, cgords, Arn.
— — testes, *Agn.* Apis. Arg. *Arn. Aur.*
Bar-m. Canth. Chin. *Clem.* Con.
Cop. *Dig.* Elaps. *Iod.* Kali-c. Merc-sulph.
Mez. Millef. Ntr-c. *Nitr-ac. Nux.*
Ol-an. Phosp-ac. Plb. *Puls. Rhod.*
Spong. Sulph. Tart. Zinc.
— — — left, Brom. Mez. Ocim. Pod. Rhod.

20. MALE SEXUAL ORGANS.

Swelling of testes, right, Arg. Aur. Clem.
— — — — lower part of, Aur.
— — — after gonorrhoea, Rhod.
— bluish red, *Arn.* Ars.
— dropsical, Dig. Lyc.
— hard, *Agn Arn.* Merc. Nux. Phosp-ac. Sabin *Spong.*
— hot, Arn. Kali-c. Puls.
— oedematous, Arn. Graph. Lyc. Nux. Puls. Rhod. Sil. Sulph.
— painful, Arn. Ars. Aur. Canth. Laur. Lyc. Merc. Nitr-ac. Nux. Ol-an. Plb.
— from a bruise, Con.
Tearing, in glans, Colch. Euph. Kali-c. Pareria.
— — penis, Kali-c. Mez.
— — spermatic chord, Bell. Colch. Puls.
— — testes, Euph. Puls. Staph.
Tension, in genitals, Graph.
— — glans, Kali-c.
— — penis, Arn. Kali-c.
— — scrotum, Arn.
— — spermatic chord, Cannab. Phosp-ac.
Thickening of the prepuce, Elaps. Lact.
— — — scrotal skin, Carb-veg. Clem. Rhus.
— — — epididymus, Sulph.
Throbbing, of glans, Rhod.
— — penis, Cop.
— — spermatic chord, Amm-m.
Tingling, crawling, tickling, of genitals, Mosch. Selen.
— of the frenum, Phosp-ac.
— glans, Merc. Spig. Tart.
— crawling prepuce, Merc. Phosp-ac.
— scrotum, Acon. Lachn. Selen.
— testes, Euphr. Merc.
To touch the genitals, inclination to, Bufo.
Turning about in testes, sensation of, Sabad.
Twitching in penis, Mez.
— — spermatic chord, *Mang.* Plb.
Ulcers, on glans, Ars. Cor-r. *Merc.* Nitr-ac. Sep. Sulph.
— prepuce, Arg-n. Ars. Caust. Cor-r. Hep. *Merc.* Nitr-ac. Sep. Sulph. Thuj.
— elevated, lead colored, sensitive edges, Nitr-ac.
— flat, red, Cor-r.
— chancre, Arg-n. Lac-can. *Merc.*
— — like, Hep. Lac-can. *Merc. Nitr-ac.* Thuj.
— deep, Nitr-ac. Sulph.
— mercurio, syphilitic, Lach.
Ulcerous pain in prepuce, *Igt.*
Voluptuous irritation of genitals, Amb. Ang. Chenop. Graph Plb. (compare Itching, voluptuous.)
Warmth, sensation of, in genitals, Meph. Sulph-ac.
Warts on prepuce, bleeding when touched, Cinnab.
Wasting of testes, Agn. Caps. Caust. Iod. Kali-jod. Zinc.
Weakness of genitals, *Agn.* Berb. Hep. Mang. Mur-ac. Sep. Sulph.
— after stool or urination, Calc-ph.

21. Female Sexual Organs.

Abortion, Acon. Actea-r. Aletris. Aloe. Apis. Arn. *Asar.* Bell. Bry. *Calc.* Camph. *Cannab.* Canth. Carb-veg. Cauloph. Cham. Chin. Cinnam. Cocc. Con. Creos. *Croc.* Dulc. Eugen. *Ferr.* Gels. Hyosc. Igt. Iod. *Ip.* Jatr. Kali-c. *Lyc.* Merc. Nitr-ac. Nux-m. Nux. Op. Phosp. Plat. Plb. Pod. Puls. Rat. Rhus. *Sabin* Sec-c. *Sep. Sil.* Stram. *Sulph.* Verat. Viburn. *Zinc.*
— disposition to, Actea-r. Aletris. Lyc. Ntr-c.
— after fright, Gels.
— in third month, Apis. Sabin. Sec-c. Thuj.
— with convulsions, Cannab.
— — distention of uterus. Sec-c.
— — varices on pudenda, Carb-veg. Lyc. Zinc.
After pains, too long, *Arn.* Bell. Bry. Calc. Cham. Cupr. Ferr. Kali-c. Ntr-m. Nux. Op. *Puls.* Rhus. Ruta. Sabin. Sec-c. Sep. Sulph.
— painful and strong, Acon. Arn. Calc. *Cham. Coff. Nux.* Pod. *Puls.* Rhus. Sec-c.
— to thighs, Lac-can.
— return when nursing the child, Arn.
Apthae, Carb-veg.
Biting in genitals, Staph. Thuj.
Bloatedness of uterus, as if filled with wind, Phosp-ac.
Blood, congestion of, to genital, Aletris. Ambr. Bell. Bry. *Chin. Croc. Hep.* Lac-can. *Merc. Nux.* Plat. Sabin. Sec-c. Sulph.
— discharged during the intervals, Ambr. Arn. *Bell. Bov.* Bry. Calc. *Cham.* Chin. Cocc. Coff. Croc. Hep. Ip. Kali-c. Mgn-s. Phosp. Rhus. Sabin. Sec-c. Sil.
— during lactation, Calc. Pallad. Sil.
— at new or full moon, Croc.
— during pregancy, Cocc. Creos. Kali-c. Phosp. Rhus. Sec-c.
— — green red fluid, Sep.
— discharge of, during and between the catamenia, acrid, Amm-c. Ars. Bov. Canth. Cham. Kali-c. Ntr-s. Nitr. Rhus. Sass. Sil. Sulph.
— black, dark, Actea-r. Aletris. Amm-c. Ant. Arn. Asar. Bell. Bism. Bry. Cact.
Canth. Cham. Chin. Creos. *Croc.* Cycl. Elaps. Ferr. Ham. Igt. Lach. Mgn-c. Mgn-m. Mgn-s. Nitr-ac. *Nitr.* Nux. Nux-m. Ol-an. Plat. Puls. Sabad. Sabin. Sang. Sec-c. Selen. Sep. Stram. Sulph. Trill. Xanthox. Zing.
Blood, black like ink, Nitr.
— brown, Berb. Bry. Calc. Carb-veg. Mgn-c. Rhus.
— bright-red, Arn. *Bell.* Brom. Cinnam. Diad. Dulc. Hyosc. Ip. Lac-can. Lachn. Led. Phosp. Rhus. *Sabin.* Sec-c.
— — stringy, Lac-can.
— burning, Sil.
— clotted, coagulated, Actea-r. Aletris. Amm-c. Apocyn. Arn. Bell. Caust. Cham. Chin. Cocc. Croc. Cycl. Ferr. Fluor-ac. Hyosc. Igt. Ip. Kali-c. Mgn-m. Ntr-s. Plat. Puls. Rhus. Sabin. Stram. Stront. Trill. Ustil. Viburn. Zing.
— — black, Chin. Ferr. Nux-jug. Sabin.
— first dark, then watery, Thuj.
— excoriating, acrid. Amm-c. Carb-veg. Kali-c. Ntr-s. Sass. Sil. Sulph.
— — corroding the limbs, Ntr-s. Sil. Sulph.
— fetid, Bell. Bry. Carb-an. Caust. Cham. Croc. Kali-c. Sabin.
— flesh-colored (like the washings of meat) Apocyn. Stront.
— grayish serum, Berb.
— hot blood, Bell. Bry.
— itching, Petr.
— by jerks, Cham. Puls. Sabin.
— lumpy, Arn. Bell. Caust. *Cham.* Ferr. Mgn-m. Plat. Puls. Rhus. Sabin. Stram. Stront.
— mucus, Cocc. Lachn. Puls. Sulph-ac.
— — menses of gray mucus, or brown blood, Berb.
— — bloody mucus during pregnancy, Cocc.
— too pale, Alum. *Bell.* Berb. Borax. Carb-veg. Ferr. *Graph.* Hipp-m. Prun. Puls. Sabin. Sacch. Sulph. Tilia.
— pitch-like, Mgn-c.
— putrid odor, Igt.
— sour-smelling, Carb-veg. Sulph.
— stringy, Croc.
— — red, Lac-can.
— thick, Cact. Fluor-ac. Mgn-s. Nux-m. Plat. Puls. Sulph.

21. FEMALE SEXUAL ORGANS.

Blood thin, Laur. Puls. Sabad.
— tough, Croc.
— viscid, Lachn. Mgn-c. Xanthox.
— watery, Berb. Dulc. Laur. Phosp. Puls. Tart.
Boring pain in left ovary, worse during menses, Zinc.
— — — — ameliorated during menses, Thuj.
Burning in genitals, *Ambr.* Amm-c. Ars. Berb. Bry. Calc. *Carb-veg.* Caust. Cham. Creos. Kali c. Lac-can. Lach. Lil-tigr. Lyc. Merc. Nitr-ac. Nux. Petr. Sulph. Thuj. Tilia.
— — uterus, Bry.
— — vagina, Berb.
Cancer of uterus, Apis. *Ars.* Aur. Calc. *Carb-an.* Chin. Clem. Cocc. *Con. Creos.* Graph. *Hydrast.* Iod. Lact. Lyc. Mgn-m. Merc. Murex. Nitr-ac. Phosp. Phyt. Rhus. Sabin. Sec-c. *Sep.* Sil. Staph. Sulph. Thuj.
Coition, aversion to, *Caust.* Kali-c. Ntr-m. Petr.
— absence of enjoyment in, Berb. Ferr. Ferr-m.
— disposition for, Creos. Hyosc. Kali-c. Murex. Sabin. Sulph-ac.
During coition, pain in vagina, Berb. Creos. Ferr-m. Kali-c. Lyc.
— — burning, followed, next day by dark blood, Creos.
After coition, nodosity in cervix and swelling of parts, Creos.
Constriction of uterus, sensation of, Cact. Murex.
Contraction, Actea-r. Bell. Cact. Igt. Lac-can. Murex. Ntr-m. Nux. Sabin. Sep. Thuj.
— hour-glass, Bell. Cham. Cocc. Con. Cupr. Hyosc. Kali-c. Nux. Plat. Puls. Rhus. Sec-c. Sep. Sulph.
Corrosion, Kali-c. Lyc.
Cutting in left labia, Ocim-c.
— — os uteri, Murex. Puls.
Darting pains from left labia through uterus to right ovary, Bell. Lac-can. Phosp. Thuj.
Deformed os uteri, Ntr-c.
Digging, Con.
Distension of uterus, meteoristic, Phosp-ac.
Drawing, Mosch.
— in uterus, Puls.
Dropsy of uterus, Aesc-hipp. Apis. Ars. Bell. Brom. Bry. Calc. Camph. Canth. Chin. Colch. Con. Dig. Dulc. Ferr. Ham. Hell. Kali-c. Lact. Led. Lyc. Merc. Phosp. Rhus. Sep. Sulph.
— — ovaries, Apis. Bell. Bry. Calc. Carb-an. Coloc. Creos. Graph. Kali-brom. Kali-c. Lach. Lil-tigr. Merc. Ntr-s. Phosp. Plat. Pod. Rhod. Rhus. Sabin.

Dryness of vagina, Bell. *Lyc.* Ntr-m.
— — uterus, Murex.
Eruption, Agar Apis. Bapt. Bry. Calad. Calc. Canth. Carb-veg. Cauloph. Coff. Collin. Con. Creos. Croton. Dulc. Ferr. Graph. Ham. Hydrast. Kali-c. Lyc. Merc. Ntr-nitr. Nitr-ac. Nux. Petr. Plat. Sep. Sil. Staph. Sulph. Tart. Thuj. Zinc.
— from menstrual blood, Kali-c.
— fretting, gnawing, Nux.
— itching, Nux. *Sep.*
— moist, Sep.
— with nodosities, Merc.
— pimples, Agar. Graph. Merc. Sulph. Tart.
— pustules, black, Bry.
— scabby on labia, Kali-jod.
— vesicular, Graph.
Extension, sensation of, Murex.
Flatus, from vagina, Brom. Lac-can. Lyc. Nux. Sang.
Foetus, violent motions of, Lyc. Op.
— — — painful, Arn. Sil.
As if foetus lay cross-wise, which gives pain, Arn.
Fullness, sense of, Aloe. Chin.
Gangrena uteri, Acon. Apis. Ars. Bell. Carb-veg. Chin. Creos. Sec-c.
— vaginae, Apis. Ars. Bell. Calc. Chin. Creos. Lach. Sec-c Sulph-ac.
Gnawing, Kali-c. Lyc.
Hair of vulva falling off, Ntr-m.
Heat, Merc. Nux. Sep.
— flushes of, and sweat, at climacteric. Sulph-ac.
Heaviness, sensation of, Aletris, Aloc. Chin. Lac-can. Murex Nux. Palad.
— — in uterus, Gels.
— — — vagina, during colic, Murex.
Herpes on genitals, Dulc. Petr.
Induration of uterus, Alnus. *Aur. Bell. Chin.* Iod. Mgn-m. Murex. Ntr-c. Pallad. Plat. Sep.
— — ovaries, Con.
— — right, Pallad.
— — vagina, Bell. Calc. Chin. Clem. Con. Ferr. Lyc. Mgn-m. Merc. Petr. Puls. Sep. Sulph.
Inflammation of labia, Acon. *Ambr.* Calc. Carb-vea. Con. Creos. Ferr. Kali-c. Merc. Nitr-ac. Nux. *Sep.* Staph. Sulph. *Thuj.*
— — left, Bry.
— — ovaries, Acon. Actae-r. Ambr. Ant. *Canth.* Chin. Iod. Merc. Staph.
— — right, Aesc-hipp. Apis. Ham.
— — left, Lil-tigr.
— — uterus, *Acon.* Apis. Ars. Aur. *Bell.* Bry. *Canth.* Carb-an. Cham. *Coloc.* Con. Hyosc. Iod. Kali-c. Lac-can. Lach. Lyc. Merc. *Nux. Puls.* Rhus. Sec-c. Sep. Sil. Sulph. Verat.
— — after parturition, Sabin.
— of vagina, Cocc-c. Merc.

21. FEMALE SEXUAL ORGANS.

Itching, Agar. *Ambr.* Amm-c. Ars. Calad. Calc. *Carb-veg.* Caust. Coff. *Con.* Creos. Croton. Elaps. Eupat. Kali-c. Lac-can. Lach. Lyc. Merc. *Ntr-m* Ntr-s. Nitr-ac. *Petr. Sep. Sil.* Staph. Sulph. Tarant. Thuj. Zinc.
— of ovaries, Prun.
— voluptuous, Coff. Creos. Plat.
Labor pains, (compare Throes.)
Leucorrhœa, in general, Acon. Agn. Aloe. *Alum.* Ambr. *Amm-c.* Amm-m. Anac. Ant. Ars. Bar-c. Bell. Borax. Bov. *Calc.* Cannab. Canth. Caps. *Carb-an. Carb-veg Caust.* Cham. *Chin.* Cinnab. *Cocc.* Coff. *Con.* Cop. *Creos.* Dros. Ferr. Gels. Gran. *Graph.* Hep. Hydrast. Hyper. Igt. Iod. Kali-c. Kali-jod. Lach. Laur. Lept. Lil-tigr. *Lyc. Mgn-c. Mgn-m.* Mgn-s. *Merc.* Merc-cor. Mez. Millef. Murex. Mur-ac. *Ntr-c.* Ntr-m. Ntr-s. Nicc. Nitr-ac. Nitr. Nux. Ol-an. Petr. *Phosp.* Phosp-ac. Phyt. Plat. Plb. Pod. Prun. *Puls.* Ran-b. Ran-sc. Rat. Ruta. *Sabin.* Sass. Sec-c. *Sep. Sil.* Stann. Stront. *Sulph.* Sulph-ac. Tabac. Thuj. Viol-tr. Zinc.
— acrid, *Alum.* Amm-c. Anac. Ant. Ars. Borax. *Bov.* Carb-veg. Chin. *Con.* Creos. Ferr. Fluor-ac. Igt. Iod. Kali-jod. Lach. Lyc. Merc. Ntr-m. Nitr-ac. Phosp. Phosp-ac. Prun. Puls. Ran-b. Sabin. Sep. *Sil.* Sulph-ac. (compare Excoriating).
— albuminous. Amm-c. Amm-m. Borax. Bov. Mez. Petr. Plat.
— biting, smarting, Alum. Ant. Carb-an. Cham. Con. Hep. Laur. Mgn-c. Merc. Phosp. Sulph.
— blistering, Phosp.
— bloody, Ars. Bar-c. Chin. Cocc. Coff. Creos. Lyc. Murex. Nitr-ac. Sep. Sil. Sulph-ac. Tart. Zinc.
— bluish, Ambr.
— brown, Amm-m. Berb. Nitr-ac.
— burning, Amm-c. *Calc.* Canth. Carb-an. *Caust. Con.* Creos. Kali-c. Mgn-s. Phosp. Puls. Sulph. Sulph-ac.
— corroding, Ars. Creos. Iod. Kali-jod. Lyc Mez. Ruta. Sil. Sulph.
— — the linen, Iod.
— debilitating, Creos. Stann.
— excoriating, Alum. Amm-c. Anac. Ars. *Bov.* Carb-veg. Cham. Chin. Cocc. Con. Creos. Ferr. Igt. Kali-jod. Lyc. Merc. Mez. Phosp. Prun. Ran-b. Ruta. Sep. *Sil.* Sulph. Sulph-ac.
— fetid, Caps. Creos. Ntr-c. Nitr-ac. Nux. Sabin. Sep.
— flesh-colored (like the washings of meat), Alum. Cocc. Nitr-ac. Sep.
— glairy, Mez. Petr.
— greenish, Bov. Carb-veg. Lach. Merc. Murex. Ntr-m. Nitr-ac. Sep.
Leucorrhoea itching, Alum. Anac. *Calc.* Chin. Creos. Kali-c. Merc. Ntr-m. Phosp-ac. Sabin. Sep.
— jelly-like, transparent, Pallad.
— long continued, Creos. Mez.
— malignant, *Mez.*
— mild, Ferr. Puls. Ruta.
— milky, Amm-c. Calc. Carb-veg. Con. Creos. Ferr. Lam. Lyc. Phosp. Puls. Sabin. Sep. Sil. Sulph. Sulph-ac.
— mucus, Ambr. Amm-m. Bar-c. Borax. Bov. Calc. Cocc. Cocc-c. *Dict.* Graph. Kali-jod. Laur. Lach Mgn c. Mez. Nitr-ac. Nux. Ol-an. Plat. Pod. Sass. Seneg. Sep. Stann. Staph. Sulph. Sulph-ac. *Zinc.*
— ochre-colored, Phosp.
— painful, Sep. Sulph.
— painless, Amm-c. Calc. Carb-veg. Lam. Puls. Sil. Sulph.
— profuse, Agar. *Graph.* Iod. Lach. Lam. Lyc. Petr. Phosp.
— purulent, Chin. Cocc. Igt. Merc. Sep.
— putrid, smelling, Colch. Coloc. Creos. Lach. Ntr-c. Nitr-ac. Nux. Sabin. Sep.
— rasping, Alum. Hep.
— reddish, Lyc. Nitr-ac. Sep.
— ropy, Hydrast. Kali-b.
— salt, smarting like, Sulph.
— by shocks, discharged, Calc. Graph. Sil.
— stiffening the linen, Alum. Creos Lach. Nitr.
— suppressed, Sacch.
— thick, Ambr. Ars. Bov. Carb-veg. Mgn-s. Ntr-c. Ntr-m. Murex. Pod. Puls. Sabin. Tong. *Zinc.*
— thin, Graph. Kali-jod. Nicc. Nitr. Ol-an. Puls.
— tough, Acon. *Dict.*
— transparent, Alum. Ntr-m. Pallad. Pod. Stann.
— from uterus, thick, bloody, purulent, Cop.
— — vagina, Caps. Creos. Merc. Plb.
— viscous, Borax. Bov. Mez. Sabin. Stann.
— watery, Alum. Amm-c. Ant. Carb-an. Cham. Chin. Ferr. Graph. Kali-jod. Mgn-c. Mgn-m. Merc. Merc-cor. Mez. Murex. Nicc. Puls. Sep. Sil. Sulph-ac. Tabac.
— weakening, Stann.
— white, Borax. Gels. Graph. Lam. Mgn-c. Ntr-m. Nitr. Sulph.
— yellow, Acon. Alum. Ars. Carb-an. Carb-veg. Cham. Cinnab. Con. Creos. Fluor-ac. Hydrast. Kali-b. Kali-c. Kali-ferr-cyn. Kalm. Lyc Merc-cor. Ntr-c. Ntr-m. Nux. Phosp. Phosp-ac. Puls Sabin. Sep. Sil. Stann. Sulph.
— yellow staining, Carb-an. Nux. Prun.
— in day-time only, Alum. Plat. Sep.

21. FEMALE SEXUAL ORGANS.

Leucorrhœa before full moon, aggravated, Lyc.
— morning, when rising, Carb-an.
— at night, Ambr. Caust. Merc. Nitr-ac.
— abdomen, pain in, preceded by, Con. Kali-c. Lyc. Mgn-m. Merc. Ntr-c. Ntr-m. Puls. Rat. Sil. Sulph. Zinc.
— with ammorrhœa, Apis. Ruta. *Sabin.*
— before catamenia, Alum. Bar-c. *Calc.* Carb-veg. Chin. Cocc. Creos. Graph. Lach. Pallad. Puls. Ruta. Sep. Sulph. Zinc.
— during catamenia, Alum. Graph. Iod. Puls. Zinc.
— after catamenia, Alum. Bov. Cocc. Creos. Graph. Merc. Nitr-ac. Pallad. Phosp-ac. Puls. Ruta. Sulph. Tabac. Zinc.
— — cessation of catamenia, Ruta. Sang.
— in place of catamenia, Cocc.
— at climacteric period, Sang.
— after coition, Ntr-c.
— colic, preceded by, Mgn-c. Mgn-m.
— when exercising, Mgn-m. Mgn-s.
— by hysteric cramps, preceded, Igt. Mgn-c. *Mgn-m.*
— after a meal, Cham.
— in morning, when rising, Carb-an.
— when standing, Ars. Carb-an.
— with stool, Murex. Tong.
— after stool, Mgn-m.
— before urinating, Creos.
— after urinating, Amm-m. Canth. Nicc. Sep.
— — ceasing, Ntr-c.
— when walking, Ntr-m. Sass. Stront. Tong.
— — passing water, Amm-m. Calc. Sil. Tong.
— — wind, Ars.
Leucorrhœa, attended by, abdomen, distention of, Amm-m. Graph. Sep.
— — painfulness of, Lyc. Puls. Sil.
— — labor-like pains in, Dros.
— — spasms in, Igt. Mgn-c. Mgn-m.
— colic, Alum. Amm-m. Bell. Con. Kal-c. Lyc. Mgn-c. Mgn-m. Merc. Ntr-c. Ntr-m. Puls. Rat. Sil. Sulph. Zinc.
— countenance, yellow, Ntr-m.
— debility, Creos.
— diarrhœa, Ntr-m.
— dreams, lascivious, Petr.
— fatigue, Alum.
— genitals, stitches in, Sep.
— headache, Ntr-m.
— legs, soreness of, Mgn-s.
— navel pain about, Amm-m.
— sacral region, pain in, Kali-b. Kali-c. Mgn-s. Nitr.
— shooting in parts, Sep.
— trembling, Alum.
— vagina, pressing in, Cinnab.
— weakness in back, Graph.
Lochia, abnormal, Chin. Hep.

— turning bloody again, Cauloph. Rhus. Sec-c.
— blackish, clotted, Plat.
— blackish, lumpy, offensive and exoriating, Creos.
— too copious, Bry. Calc. Carb-an. Coff. Croc. Hep. Milleff. Plat. Puls. Rhus. Sec-c.
— dark, stringy, Croc.
— fetid, Acon. Bapt. Bell. Carb-an. Creos. Nux. Rhus. Sec-c. Sep. Stram.
— too long-continued, Calc. Cauloph. Chin. Rhus. Sec-c.
— milky, Calc.
— too small, Acon. Bell.
— suppressed, Acon. Bell. Bry. Cham. Coloc. Dulc. Hyosc. Millef. Nux. Op. Plat. Puls. Sec-c. Verat. Zinc.
— — after vexation, Coloc.
— — with delirium, Verat.
— too thin, Carb-an.
Lump, hard, in neck of uterus, ulcerative, pain during coition, Creos.
Menopause, Cocc. Igt. Lach. Puls. Sang. Sep. Sulph. Sulph-ac.
Metrorrhagia, Acon. Aloe. Amm-c. Anac. Ant. Apis Apocyn. Arg-n. Arn. Ars. *Bell. Bry. Calc.* Canth. Carb-veg. *Cauloph.* Caust. *Cham.* Chin. Cina. Cinnam. Cocc. *Coff. Cop.* Creos. *Croc. Diad.* Erig. *Ferr.* Ham. *Hyosc.* Igt. Iod. *Ip.* Led. Lyc. Mgn-m. Merc. *Millef.* Murex. Ntr-c. Ntr-ac. Nux-m. *Nux.* Phosp. *Plat.* Prun. *Puls.* Rat. Rhus. Ruta. *Sabin.* Sang. Scill. *Sec-c.* Sep. *Sil. Stram.* Stront. Sulph. Sulph-ac. Trill. Vinca.
— after abortion, *Plat.*
— of black blood, Arn. Bell. Cham. Chin. Croc. Ferr. Igt. Plat.
— — pale blood, with fainting and convulsions, Hyosc.
— — thin blood, becoming more watery, the longer it lasts, Prun.
— flow intermits, then freshens up, (chronic hemorrhage), Creos. Sulph.
— discharge now stopping, then stronger again, Puls.
— in aged females, Merc.
— after abuse of chamomilla, Chin. Igt.
— at climacteric, Ustil.
— after delivery, Bell. Cham. Chin. *Cinnam.* Croc. Ip. Nux. Phosp-ac. *Plat. Sabin.*
— when exercising, discharge, Sec-c.
— after every stool, Amm-m. Ind.
— with abdomen, distension of, Hep.
— — painfulness of. Ferr. Sabin.
— — bearing down towards genitals, *Bell. Cham.* Nitr-ac. Rhus. Sabin.
— — congestion of the blood and red face, *Ferr.*
— — breathing oppressed, Ip.

21. FEMALE SEXUAL ORGANS.

Metrorrhagia with excitability of sexual system, Plat.
— — fainting and convulsions, Chin.
— — with headache and pain in sacral region, Bell. Bry.
— — — spasms, Hyosc.
— — unconsciousness, heavy sleep and tingling in limbs, Sec-c.
Moles, escape of, Canth.
Neuralgia, vaginae, Bell. Calc. Canth. Chin. Creos. Ferr. Kali-c. Lyc. Merc. Nux. Puls. Rhus. Sep. Sulph. Thuj.
— uteri, Bell. Carb-an. Cham. Con. Croc. Ferr. Gels. Kali-c. Nux. Op. Plat. Puls. Flus. Sabad. Sec-c. Sep. Sulph.
Nymphomania Ant. Bell. Calc. Canth. Carb-veg. Chin. Coff. Graph. Grat. Lach. Merc. Mosch. Murex. Ntr-c. Ntr-m. Nux. Op. Phosp. Plat. Puls. Sabin. Sil. Stram. Verat. Zinc.
Ovaries, pain in, Apis. Coloc. Lach. Pod.
— — — as if dislocated, tender on pressure, Apis.
Ovaritis, Pod. (compare Inflammation.)
— right, Aesc-hip. Apis. Bell. Ham. Lac-can. Lyc. Pallad.
— left, Arg. Caps. Graph. Lac-can. Lach. Led. Thuj. Zinc. Zizia.
Painfulness, Staph.
Placenta adherent, Actea-r. Bell. Canth. Cris. Puls. Sabin. Sec-c. Sep.
Pressing down, towards genitals, Aloe. Ant. Apis. Arg. Asa-f. Bell. Borax. Calc. Cham. Chin. Cocc. Con. Croc. Graph. Hydroph. Ip. Kali-c. Lac-can. Lyc. Mang. Mgn-c. Mosch. Murex. Mur-ac. Ntr-c. Ntr-m. Nitr-ac. Nux. Pallad. Plat. Rat. Rhus. Sabin. Sep. Sulph. Tarant. Thuj. Tilia. Ustil. Zinc.
— as if menses about to commence, Cina. Croc. Kali-c. Lam. Mgn-c. Mosch. Mur-ac. Puls Sep. Stann. Tilia.
— from groins through hip to back, Plat.
— when standing, Bell. Rhus.
— with oppression of breathing, Sep.
Prolapsus, of uterus, Alum. Arg. Aur. Bell. Calc. Canth. Carb-an. Cham. Con. Creos Croc. Ferr. Ferr-jod. Ferr-m. Hydroph. Iod. Kali-c. Lac-can. Lil-tigr. Merc. Millef. Murex. Nux-m. Nux. Op. Pallad. Plat. Pod. Puls. Rhus. Sabin. Sec-c. Sep. Stann. Sulph.
— after lifting, Agar.
— with pain in sacrum, Pod
— of vagina, Creos. Ferr. Merc. Nux. Ocim-c. Sep.
Pulsating in uterus and ovaries, Cact.
Pulsative pains, Merc. Murex.
Pus discharge, from parts, Calc.
Pustules, black, on pudenda, Bry.
Puerperal fever, Acon. Arn. Ars. Bell. Bry. Cham. Coff. Coloc. Hyosc. Ip. Merc. Nux. Plat. Puls. Rhus. Sec-c. Stram.

Tilia. Verat.
— with fulness of the mammae, Bry.
Redness of pudenda, Ars. Calc. Merc. Sep. Tilia.
Rigidity of, os uteri, Acon. Actea-r. Bell. Cauloph. Gels. Lob.
— cervex uteri, Gels.
Rubbing, pain in right ovary, ameliorated by, Pallad.
Scirrhus of uterus, Aur. Bell. Carb-an. Chin. Clem. Cocc. Con. Mgn-m. Phosp. Rhus. Sep. Staph.
Sensitiveness, tenderness, Ambr. Arn. Canth. Coff. Plat. Puls. Rhus. Sec-c. Staph. Tilia. Zinc.
— painful, Merc. Nux. Staph.
Sexual passion, excited, Ars. Bell. Canth. Chin. Cinnam. Coff. Grat. Lac-can. Lach. Mosch. Murex. Nux. Plat. Sabin. Verat. Zinc.
— — in lying-in women, Bell. Chin. Grat. Plat. Verat. Zinc.
— diminished, Bar-c. Bell. (compare Aversion to coition and Sect. 20.)
Sinking down, as if uterus were, with pain and weakness, Pallad.
Smarting pain, Cham. Creos. Ferr-m. Kali-b. Staph. Thuj.
Softness of uterus, Op.
Soreness (excoriation) of pudenda, Ambr. Berb. Carb-veg. Caust. Graph. Hep. Kali-b. Lyc. Meph. Merc. Ntr-c. Nitr-ac. Petr. Sep. Sulph. Thuj. Tilia.
— — and moisture, Petr.
— of uterus, Tilia.
— between the thighs, Amm-c. Caust. Creos. Graph. Hep. Lyc. Ntr-c. Nitr-ac. Petr. Sep.
— and rawness of vagina, Kali-b.
— pain, as from excoriation, Berb. Ferr-m. Rhus. Thuj.
Spasms of vagina, Bell. Cocc. Igt. Merc. Nux. Plat. Puls
Spasmodic pain, in genitals, Creos. Igt. Nux. Thuj.
Squeezing pain in cavity of pelvis, Bar-m.
Sterility, Agn. Amm-c. Borax. Calc. Cannab. Caust. Cic. Con. Croc. Dulc. Ferr. Filix. Graph. Hyosc. Merc. Ntr-c. Ntr-m. Phosp. Plat. Ruta. Sep. Sulph. Sulph-ac.
— from excessive sexual desire, Phosp.
— with want of sexual desire, Ang.
— with catamenia too copious, Calc. Merc. Millef. Ntr-m. Phosp. Sulph. Sulph-ac.
— — early, Calc. Ntr-m. Sulph. Sulph-ac.
— — retarded, Caust. Graph. Phosp.
— — too small, Amm-c.
— — suppressed, Agn. Con.
Stinging, stitches, Apis. Bell. Borax. Calc. Cannab. Con. Creos. Kali-c. Merc. Murex. Nitr-ac. Pallad. Phosp. Rhus. Sep. Staph. Thuj.

21. FEMALE SEXUAL ORGANS.

Stinging from abdomen to vagina, Ars.
— — perineum, deep into genitals, Berb.
— deep into vagina, Sabin.
— in vagina, upwards, Berb. Creos. Mur-ac. Nitr-ac. Phosp. Rhus. Sep.
Stitches in ovaries, Ambr. Bry. Coloc. Lil-tigr. Staph.
Swelling of genitals, Kali-b. Meph.
— — labia maj., Merc-acet. Pod.
— — os uteri, Canth. Iod. Nux. Sec-c.
— — ovaries, Apis. Iod. Graph.
— — — right, Pallad.
— — — left, Graph. Lach.
— — pudenda, Ambr. Amm-c. Bry. Calc. Cannab. Carb-veg. Lach. Meph. Merc. Ocim-c. Sec-c. Sep. Thuj.
— — vagina, Merc.
Tearing in genitals, *Phosp.*
Tenderness of vagina, Berh. Bry. Calc. Ferr. Graph. Merc. Nux. Plat. Sec-c. Thuj.
Tension in uterus, as from a tight bandage, Hyper.
Tingling, pricking, voluptuous, *Plat.*
Throes, labor pains.
— like labor pains, Asa-f. Bell. Cham. Cina. Creos. Iod. Kali-c. Ntr-m. Plat. Puls. Sec-c. Sep. Sulph-ac.
— from back to thighs, Kali-c.
— ceasing, Arn. *Bell.* Borax. Camph. Carb-veg. Cham. Chin. Cocc. Graph. Igt. *Kali-c.* Lyc. Mgn-m. Ntr-m. Nux. *Op.* Plat. *Puls.* Ruta. *Sec-c.* Sep. Sulph. Thuj.
— distressing, Aur. Bell. *Cham. Coff.* Con. *Gels. Kali-c.* Lyc. Nux. Sec-c. *Sep.*
— drawing into legs, Aloe.
— false, *Bell.* Kali-c. Nux-m. Nux. *Op. Puls.*
— too long, Puls.
— running upwards, Gels.
— spasmodic, *Bell.* Caust. Cham. Cocc. Cupr. Gels. *Hyosc.* Igt. Ip. Kali-c. Nux-m. Nux. *Op. Puls.* Sec-c. Sep. Stann.
— spasms instead of, Bell. Cham. Cic. Hyosc. Igt.
— desire for stool with every pain, Nux.
— too strong, Acon. Bell. Cham. *Coff.* Con. Nux. *Puls.* Sec-c.
— suppressed and wanting, Cact. Carb-veg. *Op.* Puls. *Sec-c.*
— weak, powerless, *Actea-r.* Bell. Cannab. Carb-veg. *Cauloph.* Cham. Chin. *Gels.* Kali-c. Ntr-m. Nux-m. Nux. Op. *Puls.* Ruta. Sec-c. Sep. Thuj.
Throbbing in uterus, Murex.
Ulcers, *Arg-n. Ars. Asa-f.* Bell. Bry. Calc. Carb-veg. Con. Hep. *Lach. Lyc. Merc.* Nitr-ac. *Nux.* Phosp. Phosp-ac. *Puls.* Rhus. Sep. *Sil.* Staph. Sulph. Thuj. (compare Sect. 20.)

Uterine cramps, Caust. Cocc. *Con. Igt. Mgn-m.* Ntr-m. Nux. Sep. Stann.
— extending to thighs, Mgn-m.
Uterus feels as if open, Lach.
— pain in, from pessary, Nux-m.
Varices on pudenda, Calc. Carb-veg. Lyc. Nux. Zinc.
Voluptuous itching and tingling, Coff. Creos. Plat.
Warts on os uteri, Sec. *Thuj.*
Weight at uterus, at vagina, after hysteric attacks, Elaps.
Wind discharge from vagina, Brom. Lac-can. Lyc. Nux-m. Nux. Sang.
Catamenia, too copious, Acon. Agar. Aloe. Ambr. Amm-c. Amm-m. *Ars.* Bar-c. *Bell.* Borax. Bov. Brom. Bry. *Calc.* Cannab. *Canth. Carb-veg. Caust. Chelid. Chin.* Cina. Cocc-c. Creos. Croc. Cycl. Diad. Dulc. Ferr. Fluor-ac. Grat. Gum-gut. *Hyosc.* Igt. Iod. Ip. Kali-jod. Lachn. Laur. Led. *Lyc.* Mgn-c. *Mgn-m.* Mgn-s. *Merc.* Merc-cor. Millef. *Mosch.* Murex. Mur-ac. Ntr-c. Ntr-m. Nitr-ac. Nitr. Nux-jug. Nux-m. *Nux. Op. Phosp.* Phyt. *Plat.* Prun. *Rat.* Rhod. Rhus. Ruta. Sabad. *Sabin. Samb. Sec-c.* Sep. *Sil.* Spong. Stann. Stram. *Sulph. Sulph-ac.* Tabac. *Verat.* Vinca. Zinc.
— — mania from, Sep.
— — when walking in afternoon, Ntr-s.
— too early, Aloe. Alum. *Ambr.* Amm-c. *Amm-m.* Arn. *Ars.* Asa-f. Asar. Bar-m. Bell. Borax. *Bov.* Brom. Bry. Bufo. *Calc. Canth. Carb-an. Carb-veg. Caust. Cham.* Chin. *Cina.* Clem. *Cocc.* Cocc-c. Colch. Coloc. Con. Creos. *Croc.* Cycl. Diad. Ferr. Fluor-ac. Graph. Grat. Gum-gut. Hipp. Hyosc. Igt. Ind. Iod. Ip. Kali-b. *Kali-c.* Kalm. Lach. Lachn. Lam. Laur. Led. Lyc. Mgn-c. *Mgn-m. Mgn-s.* Mang. Merc-cor. Mez. Mosch. Mur-ac. Ntr-c. *Ntr-m.* Nicc. Nitr-ac. Nitr. Nux-jug. Nux-m. *Nux. Ol-an.* Par. *Petr. Phell. Phosp.* Phyt. *Plat.* Prun. Puls. Rat. *Rhod. Rhus* Ruta. Sabin. Sang. Sass. Sep. *Sil.* Spong. Staph Stront. *Sulph. Sulph-ac.* Tart. Thuj. Tong. *Verat.* Zinc. Zing.
— only in daytime, Caust. Puls.
— irregular, Cocc. Iod. Nux-m. Ruta.
— during lactation, Calc. Pallad. Sil.
— only when moving about, Lil-tigr.
— — asleep, Mgn-c.
— too late, Acon. Ang. Amm-c. Bell. Bov. Carb-an. *Caust.* Chelid. Cic. Cocc. Con. Cupr. Dros. Dulc. Ferr. *Graph.* Hep. Hyper. Igt. *Iod. Kali-c.* Kalm. Lach. Lith. Lyc. *Mgn-c.* Mgn-s. Merc. Ntr-c. *Ntr-m. Ntr-s.* Nicc. Nitr. Nitr-ac. Nux-m. Petr. Phosp. *Puls.* Sabad. Sabin. Sass. Sep. Sil. Stront. Sulph. Sulph-ac. Tabac. Tereb. Tilia. Valer. Zinc.

21. FEMALE SEXUAL ORGANS.

Catamenia, too late in ill-tempered fat women, Dulc.
— — long, *Acon.* Asar. Bar-c. Bry. Canth. Chelid. Chin. Coff. Creos. Croc. Cupr. Diad. Ferr. Grat. Igt. Kali-c. Lyc. Merc. Mez. *Ntr-m.* Ntr-s. Nux-jug. *Nux. Phosp. Plat.* Puls. *Rat.* Rhus. Sabad. Sabin. *Sec-c.* Sep. *Sil.* Sulph-ac.
— ceasing on lying down, Cact.
— more profuse in morning, less at night, Bov.
— more profuse at night, Amm-m.
— regular periods, at, but lasting only one hour, Euphr.
— retarded, first time in young females, Agn. Amm-c. Bry. *Calc. Caust.* Chelid. Cocc. Con. Dig. Dulc. Ferr. *Graph. Kali-c.* Lach. Lyc. Mgn-c. Ntr-m. Petr. *Puls.* Sabin. Sep. Sil. *Sulph.* Valer.
— too weak, scanty, *Alum. Amm-c.* Asa-f. Bar-c. Berb. Bov. Carb-veg. Caust. Cic. *Con.* Cocc. Croton. Dulc. Ferr. *Graph.* Hep. *Kali-c.* Kalm. Lach. Lam. Lith. *Lyc.* Mgn-m. Mgn-s. Mang. Merc. *Ntr-m.* Ntr-s. Njcc. Nux. Ol-an. Petr. *Phosp.* Puls. Sabad. Sacch. Sass. Sep. *Sil.* Staph. *Sulph.* Tereb. Thuj. Tong.
— — with bleeding of anus, Lach.
— too short, Alum. Amm-c. Bar-c. Berb. Bov. Con. Dulc. Graph. Merc. Nicc. Phosp. Plat. Puls. Sulph. Stront. Tilia.
— suppressed, amemorrhoea, Acon. Actea-r. *Agn.* Aletris. Amm-c. Ars. Bar-c. Bell. Berb. Brom. *Bry.* Calc. Caust. Cham. Chin. Cocc. *Con.* Cupr. Dros. *Dulc.* Ferr. *Gels.* Glon. *Graph.* Hyosc. Iod. *Kali-c.* Kali-jod. Kalm. Lach. Lil-tigr. *Lyc.* Mgn-c. Mgn-m. Merc. Mez. Millef. *Ntr-m. Nitr-ac. Nux-m.* Nux. Op. Phosp. Plat. Pod. *Puls. Rhod.* Sabad. Sabin. Sang. Sec-c. *Sep. Sil.* Staph. Stram. *Sulph.* Valer. *Verat. Zinc.*
— — for a long time, *Lyc.* Sil.
— — from a cold, Dulc. Puls.
— — after fright, Acon. Lyc.
— — in plethoric individuals, Calc.
— — — young people, with bearing down in hypogastric, and sacral regions, pain from motion, and ameliorated in lying down, Pod.
— — with pain in abdomen, Agn. Mgn-c.
— — — backache, Ars.
— — — bleeding at anus, Graph.
— — — chilliness and pain in back. Puls.
— — — congestion to head, Apis.
— — — convulsions, Gels.
— — — dropsy, Kali-c.
— — — epistaxis, *Bry.* Cact. Puls.
— — — haemorrhoids, Phosp. Sulph.
— — — milk in breast, Lyc. Puls.
— — — painfulness of breast, and genitals, Zinc.
— — — restlessness, Nicc.
— — — toothache, Lach.
Before catamenia, disorders in general, Alum. Iod.
— abdominal cramps, Carb-veg. Cham. Hyosc. Ol-an. Sulph.
— — distension, Creos.
— — heaviness, Puls.
— — pains, Alum. Amm-c. Bar-c. Bell. Calc. Caust. Cham. Hyosc. Lach. Mgn-c. Nitr. Plat. Puls. Sep.
— — swelling and bloatedness, Cycl. Lyc.
— anorexia, Bell.
— anxiety, anxiousness, Amm-c. Cocc. Nitr-ac. Strann.
— asthma, Sulph.
— back, pain in, Asar. Borax. Nitr. Nux-m. Spong.
— blood, congestion of, Cupr. Merc.
— chilliness, Calc. Kali-c. Lyc. Puls.
— constipation, Grat. Sil.
— cough, Sulph.
— — fatiguing, Graph.
— cramps, hysteric, *Hyosc.*
— diarrhoea, Apis. Bov. Lach. Sil. Verat.
— dolefulness, *Ntr-m.* Stann.
— dreaming much, Alum.
— epistaxis, Lach. Sulph. Verat.
— eructations, Creos. Lach. Mgn-c.
— eruption, itching, on forehead, Sass.
— face pale, Puls.
— flatulence, Cocc. Lac-can.
— genitals, contraction in, Chin.
— — chafed, Sep.
— — — thighs, Lac-can. Sil.
— — itching, Sulph.
— — pain in, Chin. Plat.
— — pressure in, Plat.
— giddiness, Cact. Kali-b. Lach. Puls. Verat.
— groins, pain in, Tart.
— gums swollen, Bar-c.
— headache, Alum. Calc. Carb-veg. Cupr. Ferr. Gels. Lach. Ntr-c. Ntr-m. Nux-m. Puls. *Sulph. Verat.*
— head congestion to, Hipp-m. Merc.
— — heat in, Con.
— head, tearing in forehead, Cinnab.
— hearing, hardness of, Creos.
— heart palpitation of, Cupr. Iod. Spong.
— — pains at, Lith.
— heat, dry, Merc.
— hunger, Mgn-c.
— hysteric, fits, Creos. *Hyosc.*
— irritability, Creos. Ntr-m.
— itching of vulva, Carb-veg. Merc.
— labor-like pains, Cycl. Mosch. Plat.
— langor, Iod. Nux-m.
— to laugh, disposition, Hyosc.
— legs, heavy, Bar-c.
— leucorrhoea, Alum. Bar-c. *Calc.* Carb-veg. Chin. Puls.
— liver, pain in, Con. Nux-m. Puls.

21. FEMALE SEXUAL ORGANS.

Before catamenia, malar bone, pain in, Stann.
— mammae, painful, Calc. Con.
— — swollen, Calc. Kali-c. Murex.
— melancholy, Lyc.
— nausea, Puls.
— night-mare, Sulph-ac.
— night-sweat, Verat.
— pains in general, Alum.
— — — left ovary and iliac region, Thuj.
— perspiration, Thuj. Verat.
— rash, Dulc.
— restlessness, Con. Creos. Sulph.
— ringing in ears, Ferr.
— sacral region, pain in, Amm-c. Bar-c. Caust. Lach. Mgn-c. Nux-m. Nitr. Puls.
— sadness, Caust. Lyc. Ntr-m. Stann.
— sight confused, Bell.
— stomach, pain in, Lach. Nux-m. Puls. Sulph.
— stretching, Puls.
— — tinkling in ears, Ferr
— toothache, Bar-c. Sulph.
— ulcers, bleeding, Phosp.
— urethra, discharge from, Lach.
— urinate, frequent desire to, Kali-jod. Phosp. Sulph.
— vexed mood, Ntr-m.
— vomiting, Creos. Puls.
— water-brash, Nux-m.
— weakness, Iod. Nux-m.
— weeping, Con. Phosp.
— yawning, Puls.
At commencement of catamenia, abdominel pain, Graph. Lyc.
— back, pain in, Phosp.
— chest, pain in, Lach.
— chills, Verat.
— coldness of body, Sil.
— colic, commencing in left ovary, Lach.
— — commencing in right ovary, Apis.
— cramps, Plat. Zinc.
— diarrhœa, nausea, chilliness, Verat.
— furor, Acon.
— right groin, soreness in, and urging to urinate, Sass.
— heart, pain at, Lith.
— itching in old herpes, Carb-veg
— langor, Phell.
— legs, heavy and sore, Lach. Phell.
— nausea, Verat.
— sacral region, pain in, Asar. Lach.
— sadness, Ntr-m.
— urinate, frequent urging to, Kali-jod.
— vomiting, Phosp.
During catamenia, abdominal cramps, Amm-c. Cham. Chin. *Cocc. Con.* Cupr. *Graph.* Hipp-m. Igt. Lach. Mgn-m. Ntr-m. Nitr-ac. Nux. Ol-an. Op. Plat. *Puls.* Sep. Sulph.
— — cutting, Amm-m. Bar-c. Bell. Calc. Cannab. Carb-veg. Caust. Con. Kali-b. Phosp. Plat. Sil.
— — digging, Ntr-s.

— distension, Alum. Berb. Carb-an. Cocc. Lachn. Mgn-c. Ntr-c. Nicc. Nitr-ac. Zinc.
— — fermentation, Phosp.
— — pain, *Alum. Amm-c. Amm-m.* Bar-c. Bell. Bov. Brom. *Calc.* Carb-veg. Caust. Cocc. Con. Creos. Graph. Igt. Jatr. Kali-c. Lach. Laur. Lyc. Mgn-c. Merc. Millef. Mosch. Ntr-c. Ntr-s. Nicc. Nitr. Nux. Ol-an. Phosp. Plat. Puls. Rat. Sass. Sil. Stann. Stram. Stront. Sulph. Sulph-ac. Zinc.
— — tension, Nicc.
— — anus, bleeding, Amm-m. Graph. Hydroph.
— — soreness, Berb.
— anxiety, Bell. Igt. Kali-jod. Merc. Ntr-m. Nitr-ac. Sil. Zinc.
— aversion to life, Berb.
— back, pain in, Aloe. Amm-c. *Amm-m.* Berb. Brom. Calc. Carb-an. Carb-veg. Caust. Kali-c. Kalm. Lyc. Mgn-c. Mgn-m. Mgn-s. Nicc. Nitr. Phosp. Pod. Prun.
— — griping, Bell. Calc. Carb-veg. Phosp.
— beaten, pain as if, Berb. Bry. Graph. Nux-m. Nux. Sep.
— blood, congestion to head, Bell. Calc. Cham. Chin. Cinnab. Glon. Mgn-c. Sulph.
— buzzing in ears, Verat.
— catarrh, Graph.
— cheek swollen, Graph.
— chest, congestion to, Glon.
— — cramps in, Chin.
— — pain in, Berb. Graph. Puls.
— chills, Amm-c. Berb. Carb-an. Cast. Creos. Graph. Kali-jod. Mgn-c. Ntr-c. Ntr-m. Ntr-s. Nux. Phosp. Puls. Sep. Sulph. Verat. Zinc.
— consciousness, loss of, Chin.
— constipation, Creos. Kali-c. Ntr-s. Sil.
— coryza, Graph. Kali-c.
— cough, Coff. Zinc.
— — fatiguing, Graph.
— delirium, Hyosc. Lyc.
— diarrhœa, Alum. Amm-c. Amm-m. Bov. Caust. Creos. Kali-jod. Mgn-c. Plat. Verat.
— dolefulness, Sep.
— dreaming much, Alum.
— earache, Aloe. Kali-c.
— epilepsy, Arg-n. Sulph.
— epistaxis, Lach. Ntr-s. Sep. Sulph. Verat.
— eruption between legs, Kali-c. Sil.
— exhaustion, Berb.
— eyes burning of, Nicc.
— — convulsion of, Chin.
— eyelids, upper, twitching of, Ntr-m.
— face bloated, Chin.
— — jaded, Berb.

21. FEMALE SEXUAL ORGANS.

During catamania, face pale, Cast. *Mgn-c.* *Mgn-m.* Puls.
— — yellow, Caust.
— faintness, Berb. Glon. Igt. Nux.
— feet, painful, Amm m.
— — swollen, Graph. Lyc.
— fever, Amm-c. Calc. Phosp.
— flatus, discharge of, Brom. Creos. Nicc.
— gaping, Bell.
— gastric complaints, Kali-c.
— genitals, burning, Sil.
— — chafing of, Sil.
— — fulness, sensation of, Puls.
— — pressing pain and urging sensation, Amm-c. Bell. Berb. Borax. Con. Kali-b. Mosch. Nitr-ac. Nux-m. Plat. Puls. Sep. Sil. Sulph.
— — sensitiveness, Plat.
— — stinging, Sulph-ac.
— — tearing, Amm-c.
— giddiness, Caust. Kali-b. Verat.
— groins, pain in, Borax.
— — pressure and stitches in, Borax.
— gums, affections of, Merc. Phosp.
— hæmoptisis, Phosp.
— headache, Alum. Berb. Borax. Bov. Bufo. Calc. Carb-veg. Cast. Creos. Glon. Graph. Hyosc. Igt. Kali-b. Kali-c. Lach. Laur. *Lyc.* Mgn-c. Ntr-c. Ntr-m. Ntr-s. Nux. Ol-an. Phosp. Plat Puls. Sep. Stann. Sulph. Verat.
— — amelioration of, Bell.
— — — by cold water, Aloe.
— head, heat of, Calc. Igt. Kali-jod.
— — heaviness in, Mgn-s.
— hearing, hardness of, Creos.
— heart, palpitation of, Alum. Igt. Iod. Phosp.
— hoarseness, Graph.
— humming in ears, Borax. Creos. Verat.
— hysterical spasms, Lach. Puls.
— inguina chafed, Bov. Sass.
— — pain in, Mgn-s.
— itching of body, Kali-c.
— — between thighs, Kali-c.
— — of vulva, Zinc.
— jerks, Chin.
— laughing, Hyosc.
— legs blue, from varices, Ambr.
— — heavy, Zinc.
— — painful, Ambr. Con. Spong. Stram.
— — pains drawing in, from navel, Nux-m.
— — weak, Sulph. Zinc.
— limbs, painful, Bry. Graph. Nux-m.Sep.
— — drawing in, Spong.
— — heaviness, Zinc.
— — sore, as if beaten, Phosp. Sep. Verat.
— lips, swelling of, Phosp.
— liver, pain in, Phosp-ac. Puls.
— to lie down, necessity, Amm-c. Igt.
— mammae, burning in, Ind.
— — swelling and soreness of, Con.
— melancholy, Ntr-m. Sep.
— nausea, Borax. Calc. Graph. Kali-b. Mgn-c. Nux. Puls.
— — with inclination to vomit, Verat.
— odor of body, goatish, Stram.
— right ovary, swollen, sharp, cutting, stinging pain in, Apis.
— pains in general, Alum. Ars. Canth. Croc. Mgn-c. Ntr-c.
— peevish, Berb.
— palate, burning in, as if sore or raw, Ntr-s.
— pale appearance of objects, Sil.
— photophobia, Igt.
— pressure towards the parts, Bell. Berb. Lach. Nitr-ac. Plat.
— — and stitches in groins, Borax.
— — crampy, relieved by pressure and lying down, Igt.
— quarrelsome, Amm-c.
— restlessness, Plat. Sulph.
— sacral region, pain in, *Amm-c.* *Amm-m.* Berb. Borax. Calc. Carb-veg. Cast. Creos. Kali-b. Lob. Lyc. Mgn-c. Mgn-m. *Ntr-c.* Nitr. Ol-an. Phosp. Prun. Puls Rat. Sass. Sulph.
— sadness, Amm-c. Mur-ac. Nitr-ac.
— scrobiculus, pit of stomach, pain in, Sass.
— senselessness, Chin.
— shivering, Berb.
— sleep, restless, Alum. Kali-c.
— soreness between the thighs, Graph. Kali-c.
— — excoriation, Bov. Sass.
— sour taste of mouth, Lyc.
— spasms, Sec-c.
— stinging, sharp, and cutting pain in swollen right ovary, Apis.
— stomach, cramp of, Puls.
— — to sacrum, pain, Borax.
— — pain in, Borax. Sass.
— stool, urging to, Op. Puls.
— sweat, Hyosc.
— — at night, Bell.
— syncope, fainting, Lyc.
— taciturnity, Mur-ac.
— talkativeness, Stram.
— taste salt, Merc.
— tearing pain through the whole body, Berb.
— teeth, dullness of, Merc.
— tibia, tearing pain in, Sep.
— thirst, Bell. Mgn-s. Verat.
— timid, low-spirited, Caust.
— tongue dry, burning, with deep-colored spots, Merc.
— toothache, Amm-c. Bov. Calc. Carb-veg. Cham. *Graph. Kali-c.* Lach. Laur. Mgn-s. Ntr-m. Nitr-ac. Phosp. Sep.
— tremor, Hyosc.
— ulcers, growing worse, Graph.
— to urinate, urging, Puls. Sass.

During catamenia urine, flow of, Hyosc.
— uterus, constriction as of, Murex.
— varies distended, Ambr.
— — pain in, Graph.
— vision obscured, Sep.
— — uncertainty of, and entire invisibility of right half of objects, second day of menses, Lith.
— vomiting, Amm-c. Amm-m. Carb-veg. Kali-c. Lyc. Phosp. Puls.
— — sour, Lyc.
— weakness, Alum. Borax. Bov. Calc. Carb-an. Cast. Caust. Graph. Igt. Iod. Kali-c. Lyc. Mgn-c. Mgn-m. Nicc. Nitr. Nux. Ol-an. Petr. Phell. Phosp.
— weariness of life, Berb.
— weight above pubes, Bar-c.
— whining, Lyc. Plat.
After catamenia, disorders in general, Borax. Iod.
— anxiety, Phosp.
— chills, Graph. Nux. Puls.

After catamenia colic, Borax. Graph. Kali-c. Lach. Puls.
— diarrhoea, Graph. Lach.
— eyes, livid-bordered, Phosp.
— face, livid, Verat.
— — pale, Puls.
— genitals, bearing down towards, Chin. Creos.
— gnashing the teeth, Verat.
— headache, Berb. Lach. Ntr-m. Puls.
— heart, palpitation of, Iod.
— itching of nose, Sulph.
— legs, lassitude of, Creos.
— leucorrhoea, Alum. Merc. Phosp-ac.
— nausea, Puls.
— sacral region, pain in, Puls.
— sobbing, and moaning, Stram.
— toothache, Calc. Mgn-c. Phosp.
— urinate, frequent desire to, Puls.
— uterine cramps, Chin.
— vertigo, Puls.
— weakness, Alum. Berb. Iod. Nux. Phosp. Plat.

22. Coryza.

Catarrh, epidemic, Anac. Ars. Bell. Bry.
Camph. Carb-veg. Caust. Chin. Creos.
Dulc. Lob. Lyc. *Merc.* *Nux.* Puls.
Rhus. Sabad. Seneg. Spig.
— of aged persons, Poth.
Coryza in general, Alum. *Amm-c. Amm-m.*
Chenop. Chin. Cocc. Diad. Dig. Graph.
Ip. Lyc. Mgn-c. Ntr-m. Nitr. Ol-an.
Petr. Sang. *Sulph.* Tereb. Teucr.
— of almost any kind, *Amm-c. Lyc.*
— chronic, long continued, Alum. Amm-c.
Anac. Calc. Canth. Coloc. Lyc. Ntr-c.
Puls. Sil.
— constant, Calc. Ntr-c. Sil.
— every other day, Ntr-c.
— suppressed, Ambr. Chin. Puls.
— incomplete, Lach,
— one sided, *Hep.*
— in morning, Dig.
— after a cold, Ntr-c. Spig.
— when becoming cold, Graph.
— indoors, Acon.
— from draft of air, Elaps. Ntr-c.
— after perspiration, relieved, Ntr-c.
— — becoming wet, Sep.
— with discharge, All-cep. Alum. Amm-m.
Anac. *Arg. Ars.* Aur. Bad. Bar-c. Bell.
Berb. Bov. Brom. Bry. Calc. Carb-an.
Carb-veg. Caust. Cham. Chenop.
Cimex. Cina. Cinnab. Clem.
Colch. Coloc. Con. Cor-r. Creos.
Croton. Cupr. Cycl. Dros. Dulc. Eupat.
Euphr. Fluor-ac. Gels. Graph. Hep.
Igt. Jac-cor. Kali-b. Kali-c. Kali-chl.
Lach. Lyc. Mgn-s. Meph. *Merc.*
Merc-cor. Merc-sulph. *Mez. Ntr-c.*
Ntr-m. Nitr-ac. Nux. Osm. Par. Petr.
Phell. Phosp. Phosp-ac. Plb. *Puls.*
Rhus. Rumex. Sabad. Scill. Selen.
Sep. *Sil.* Spig. Staph. *Sulph. Tart.*
Thuj. Zinc.
— alternating with dry coryza, Alum. Bell.
Euphr. Nux. Par.
— frequent, Sil. Thuj.
— one-sided, Alum. Bell. Rhod. Staph.
— worse in left nostril, Bad.
— relieving headache, Kali-b. Lach.
— — obstruction of nose, Sil.
— — — — ears, Lach.
— in daytime with dry coryza in evening,
Calc. Euphr. Nicc. Nux.

Coryza in morning, Berb. Nux. Puls. Scill.
— at noon, Cina.
— in evening, Carb-veg. Iod. Lach. Lith.
Rumex. Selen.
— at night, Caust.
— in open air, Coloc. Iod. Kali-b. Lith.
Merc. Plat. Puls. Sulph. Teucr. Thuj.
— — relieved, All-cep.
— — house, Nux.
— on coming into warm room, All-cep.
— without discharge, Acon. Alum. Ambr.
Amm-c. Amm-m. Aur. *Bry. Calc.*
Camph. *Caps. Carb-an.* Carb-veg.
Caust. Cham. Chelid. Chin. Creos.
Dulc. *Graph.* Hep. Igt. *Ip. Kali-c.*
Kali-chl. Lach. *Lyc.* Mgn-c. Mgn-m.
Mang. Merc. Mosch. *Ntr-m.* Ntr-s.
Nitr-ac. *Nux.* Ol-an. Op. *Par. Phosp.*
Plat. Psor. Rat. Sabin. Sacch. Samb.
Sass. Sep. Sil.; Spong. Stann. Sulph.
Sulph-ac. Thuj. Verb.
— alternating with discharge, Alum. Bell.
Euphr. Lach. Mgn-c. Nux. Par. Phosp.
Zinc.
— chronic, long-continued, *Bry. Ip.* Ntr-m.
— constant, Caust.
— one-sided, Alum. Lyc. Plat. Sabad. Sep.
Stann. Sulph-ac.
— in nursing, infants, Nux.
— — daytime, Caust.
— — morning, Calc. Carb-veg. Con. Iod.
Lach. Ntr-m. Nux.
— — evening, with discharge in daytime,
Euphr. Nux.
— at night, Calc. Caust. Mgn-m. Nicc.
Nux.
— in evening, Puls.
— — cold air, worse, Dulc.
— — open air, commencing to run, Thuj.
— — room; Sulph.
— attended by, back aching in, Cinnab.
Kali-c.
— beaten, pains as if, Hep.
— breathing obstructed, Bov. Calc.
Kali-c. Lact.
— catarrh, Acon. Graph. Igt. Mang. Spig.
Sulph.
— cheeks, cold, Ntr-c.
— chest oppression of, Calc. Graph.
— — pain in, Bell. Mgn-s. Mez. Ol-an.
Phosp-ac. Sang. Sulph. Zinc.

22. CORYZA.

Coryza, chest, rawness of, Carb-veg. Creos. Mez.
— chilliness, Arg-n. Chenop. Ntr-c. Puls. Spig. Sulph.
— coldness, felt up to knees, Chenop.
— cough, All-cep. Alum. Ambr. Bar-c. Bell. Canth. Euphr. Igt. Lyc. Ntr-c. Nitr-ac. Phosp-ac. Sang. *Spong.* Sulph. *Thuj.*
— — at night, Caust.
— diarrhœa, followed by, Sang.
— ear-ache, Lach.
— epistaxis, Puls.
— eye-brows, pressing in, Ars.
— eyes, protruded, Spig.
— fever, Lach. Merc. Ntr-c. Spig.
— gaping, Carb-an.
— griping, alternately, Calc.
— hands cold, Ntr-c.
— headache, Acon. All-cep. Arg-n. Ars. Bell. Bry. Calc. Caust. Cina. Euphr. Graph. Hep. Igt. Kali-c. Lach. Lyc. Merc. Nitr-ac. Nux. Sep. Spig. Thuj.
— head, confusion of, Bov. Euphr. Lyc. Phosp.
— — heat of, Lyc. Nux.
— — heaviness and weariness at vertex, forehead and eyes, Jac-cor.
— heart, anguish at, Anac.
— heat, All-cep. Spig.
— hoarseness, Ars. Carb-veg. Caust. Dig. Graph. Kali-c. *Nitr-c.* Ntr-ac. Petr. Phell. *Sep.* Spig. *Spong.* Sulph. Tellur. *Thuj.*
— hysterical excitement, Igt.
— lachrymation, Chin. Euphr. Lach. Sang. Staph.
— legs, straining in, Anac.
— limbs, pain in, Sep.
— lips, eruption on, Mez.
— to lie down, necessity, Graph.
— mouth, dryness, Nux.
— nausea, Graph.
— nose, bleeding at, Ars.
— — burning, Ars. Calad. Cina. Mez.
— — obstruction, Brom. Cham. Lach. Ntr-s. Nitr. Nux. Par. Phell. Rat. Rhod. Teucr. Tong.
— — one-sided, Rhod. Staph.
— — scraping, Nux.
— — tingling, Caps. Carb-veg. Tilia.
— nostrils, inflamed, Hep. Lach. Mang. Phell.
— — ulcerated, Brom. Calc. Cocc. Lach. Nitr-ac. Scill. *Staph.* Tart.
— phlegm, hawked up, Colch.
— sleeplessness, Ars.
— smell, loss of, Amm-m. Carb-an. *Mgn-m.* Mgn-s. Merc-cor. Mez. Ntr-m. Nitr. *Puls.* Rhod. Sulph-ac. Tart.
— — increase of, Kalm.
— stench, from the nose, Bell.
— taste, loss of, Mgn-m. Ntr-m. Puls. Psor. Rhod. Tart.

— thighs, lameness of, Cinnab.
— thirst, Diad. Ntr-c.
— throat, pain in, Nitr-ac. Phosp. Phosp-ac.
— — roughness in, Caust. Tilia.
— — scratching in, Hep. Nux.
— — sore, Laur.
— toothache, Chin. Lach.
— urine, flow of, Verat.
— voice, deep and hollow, Bar-c.
— — not clear, Mgn-s.
— to weep, disposition, Spig.
Dryness of the nose, Agar. Aloe. Ambr. Ars. Bar-c. *Bell.* Berb. Bry. *Calc. Cannab.* Cimex. Cocc-c. Cor-r. Croton. Dros. Dulc. Graph. Hipp-m. Hydroc-ac. Hyosc. Hyper. Igt. Kali-b. Kali-c. Lach. Lact. Lyc. Mgn-m. Meph. Merc. Mez. *Ntr-m.* Nicc. Nitr-ac. Nux-m. Nux. Ol-an. Op. Petr. *Phosp.* Phosp-ac. Rat. Rhod. Rhus. Sabad. Seneg. *Sep. Sil.* Spig. Sticta. *Sulph.* Tabac. Zinc. Zing.
— — right nostril, Gum-gut.
— chronic, Amm-c.
— painful, Calc. Sep.
— at night, Nux. Sil.
— on walking in open air, Ant.
— with heat in it, Cannab. Clem.
— — sneezing, Rat.
— sensation of, Anac. Con. Mez. Petr. Phosp. Seneg. *Sil. Verat.*
— compels blowing nose, there is no discharge, Kali-b. Lach. Sticta.
Fulness, sensation of, in nose, Laur. Par.
Grippy, influenza, Acon. Ars. Bell. Bry. *Camph.* Carb-veg. Caust. Chin. Creos. Lob. Lyc. *Merc. Nux.* Puls. *Rhus.* Sabad. Seneg. Spig.
Mucus (with or without coryza), quality,
— acrid, All-cep. Alum. Amm-c. Amm-m. *Ars.* Arum-trif. Cast. Ferr. Kali-b. Kali-jod. Lach. Lyc. Mgn-c. Mgn-m. Merc. Mez. Mur-ac. Nitr-ac. Nux. Phosp. Scill. Sil. (compare Excoriating.)
— — tears not, All-cep.
— biting, Ars.
— bloody, Arg. Ars. Caust. Chin. Clem. Cocc. Creos. Dros. Ferr. Ip. Kali-c. Lac-can. Laur. Lyc. Ntr-m. Nitr-ac. Nux. Par. Phosp. Phosp-ac. Puls. Sep. Sil. Sulph. Sulph-ac. Thuj. Zinc.
— brownish, Thuj.
— burning, All-cep. Alum. Amm-c. *Ars.* Arum-trif. Brom. Calc. Chenop. Cina. *Cinnab.* Con. Creos. Kali-jod. Merc. Mez. Puls. Sulph.
— dries quickly, forming scabs, Sticta.
— excoriating, All-cep. Amm-c. Amm-m. Ars. Arum-trif. Brom. Euphr. Gels. Kali-b. Kali-jod. Lac-can. Lyc. Mgn-s. *Merc.* Mez. Mur-ac. Nitr-ac. Sil. Staph. (compare Acrid.)

22. CORYZA.

Mucus fetid, Asa-f. Aur. Calc. Caust. Graph. Hep. Kali-c. Led. Mgn-m. Merc. Ntr-c. *Puls.* Rhus. Thuj.
— gelatinous, Selen.
— like glue, Merc-cor.
— gray, Ambr. Ars. Carb-an. Chin. Lyc. Nux. Sep.
— greenish, Ars. Asa-f. Arn. Berb. Borax. Carb-veg. Creos. Ferr. Graph. Kali-b. Kali-c. Led. Merc. Ntr-c. Nitr-ac. Nux. Par. Phosp. *Puls.* Rhus. Sep. Stann. Thuj.
— hard crusts, Alum. Bry. Ntr-c. Sep. Sil.
— hard plugs, forming, Sep. *Sil.*
— — elastic plugs (clinkers) Kali-b.
— — fetid clots from one nostril, Ntr-c.
— indurated, Bry. Con. Kali-b. Ntr-c. Sil. Stront. Sulph.
— purulent, Arg-n. Asa-f. Aur. Berb. *Calc.* Chin. Cina. Con. Creos. Ferr. Ip. Kali-c. Lach. Led. Lyc. Mgn-m. Ntr-c. Nitr. Nitr-ac. Petr. Phosp. Phosp-ac. Puls. Rhus. Sabin. Sep. Sil. Stann. Staph. Sulph.
— like pus, smelling, Gum-gut.
— putrid-smelling, Graph.
— reddish, Par.
— tallow, like, Cor-r.
— thick, All-cep. Amm-m. Bar-c. Carb-veg. Cor-r. Euphr. Graph. Kali-b. Lyc. Mur-ac. Ntr-c. Ntr-m. Phosp. Phosp-ac. Plb. Puls.
— — clean, if it ceases, headache, Kali-b.
— tough, viscid, Ars. Bov. Cannab. Canth. Cham. Colch. Dros. Kali-b. Mez. Mur-ac. Ntr-c. Par. Phosp. Plb. Ran-b. Samb. Selen. Stann.
— watery, Agar. All-cep. Amm-c. Amm-m. Ars. Bov. Brom. Carb-veg. Cast. Cham. Chenop. Cinnab. Colch. Elaps. Euphr. Gels. Graph. Kali-b. Kali-jod. Kobalt. Lac-can. Lach Mgn-s. Mgn-m. Merc. Mez. Mur-ac. Nitr-ac. Par. Plb. Puls. Ran-sc. Scill. Sulph. Sulph-ac. Tereb.
— white, Berb. Sabad. Spig.
— yellow, Ant. Ars. Berb. Bov. Calc. Cic. Cinnab. Creos. Graph. Kali-c. Lyc. Mgn-m. Mgn-s. Mez. Mur-ac. Ntr-c. Nitr-ac. *Phosp.* Puls. Sabin. Sang. Seneg. Sep. Spig. Stann. Sulph.
— yellow-green, Kali-b. Kali-c. Ntr-c. Par. Phosp. Puls. Thuj.
— discharge of, without coryza, Agar. Anac. Calc-phosp. Carb-veg. Cast. Caust. Creos. Croton. Euph. Euphr. *Graph.* Mgn-m. Merc-jod. Nitr-ac. Par. *Phosp.* Ran-b. Ran-sc. Rhus. Sulph-ac. Tereb. Therid.
— lumps of dirty yellow mucus from posterior nares, Cinnab.
— secretion increased, Bar-c. Brom.

Euphr. *Iod.* Phosp. Plb. Ran-sc. Rhod. Sabad. Spig.
— in open air, Rhod.
Obstruction of the nose, Alum. *Ambr.* Amm-c. *Amm-m.* Anac. Ant. *Arg.* Ars. Arum-triif. Aur. Bov. Bry. Calad. *Calc.* Cannab. *Carb-an. Carb-veg.* Cast. *Caust.* Chelid. Cic. Cina. Con. Croton. Cupr. Dulc. Elaps. Fluor-ac. *Graph.* Grat. Igt. Iod. *Ip.* Kali-b. Kali-c. Kali-jod. Kobalt. Lac-can. Lach. Laur. *Lyc.* Mgn-c. Mgn-m. *Mang.* Mez. Mur-ac. Ntr-c. Ntr-m. Nicc. *Nitr-ac.* Nitr. *Nux-m.* Nux. Ol-an. Op. Par. Petr. Phell. Phosp. Phosp-ac. Plb. Puls. Ran-b. Rat. Rhod. Sabad. Samb. Sass. Selen. *Sep. Sil.* Spig. Stann. Staph. Sticta. Stram. *Sulph.* Tabac. Teucr. Verb. Zinc. Zing.
— chronic, Bry. Con. *Sil. Sulph.*
— one-sided, Alum. Chelid. Igt. Nux-m. *Rhod.* Staph. *Sulph.* Sulph-ac. Teucr.
— — right, Brom. Lac-can. Nicc. Sticta. Teucr.
— — left, Nux-m.
— in morning, Arn. Con. Kali-b. Lach. Lith. Par. Rhod.
— — evening, Carb-veg. Cina. Euphr. Puls.
— at night, *Amm-c.* Calc. Lyc. Mgn-c. Mgn-m. Nux. Phell.
— — — moist by day, Calc. Phell.
— in nursing infants, Nux. Samb.
— from pus, Calc. Lach. Led. Ntr-c. Puls. Sep.
— when reading aloud, Verb.
— in a room, Puls. Ran-b.
— with nasal pain, biting, Arg.
— — sore, Ambr. Ran-b.
Ozoena, Arg. Asa-f. Aur. Con. Kali-b. Lach. Lyc. Merc. Puls. Sep.
Sneezing, Agar. All-cep. Alum. Ambr. Anac. Bad. Bell. Borax. Brom. Bry. Bufo. *Calc.* Calc-phosp. Carb-an. Carb-veg. Caust. Chenop. Chin. Cic. Cina. Cist. Cocc-c. Con. Creos. Croc. Cycl. Eupat. Euph. Euphr. Ferr-m. Gels. Grat. Hep. Jac-cor. Kali-b. Kali-c. Kali-chl. Lac-can. Lach. Lact. Meph. Merc. Merc-sulph. Mez. *Ntr-m.* Nicc. Nitr-ac. Nux. Phosp. Prun. Puls. Ran-sc. Rat. Rhus. Rumex. Sabad. Sacch. Scill. Sep. Sil. Staph. *Sulph.* Tar. Tart. Teucr. Therid. Verat.
— without coryza, Acon. Con. Hell. Kali-c. Sep. Sil. Sulph.
— spasmodic, Arn. Calc. Con. Hell. Lach. Ntr-m. Rhus. Sil. Staph. *Stram. Sulph.*
— strong and frequent, Con. Kali-c. Sil.
— violent, Acon. Ars. Bruc. Bry. Rhus. Sabad.
— in daytime, Gum-gut.

Sneezing in morning, Caust. Cimex. Creos. Nux-m. Puls.
— — evening, Puls.
— with coryza, Arg. Arg-n. Ars. Calad. Calc. Carb-an. Cham. Chin. Cist. Clem. Creos. Cycl. Dros. Gels. Kali-c. Kali-chl. Lach. Ntr-m. Nux. Osm. Scill. Sep. Staph. Tart. Tilia.
— without coryza, Acon. Con. Hell. Kali-c. Sep. Sil. Sulph.
— in sleep, Nitr-ac.
— — sunshine, Merc-sulph.
— constant, on entering a warm room, All-cep.
— with chilliness, Ox-ac.
— — epistaxis, Con.
— — soreness of larynx, Chenop.

— — nausea, Sulph.
— — pain in abdomen, Acon.
— — — chest, Acon. Cina. Grat. Seneg.
— — — head, Cina.
— — — hypochondria, Grat.
— — — nape of neck, Amm-m.
— — tingling in nose, Ferr-m. Pæon. Plat. Teucr.
— — stinging in the side, Acon. Borax. Grat.
— gives relief, Lach. Thuj.
— sneeze, constant desire, Anac.
— ineffectual efforts, Acon. Carb-veg. Caust. Laur. Ntr-m. Nitr-ac. Mez. Phosp. Plat. Plb. Sil. Zinc.
Ulceration of nostrils, at night, Lyc.

23. Larynx and Trachea.

Acridity of larynx, Chenop.
Adhesion in chest, Bar-c. Bell. Ntr-m. Sep.
Angina mucosa, Seneg.
Aphonia, Ant. Bar-c. *Bell.* Cannab. Carb-an. Carb-veg. *Caust.* Dros. Eupat. Hep. Kali-c. Lach. *Merc.* Merc-cor. Ntr-m. Nicc. Nux-jug. *Phosp.* Plat. Plb. Puls. Rhus. Spong. Sulph. Verat.
— at night, Carb-an. Carb-veg.
— in cold and damp weather, Carb-veg. Sulph.
— from being overheated, Ant.
— when talking, Carb-veg. Rumex. Spong.
Asthmatic affection, Asa-f.
Ball, sensation of, Lach.
Blood, hawked out, Sabad. Zinc. (compare Sect. 24).
Body, as of a soft, lodged in larynx, Dros.
Bruised as if, Ruta.
— in larynx, Rumex.
Burning, *Amm-m.* Ars. Bar-c. Canth. Caust. Cham. Chenop. Cycl. Gels. Graph. Hydroc-ac. Iod. Lach. Lact. Lyc. Mgn-m. Merc. Merc-cor. Mez. Par. Phosp. Rumex. Seneg. Sep. Spong. Staph. *Tong.*
— in trachea, Iod. Mez. Phosp. Zinc.
— — larynx, Ars. Cham.
— when lying down, Seneg.
Catarrh, Acon. Alum. Amm-c. Arn. Bar-m. Bell. Calc. Camph. Cannab. Canth. Carb-an. *Carb-veg.* Caust. *Cham.* Chin. *Coff.* Con. Creos. Croton. Dros. Dulc. Ferr. Graph. Hyosc. Igt. Ip. *Kali-c.* Lob. Lyc. Mang. Meph. Merc. Ntr-m. *Nux-m. Nux.* Phell. Phosp. *Rhod.* Spig. Stann. Sulph. Tart. Verat. Verb.
— — aged persons, Poth.
— — the bronchia, Cannab. Chin. Croton. Hyosc. Lob.
— — — chest, Arn. Carb-veg. Croton. Nux. Verat.
— — — — and bronchia, Alum. Cannab. Dulc. *Hyosc.* Ntr-m. Verb.

— of the trachea, Calc. Cannab. Chin. Nux-m.
— chronic, Calc. Cannab. Caust. Creos. Dros. Dulc. Lob. Lyc. Meph. Merc. Phell. Stann.
— in evening, Carb-an.
— at night, Carb-an. Spig.
— in children, *Cham.*
— after a cold, *Cham.*
— — measles, Carb-veg.
— with chills, Spig. Sulph.
— — coryza, Caust. Graph. Igt. Mang. Spig. Sulph.
— — cough, Bell. Caust. Con. Ferr. Merc. Phosp. Puls. Spig. Sulph.
— — eyes protruded, Spig.
— — fever, Spig.
— — headache, Spig.
— — hoarseness, Canth. Carb-veg. Caust. Nux. Phosp. Spig. Verb.
— — sore throat, Carb-veg.
— — suffocative fits, *Coff.*
— — to weep, disposition, Spig.
Choked, readily, when swallowing, Acon. Bell. Kali-c. Meph. Rhus.
Clear the throat, constant desire to, Croton.
Coldness, sensation of, when breathing, Arn. Brom. Camph. Chin. Cist. Rhus. Sulph.
Constriction, Asar. *Bell. Calad.* Camph. Canth. Cham. *Cocc.* Coloc. Dros. *Hell.* Igt. *Ip.* Lach. Laur. Mang. Meny. *Mosch. Nux-m.* Ol-an. Ox-ac. Phosp-ac. *Plb.* Poth. *Puls.* Rhus. *Sass.* Sil. Spong. Verat.
— in larynx, Ars. Carb-an. Laur. Nux. Stram. Verat.
— — trachea, Ars. Bell. Cham. Chelid. Hyosc-ac. Ip. Lach. Mosch. Puls. Sass. Spong. Verat.
— when lying down and at night, Puls.
— — walking, Rhus.
Contractive pain, Brom. Dros. Igt. Iod. Phosp-ac. Stram. Staph. Thuj. Verat.
— when speaking, Dros.

23. LARYNX AND TRACHEA

To cough, irritation, Bry. Chenop. Chin-sulph. Coff. Colch. Dros. Ferr. Kali-b. Lact. Lob. Mez. Nux. Stann. Stront. Sulph. Tart.
— when breathing, Kali-b. Meny.
Croup, Acon. Asa-f. Asar. Bell. Brom. Cham. Chin. Dros. *Hep.* Iod. Kali-b. *Phosp. Samb.* Sang. *Spong.* Tart.
— membranous, Acon. Amm-c. Asar. Bell. Brom. Cham. Hep. Iod. Kali-b. Phosp. Samb. Spong. Tart.
— before midnight, aggravated, Spong.
— after midnight, aggravated, Hep.
— with swelling under larynx, Hep.
Cutting pain, Arg. Canth. Hipp-m. Nitr.
Cynanche tonsillaris, Kali-chl.
Drawing sensation, Borax. Caust. Chin. Hydroc-ac. Iod. Sulph.
Dryness, Ant. Carb-veg. Chin. Dros. Gels. Ferr. Hyosc. Kali-b. Kali-chl. Lact. Lob. Ntr-c. Ntr-m. Nicc. Rhod. Sep. Stann. Tart. Tereb.
— larynx, Kali-chl. Laur. Nicc. Rhus. Sabad. Sep. Verb.
— trachea, Dros. Laur. Mez. Ntr-m. Phosp. Rhus. Spong Verb.
Dryness sensation of, Caust. Kali-b. Laur. Ntr-m. Par. Sep. Stann. Teucr.
Eruption or granular secretion, in trachea, with tracheal cough, Ambr.
Flapping sensation in larynx. Lach.
Heat in the chest, Bar-m.
— when exercising in open air, Ant.
— — larynx, Iod. Merc-sulph. Phyt.
— — trachea, Chelid.
Hoarseness, Acon. Alum. Ambr. *Amm-c. Amm-m.* Ang. Arn. Ars. *Bar-c.* Bell. Berb. *Bov.* Brom. *Bry.* Calc. Calc-caust. *Canth.* Caps. Carb-an. *Carb-veg. Caust. Cham. Chin.* Cic. Cina. Cocc-c. Coff. Colch. Creos. Crotal. Croton. Cupr. *Dig. Dros.* Dulc. Ferr. Gels. Graph. *Hep.* Hydroc-ac. Hydroph. Hyper. Iod. Kali-b. *Kali-c.* Kali-chl. *Lach.* Lact. Laur. Led. *Lyc.* Mgn-c. Mgn-m. *Mang.* Meny. *Merc.* Merc-cor. Merc-sulph. *Mez.* Murex. *Mur-ac. Ntr-c. Ntr-m.* Nicc. *Nitr-ac.* Nitr. Nux-jug. *Nux-m. Nux.* Ol-an. *Op.* Ox-ac. *Par. Petr.* Phell. *Phosp. Phosp-ac.* Plb. *Puls. Rhod.* Rhus Rhus-rad. Sabad. Samb. Sec-c. Selen. *Seneg. Sep.* Sil. Spig. *Spong.* Stann. Staph. Stront. *Sulph. Sulph-ac. Tart.* Thuj. Tilia. *Tong. Verb.* Verat. Vinca. Zinc.
— chronic, Bar-c. *Calc. Carb-veg. Caust.* Cupr. Dros. *Mang. Mur-ac. Phosp.* Plb.
— clergyman's aggravated by talking, Arum-trif.
— painful, Kali-brom.
— painless, Calc. Par.
— — periodical, Par.
— sudden, Alum. Nux-m.

Hoarseness in morning, Acon. Apis. Ars. *Bov.* Calc. Carb-an. Carb-veg. Cast. Caust Colch. Creos. *Dig.* Eupat. *Iod.* Lachn. Lact. Mgn-m. Mang. Ntr-m. Nicc. Nux. Phosp. Sulph.
— — afternoon, Alum.
— — evening, Alum. Brom. *Carb-veg.* Caust. Cinnab. Graph. Lach. Lact. Kali-b. Mgn-c. Nicc. Rumex. Sulph. Thuj.
— — — in bed, Nux.
— at night, Carb-an. Spig.
— periodical, Nux.
— every year, at same time, Nicc.
— in open air, Mang.
— — children, Cham.
— after a cold, Bry. *Cham.*
— after measles, Bry. Carb-veg. Dros.
— in moist cold weather, Carb-veg. Sulph.
— from mucus, Ang.
— — — in trachea, Ang. Chin.
— — — tenaceous, Cham.
— — — tough, in larynx, Bar-c. Chin.
— from reading aloud, Sacch. Verb.
— when singing, Selen.
— after a night-sweat, Dig.
— by talking aggravated, Arum-trif. Carb-veg. Nitr-ac. Staph.
— when walking against the wind, Nux-m.
— with burning, in larynx, Amm-m.
— — chest, pain in, Sulph.
— — chills, Ntr-c. Nux.
— — constipation, Nux.
— — coryza, Ars. Carb-veg. Caust. *Dig.* Graph. Kali-c. *Ntr-c.* Nitr. *Nitr-ac.* Petr. Phell. Sep. Spig. *Spong.* Sulph. Sulph-ac. *Thuj.*
— — cough, *Ambr.* Amm-m. Bry. Carb-an. *Dros.* Dulc. Kali-jod. Mgn-m. Mang. Merc. Ntr-c. Ntr-m. Nitr. Nitr-ac. Phosp. Seneg. Spong. Thuj.
— — — dry, Con. Sep. Sil.
— — — — from tickling in throat, Ambr. Dros. Merc. Ntr-c. Phosp. Sep. Spong.
— — ears obstruction of, Meny.
— — fever, Ntr-c.
— — headache, Nux.
— — to lie down, inclination, Cupr.
— — mouth, dryness of, Op.
— — mucus in trachea, Lact. Ntr-m. Tilia.
— — to perspire, disposition, Bry.
— — sneezing, Kali-c.
— — sore throat, Acon. Carb-veg. Nitr-ac.
— — to speak a loud word, inability, Amm-c. Carb-veg. Cupr. Dig. Graph. Hep. Ntr-c. Nicc. Nitr-ac. Ol-an. Par. Phosp. Puls. Sep.
— — stitches and burning in larynx, Cham.
— — to swallow almost inability, Acon. Bell. Phosp.

23. LARYNX AND TRACHEA.

Hoarseness with throat dryness of, Gels.
— — tongue, dryness of, Op.
Hot vapor rising from throat, Rhus.
Husk, sensation of, Berb.
Inflammation of bronchia, Acon. Ars. Bry. Cact. Calc. Carb-veg. Caust.Chin. Cist. Dig. Dros. Gels. Hep. Iod. Kali-b. Lach. Led. Lyc. Mang. Merc. Nitr-ac. Nux. Par. Phosp. Samb.Spong.
— — larynx, Acon. Bell. Cham. Dros. Hep. Hydroc-ac. Iod. Ip. Merc. Phosp. Seneg. Spong.
— — trachea, Acon. Ars. *Bell.* Bry. Canth. Carb-veg. Cham. Chin. Dig. Dros. Hep.*Iod.* Ip. Lob. *Mang.* Nux. *Samb.* Spong. Verat.
Itching larynx, Fluor-ac.
— trachea, Ambr. Nux.
Lacerating pain, Borax. Igt.
Leaf closing up trachea, like a, Mang.
Movement up and down, of larynx, Lyc.
Mucus, accumulated, Aeth. *Ambr.* Amm-c. *Ang.* Arg. Arn. Ars. Arum-trif. Aur, Bar-c. Bell. Bov. Bry. Calc. Camph. Cannab. Caps. Caust. Cham. Chin. Cina. Cocc. Cocc-c. Creos. Croc. Croton. Cupr. Dig. Dros. Dulc. Ferr. Hyosc. Iod. Kali-b. Lach. Laur. Lyc. Mgn-m. Ntr-m. Nux. Oleand. Osm. Ox-ac. Par. Phell. Plb. Rumex. Samb. *Seneg. Stann.* Staph. Sulph. Tart.
— in larynx, Croton. Hyosc. Phosp. Phosp-ac. Samb. Seneg. Verb.
— in trachea, Cham. Chin. Cupr. Dros. Dulc. Hep. Hyosc. Phosp-ac. Seneg.
— — chest, Arg. Aur. Bar-c. Bell. Brom. Calc.Canth.Cham.Cupr.Dulc.Euphr. Graph. Hep. Hipp-m. Iod. Ip. Lyc. Ntr-m. Nux. Sacch. Seneg. Staph. Sulph. Tart. *Zinc.*
— — morning, Caust. Ntr-m.
— — evening, Croton.
— when ascending steps laughing, stooping, Arg.
Mucus, ejected with difficulty, Aur. Canth. Croton. Mosch. Staph.
— — easily, Arg. Dig. Stann.
— hangs like a string in pharynx, with hawking and straining to vomit, on sneezing, mucus becomes looser, Osm.
— hardened, Iod.
— hardened and soft, alternately yellow-green or gray, Dros.
— hawked up, Agar. Amm-m. Ant. Bism. Calc. Caust. Carb-an. Chenop. Cina. Con. Croc. Croton. Ferr-m. Hep . Iod. Kali-b. Kali-c. Lam. Laur. Lyc. Meph. Ntr-m. Osm. Par. Petr.*Phosp.*Phosp-ac. *Plat.* Plb. Rhod. Rhus. Selen. Seneg. *Sep.* Stann. Tar. *Teucr.* Thuj.
— loosened as if could not be, Alum.

Mucus, lumpy, Ox-ac. Plb.
— with lumps of blood, Selen.
— rattling, Alum. Amm-c. Aspar. Bell. Calc. Cham. Chin. Iod. Lyc. · Tart. (compare Rattling.)
— — in trachea, Cham. Cina. Cupr. Hep.
— stringy, accumulates in trachea, Asa-f.
— tenacious, in trachea, Ang.
— thick, Ambr. Ox-ac. Sang.
— tough, Ars. Bar-c. Bov. Canth. Cham. Cina. Dig. Hep. Nux. Ol-an. Plb. Sep.
— yellowish-green, Plb.
— yellowish-white, with black lumps in centre, Ox-ac.
— in morning, Ambr. Caust. Ntr-m. Petr. Phosp. Rhus. Sep.
Numbness, sensation of, Acon.
Obstruction sensation of, Lob. Mang. *Spong.* Verb.
— as if narrow impeding breath, Alum.
— tightness, Bar-c. Carb-veg. Graph. Kali-b. Ntr-m. Teucr. Verat. Verb.
— — in larynx, Chin. Lach.
Painfulness, in general, *Bell. Cist.* Graph. *Hep.* Iod. Lact. Phosp. Puls. Thuj.
— of trachea, Igt.
— — a soft body lodged in larynx, Dros.
— like a small spot in larynx, Hep.
— preventing talking, Nicc. Phosp.
— when breathing, Bell. Hep.
— — coughing, Arg. Bell. Borax. Bry.
— after reading, Nitr-ac.
— when singing, Spong.
— — sneezing, Borax.
— from talking, Amm-c. Arg. Bell. Bry. Carb-veg. Hep. Nitr-ac. Phosp. Spong. Sulph. Sulph-ac.
— — aggravated, Bry. Nicc.Nitr-ac.Phosp.
— — tobacco smoking, aggravated, Bry.
— when touching the throat, Acon. *Bell.* Bry. Cic. Gum-gut. Hep. Lac-can.Lach. Mez. Nicc. Phosp. *Spong.* Sulph. Teucr. Zinc.
— — turning the throat, Lach. *Spong.*
Palsy, of epiglottis, Acon. Gels.
Phthisis, laryngea, Calc. *Carb-veg. Caust. Dros.* Hep. Mang. Merc. Phosp. *Spong.* Sulph.
— trachealis, *Ars.* Calc. *Carb-veg.* Caust. Chin. Coloc. Con. *Dros.* Hep. Iod. Lyc. *Mang.* Nitr-ac. Nitr. Seneg.Spong. *Stann.*
Piercing pains in larynx, Cham. Kali-c. Nitr-ac. Phosp.
— — trachea, Kali-c. Nitr-ac.
Plug, sensation of, Ant. Bell. Dros.Kali-c. Lach. *Spong.* Sulph.
Pressure, Croton. Zinc.
Rattling in trachea. Bell.Carb-an.Carb-veg. Caust. Euphr. Hep Hyosc. Ip. Laur. Ntr-m. Puls. Samb. Scill. Sep. Sil. Tart.

23. LARYNX AND TRACHEA.

Rawness, Alum. Ang.
— in trachea, Nux.
Rending, tearing in larynx and trachea, Staph.
Roughness, Agar. Ambr. Anim-c. Anac. Ant. Ars. Borax. Bov. Brom. Calc. Canth. Caps. Carb-veg. *Caust.* Chenop. Chin. Cist. Cocc-c. Coff. Colch. Creos. Dig. Dros. Ferr. Gels. Graph. Hep. Hipp. Hydroc-ac. Iod. Kali-c. Kali-jod. Lach. Lact. *Laur.* Lyc. Mgn-m. *Mang.* Meny. Merc-sulph. Mur-ac. Ntr-c Nitr-ac. Nitr. Nux-m. Ol-a 1. Ox-ac. Pat. Phell. *Phosp.* Phosp-ac. *Plb.* Prun. Puls. Rhod. Rhus. Sabad. Sacch. Sang. *Seneg.* Sep. Sil. *Stann.* Stront. *Sulph. Sulph-ac.* Verat. Zinc.
— in larynx, Carb-an. Creos. Dros. Ferr. Hep. Kali-c. Laur. Mgn-m. Mgn-s. Rhod. Sabad. Seneg. Sep. Spong. Sulph-ac.
— trachea, Carb-an. Creos. Dros. Hep. Kali-c. Lam. Phosp. Seneg. Sep. Spong. Verb.
— chest, Ntr-c. Nitr-ac. Zinc.
— chronic, *Mang. Phosp.*
— in morning, Zinc.
— after meals, Anac. Zinc.
— by coughing, ameliorated, Nicc.
— from reading aloud, Lact.
— after talking, Lyc. Staph.
Scraping, Anac. Chenop. Cocc. Cycl. Dros. Graph. Hep. Hipp-m. Laur. Nux.
— in larynx, Sabad.
— trachea, Ambr. Creos.
Scratching, Alum. Bov. Calc. *Graph. Laur.* Lyc. Nitr-ac. Nitr. Nux. Verat.
Sensitiveness of larynx, Bell. Graph. Hep. Lach. Spong. Sulph.
— to cold air, Hep.
Shocks, in trachea, Bry. Cina.
Skin, like a, in larynx, Lach. Phosp. Thuj.
Smarting, Gymnoc. Zing.
Smoke, sensation of, in larynx, Bar-c.
Snoring in trachea, Cham. Chin. Hyosc. Ntr-m. Stann. Sulph.
Sore pain, Ambr. *Arg.* Bov. Brom. Bry. Carb-veg. Caust. Chin. Graph. Igt. Iod. Lach. Phosp. Puls. Rumex. Seneg. Sil. Sep. Sulph.
— in larynx, Ambr. Brom. Carb-an. Carb-veg. Chin. Igt. Kali-c. Ntr-m. Sep. Stann.
— trachea, Ambr. Ant. Bry. Carb-an. Carb-veg. Caust. Chin. Kali-c. Ntr-m. Nux. Phosp. Sep. Stann. Sulph. Zinc.
Spasm, Acon. Laur. Meny. *Nux.* Verat.
— of larynx, Bell. Laur.
— at night, Ol-an.
— on expiration, Chelid.
Stinging, stiches, Ang. Bar-c. Borax. Canth. Caps. Chenop. Chin. Croc. Dros. Hydroc-ac. Hyosc. Kali-c. Kobalt. Laur. Menz.

Merc-cor. *Nitr-ac.* Oleand. Phosp. Sulph-ac. Thuj. Tilia. Zinc.
Stoppage, sensation of, Rhus, Spong. Verb.
Suffocation, pain with danger of, Bell. Hep. Lach. Seneg.
Swallows constantly when talking, Staph.
Swelling, sensation of, Hydroc-ac. Ip. Laur. Ox-ac. Sang. Sulph.
— — — right side, Chelid.
— — — below larynx, Hep.
— — — as if cold air could not pass, Chelid.
Tension, Lach. Nitr.
Throbbing in larynx, Chelid. Lach.
Tickling, Brom. Carb-veg. Cham. Chenop. Colch. Ferr. Iod. Hipp. Kali-b. Merc. Nux. Osm. Ox-ac. Sang. Stann. Zinc. (compare Sect. 24.)
— in larynx, All-cep. Iod. Stann.
— trachea, Creos. Iod.
Tied around, with a napkin, as if, in trachea, Chelid.
Tingling, crawling, *Arn. Carb-veg.* Colch. *Dros.* Iod. Laur. Lyc. Mgn-m. *Stann.* Sulph. *Thuj.*
— in trachea, Creos.
— at night, Lyc.
Torn loose, sensation as if something in trachea were, Calc.
Ulcerous pain of larynx, Ambr. Calc. Carb-veg. Caust. Gels. Ip. Kali-b. Sacch.
Valve, like a, in larynx, Spong.
Voice, altered, Murex. Nux-*m.* (compare Sect. 10.)
— barking, Bell. Brom. Dros. Nitr-ac. Spong. Stann. Stram.
— cracked, Dros.
— — when singing, Graph.
— croaking, Acon.
— crowing, Ars. Chin. Cina. Samb.
— deep, Ambr. Anac. Ant. *Chin.* Dig. Dros. Hep. Iod. Laur. Mgn-m. Nux. Par. Sacch. Samb. Spong. Stann. Sulph. Verat. Verb.
— — in moist, cold air, Sulph.
— failing, momentarily, *Alum.* Dros. Spong.
— feeble, Amm-caust. Ant. Bar-c. Bell. Cannab. Crotal. Hep. Lyc. Tart. (compare Weak.)
— from weakness of vocal organs, after anger, Staph.
— high, Acon. Ars. Cupr. Dros. Rumex. Stann. Stram.
— hissing, Phosp.
— hollow, Acon. Ant. Bar-c. Bell. Canth. Carb-veg. Caust. Cham. Chin. Creos. Croton. Dig. Dros. Hep. Igt. Ip. Lach. Led. Lyc. Mgn-s. Phosp. Puls. Samb. Sec-c. Spong. Stann. Staph. Thuj. Verat. Verb.
— husky, Camph. Caust. Chin. Croc. Graph. Hyosc. Mang. Merc. Rumex. Sabad. Selen. Spong.

23. LARYNX AND TRACHEA.

Voice husky or weak, Chin. Lyc.
— indistinct (voilè) Chenop.
— lost, Cannab. Carb-veg.
— — at night, Carb-an. Carb-veg.
— low, Ang. Ant. Canth Cham. Chin. Hep. Igt. Lyc. Puls. Sec-c. Spong. Staph. Verat.
— for singing is higher, after hawking up mucus, Stann.
— nasal, Aur. Bell. Bry. Lach. Merc. Phosp. Rumex. Sang. Staph.
— — catarrhal, Kali-jod. Phosp-ac.
— powerful, Hydroc ac.
— rough, Ant. Bell. Brom. Bry. Caust. Chin. Dig. Dros. Hep. Iod. Mang. Meny. Nux. Phosp. Plb-acet. Puls. Seneg. Spong. Stann. Sulph.
— — with nasal sound, Bell.
— — from mucus in larynx and trachea, Hyosc.
— — going off by hawking, Chenop.
— shrieking, Cupr. Stram.
— soft, Igt.
— squeaking, Stram.
— swallows constantly when talking, Staph.
Voice timid, Agn. Canth. Laur.
— tremulous, Acon. Ars. Canth. Igt. Merc. Phosp.
— uncertain and changing continually Arum-trif.
— — variable, Ars. Lach.
— unsonorous, Agn. Calad. Canth. Chin. Dros. Hep. Spong.
— weak, low. Amm-caust. Ang. Ant. Canth. Carb-veg. Caust. Daph. Gels. Hep. Igt. Lach. Lam. Laur. *Lyc*. Nux. Op. Par. Phosp. Prun. Puls. Spong. Stann.
— wheezing, Bell.
— whistling, Acon. Ars. Brom. Chin. Creos. Hep. Laur. Sabad.
Weakness, sensation of, *Canth*. Caust.
— cannot talk, from, Hep.
— in chest, inability to speak long, pain, Phosp-ac.
— when reading aloud, Cycl.
— — talking and breathing, Canth.
Wheezing in larynx, and painfulness of a small spot, Hep.

24. Cough.

Asthmatic cough, Asa-f. Cham. *Hep.* Kali-c. Sabad. Samb. Sulph-ac.
Autumnal cough, Verat.
Barking cough, Acon. All-cep. Bell. Brom. Clem. Cocc-c. Dros. Hep. Hipp. Lact. Nitr-ac. Phosp. Rumex. *Spong.* Stann. Stram.
— — evening, Nitr-ac.
— — day and night, *Spong.*
Blood coughed up, *Acon.* Aloe. Amm-c. Anac. *Arn.* Ars. Bell. *Bry.* Cact. *Calc.* Carb-veg. Cham. *Chin.* Cina. Cist. *Con.* Cop. Creos. Croc. Cupr. Daph. Diad. *Dig.* Dros. Dulc. Eugen. Euphr. *Ferr.* Ham. Hep. Hydroc-ac. Hyosc. Iod. Ip. Kali-b. Kali-jod. Lach. *Laur.* Led *Lyc.* *Mgn-c.* Mgn-m. Mang. *Merc.* Merc-cor. *Mez. Millef.* Mur-ac. Ntr-c. *Ntr-m.* Nitr-ac. *Nitr.* Nux-m. Nux. *Op. Phosp.* Phosp-ac. *Plb.* Puls. *Rhus.* Ruta. Sabad. Sabin. Sang. Scill. Sec-c. Selen. Sep, Sil. Staph. *Sulph Sulph-ac. Zinc.*
— black, Dig. Dros. Elaps. Nitr-ac. Phosp-ac. Puls. Rhus. Zinc.
— bright-red. Acon. Arn. Ars. Bell. Dros. Dulc. Hyosc. Ip. Kobalt. Led. Merc. Millef. Nitr. Phosp Rhus. Sabad. Sil. Zinc.
— brown, Bry. Carb-veg. Rhus.
— chronic, *Rhus. Sulph-ac.*
— clotted, coagulated, Acon. Arn. Bell. Cham. Chin. Dros. Hyosc. Mgn-m. Nux. Puls. *Rhus.*
— — brown, Bry.
— dark, Ant. Carb-veg. Cham. Chin.Croc. Cupr. Mgn-c. Mur-ac. Nux. Puls. Sep. Sulph. Sulph-ac.
— foaming, Arn. Dros. Led. Phosp. Sil.
— pale, Arn. Bell. Dulc. Hyosc. Led. Phosp. Rhus. Sabin. Sec-c. Sil.
— pus, mixed with, Chin.
— in morning, Ferr. Selen. Sep.
— — evening, Sep.
— at night, Arn. Ars. *Ferr.* Rhus.
— from least exertion, Ip.
— from violent exertion of lungs, Urt-ur.
— after hemorrhage from lungs, Plb.
— sea-bathing, brought on by, Mgn-m.
— with spasms, Hyosc.
— — suppressed menstruation, Puls.
Chronic cough, *Bell. Dros.* Igt. *Iod. Lyc.*

Ntr-m. Phosp. Sep. *Spong.* *Sulph.* Sulph-ac.
Clear ringing, Acon. All-cep. Ars. Dros. Stram.
Concussive, shaking cough, *Anac.* Ant. Ars. Bell. Caust. Chin. Hyosc. Igt. Ip. Lach. Lyc. Merc. Nitr-ac. Oleand. *Puls.* Rhus. Seneg. Sep. Sil.
Cough in general, *Alum.* Amm-c. Ars. Bell. *Caps. Cham.* Con. Cor-r. Graph. Kali-c. Led. Lyc. *Nux.* Petr. *Phosp. Sep. Sil. Sulph.*
— commencing with dyspnœa, Bry. Led.
— — gasping for breath, Cor-r.
— — stomach-ache, Bell.
— — whining, Arn. Bell.
Cough excited and aggravated by agitation, mental, Cist,
— an acrid fluid, sensation of, through posterior nares, Kali-b.
— ascending steps, Bar-c. Iod. Mgn-c. Mgn-m. Merc. Nitr. Scill. Seneg. Sep. Spong. Stann. Staph. Zinc.
— after bathing, Ant. Calc. Nitr-ac. Rhus.
— in bed, and after going to bed, (compare Sect. 34.)
— breath, want of, Euph. Guaj. Hep.
— chest, burning in, Euph. Phos.
— — congestion to, Bell.
— — constriction of, Mosch. Samb. Stram.
— — creeping in, Creos. Rhus. Scill.
— — dryness in, Lach. Merc. Puls.
— — irritation in general, Bell. Dros. Euph. Merc. Petr. *Phosp.* Spong. Stann. Sulph-ac.
— itching in, Cocc-c. Con. Phosp. Puls.
— — mucurs accummulated, Ars. Euphr. Stann.
— — oppression of, *Cocc.*
— — roughness and scraping in, Creos. Grat. Nitr. Phosp-ac. Puls.
— — spasm in, Samb.
— — tickling in, Bov. Cham. Con. Euph. Igt. Iod. Lach. Merc. Mez. Mur-ac. *Phosp.* Phosp-ac. *Rhus.* Scill. Sep. Stann. Sulph. *Verat.* Verb. Zinc.
— close thinking, *Nux.*
— coal gas, Arn.
— coffee, Caps. Caust. Cham. Igt. Sulph-ac.
— coldness, Arn. Ars. Carb-veg. Caust

24. COUGH.

Hep. Kali-c. Mosch. Mur-ac. Nux. Rhus. Sabad. Spong.
Cough excited by cold air, All-cep. Ars. Aur. Bar-c. Bry. Carb-an. Caust. Cham. Cina. Cist. Cupr. Hep. Hyosc. Ip. Kali-c. Mez. Nux. Phosp. Phosp-ac. Rhus. Rumex. Sep. Sil. Spong. Stram. Sulph.
— — drinks, Amm-m. Calc. Carb-veg. Dig. Hep. Kali-c. Lyc. Rhus. Scill. Sil. Staph. Sulph. Sulph-ac. Verat.
— — food, (compare Sec. 34.)
— — room, Carb-veg.
— — a part becoming, Hep. Sil.
— — the feet getting, Bar-c.
— taking cold, Bry. Cham. Dros. Hep. Hyosc. Ip. Lob. Ntr-c. *Nux-m.* Nux. Op. Rhus. Sep. Sil.
— — in water, *Nux-m.*
— drinking, Acon. Ars. Bry. Calc. Carb-veg. Chin. Cina. Cocc. Dig. Dros. Ferr. Hep. Hiop-m. Hyosc. Lach. Laur. Lyc. Meph. Ntr-m. Nux. Op. Phosp. Psor. Rhus.
— — rapidly, Sil.
— dry, cold air, Acon. Cham. Samb.
— after eating and drinking, Bry.
— expiration, Carb-veg. Caust. Creos. Nux. Phosp-ac. Staph.
— fasting, Kali-c. Murex. Staph.
— a hair, sensation of on tongue, Sil.
— becoming heated, Ant. Dig. Iod. Kali-c. Sil.
— after becoming heated, Acon. Bry. Kali c. Mgn-c. Rhus. Zinc.
— inhaling, Con. Kali-b. Meny. Meph. Merc-jod. Verb.
— keeping back the breath, Nitr.
— larynx, irritation, in general, Acon. Asar. *Calad.* Cocc. *Coloc.* Dros. Hep. Kali-jod *Merc.* Mez. Par.
— — pain, Acon. Ang. Bry. Calad. Euph. Hep. Spong.
— — burning, Acon. Mgn-s. Seneg.
— — crawling, Carb-veg. Caust. Creos. Iod. Led. Rhus. Stront. Tart.
— — dryness, Carb-an. Con. Dros. Laur.
— — itching, Con.
— — mucus, Caust. Croton. Dulc. Euphr. Kali-b.
— — pressure, Lach.
— — roughness, Bar-c. Carb-an. Creos. Dig. Sabad.
— — spasm. Cupr.
— — tickling, Acon. All-cep. Alum. Ambr. Amm-c. Amm-m. Ang. Bar-c. Bell. Brom. Bry. Calc. Caust. Cham. Cinnab. Cocc-c. Colch. Coloc. Con. Croton. *Dros.* Gum-gut. Hep. Iod Ip. Kali-b. Kali-c. Kalm. Lac-can. Lach. Lact. Laur. Lob. Led. Mgn-c. Mgn-m Merc. Mez. Ntr-m. Nux. Oleand. *Phosp-ac.* Prun. Rhus. Scill.

Seneg. Sep. Spong. Stann. Staph. *Sulph.* Tart. Teucr. Zinc. (conpare Throat and throat pit.)
Cough excited by larynx, tickling as from sugar, Bad.
— — — unsupportable, Kali-b.
— — — low in larynx, Ang.
— — — to the lung, Sticta.
— laughing, Arg. Ars. Bry. Chin. Cupr. Dros. Kali-c. Lach. Mang. Mur-ac. Nitr-ac. Phosp. Stann. Zinc.
— lying down, All-cep. Apis. Ars. Bell. Cinnab. Con. Creos. Croton. Dros. Ferr. Hep. *Hyosc.* Lact. Lith. Mgn-c. Meph. Merc. *Mez.* Nicc. Nitr-ac. Nux. Par. Petr. Phosp. Phosp-ac. Puls. Rumex. Sabad. Sang. Stann. Sulph.
— — on back, Amm-m. Iod. Nux. Phosp. Sil.
— — — ameliorated, Acon.
— — with head low, Amm-m. Chin. Puls. Samb. Spong.
— — on side, Bar-c. Carb-an. Creos. Kali-c. Lyc. Merc. Phosp. Puls. Seneg. Sep. Stann. Sulph.
— — left side, Bar-c. Eupat. Ip. Kali-c. Lyc. Merc. Par. Phosp. Rumex. Seneg. Sep.
— — right side, Amm-m. Carb-an. Cina. Stann.
— manual labor, Led. Ntr-m.
— after measles, Ant. Bry. Con. Dros. Hyosc. Igt. Nux.
— meditation, Arn. Cist. Igt. *Nux.*
— motion, Arn. Bar-c. Bell. Brom. Bry. Carb-veg. Creos. Dulc. Eupat. Ferr. Iod. Ip. Kali-c. Laur. Led. Lyc. Merc. Mez. Mosch. Mur-ac. Ntr-m. Nux. Phosp. Scill. Sil. Spong. Staph. Sulph-ac. Verat.
— after motion, Ars. Zinc.
— — of arms, Ars. Calc. Ferr. Kali-c. Led. Ntr-m. Nux.
— — right arm, Lyc.
— bending body forwards, Dig.
— — — backwards, Cupr.
— nitric acid, *Mez.*
— noon, (compare, Sect. 34.)
— œsophagus, tickling in, Arn.
— odors, strong, Phosp.
— old age, (compare Sect. 34.)
— pen air, Alum. Ars. Bar-c. Calc. Carb-veg. Cham. Cina. Dig. Lach. Mosch. Nitr-ac. Nitr. Nux. Phosp. Seneg. Sil. Spig. Staph Sulph. *Sulph-ac.*
— — going out into, Bry. Ip. Rumex. Scill.
— overheating, Nux-m. *Thuj.*
— playing, piano, Ambr. Calc. Cham. Creos. Phosp-ac.
— reading, Cina. Mang. Meph. *Nux.* Phosp.
— — aloud, Ambr. Mang. Meph. Nitr-ac. Phosp. Stann. Verb.

24. COUGH.

Cough excited by respiration, Cina. Merc. Op. Scill. Sulph.
— — deep, Acon. Amm-c. Arn. Bell. Brom. Bry Carb-an. Chin. Cina. Con. Cupr. Dulc. Euphr. Graph. Kali-c. Lyc. Mgn-m. Mez. Mur ac Ntr-m. Nitr-ac. Scill. Seneg. Sep. Sil. Stram.
— in room, Arg. Mgn-c. Mgn-m. Ntr-m.
— scrobiculus, pressing on it, Calad. Kali-b.
— — tickling in, Igt. Lach. Ntr-m. Phosp-ac.
— shrieking and weeping in children, Arn. Cham. Tart.
— singing, Dros. Phosp. Spong. Stann.
— sitting, Alum. Euphr. Ferr. Guaj. Kali-c. Mgn-m. Ntr-c. Phosp. Phosp-ac. Puls. Sabad. Sep. Zinc.
— — ameliorated, Puls. Sang,
— — bent, Stann.
— — erect, Kali-c. Ntr-m Spong.
— — long in same position. Cocc-c. Phosp-ac.
— before sleep, Merc.
— in sleep. (compare Sect 34.)
— smoke, Euphr.
— sneezing, Seneg.
— in spring, Ambr. Verat.
— standing, erect, Acon. Stann. (compare Sect. 34.)
— stimulants, Arn. Ferr. Igt. Lach. Led. Stann. Stram. Zinc.
— stooping, (compare Sect. 34.)
— sulphur-vapor, sensation of, in throat, Ars. Bry. Chin. Igt. Ip. Kali-chl. Lach. Par. Puls.
— sun. hot, (compare Sect. 34.)
— swallowing, Op.
— a swallow of water relieves, Caust.
— talking, Acon. Ambr. Anac. Arn. Bar-c. Bell. Bry. Calc. Carb-veg. Caust. Cham. Chin. Dig. Dulc. Euphr. Hep. Igt. Iod. Lach. Mgn-m. Mang. Meph. Merc. Mez. Mur-ac. Ntr-m. Nitr-ac. Phosp. Phosp-ac. Rhus. Scill. Sil. Spong. Stann. Stram. Sulph. Sulph-ac. Verb.
— tight clothing, Stann.
— trachea, irritation in general, Bry. Ferr-m. Kali-jod. Sulph.
— — creeping, Anac. Arn. Carb-veg. Caust. Creos. Rhus.
— — feather in, Rumex.
— — heat Chelid.
— — mucus, Caust. Cina. Cupr. Dulc. Euphr. Hyosc. Scill.
— — tickling, Acon. Amm-m. Arn. Bry. Caust. Cina. Coloc. Euph. Ferr. Gymnoc. Hyosc. Lach. Lact. Ntr-m. Nicc. Nitr-ac. Nux. Phosp. Phosp-ac. Psor. Rhus. Sang. Seneg. Sep. Sil. Teucr.
— — pain, Ang. Bry. Euph. Grat. Ip.

Cough excited by trachea burning, Aco. Ars.
— throat,(larynx and trachea,) contraction of, Ars. Lach.
— — dryness, Carb-an. Lach. Laur. Mang. Petr. Puls. Stann.
— — feather dust, sensation of. Amm-m. Bell. Brom. Calc. Chelid. Cina. Dros. Hep. Igt. Phosp-ac. Sulph.
— — irritation, Acon. Ambr. Ant. Ars. Asa-f. Asar. Bar-c Bell. Brom Bry. Calad. Carb-veg. Caust. Cham. Chenop. Chin. Cocc. Coloc. Con. Croc. Dros. Ferr. Hep. Hydroc-ac. Hyosc. Kali-c. Kali-jod. Laur. Mgn-c. Mgn-m. Merc. Mez. Ntr-m. Nicc. Nitr-ac. Par. Phosp-ac. Rhus. Sep. Sil. Staph. Stront. Tart. Teucr. Verat. Verb. Zinc.
— — — at bifurcation, Kali-b.
— — — as from smoke, Cocc.
— — — itching. Con. Nux. Puls.
— — — pain, Acon. Ang. Arg. Brv. Calad. Euph. Grat Hep. Sass. Spong. Stann.
— — pressure, Rumex.
— — roughness, Bar-c. Carb-an. Carb-veg. Caust. Creos. Con. Dig. Graph. Kali-jod. Laur. Mang. Ol-an. Puls. Rhod. Sabad. Sass. Stront.
— — scraping, Kalm.
— — scratching, Creos. Dig. Petr. Puls.
— — smothering, Lact.
— — stinging. Arg-n.
— — stitches, Cist.
— — sulphur-vapor, sensation of, Ars. Brom. Bry. Carb-veg. Chin. Igt. Ip. Kali-chl. Lyc. Mosch. Par. Puls.
— — tearing, Cist.
— — tickling, Cinnab. Coloc. Stann.
— throat-pit, burning, Ars.
— — constringing, sensation, Igt.
— — tickling, Bell. Cham. Cinnab. Coloc. Lac-can. Rhus-rad. Rumex. Sang. Sil.
— thyroid body, cutting, Arg-met.
— tobacco smoking, Acon. Brom. Bry. Carb-an. Cham. Cocc-c. Coloc. Dros. Euphr. Ferr. Hep. Igt. Iod. Lach. Mang. Nux. Petr. Spong. Staph. Sulph ac.
— tongue, sensation of a hair on, Sil.
— ulcers in throat, Lach.
— violin playing, Kali-c.
— walking, Dig. Ferr. Iod. Lach. Ntr-m. Rumex.
— — in open air, Acon. Ars. Carb-veg. Cina. Dig. Ferr. Ip. Lyc. Nux. Phosp. Phosp-ac. Seneg. Spig. Staph. Stram. Sulph. Sulph-ac.
— — — rapidly, Merc. Ntr-m. Scill. Seneg. Sil. Stann.
— — after walking rapidly in the open air, Sep.
— warm air, (compare Sect. 34.)

24. COUGH.

Cough excited by warmth, entrance into, All-cep. Bry. Cocc-c. Ntr-c. Verat. Verb.
— warm room, Ambr. Arn. Bry. Dig. Ip. Laur. Lyc. Mez. Puls. Seneg. Verat.
— — going into, from open air, Acon.
— becoming warm in bed, Dros. Nux-m. Puls. Tart. (compare Sect. 34.)
— warm food and drinks, Kali-c. Mez. Stann.
— — drinks, Ambr. Laur. Mez. Stann. Tart.
— water and washing, (compare Sect. 34.)
— weather, change of, Lach. Nitr-ac. Phosp. Sil. Verat. Verb.
— weeping, in children, Arn. Bell. *Cham.* Dros. Ferr. Hep. Lyc. Phosp. Verat.
— wind, (compare, Sect. 34.)
— winter, Acon. Cham. (compare Sect. 34.)
— yawning, Arn. Cina. Mur-ac. Nux. Staph.
Cough attended by, abdomen, pain in, Ars. Bell. Coloc. Con Ip. Lyc. Phosp. Scill. Stann. Sulph.
— — soreness in, Croton. Hyosc. Nux.
— — shaking of, Creos.
— — shooting pain, Bell. Chin. Lach. Sep. Staph.
— abdominal region, pain in, Verat.
— anxiety, *Acon.* Cina *Coff. Hep.* Iod. Rhus.
— — nocturnal, Acon.
— aphonia, Phosp.
— appetite loss of, Pod.
— arm pain in, Dig.
— back stinging in, *Bry.* Merc. Nitr-ac. Sep.
— bladder pain in, Caps.
— — pressure on, Scill.
— blood, congestion of, Arn.
— breath obstructed (asthma,) Acon. Alum. Amm-m. Anac. Arn. Ars Bell. Calad. Calc. Caust. Cina. Con. Creos. *Cupr.* Dolich. Euphr. Ferr. Ip. Lach. Led Lyc. Merc. Mur-ac. Ntr-s. Nicc. Nitr-ac. *Nux-m.* Op. Phell. Puls. Scill. Sep. Spig. *Tart.* Verat. Zinc.
— breath offensive, Ambr. Arn. Caps. Dros. Graph. Mgn-s. Mez. Plb. Sep. Stann.
— — panting, Mur-ac. Sulph-ac.
— catarrh, Bell. Puls.
— cervical glands, pain in, Ntr-m.
— chest, as if beaten, sensation, Arn. Ferr. Verat. Zinc.
— — — blood, congestion of, Bell. Sabin.
— — — burning, Ambr. Carb-veg. Caust. Iod. Mgn-m. Spong. Zinc.
— — — from larynx to pit of stomach, Mgn-s.
— — — — in sternum, Clem.
— — — as if bursting, pain, Bry Merc. Zinc.

Cough with, chest with coldness in, Zinc.
— — contraction, constriction, **Ars.** Lach. Sulph.
— — cutting, *Nitr.*
— — dryness, Kali-chl.
— — heaviness, Amm-c. Calad.
— — hoarseness, Phosp.
— — mucus accumulated, Ars. Bar-c. Cham. Ntr-m.
— — muscles of, pain in, Hyosc.
— — oppression of, Amm-c. Asar. Cocc. Con. Graph. Grat. Iod. Lach. Lact. Mur-ac. Ntr m. Nicc. Rhod. Rhus. Seneg. Stann. Verat.
— pain in general, Ambr. Ars. Bell. Brom. Calc. Carb-veg. Chin. Creos. Dros. Iod. Kali-b. Ntr-m. Nitr. Phosp-ac. Rhus. Sang. Sulph. *Verat.* Zinc.
— pressure, Borax. Chin. Cor-r. Iod. Sil. Sulph.
— — qualmish, Rhus.
— — rasping, smarting, Dig. Lyc. Phosp.
— — rattling, *Amm-m.* Ang. Arg. Bell. Calc. Caust. Chom. Hep. Ip. Lyc. Nitr-c. Ntr-m. *Nux.* Sep. Tart.
— — rawness, soreness, Ars. Calc. Carb-veg. Caust. Ferr. Lach. Mgn-m Mgn-s. Meph. Merc. Ntr-s. Nitr-ac. Nux-m. Nux. *Phosp.* Psor. Sep. Sil. Spig. Spong. *Stann.* Sulph. Zinc.
— — — after the cough, Stann. Zinc.
— — scraping, Creos. Ruta.
— — snoring, Ntr-m. Nux. Sep. Tart.
— — softness, sensation of, Rhus.
— — spasm, Kali-c.
— — stinging, stitches, *Acon.* Amm-m. Arn. Ars. Bell. Borax. *Bry.* Cannab. Carb an. Chin. Clem. Con. Dros. Ferr. Iod. Kali-b. Kali-c. Lach. Merc. Ntr-m. Ntr-s. Nitr-ac. *Nitr. Phosp.* Psor. Puls. Rhus. Sabad. *Scill.* Seneg. Sep *Sulph.* Zinc.
— — — in sides, Acon. Bry. Phosp. Puls. Scill.
— — under sternum, Petr.
— — ulcerative pain, Rat. Staph.
— — weakness, Psor. Sep.
— chills, Creos. Grat.
— constipation, Nux. Pod. Sep.
— convulsions, Hyosc. Meph.
— coryza, Acon. Alum. Ambr. Ars. Bar-c. Bell. Calc. Canth. Carb-an. Caust. Cimex. Con. Dig. Euphr. Graph. Ign. Kali-c. Kali-chl. Lach. Lyc. Mgn-c. Meph. Merc. Ntr c. Nitr. Nitr-ac. Phosp. Phosp-ac. Rhus. Rumex. Sang. Sep. Spong. Sulph. Sulph-ac. Thuj.

24. COUGH.

Cough, diarrhœa, followed by, Sang.
— with dysecoia, Chelid.
— earache. *Caps.*
— emaciation, Hep. Iod. Lyc.
— eructation, *Ambr.* Verat.
— eyes, pain in, Lach.
— — sparks from, Kali-c.
— — stitches over one eye, Phosp.
— face, bloated, Meph.
— — blue, Dros. Ip. Op. Verat. (compare Hooping cough.)
— — flushed, Eupat.
— — hot, Amm-c. Bell. Ip. Sulph.
— — pale, Cina.
— — red, Bell. Con. Ip. Kali-c.
— circumscribed redness of cheeks, Sang.
— fetid air exhaled, when coughing, Caps.
— fever, evening, Con. Creos. Hep. Iod. Lyc. Sulph.
— fingers, twitching of, Osm.
— to be frightened, liability, *Acon.*
— groins, pain in, Bo ax.
— hands, coldness of, Rumex.
— — hot and moist, Tart.
— headache, Acon. Alum. Ang. Anac. *Arn.* Bell. *Bry.* Cact. Calc. *Caps.* Carb-veg. Chin. Con. Hep. Ip. Lach. Lyc. Mang. Merc. Ntr-m. Nitr-ac. Nitr. Nux. Phosp. Phosp-ac. Puls. Rhus. Sabad. Sass. Scill. *Sulph.* Verat.
— — congestion of blood, Anac. Bell.
— — as if bursting, sensation, Bry. Cact. *Caps.* Merc. Ntr-m. Nux. Phosp. Phosp-ac. Sulph.
— — jerks, Ars. Calc. Ip. Lach. Mang. Ntr-m. Rhus. *Spig.*
— — perspiration, Ip. Tart.
— — stinging, Bry.
— hearing, loss of, Chelid. Seneg.
— heart, palpitation of, Arn. Calc. Phosp.
— heat, Ars. Creos. Lach. Scill.
— hiccough, Tabac.
— hoarseness, *Ambr.* Amm-c. Bry. Calc. Cham. *Dros.* Dulc. Lach. Laur. Lyc. Mang. *Merc.* Ntr-c. Ntr-m. Nitr-ac. *Phosp.* Rumex. Seneg. Sil. Spong. Sulph. Thuj.
— hyphochondria, pain, in, Ambr. Amm-m. Arn. Ars. Bry. Dros. Hell. Lach. Lyc.
— the more irritation, the longer he coughs, Igt. Teucr.
— ischiatic pain, Ars. Bell. Caust. Kali-b. Sulph.
— lachrymation, Eupat. Sabad.
— legs or knees, pain in, Caps.
— loathing, Ip.
— mouth, bleeding, Dros. Ip. Nux.
— — painful, Mgn-s.
— — stench of, Caps.
— — taste, as after blood, Amm-c.

Cough with, mouth coppery, metallic taste, Cocc.
— — — nauseous, Caps.
— — — sour, Cocc.
— — water in, Lach.
— nape of neck, pain in, Alum. Bell.
— nausea, Phosp-ac. Scill. Sep.
— — with retching, Verat.
— nose-bleed, Dros. Ind. Ip. Merc. Nux. Puls.
— occiput pain in, Ferr. Merc.
— perspiration, Ars. Cinnex Rhus. Sabad.
— pregnancy, Con. Nux-m.
— restlessness, Acon. Coff. Samb.
— sacral region (loins), pain, Amm-c. Merc. Nitr-ac. Sulph.
— salivation, Verat.
— scrobiculus, pain in, Amm-c. Ars. Bry. Lach. Phosp. Thuj.
— shoulders, pain in, Chin. Dig. Puls.
— — left, Ferr.
— — pain between, Kali-b.
— sight, cloudiness of, Sulph.
— to sit up, necessity, Ars. Hyosc. Puls.
— sleep, Creos.
— sleeplessness, Creos. Nitr.
— stitches in side, *Acon.* *Bry.* Phosp. *Scill.*
— — in right side, lower part, Kali-c.
— — liver, Ntr-m.
— — left lung, Rumex.
— sneezing, *Bell.* Bry. Osm.
— snoring, Arg. Bell. Caust. Ip. Ntr-c. Ntr-m. Nux. Puls. Sep. Tart.
— starting in sleep, Cina. Hep.
— sternum, pain in, Amm-c. Bell. Chin. Mez. Sep. Sil.
— stitches in, has to press it with hands, Bry.
— stiffness of body, Cina. Ip.
— stomach, coldness in, Lact.
— — jerks in, Ip.
— — pain, Bell. Ip. Lyc. Nitr-ac. Phosp. Rhus. Rumex. Sabad.
— — — before an attack, Arn. Bell. Cham. Tart.
— — as if turning, Puls.
— — weakness of, Lyc.
— sweat at night, Lyc.
— testicles, pain in, Zinc.
— thirst, Bry. Cocc-c. Samb.
— throat (larynx and trachea), dryness of, Kali-chl. Merc. Osm.
— — — and burning, Phosp.
— — pain, Caps. Carb-an. Chin. Hep. Lach. Mgn-s. Nux. *Phosp.*
— — rawness, Arg. Carb-veg. Chin. Kobalt. Ntr-m. Rumex. Sep.
— — roughness, Creos. Gels. Kali-c. Ntr-s. Phosp. Seneg.
— — soreness, Ambr. Amm-c. Caust. Chin. Kobalt. Lyc. Mgn-s. Ntr-m. Nitr-ac. Nux-m. Phosp. Rumex.

24. COUGH.

Cough, with throat stinging, stitches, Carb-veg. Kali-c. Merc. Nitr-ac. Nux.
— — tickling, *Ambr.* Anac. Borax. Creos. Rat. Spong.
— trachea, coldness in, Brom. Sulph.
— tremor, Phosp.
— unconsciousness, Cina.
— urination, involuntary, Ant. Bell. Bry. Caust. Colch. Creos. Ip. Ntr-m. Phosp-ac. Puls. Scill. Sep. Spong. Staph. Verat.
— vertigo, Calc.
— vomit, inclination to, Ars. Bell. Caps. Cimex. Cina. Dros. Hep. Ip. Kali-b. Kali-c. Lach. Merc. Nux. Petr. Phosp-ac. Puls.
— vomiting, Anac. Arn. *Bry.* Calc. Caps. Carb-veg. Daph. Dig. Dros. Ferr. Ind. *Ip.* Kali-c. Lach. Millef. Ntr-m. Nitr-ac. Nux. *Phosp-ac. Puls.* Rhus. Sabad. Sep. Sil. *Sulph. Tart.* Verat.
— — bilious, Chin.
— — bitter, Arn. Calc. Caps. Carb-veg. Daph. Hep. Lach. Ntr-m. *Sep.* Sil. Sulph.
— — of ingesta, Anac. *Bry.* Dig. Dros. Eugen. Ferr. Ip. Lach. Meph. *Phosp-ac.* Rhus. Sil. Stann. *Tart.* Verat.
— — mucus, Dros. Sil.
— — — morning, Kali-c. Sulph.
— — — evening, Ind. *Mez.* Rhus.
— — at night, *Ip. Mez.*
— — after drinking, Bry.
— — — eating, Anac. *Bry.* Dig. *Tart.*
— vomiturition (retching), Bell. Carb-veg. Chin. Creos. *Dros. Hep. Ip.* Kali-c. Merc. Mez. Ntr-m. Nux. *Puls.* Scill. Sep. Stram. *Sulph.*
— water-brash, Bry.
— weakness, Verat.
— weeping. Arn. Bell. Cina. Hep. Samb. Tart.
Cough ending with anxiousness, obstruction of breath, pale face, and whimpering, Cina.
— chest, coldness in, Zinc.
— — gurgling in, Mur-ac.
— — soreness of, Stram. Zinc.
— eructation and regurgitation, Sulph-ac.
— sneezing, Alum. Bell. Bry. Hep.
— somnolency, Tart.
— vomiting, Hyosc.
— weeping, Hell.
— yawning and sleepiness, Anac.
Cough relieved after breakfast, Kali-c.
— drinking, Spong.
— — cold water, Caust. Cupr.
— eating, Ferr.
— flatus, discharge of, Sang.
— deep inspiration, Verb.

Cough relieved, lying, down, Mang.
— change of position, Cocc-c. Igt.
— — — — from left to right side, Thuj.
— putting the hand against the chest, Creos. Croc. Dros.
— rising, Led. Puls. Sulph.
— sitting up, Hyosc. Ntr-m. Nicc. Puls. Sang.
— suppressing, cough, Igt.
— a swallow of water, Cupr.
— getting warm in bed, Cham.
— inhaling warm air, Rumex.
To cough, irritation, felt, in abdomen, Ambr. Verat.
— — bronchia, with soreness and heat, Euphat,
— — chest, Ars. Bov. Cham. Dros. Euph. Grat. Merc. Nitr. *Phosp.* Phosp-ac. Puls. *Rhus.* Sep. Spong. Stann. *Verat.*
— — larynx, Ang. Asar. *Calad.* Cocc. Coff. Colch. *Coloc.* Dros. Hep. Ip. Laur. Lith. Meny. Merc. Oleand. *Phosp-ac. Rhus.* Scill. *Seneg. Sep.* Stann. *Sulph.*
— — scrobiculus, pit of stomach, Bar-c. Bry. Cham. Guaj. Hep. Lach. Ntr-m. Nitr-ac. Phosp-ac.
— — stomach, Bell. Bov. Puls. Sep.
— — the throat, *Ambr.* Amm-c. Anac. Bov. Bry. Calc. Carb-an. Carb-veg. Caust. Chenop. *Con.* Graph. Kali-c. Laur. Mgn-c. Mgn-m. Mang. Mez. *Ntr-m.* Nux. Ol-an. Petr. Puls. Rhod. Sabad. Sass. Stront. Tabac.
— — throat pit, Bell. *Cham.* Croc. *Igt.* Iod. Lac-can. Phosp-ac. Rhus-rad. Rumex.
— — thyroid body, Mgn-c.
— — tongue, Sil.
— — trachea, Arg. *Arn.* Bry. *Euph.* Ferr. Grat. Ip. Kali-jod. *Rhus.* Seneg. Sep. Stront.
Croupy cough, Brom.
Crowing cough, Ars.
— — with inspirations, Cor-r.
Day and night cough, Bell. Bism. Cupr. Dulc. Euph. Igt. Lyc. Ntr-m. Nitr-ac. Spong. Stann. Sulph.
Every other day, cough, Anac. Lyc.
— third day, cough, Anac.
Deep cough, Ambr. Ang. Ant. Ars. Dig. Hep. Lach. Petr. Samb. Sil. Spong. Stann. *Verat. Verb.*
Diurnal cough, Amm-c. Arg. Brom. *Calc.* Chinin. Cic. Euphr. Ferr. Hep. Lach. Laur. Nitr. Nitr-ac. Phosp. Stann. Staph.
— — forenoon, Rhus. Sabad. Sep. Staph. Sulph-ac.
— — afternoon, All-cep. Bad. Chin. Mosch. Mur-ac. Nux. Staph. Sulph. Thuj. Zinc.

Dry cough, *Acon. Alum. Amm-c. Amm-m.*
Ang. Ars. *Bar-c. Bell.* Berb. Bov.Brom.
Bry. Calc. Cannab. *Carb-an.* Caust.
Cham. Chenop. Chin. *Cina.* Cinnab.
Cocc. *Coff.*Coloc.*Con.* Cop. Cieos. *Croc.*
Cupr. Dig. *Dros.* Euph. Ferr-m.
Fluor-ac. Gels. Grat. Guaj. *Hep. Hyosc.*
Hyper. *Igt. Iod. Ip.* Kali-b. *Kali-c.*
Kali-jod. Lachn. *Lact.* Laur. Lyc.
Mgn-m. Mgn-s. Mang. *Merc. Mez.*
Murex. Nitr-ac. *Nitr. Nux-m.* Nux.
Ol-an. Op. Petr. Phell. *Phosp.* Plat.
Plb. Pod. Psor. Puls. Rat. Rhod. Rhus.
Rhus-rad. Sabad. Sacch. *Sabin.* Samb.
Scill. Seneg. *Sep.* Sil. Spig. Spong.
Stann. Stront. Sulph. *Sulph-ac. Tabac.*
Teucr. *Verat. Verb.* Zinc. Zing.
— — which ends in raising black blood,
 Elaps.
— — causes vomiting, Cocc-c.
— in morning, *Alum.* Amm-m. Ant.
 Chin. Grat. Gymnoc. Lyc. *Mgn-s.*
 Ntr-s. Rhod. Scill. Stann. Sulph-ac.
— — aggravated, Stann.
— in evening, Ars. Bar-c. Calc. Caps.
 Ferr. Hep. Kali-c. *Mgn-m* Merc. Ntr-c.
 Nux. Petr. Phosp-ac. *Rhus. Sep. Stann.*
 Sulph. Tabac.
— at night, *Acon. Bell.* Bry. *Calc.* Caps.
 Carb-veg. Cham. Chin. Grat. Kali-c.
 Mgn-c. Mgn-m. Mgn-s. *Merc. Mez. Nux.*
 Ol-an. *Petr.* Rhod. *Rhus.* Sabad. Scill
 Sulph. *Verat. Verb.* Zinc.
— — 3 A. M., Amm-c. Kali-c.
— — aggravated, Cham. Op. Stront.
— after a cold, Nux-m.
— from cold air, Ars. Phosp.
— after drinking, Ars, Phosp.
— from violent exercise, Ox-ac.
— after gonorrhoea suppressed, Benz-ac
 Selen.
— when lying down, Cinnab. Hyosc. Lyc.
 Nitr-ac. Puls. Sabad. Sang. Sulph.
— after measles Cham. Hyosc. Igt.
— from reading aloud, Phosp.
— when smoking tobacco, Hell.
— from talking, Mang.
— with expectoration, in morning, Euph
 Kali-c. Nux. Phosp-ac.
— in forenoon, Alum.
— — afternoon, Amm-m.
Evening cough, All-cep. Ambr. *Amm-m.*
 Anac. Ant. Apis. Arn. Ars. Bad.
 Bar-c. Bell. Bism. Bry. *Calc.* Caps
 Carb-an. *Carb-veg.* Caust. Cham Chin.
 Cina. Croton. Dros. Eugen. Eupat
 Euphr. Ferr. *Fluor-ac.* Graph. *Hep.* Igt.
 Ind. *Iod.* Lach. Laur. Led. Lith. Lyc.
 Mgn-c. Mgn m. Merc. Mez. Mosch.
 Mur-ac. Ntr-m. *Nitr-ac.* Nux-m. *Nux*
 Petr. *Phosp.* Phosp-ac. *Puls. Rhus.*
 Rumex.Sang Seneg *Sep.*Sil Spong *Stann*
 Staph. Sticta. *Sulph.* Sulph-ac. Tabac.

Verat. Verb. Zinc.
Evening cough from 4 to 6 o'clock, Lyc.
— about bed-time and for a while in bed,
 Dolich.
— in bed, Agn. Amm-c. Anac. Ars. Bell.
 Calc. Caps. Carb-veg. Creos. *Dros.*
 Graph. Hep. Hyosc. Igt. Ind. Mgn-c.
 Merc. Ntr-m. Nicc. Nux-m. Nux. Par.
 Petr. Puls. Rhus. Ruta. Sep. Staph.
 Verb.
In the evening, increased, *Caps.* Spong.
— — after lying down, Euphr. Lach.
 Nitr-ac. Staph. Thuj.
— — to midnight, Hep.
Exhausting cough, Chelid.
Expectoration, Ambr. Amm-c. Ang. Arg.
 Ars. Asar. Bell. Bism. Borax. Bry.
 Calc. Cannab. Carb-an. Carb-veg Caust.
 Chin. Cic. Cocc-c. Con. Creos. Cupr.
 Dros. *Euphr.* Ferr. Iod *Kali-c.* Led.
 Lyc. Mgn-c. Mgn-m Mgn-s. Merc.
 Ntr-c. Ntr-m. Ntr-s. Op. Par. *Phosp.*
 Phosp-ac. *Puls.* Rhod. Ruta. Sabad.
 Sabin. Scill. *Seneg. Sep. Sil.* Spong.
 Stann. Staph. *Sulph.* Sulph-ac. Tart.
 Thuj. Verat. Zinc.
— day and night with, Dulc.
— — — without, Acon. Ars. Bell.
  Brom. Creos. Laur. Mosch.
  Stram. Verb.
— with, night without, Acon. Anac.
 Ars. Bry. Calc. Carb-an. Caust.
 Cham. Chin. Con. Graph. *Hep.*
 Hyosc. Kali-c. Lach. Lyc. Mgn c.
 Mgn-m. *Merc.* Nitr-ac. Nux.
 Phosp. *Puls.* Sabad. Samb. *Sil.*
 Stront. Sulph. Verat. Zinc.
— night with, day without, Caust. Hep.
 Rhod. Sep. Staph.
— in evening. Arn. Bar-c. Bov. Chin.Cina.
 Croton. Dig. Igt. Iod. Nux. Ruta.
— — loose, and at night, in morning
  generally swallowed, Caust.
— morning, Acon. Alum. Ambr. Ang. Ant
 Bar-c. Bry. Calc. Carb-veg. Cupr. Dros.
 Euph. Euphr. Ferr. Hep. Ip. Kali-c.
 Lach. Lyc. Mgn-c. Mgn-m.Mez.Mur-ac.
 Ntr-m. Nitr-ac. Par. Phosp. Phosp-ac.
 Puls. Scill. Seneg. Sep. Spong. Stann.
 Sulph. Sulph-ac. Tart. Zinc Zing.
— acrid, Anac. Caust. Merc. Nitr-ac.Rhus.
 Sil.
— albuminous, Ars. Asa-f. Bar-c. Chin.
 Cocc-c. Ferr. Laur. Seneg. Stann.
— bitter, Ars. Cham Ci-t. Dros. Lyc.
 Merc. Ntr-c. Nitr-ac. Nux. Puls. Sep.
 Verat.
— bloody. (compare Blood coughed up.)
— black, Chin. Kali-b. Lyc Rhus.
— with blackish grains, Chin.
— blood-streaked, Arn. *Borax.* Bry. Chin.
 Ferr. Ip. Laur. Phosp. Sabin. Sep.Zinc.
— with bloody points, Laur.

24. COUGH.

Expectoration, brownish, Carb-veg.
— cannot be raised, must be swallowed, Arn. Cannab. *Caust.* Con. Dros. Kali-c. Lach. Mur-ac. Osm. Sep. Spong.
— old catarrh, tasting like, Igt. Mez. Puls. Sulph.
— old cheese, tasting like, Thuj.
— cold, Bry. Nux. Phosp. Rhus. Sulph.
— cold mucus, tasting flat, Bry.
— in consumptives, if worse they expectorate less, Sep.
— from deep in lungs, Chelid.
— difficult, Ars. Bar-c. Bry. Caust. Chin. Cina. Cocc-c. Con Cor-r. Cupr. Dig. Euph. Igt. Kali-c. Lach. Mgn-m. Osm. Par. Scill. Sep. Stann. Sulph. Zinc.
— dust, as if mixed with, Phosp.
— easy, Arg. Creos. Dulc. Euph. Ruta. Verat.
— fetid, Ars. Calc. Carb-veg. Cocc. Cop. Guaj. Led. Lyc. Ntr-c. Nitr ac. Phosp-ac. Puls. Sacch. Sang. Sil. Stann. Sulph.
— flat-tasting, Anac. Ant. Bry. Calc. Chin. Euphr. Igt. Kali-c. Lyc. Ntr-m. Par. Puls. Rhus. Sep. Staph. Sulph. Tart.
— flying forcibly out of mouth, Bad. Chelid.
— frequent, Agar. Asar. Chenop. Cina. Daph. Euph. *Euphr.* Hep. Iod. Lact. Laur. Lyc. *Puls.* Ruta. Samb. *Seneg. Sep.* Sil. *Stann* Sulph Verat.
— frothy, Ars. Daph. Ferr. Kobalt. Lach. Nux. Op. Phosp. Puls. Sil
— gelatinous, Arg. Arn. Bar-c. Dig. Ferr. *Laur.*
— gray, Ambr. Anac. Ars. Calc. Carb-an. Chin. Cop. Dros. *Lyc.* Nux. Rhus. Sep. Thuj.
— greasy tasting, Alum. Caust. Mgn-m. Mur-ac. Puls. Sil.
— greenish, Ars. Calc. *Cannab.* Carb-an. Carb-veg. Cop. Creos. Dros. Ferr. Hyosc. Kali-b. Kali-jod. Led Lyc. Mgn-c. Mang. Ntr-c. *Par.* Phosp. *Puls.* Rhus. *S p* Sil. *Stann. Sulph. Thuj.*
— herby-tasting. Ca'ad. Nux. Phosp-ac.
— indurate l. Bry. Con. Iod. Kali-c. Ntr-c. Phosp. Sep. Sil. Spong. Stront. Sulph. Thuj.
— infrequent. Acon. Alum. Arn. Bell. Igt.
— in lumps, Agar. Arn. Ars. Hep. Mang. Thuj.
— metallic-tasting, Nux. Rhus. Zinc.
— milky, Ars. Puls. Sep. Sil. Sulph.
— by mouthfuls at a time, light-rust color. Lyc.
— mucus, Acon. Ambr. Anac. Ang. Ant. Arg. Arn. Ars. Asar. Bar-c. Bell. Bism. Bry. Cact. Calc. Carb-veg. Caust. Cham. Chenop. Chin. Cina. Cocc c. Con. Cop. Creos. Cupr. Dig. *Dulc.* Eugen. Ferr. Hep Hyosc. Igt. Iod. Kali-b. Kali-c. Kobalt. Lach. Laur. Lyc. Mgn-c. Mgn-m. Mang. Merc. Mez. Mur-ac. Ntr-m. Nicc.

Nux. Op. Par. Phell. *Phosp.* Phosp-ac. Plb. *Puls.* Rhus. Ruta. Sabad Sabin. Samb. *Scill.* Selen. *Seneg. Sep. Sil.* Spong. *Stann.* *Staph.* Sulph. Sulph-ac. *Tart. Thuj.* Verat. Zinc.
Expectoration mucus, bluish lumps of, Kali-b.
— — with blood mixed, Acon. Alum. Anac. Ant. Arn. Ars. *Borax. Bry.* Cact. Calc. Chin. Cina. Con. Cupr. D.g. Dulc. Eugen. Euphr. Ferr. Hep. Iod. Ip. Kali-b. Kali-c. Kobalt. Lachn. Lyc Mgn-m. Merc. *Ntr-m.* Op. Phosp. Sabin. Scill. Sulph-ac. Zinc.
— — in globules, with blood, Selen.
— — profuse ropy, adhering to larynx, Cocc-c. Kali-b. Lob. Sticta.
— — thick, Calc. *Dulc.* Phosp. *Puls.* Scill. Seneg. Sep. Sil. Stann. Sulph. Tart. Thuj.
— — tough, Cist. Iod. *Seneg.* Stann. Zinc.
— muddy, like pus, flies like batter, Phosp.
— nauseous, Dros.
— offensive, smelling, Ars. Calc. Carb-veg. Con. Cop. Cupr. Guaj. Hep. Igt. Led. Lyc. Mgn-c. Mgn-m. Merc. Ntr-c. Nitr-ac. Phosp-ac. Sang. Scill. Seneg. Sep. Sil. Stann. Sulph.
— onions, tasting like, Asa-f.
— pellucid, Ars. Ferr. Laur. Seneg. Sil.
— profuse, Agar. Dulc. Euphr. Iod. Laur. Lyc. Puls. Seneg. Sep. Stann. Sulph.
— purulent, Anac. *Ars. Bry. Calc. Carb-an.* Carb-veg. *Chin.* Con. Cop. Cor-r. Creos. Dros. Dulc. Ferr. Graph. Guaj. Hep. *Kali-c.* Led. Lyc. Mgn-c. Mgn-m. Merc. Ntr-c. Ntr-m. Nitr-ac. Nitr. *Phosp. Phosp-ac. Plb.* Rhus. Sec-c. Sep. *Sil.* Stann. *Staph. Sulph.* Zinc.
— putrid, Arn. Ars. Calc. Carb-an. Carb-veg. Cham. Con. Cop. Creos. Cupr. Ferr. Guaj. Iod Ip. Lyc. Merc. *Ntr-c.* Nux. Phosp-ac. *Puls.* Rhus. Samb. Sep. Sil. Stann. Sulph. Verat. Zinc.
— reddish, Bry. Cocc-c. Phosp. Scill.
— rust-colored, Phosp. Scill.
— salty, Ambr. *Ars.* Bar-c. *Carb-veg.* Chin. Dros. Hyosc. Lach. *Lyc.* Mgn-c. Merc. Mez. Ntr-c. Ntr-m. Nitr-ac *Phosp. Puls.* Rhus. Samb. *Sep.* Sil. Stann. Sulph. Sulph-ac. Tart. Therid. Verat.
— scanty, Acon. Ars. Cham. Cupr. Dig. Samb. Sang. Spong.
— — tenacious, round lump, cherry-colored, Acon.
— soft, fetid tubercles, color of peas, Mgn-c.
— sour, Ambr. Bell. Calc. Carb-an. Carb-veg. Chin. Cocc-c. Croton. Ferr. Hep. Kali-c. Lach. Lyc. Mgn-m. Ntr-m. Nitr-ac. Nux. Phosp. Phosp-ac. Puls. Rhus. Sep. Spong. Stann. Sulph. Sulph-ac. Tart. Verat.

24. COUGH.

Expectoration like boiled starch, Arg. Dig.
— stringy, Asa-f. Cocc-c. Kali-b.
— suppressed expectoration restored, Sacch.
— sweetish, Anac. Calc. Chin. Dig. Ferr. Hep. Ip. Kali-b. Kali-c. Lyc. Nux. *Phosp.* Plb. Puls. Sabad. Samb. Scill. Sep. *Stann.* Sulph. Sulph-ac. Zinc.
— tasteless, Cina. Dulc
— thick, Arg. Calc. Creos. Kali-b. Kobalt. Op. Phosp. Ruta. Stann. Sulph.
— like tobacco-juice, Puls.
— tough, viscid, Ant. Arg. Ars. Bad. Bar-c. Bov. *Cannab.* Carb-veg. Cham. Chin. Cist. Cocc-c. Iod. Kali-b. Kali-c. Kobalt. Mgn-c. Mgn-m. Mez. *Par. Phosp.* Phosp-ac. Ruta. Sabad. Samb. Seneg. Sep. Sil. Spong. *Stann. Staph.* Tart. Verat. Zinc.
— tough, hard to separate, round lumps, brick shade, Bry.
— watery, Arg. Carb-veg. Cham. Euphr. Graph. Lach. Mgn-c. Mgn-m. Merc. Mur-ac. Stann. Sulph-ac.
— white, Ambr. Amm-m. Arg. Carb-veg. Cina. Cocc-c. Creos. Croton. Kali-b. Kobalt. *Lyc.* Nicc. Phosp. Phosp-ac. Scill. *Sep.* Sulph.
— yellow, Acon. Ambr. Amm-m. Anac. Ang. Ars. Bad. Bar-c. *Bry. Calc.* Carb-veg. Cocc-c. Con. Cor-r. Creos. Dig. Dros. Eugen. Iod. Kali-b. Kali-c. *Lyc.* Mgn-c. Mgn-m. Mang. Merc. Mez. Mur-ac. Ntr-c. Ntr-m. Nitr-ac. Nux. Phosp. Phosp-ac. *Puls.* Ruta. Sabad. Seneg. Sep. Sil. Spong. Stann. *Staph. Sulph.* Sulph-ac. Thuj. Vera:. Zinc.
— lemon-yellow, Kali-c. Lyc. Phosp. Puls.
— easier when turning from left to right side, Kali-c. Lyc. Phosp. Sep. Thuj.
Fatiguing cough, Rumex. Sang.
First cough the most violent, Aut.
Frequent cough, Lob. Sang.
Gasping for breath, cough commencing with, Cor-r.
Hectic cough, Borax. Nux. Phosp. Puls. Sil. Stann.
— from suppressed intermittent fever, Eupat.
Hoarse cough, Acon. Agar. Agn. All-cep. Ars. Asa-f. Berb. Bov. Brom. Cannab. Carb-an. Carb-veg. Caust. Cham. Chenop. Chin. Creos. Eupat. Graph. *Hep.* Hydroc-ac. Kali-c. Lact. Laur. Lyc. Merc. Mur-ac. Ntr-c. Ntr-m. Nitr-ac. Nux. Puls. Rhod. Rumex. Samb. Seneg. Verat. *Verb.*
— from a cold, Ntr-c.
— after measels, Igt. Nux.
Hollow cough, Acon. Bell. Brom. Carb-veg. Caust. Chelid. Cina. Creos. Dig. Euph. Igt. Ip. Lact. Led. Mgn-c. Merc. Merc-cor. Op. Phosp. Samb. Sil.

Spig. *Spong.* Stann. Staph. *Tart. Verat. Verb.*
Hooping cough, Ambr. Anac. Ant. Arn. Ars. Bar-c. *Bry. Carb-an.* Carb-veg. Cham. Chin. Cina. Cocc-c. Con. Cor-r. Cupr. Dros. Dulc. Euphr. Hep. Hyosc. Igt. Ind. Ip. *Led.* Lyc. Meph. Mez. Mur-ac. Ntr-m. Nux. Op. Phell. Pod. Puls. *Samb.* Seneg. Sep. *Spig.* Spong. *Sulph.* Sulph-ac. *Tabac. Tart.* Verat.
— in chilren, Bry. *Samb. Sulph.*
— with shrieking and hallooing, *Samb.*
— in evening, Carb-an. Ind. Ntr-m.
— at night, Bry. Cham. Chin. Sil.
— after eating or drinking, *Bry.*
In infants, Arn. Bry. *Cham.* Samb. Sulph. *Tart.*
— — — with shrieking and whining, Arn. Cham. Tart.
Incessant, Rumex.
Infrequent, Aur. Murex.
Loose cough, without expectoration, Con. Mgn-s. Pod.
After meals, cough, Anac. Bell. Bry. Dulc. Eugen. Puls. Sep. Stann. *Tart.*
— increased, Cham. Op. (compare After meals, cough.)
During or after measles, cough, *Acon.* Chin. Cina. *Coff. Dros.* Hyosc. Igt. Nux.
Moist cough, Arn. Bry. Dulc. Eugen. Puls. Sep. Stann.
In the morning, cough, Acon. *Alum.* Amm-c. Ant. Arn. Aur. Bell. Bry. *Calc.* Carb-an. Caust. Cham. Chelid. Chin. Cina. Cocc-c. Creos. Croton. Cupr. Dig. Dros. Dulc. *Euphr.* Grat. Gymnoc. Hep. Iod. Ip. Kali-b. Kali-c. *Led.* Lyc. Mgn-c. *Mgn-s.* Ntr-c. *Ntr-m.* Nitr. Nux. Phosp-ac. *Puls.* Rhod. Rhus. Scill. Selen. Sep. Staph. Stram. Sulph. Sulph-ac. Tabac. Thuj. Verat.
— chronic, *Iod. Lyc.*
— in bed, Amm-c. Nitr. Rhus.
— at 3 o'clock, Amm-c. Kali-c. Nitr.
— after rising, Euph. Lach. Nitr-ac. Staph. Thuj.
— forenoon, Rhus. Sabad. Sep. Staph. Sulph-ac.
— increased, *Nux.* Stann.
At night, cough, Acon. Alum. *Ambr. Amm-c. Amm-m.* Arn. Ars. *Bar-c. Bell.* Bry. Calad. Calc. Caps. *Carb-an Caust. Cham. Chin.* Cocc. Cocc-c. Coff. Colch. Con. Cor-r. Dig. *Dros.* Dulc. Eugen. Graph. Grat. *Hyosc. Igt. Ip.* Kali-c. Lact. Led. *Lyc. Mgn-c. Mgn-m.* Meph. *Merc. Mez.* Nicc. Nitr-ac. Nitr. Nux. Ol-an. Par. *Petr.* Phell. Phosp. Puls. Rhod. Ruta Sabad. Sang. Seneg. Sep. Sil. Spig. Stann. Staph. Sticta. *Sulph.* Tart. *Verat. Verb.* Zinc.
— before midnight, Mez. Rhus. Spong. Stann.

24. COUGH.

Cough, at 11 P. M., Arn. Bar-c. Carb-veg. Caust. Ferr. Hep Led. Lyc. Mgn-c. Mgn-m. Mosch. Mur-ac. Nitr ac. Puls. Rumex. Sabad. Sep. Stann. Staph. Sulph. Sulph-ac. Verat. Zinc.
— — midnight, Bell. Dig. Hipp-m. Mgn-c. Mgn-m. Samb.
— — after midnight, Acon. Bell. Bry. Cham. Chin. Dig. Dros. Kali-c. Hyosc. Mgn-c. Merc. Nux. Samb. Tart.
— — to 4 A. M., Nicc.
— — at 3 A. M., Amm-c. Kali-c. Nitr.
— — — 3—4 A. M., Kali-c.
— — — 2—5 A. M., Rumex.
— — in sleep, cough, Arn. Calc. *Cham.* Hipp. Lach. Nitr-ac. Sep. *Verb.*
— — awaking him from sleep, Merc. Nitr-ac. Phosp. Rhod. Sep. Sulph.
Nightly exacerbation, *Caps. Cham.* Op. *Ntr-s.* Stront.
In old people, cough, Caust. Hyosc. Stann.
Panting cough, Mur-ac. Sulph-ac.
Paroxysms of cough, Ang. Alum. Ambr. Carb-veg. Chelid. Cor-r. Cupr. Lob.
— occasional, Bad.
— two coughs, Puls.
— — — in quick succession, Merc. Sulph.
— three coughs, Stann.
— few, Bell. Calc. Laur.
— in rapid succession, Dros. Hep. Ip. Sep. Sulph. Tart.
Periodical cough, Ars. Cocc. Cocc-c. Lach. Nux.
— painless, barking, shrieking tone, without expectoration, Stram.
— at same time every day, Lyc. Sabad.
In pregnancy, cough, Calc. Con. Phosp. Sep.
Rattling cough, only during day in room, Arg.
Rough cough, Bell. Brom. Eupat. (compare Hoarse.)
Screeching cough, Stram.
Short cough, *Acon. Alum.* Anac. Arg. Asa-f. *Bell.* Berb. Caust. *Coff.* Eupat. Hydroc-ac. Ign. Kali-c. Kali jod. Kobalt. Lach. Lact. *Laur.* Lob. Merc. Ntr-m Nitr-ac Nux. Oleand. *Petr.* Phosp. Plat. Pod. Puls. Rhus. Rumex. Sabad. *Scill.* Sticta. Sulph-ac. Teucr. Zing.
— in paroxysms, Alum. Asa-f. Bell. Calc. Carb-veg. Dros. Kali-b. Kali-c. Lact. Scill. Tart.
When sitting, cough, Alum. Ferr. Guaj. Mgn-m. Ntr-c.
— long in same position, Phosp-ac.
Soundless, Dros.
Spasmodic cough, Acon. All-cep. *Ambr.* Bad. Bar-c. *Bell.* Brom. *Bry.* Cact. Calc. *Carb-veg.* Chin. *Cina.* Con. Cor-r. Creos. Cupr. Dig. *Dros.* Ferr. Hep. *Hyosc.* Ign.

Iod. *Ip.* Kali-c. Lach. *Lact.* Laur. Led Lob. *Mgn-c. Mgn-m.* Merc. Mez. Mosch. Ntr-m. Nitr-ac. Nux. Osm. Phosp. Phosp-ac. Plb. Puls. Rhus. Scill. Sep. Sil. Staph. Stram. Sulph. Zinc.
Spasmodic cough in morning, Carb-veg. Creos. Kali-c. Puls. Sulph.
— — afternoon, *Bell.* Bry.
— — evening, Carb-veg. Ntr-m.
— at night, *Bell.* Bry. *Hyosc.* Mgn-c. Mgn-m.
— day and night, Sulph.
— in children, Bry.
— — old people, at night, from continuous tickling in throat as if the palate was too long, Hyosc.
— after eating and drinking, Bry.
— from talking, Dig.
— with vomiting, Bry. Carb-veg. Ferr. Ip. Puls.
Suffocating (choking) cough, Acon. Brom. *Bry. Carb-an.* Cham. Chin. Cocc-c. Con. Cycl. Dros. Hep. Ind. Ip. Lach. Lact. *Led.* Ntr-m. *Op.* Petr. Phell. *Samb.* Sil. *Spig.* Sulph. *Tabac. Tart.*
— in evening, *Carb-an.* Ind. Ntr-m.
— at night, *Bry.* Cham. Chin. Sil.
— after eating and drinking, Bry.
— in children, Bry. *Samb. Sulph.*
— — with shrieking and weeping, Samb.
Tickling cough, *Ambr.* Anac. Ang. *Arn.* Bell. Bov. *Bry.* Calc. Carb-veg. Caust. *Cham.* Colch. *Con. Dros. Euph.* Ferr. Ip. *Kali-c.* Laur. *Lyc.* Mgn-c. Mgn-m. Merc. Ntr-c. Ntr-m. *Nux.* Oleand. Ol-an. Petr. *Phosp.* Phosp-ac. Rhus. Rumex. Sabad. *Sabin.* Sass. *Seneg. Sep.* Sil. Spong. Stann. *Tabac.* Tart. Teucr. Thuj.
— in morning, aggravated, Thuj.
— — — evening, Merc. *Rhus.*
— — at night, Rhus.
— — day and night, Ntr-m.
Trumpet-toned cough, Verb.
Typical cough, Cocc.
Unintermitting cough, Cupr.
Vehement, tormenting cough, Alum. Amm-c. Anac. Ang. Ars Arum. Asa-f. Bar-c. Bell. Borax. Brom. *Calc.* Cannab. Carb-an. Caust. Chelid. Chin. Cina. *Cocc.* Con. Cor-r. *Croc.* Cupr. Daph. Dros. Dulc. Hep. Hydroc-ac. Ip. Lach. Lact. Led. Lob. Merc. Merc-cor. *Mez.* Mur-ac. Ntr-c. Ntr-m. Nitr-ac. Nitr. *Nux.* Op. *Phosp.* Rhod. Scill. Selen. Sep. Spig. Stann. Sulph. Verat.
Wheezing, (asthmatic,) cough, Asa-f. Brom. Cham. Creos. Cupr. Hep. Kali-b. Kali-c. Prun. Sabad. Samb. Spong. Sulph-ac.
Whistling cough, Acon. Ars. Brom. Creos. Hep. Laur.
Winter cough, Acon. Cham.
The longer he coughs the more irritation there is to cough, Ign. Teucr.

25. Respiration.

Air feels cold on inspiring, Lith.
Asthma humid, Bar-m. Zing.
— millari, *Acon.* Ars. Bell. Igt. *Ip.* Lach. Mosch. Nux. Op. Puls. Samb. (compare Suffocating fits.)
Breath, offensive, Acon. Ambr. Arn. Ars. Aur. Bry. Caps. Carb-veg. Cham. Chin Cist. Croc. Daph. Dros. Dulc. Hipp-m. Hyosc. Ip. Lach. Led. Merc. Mez. Ntr-m. Nitr-ac. *Nux.* Plb. Puls. Sass. S.p. Sulph. Verb. Zinc.
— putrid, Arn. Ars. Aur. Nitr-ac.
— sour, Nux.
Deep respiration, Agar. Ant. Arn. Bell. Borax. Bry. Calc. Calc-ph. Camph. *Caps.* Carb-veg. *Cast.* Cham. Chin. Creos. Croc. Cupr. *Dig.* Eupa. *Evon.* Glon. Hell. Hep. Hydroc-ac. Igt. Ip. Kali-c. Lach. Lachn. Lact. Lob. Merc. Mez. Mur-ac. Ntr-c. Nux. Oleand. Op. Par. Phosp. Plat. Poth. *Ran-b.* Ran-sc. Rhus. Sass. Selen. Sil. Spong. Stann. Therid. Thuj.
— from heaviness at heart, Croc.
— when sitting, Lach.
— with sense of emptiness in chest, Poth.
Difficult respiration, dyspnœa, Acon. Agar. Anim-c. Arn. Ars. Asa-f. Aur. *Bell.* Borax. *Bry.* Cact. Calc. Cannab. Canth. *Carb-veg. Cast.* Chin. Cic. *Colch.* Con. Creos. Croc *Cycl.* Elat. Euphr. Fluor-ac. *Hell* Hep. Hyosc. *Igt.* Iod. *Ip.* Kali-c Kalm. Lact. Laur. Lyc. Merc. Merc-sulph. Mez. Ntr-c. Nitr-ac. *Nux-m.* Op. Osm. Ox-ac. *Phosp.* Plat. Plb. Prun. Psor. Puls. *Ran-b.* Rat. Rhus. Sabad. Sang. Sass. Scill. Sec c. *Seneg.* Sep. Spig. Spong. Stram. *Sulph.* Tart. Tereb. Valer. *Verat.* Viol-od. Zinc.
— chronic, Osm.
— spasmodic, as if lungs could not be expanded enough, Asa-f.
— like a weight on chest, Cannab. Igt. Rheum. Sabad.
— in evening, with anxiety, *Phosp.*
— as from congestion of blood, Agar. Tereb.
— from dryness of nose, Canth.
— when lying, Asa-f.
— — sitting, Alum. Euphr. Phosp. Verat.
— — walking, Calc. Carb-veg. Cast. Con.

Igt. Lact. Mgn-c. Ntr-s. Oleand. Petr. Puls. Rhus.
Difficult respiration, accompanies diseased conditions in parts not involved in the act of breathing, Puls.
— with anxiousness, or palpitation of the heart, Amm-c. Viol-od.
— with burning in face, Stront.
— — colic, Bry.
— — emptiness in stomach, Stann.
— — fainting, Ars. Lach.
— — with feeling as if next breath would be the last, Apis.
— — heat, Cannab.
— — pain in stomach, Ars.
— — perspiration, anxious face and sleeplessness, Eupat.
— — swelling around ankles, Hep.
— — tetanic spasms, Millef.
Expirations forcible, Bell. Caps. Chin. Igt. Stram.
Inspiration difficult, Nux.
— — rapid expiration, Chin. Igt.
— effected by the two distinct efforts, Led.
— with mouth open, Scill.
— deep, Bry. Chin. Igt. Lach. Sil. Stann.
Noise produced by breathing, when inspiring, *Bell.* Caps. Cham. *Chin.* Cina. Coloc. Hyosc. *Igt.* Mgn-s. *Nux.* Puls. Rheum.
— when expiring, Mgn-s. *Nux.* Op. Tart.
— — puffing, Chin.
— — rattling, Calc.
— — snuffing, Mgn-s. Nux.
— — wheezing, Ntr-m.
— as from spasm of glottis, Kalm.
Obstructed respiration, Acon. Anac. Arn. Ars. Bar-c. Bell. Bism. *Bry.* Calc. Canth. Caps. Carb-an. Carb-veg. Caust. Cham. Cina. Cocc. Croc. Cupr. Dolich. Euphr. Grat. Igt. Laur. Led. Lyc. Merc. Ntr-m. Nitr-ac. Nux-m. *Ol-an. Op.* Plb. Puls. Ran-sc. *Ruta.* Sabad. *Samb.* Scill. Selen *Sil.* Spong. *Stann.* Stram. *Sulph.* Tart. Valer. Verat. Verb.
— as if in the back, Calc. Sass.
— — — from constriction around the abdomen, Kali-b.
— in region of stomach, Lam.
— as if in supra-sternal fossa, Cham.
— in throat, *Cham. Cocc.* Con.

25 RESPIRATION.

Obstructed respiration morning in bed, Tart.
— — evening in bed, Tart.
— at night, *Kali-c.* Selen. *Stann.*
— when ascending, Canth. Grat.
— — steps, Nitr-ac.
— from pain in chest, Brom. Caps. Croc. Plb. Ran-sc. *Ruta.* Spong. Valer. Verb.
— when coughing, Ign. Scill. Sil.
— — exercising, Stann.
— from flatulency, Carb-veg. Ol-an. Zinc.
— when lying, Samb.
— — on back, Ol-an. Sil.
— — — left side, Puls.
— during meals, Mgn-m.
— after meals, Cham.
— the pains take away the breath, Diosc.
— from change of position, better, Ol-an.
— when at rest, Sil.
— — running, Sil.
— from pain in sacral region, Selen.
— — tonic spasms of pectoral muscles, Cic.
— — stooping, Calc. Sil.
— — stitches in larynx, arrest of breathing, Hydroc-ac.
— as from sulphur vapor, Canth. Croc. *Puls.*
— when talking, Caust. Lam. Sulph.
— respiration prevented by sense of weakness in chest, Plat.
— with anxiousness Puls.
— — sense of emptiness in chest, Poth.
— — nausea, Canth. Lach.
— — palpitation of the heart, Nitr-ac. Puls.
— — sweat, Ars. Lach. Nux.
— — thirst, Lach.
— — vomiting, Lach.
— — weakness, Ars. Lach.
Oppression of the chest, *Acon.* All-cep. *Ambr.* Anac. *Ang.* Ant. Arn. Ars.*Asa-f.* Aur. Bar-m. *Bell.* Berb. Bruc. Bry. Cadm. Calad. Calc. *Camph.* Cannab. Canth. *Carb-veg.* Cham. *Chin. Cina.* Cinnab. Cocc. Coff. *Colch.* Con. Croc. Crotal. Cupr. Cycl. Dros. *Dulc.* Evon. Ferr. Graph. *Hep. Ign.* Iod. Ip. Kali-chl. Lach. Lact. Led. *Lyc.* Mgn-c. Mgn-m. Mgn-s. Merc. Merc-cor. Mez. Millef. Nitr. Nux-m. Nux. Oleand. Op. Par. Petr. Phell. *Phosp.* Phosp-ac. *Plat.* Plb. Puls. *Ran-b. Rhod. Rhus.* Sabad. Sacch. Samb. Sec-c. *Seneg. Sep.* Sil.Spig. Stann. Sulph. *Tabac. Tart.* Teucr. *Thuj.* Valer. *Verat.* Verb. *Viol-od.* Viol-tr. Zinc.
— in right side, Ox ac.
— of any kind, Phosp.
— anxious, *Acon.* Anac. Arn. Cannab. Cina. Colch. Kali-c. Nux. Op. *Phosp.* Plat. Puls. Rhus. Sabad. *Spig.* Stann. Staph. *Tabac.* Tart. Thuj. Valer. Verat.
— as if from abdomen, Caps.
— as if chest were too narrow, Oleand.

Oppression of chest, from a cold, from mucus, Dulc.
— compressing, Coloc.
— constant, Lyc.
— constringing, tightening, Acon. Agar. Ars. Aur. Bov. Camph. Canth. Carb-an. Cina. *Cocc.* Colch Dig. Dros. Euph. *Ferr.* Ip. *Laur. Led.* Mgn-c. *Mosch.* Nux-m. Phosp-ac. *Plat. Puls. Rhod.* Sa-s. Sil. *Spig.* Staph. Stram. Tabac. *Verat.*
— caused by the cough, Cocc.
— driving into the open air, Anac.
— as from flatulence, Cham.
— as if from fullness of chest, Caps.
— — — — stomach, Chin.
— painful, Ambr. Con.
— from pain in pericardial region, Cina.
— periodical, Colch. Plb.
— pressing, Ang. *Bry.* Cannab. *Colch. Mgn-s.* Ran-sc. *Rhod.* Seneg. Spig. Valer. Viol-od. *Zinc.*
— with rheumatism, Kalm.
— between scapulae, Ambr.
— from scrobiculus, proceeding, Mgn-m. Nux-m. Rhus.
— as from smoke, Cocc.
— as from sulphur-vapor, Brom. Camph. Croc.
— when turning to right side, Euph.
— in morning, Bell. Carb-an. Dig. Nux. Phosp.
— — — — bed, Mgn-s.
— — afternoon, All-cep. Elaps.
— — evening, Chin. *Phosp.* Zinc.
— — in bed, Con. Sep.
— at night, Amm-m. Berb. Calc. Coloc. Ign. Lact Mgn-s Nux. Petr. Rhus. Sep.
— during a fit of anger, Apis. Staph.
— when ascending, Apis. Ars. Canth. Cupr. Grat. Merc. Nitr. Ol-an. Stann. Zinc.
— — steps, Acon. Arg.
— from bending, backwards, ameliorated, Fluor-ac.
— when bending forwards, Seneg.
— — — ameliorated, Lach. Spong.
— in cold air, Ars. Petr. Puls.
— — — ameliorated, Cist.
— when coughing, Dros.(compare Sect. 24).
— exercising, Ox-ac. *Phosp.*
— by expectoration, ameliorated, Hipp-m.
— when lying, Asa f. Cham. Dig. Oleand. Sacch. Sep.
— — — ameliorated, Psor.
— after meals, Asa-f. Carb-an Lach. Nux. Puls Selen. *Seneg.* Sulph.
— — — ameliorated, Bell.Lac-can.Puls.
— from the pressure of clothes, Caust. Sass.
— from raising the arms, Spig.
— during rest, Sil.

25 RESPIRATION.

Oppression of chest when sitting up to write, Psor.
— — standing, Phell. Sep.
— — talking, Chin. *Dros.* Lach.
— — walking, Dig. Mgn-s. *Sep.*
— — — in open air, Lyc.
— — quickly, Ang.
— in warm room, Apis.
— with backache, Lach.
— alternating with convulsions, Igt.
— with expectoration profuse, *Sep.*
— — — checked, Sep.
— with heat, Anac.
— — numbness of arms, Tilia.
— — — — hands, Puls.,
— — pain between scapulae. Bell.
— — palpitation of heart, Grat.
— — warmth rising in chest, Plat. Tart.
— — weeping, *Ran-b.*
Paralysis of lungs, Ars. *Bar-c.* Carb-veg. Chin. *Laur.* Lyc. Op. Phosp, *Tart.*
Respiration anxious, Acon. Aeth. *Arn.* Ars. *Bell.* Bry. Camph. Cham. Coff. Creos. *Hep.* Hydroc-ac. Igt. *Ip. Laur.* Lob. Phosp. *Plat.* Plb. Puls. Rhus. Samb. Scill. Sec-c. Spong. Stann.
— asthmatic, Carb-an. Cina. Ip. Nitr-ac. Phosp. Plb.
— — from manual labor, Nitr-ac.
— — when walking quickly, Sil.
— cold, Carb-veg. Chin. *Cop.* Cor-r. Verat.
— convulsive, Cupr.
— crepitating, Bell. Carb-an. Carb-veg. Caust. Cupr. Hep. Hyosc. Ip. Laur. Ntr-c. Ntr-m. Puls. Samb. Scill. Sep. Sil. Tart.
— croaking, Cham. Lach.
— with a dry sound, Nux.
— fetid, Acon. Arn. Ars. Aur. Bry. Carb-veg. Chin. Cist. Croc. Daph. Dulc. Lach. Merc. Ntr-m. Nitr-ac. Nux. Puls. Sass. Sep. Sulph. Zinc.
— hiccoughing. Aeth.Ang.Asa-f.*Led.*Sec-c.
— — when lying down, Asa-f.
— hoarse, Hep. Kali-c.
— hot, Acon. Ant. Calc. Cham. Ferr. Mang. Ntr-m. Phosp. Rhus. Sabad. Scill. Stront. Zinc.
— hurried,quick,Acon.Ars.*Asa-f.Bell.*Bry. Carb-veg. Cast. Clem. *Cupr.* Gels. Hell. Hep. Igt Ip. Led. Lyc. Ntr-c. Ntr-m. Nux. Phosp. Puls. Rhus. *Samb.* Scill. Seneg. Sep. Sil. Spong. Stann. Sulph. Verat.
— expiration impossible, Meph.
— intermittent, Ang. Bell.Cina.Cocc-c.Op.
— interrupted, stoppage, of Ang. Ars. Bar-c. Bell. Borax. Calc. Caust. Chin. Cic.Cina.Cupr.Cycl.Daph.Euphr. Guaj. Hydroc-ac. Igt. Kali-c. Merc-cor. Nux. Op. Phosp. Plat. Plb. Puls. Samb Sass. Sil. Stann. Stram. Sulph. Therid. Verat.

Respiration, stoppage of suddenly in children, Cham.
— irregular, Ang. Bell. Cham. Cina.Clem. Cocc. Cupr. Dros Igt. Iod. Laur. Led. Mosch. Nux. Op. Puls. Sep. Tart.
— — at one time slow, at another hurried. Acon. Bell. Igt. Nux. Op. Spong.
— loud, Acon. Arn.Calc.Cham.Chin.Cina. Hep. Hyosc. Igt. Kali-c. Merc. Ntr-m. Nux. Op. Phosp. Scill. Spong. Stram. Sulph.
— — when sitting still, Ferr.
— moaning, Acon. Aeth. Ars. Bell. Cupr. Hydroc-ac.Lach Laur.Mur-ac.Puls.Scill
— painful, Chin. Led. Viol-od.
— panting, Acon. Arn. Camph. Carb-an. Chin. Cina. Cocc. Con Ip. Laur. Lob. Nitr-ac. Op. Phosp. Plb. Prun. Sec-c. Sil. Spong. Stram.
— — as from running, Hyosc.
— possible only when keeping body upright, Cannab.
— — — — head high, Chin.
— putrid, Arn. Ars. Aur. Nitr-ac.
— rattling, Brom. Bry. Cact. Cannab. Carb-an. Carb-veg. Caust. Cham. Chin. Cina. Cocc-c. Cupr. Hep. Hydroc-ac. Hyosc. Ip. Lact. Laur. Lob. Lyc. Nux-m. Nux. Op. Puls. Stann. Stram. Sulph. *Tart.*
— — when walking in open air, Ang.
— short, Acon. *Aeth.* Agar. Anac. Arn. Ars. *Bell.* Bry. Camph. Cannab. Carb-veg. Cast. Cham. Chin. Cina. Cocc. Croton. Hell. Hep. Ip. Lach. Lob. Merc. Mosch. Phosp. Plat. Prun. Puls. Sep. Sulph. Thuj.
— sighing, Acon. Bell. Bry. Calad. Carb-an. Cham. Glon. Igt. Ip. Sil. Spong. Stram.
— slow, Acon. Arn,*Bell.*Brom.Bry.Camph. Caps. *Cast.* Chin. Clem. Con. Cupr. Hell. Hep. Hydroc-ac. Hyosc. Igt. Ip. *Laur.* Merc-cor. Nux-m. Nux. Oleand. Op. Spong.
— — in sleep, Acon.
— snoring, Arn. Camph. *Cham.* Chin. *Hep.* Hydroc-ac. Hyosc. Lach Laur. Lyc. Nitr-m. Op. Petr. Stann. *Sulph.*
— sobbing, Acon. Aeth. Ang. Ant. Asa-f. Bry. Ip. Led. Ran-sc. Sec-c Sil. Stram. Therid.
— soft, Bell. Canth Hep. Oleand. Phosp. Verat. Viol-od.
— sour smelling, Nux.
— stertorous, Anac. Arn. Bell. Cannab. Carb-an. Cupr. Hyosc. *Laur.* Lyc. Op. Petr. Puls. Spong. Stann. *Tart.*
— — — in evening, in bed, Carb-an.
— — when lying on the side affected, Anac.
— superficial, Acon. Lob. Puls.
— vehement, expiration, Bell. Caps. Chin. Igt. Stram.

25 RESPIRATION. 187

Respiration weak, Ant. Igt. Laur. Phosp. Stram. Viol-od.
— wheezing, Ambr. Ars. Calad. Calc. Cannab. Carb-veg. Cham. *Chin.* Croton. Dolich. Dros. Fluor-ac. Graph. Hep. Hipp-m. Kali-c. Lach. Murex. Nitr-ac. Ox-ac. Phosp. Sabad. *Samb.* Sang. Scill. Spong. Stann. Sulph.
— — in evening bed, Nitr-m.
— whistling, Acon. Ambr. Ars. Brom. Cannab. Carb-veg. *Cham. Chin.* Coloc. Creos. Cupr. Hep. Kali-c. Laur. Phosp. Sabad. *Samb.* Sang. *Spong.* Stann. Sulph.
— whooping, Carb-an. Cina. Hyosc. Nitr-ac. Sil. Stram.
Respiration, disorders of in morning, Ambr. Bell. Carb-an. *Con.* Dig. Kali-c. Nux. *Phosp.* Tart.
— — bed, Carb-an. Con. Mgn-s. Tart.
— — evening *Ars.* Chin. Cycl. Ferr. Nux. *Phosp. Puls.* Rhus. *Stann.* *Sulph.* Tart. Zinc.
— — — bed. *Ars.* Carb-an. Chin. Con. Ferr. *Graph.* Nitr-m. *Sep.* Tart.
— — — — ameliorated, Lyc.
— — at night, Acon. Alum. Amm-m. *Ars.* Aur. Berb. Bry. *Calc.* Carb-veg. Cham. Chin. Coloc. Cupr. Daph. *Dig.* *Ferr.* Graph. Igt. Kali-c. Kali-jod. Lach. Lyc. Mgn-s. Merc. *Nux.* Op. Petr. Phosp Plb. *Puls.* Ran-b. Rhus. *Samb.* Selen. Seneg. *Sep. Stann. Sulph.*
— — during a fit of anger, Ars. Staph.
— — when ascending an eminence, Ars. Aur. Calc. Canth. Cast. Cupr. Grat. Iod. Merc. Nitr. Nux. Ol-an. Sep. Stann. Zinc.
— — — steps, Amm-c. Ang. Ars. Borax. Hyosc. Led. *Merc.* Nitr-ac. Rat. Ruta. Seneg.
— when bending forward, Seneg.
— — ameliorated, Cocc-c. Kali-c. Lach.
— as from congestion of blood, Agar. Calc. Puls. Tereb.
— from bodily exertion, Amm-c. Ars.
— pain in chest, Selen.
— in children, *Ambr.* Calc. Lyc.
— from coffee drinking, Bell.
— — cold air, Ars. Petr. Puls.
— — — ameliorated, Cist.
— after a cold, Ip.
— when coughing, Cupr. (compare Sect. 24.)
— — drinking, Bell.
— after drinking, Nux.
— as from dust, Cycl. Ip.
— when evacuating, Rhus. (compare Sect. 18).
— — exercising, *Ars.* Con. Ip. Led. *Phosp.* Puls. Spig. *Stann.* Verat.
— — moving in bed, Spig.
— from flatulency, *Carb-veg.* Ol-an. Zinc.

Respiration, disorder of, from holding back the body, Cupr.
— — labor, Bov. *Lyc.* Sil.
— — — manual, Amm-m. Bov. Nitr-m. Nitr-ac. Sil.
— — laughing, Ars. Cupr.
— on lifting the arms, Spig.
— when lying, Ars. Asa-f. Calc. Cannab. *Dig. Hep.* Lach. Nux. Oleand. Phell. *Phosp.* Puls. Samb. *Sep.* Sulph. Tart.
— — on the back, Ol-an. Phosp. Sil.
— — with head low, Chin. Colch. Hep. Nitr. Puls. Sacch.
— — on the side, Carb-an. Puls.
— — — right side, ameliorated, Spig.
— during meals, Mgn-m.
— after meals, Ars. Asa-f. Carb-an. Cham. Chin. Lach. Merc. *Nux-m.* Nux. Phosp. *Puls. Sulph.* Viol-tr. Zinc.
— with mouth open, Acon. Scill.
— from mucus accumulated, Chin. Seneg. Sep.
— in open air, Ars. Aur. Graph. Lyc. Puls. Selen. Seneg. Sulph.
— — — ameliorated, Bell.
— with the pains, Ars. *Puls.* Sil.
— periodical, Colch. Plb.
— from pressure of the clothes, Caust. Sass.
— by position, change of, relieved, Ol-an.
— when at rest, Ferr. Sil.
— retracting the shoulders, relieved, Amm-c. Ars. Calc.
— — running, Igt.
— after running, Sil.
— from p. in in sacral region, Selen.
— in scrofulous persons, *Ambr.*
— when sitting, Alum. Dig. Dros. Euphr. Lach. Phosp. *Samb.* Verat.
— — bent forward, Dig. Rhus.
— by half sitting, relieved, Spig.
— during sleep, Lach, Sulph.
— when standing, Phell. *Sep.*
— from stitches in chest, Aloe.
— — stomach, originating, Caps. Rhus.
— when stooping, Calc. Caust. Chin. Laur. Seneg. Sil. Sulph.
— as from sulphur vapor, Camph. Croc. *Puls.*
— when swallowing, *Bell.*
— — talking, Caust. *Dros.* Lam. Spig. Sulph.
— — touching the throat, *Bell.* Lach.
— — turning the throat, *Bell.*
— — walking, Agar. Ars. Bell. Carb-veg. *Con.* Led. Lyc. Nitr-s. Nux. Phell. Puls. Rhus. Selen. Seneg. *Sep.* Stann. Stront.
— — — in open air, Aur. Lyc. Selen. Seneg.
— — — quickly, Ang. Aur. Caust. Cupr. Kali-c. Merc. *Nitr-m.* Puls. Seneg. Sil.
— — against the wind, Calc. Lyc. Phosp. Psor. Selen.

25 RESPIRATION.

Respiration, disorders of, in a warm room, Ars.
— from wearing too warm clothes, Ars.
— as from weakness, Cycl.
— — a weight on the chest, Cannab. Igt. Rhus. Sabad.
— in windy weather, Ars. Calc.
— with dryness of nose, Canth.
— — desire to evacuate, Bry.
— — emptiness in pit of stomach, Stann.
— — expectoration too copious, Sep.
— — — checked, Sep.
— — humming in ears, Nux.
— — mouth open, Acon. Scill.
— — pain in pit of stomach, Nux.
— — stitches in chest and pain in hip, Ox-ac.
Short breathing, Acon. *Agar. Ambr.* Amm-c. *Anac.* Arn. Ars. *Asar.* Bell. *Bov.* Bry. Calc. Cannab. *Carb-veg.* Cast. Caust. Cina. *Con.* Cor-r. Creos. Cupr. Cycl. Dros. Euph. Euphr. Ferr. Hep. Ip. Kali-c Kalm. Lach. Lact. Led. Lyc. Mgn-c. *Merc.* Mur-ac. Ntr-c. Ntr-m. Ntr-s. Nicc. Nitr-ac. *Nux-m.* Nux. Op. Phell. Phosp. Phosp-ac. *Plat.* Plb. Pod. Prun. Psor. Puls. *Ran-b.* Rhus. *Ruta. Sabad.* Sass. Scill. *Seneg. Sep. Sil.* Spig. Stann. *Sulph.* Tabac. Tart. Thuj. Verat. Viol-od. Zinc.
— excessive, Lob.
— in morning, Kali-c.
— — afternoon, Sang.
— — evening, Cycl. Rhus.
— — — in bed, Sep.
— at night, *Sep.*
— when ascending, Cast. Scill.
— — steps, Amm-c. Hyosc. Merc. Seneg.
— in children, *Lyc.*
— as if from dust, Ip.
— when exercising, Scill. Verat.
— from expectoration, suppressed, Guaj. Tart.
— — flatulency, Zinc.
— — any labor, *Lyc.* Nitr-ac.
— — manual, *Bov.* Sil.
— when lying, Sep.
— after meals, Ars. *Nux-m.* Puls. Zinc.
— from mucus, in trachea, Selen. Thuj.
— in open air, Sulph.
— from pressure in middle of sternum. All-cep.
— during rest, Sulph.
— when sleeping, or raising oneself up, Acon.
— — standing, Sep.
— — talking. Spig.
— as from something tied around abdomen, Kali-b.
— from touching larynx, Lach.
— when walking, Carb-veg. *Con.* Ntr-s. Phell. *Sep.*
— — — open air, Sulph.

Short breathing, when walking rapidly, Igt. Merc. Nitr-m. Seneg Sil.
— as from weakness, Cycl.
— with tension in chest, Rhus.
Suffocative catarrh, Ant Bar-c. *Camph.* Iod. Op. Plb. Samb. *Sec-c.* (compare Suffocative fits.)
— fits. Acon. Anac. *Ant. Ars. Aur. Bell.* Brom. Bry. Cact. Calc. Camph. Carb-an. Carb-veg. Cham. Chin. Cina. *Coff.* Con. *Cupr. Cycl.* Dig. Dios. Ferr. *Graph. Hep.* Hipp-m. Hydroc-ac. Igt. Iod. Ip. Kali-c. Lach. Lact. Led. Merc. *Mosch.* Ntr-m. *Nux.* Op. Phosp. Plat. Pod. *Puls.* Rhod. Rhus. *Samb.* Sec-c. Sil. Spig. Spong. Stram. *Sulph. Tart. Verat.* Zinc. (compare Respiration, obstructed.)
— — in morning, Dig.
— — — in bed, Carb-an. Tart.
— — when rising relieved, Led. Puls. Sulph.
— — in evening, in bed, *Ars.* Chin. Ferr. Graph. Tart.
— — at night, Chin. *Graph.* Lact. *Nux.* Phosp. Puls. *Samb. Sulph.*
— — every six months, Sacch.
— — must bend head backwards, Hep.
— — as from constriction of lungs, Hell.
— — feeling that he cannot exhale, Meph.
— — when lying, *Hep.* Lact. Puls.
— — on moving or raising arms, Spig.
— — from accumulation of mucus in air passages, Camph.
— — as if larynx was full of mucus, Chin.
— — in room, relieved in open, Ip.
— — when touching or turning the neck, *Bell.*
— — — in larynx, Bell. Lach.
— — with burning heat of trunk, and cold extremities, Ferr.
— — — open eyes, bloated blue hands and face, and heat without thirst, Samb.
— — — opisthotous before cough, Led.
— — — restlessness and weeping, *Samb.*
Tightness of chest, asthma, Acon. *Agar.* Aloe. Alum. *Ambr. Amm-c.* Anac. Ant. Apis. Arn. *Ars.* Asar. *Aur. Bar-c.* Bar-m. Bell. Brom *Bry.* Calad. *Calc.* Camph. *Cannab. Caps.* Carb-an. Carb veg. Caust. Cham. Chelid Chin. *Cic.* Cina. Cist. Cocc. *Colch.* Coloc. *Con.* Croc. Crotal. Cupr. Daph. *Dig. Dros. Dulc. Euph. Ferr.* Graph. Grat. Hep. Hydroc-ac. Hyosc. *Igt.* Iod. Ip. *Kali-c.* Lach. Lact. *Laur. Led.* Lob. *Lyc.* Meny. Merc. Mercurial. Mez. Mosch. Ntr-c. Nitr-m. Nitr-ac. *Nitr.* Nux-m. *Nux.* Op. Par. Petr. Phell. *Phosp.* Plat. Plb. Psor. *Puls.* Ran-sc. Raph. Rheum. *Rhod. Ruta.* Sabin. Samb. Sang. *Sass.* Scill. Sec-c. Selen. Seneg. *Sep.* Sil. Spig. Spong. Stann. Stram. Stront. *Sulph. Sulph-ac.* Tart. Thuj. *Verat. Viol-od.* Viol-tr. Zinc.

Tightness, as if larynx was not wide enough, Cist.
— of any kind, *Phosp.*
— — in chest, Sabad.
— caused by dust, Poth.
— with eructations as if stomach were filled with dry food, Calad.
— humidum, Bar-m. Zing.
— periodical, Lach.
— as from sulphur-vapor, Puls.
— worse in cold weather, Apis.
— with hydrothorax, Psor.
— — redness of face, eructation and as if chest was extended, Caps.
— — — oedematous swelling of who'e body, ascites and induration of liver. Lact.
— spasmodic, Asa-f. Caust. *Cupr. It.* Kali-c. Lach. Laur. *Led.* Lob. *Mosch.* Nux. *Op.* Phosp. Phosp ac. *Plb. Puls.* Raph. *Sass. Sec-c.* Sulph. *Zinc.*
— — from stomach and scrobiculus proceeding, Caps. Ferr.
— straining across chest, Calc.
— as from fulness, Calc. Carb-veg. Phosp. Puls. Sep. Verat.
— in morning.Carb an. *Con. Kali-c.* Phos .
— — — in bed, Con.
— — evening, Ferr. Nux. *Phosp.* Puls. Stann. Zinc.
— — — in bed, Graph. Sep.
— at night, Amm m. Aur. Brv. Color. Daph. Dig. *Ferr.* Kali-c. Lach. Nux. Phosp. *Puls.* Sang. *Sep. Sulph.*
— after midnight, Ferr.
— — 3 A.M., Cupr.
— when ascending, Cupr. Merc. Stann.
— — steps, Led. *Merc.* Nitr-ac.
— — bending backwards, Cupr.
— after bodily exertion, Amm-c.
— in children and old people, *Ambr.*
— from cold air, Petr.
— with coryza, Berb.
— when coughing, Cupr.

Tightness, after drinking, Nux.
— when exercising, Led. Phosp.
— with heat in forehead, Lob.
— hysterical, Ars.
— when laughing, Cupr.
— as from a lump in pit of throat, above sternum, Lob.
— when lying, Caust. Dig. Ferr. Sep.
— — with head low, Nitr.
— — horizontally, Puls.
— from manual labor, Amm-m. Ntr-m.
— after meals, Carb-an. Lach. Phosp. Puls.
— in open air, Aur. Selen.
— — relieved, Ntr-m.
— during rest, Ferr.
— when retracting, the shoulders relieved, Calc.
— as from rapid running, Hyosc.
— in scrofulous persons, *Ambr.*
— when sitting, Caust. Dig. Ferr. Psor. Verat.
— by sitting up and bending head on knees, relieved, Cocc-c. Kali-c.
— when standing, Sep.
- can only breathe when standing, Cannab.
- when talking, Dros.
- — walking, Agar.Led. *Sep.*Stann.Stront.
- — — rapidly, Cupr. Kali-c. Merc.
- by walking and talking, relieved, Ferr.
Want of breath, Ang. Arn. Ars. Bell. Bry. Carb-veg. Chin. Cina. *Cycl.* Eupat. Ferr. Hyosc. Igt. Iod. Ip. Laur. Led, Lyc.Merc. Nitr-ac. Nux. Phosp-ac.Puls. Rhus. Scill. Seneg. Sep. Stann. Stram. Verat.
— when exercising, Ars.
- gasping, Brom. Bry. Dros. Ferr. Ip.
- cannot recover breath, Dros. Hyosc. Sep. Tart.
- as from rapid running, Hyosc.
- when talking, Lam. Phosp-ac.

26. Chest and Heart.

Abscess of lungs, Kali-c.
Adhesion of lungs, after inflamation, Ran-b.
— sensation of, Cadm. *Euph.* Kali-c. *Mez.* Nitr. Ran-b. Seneg. *Thuj.*
As if air could not penetrate deep enough, sensation, Croton.
As if lungs touched the back, sensation, Sulph.
Angina pectoris, Ang. Ars. Dig. Hep. Ip. Lach. Ox-ac. Samb. Sep. Verat.
Anxiety in chest, *Acon.* Anac. Arn. Bell. Bry. Calc. Carb-veg. Cocc. Con. Creos. Croton. Graph. Hyosc. Lam. Lyc. Ntr-m. Nitr-ac. *Nux.* Ol-an. Petr. Phosp. Puls. Rhus. Seneg. Sep. *Spig.* Spong. Stann. Sulph. Teucr. Viol-od.
— about the heart, *Ars.* Aur. Bell. Calc. Camph. Cannib. *Caust. Cham. Coff.* Croc. Cycl. Dig. *Evon.* Lyc. Merc. Mosch. *Nux. Plat. Plb. Puls.* Rhus. Sec-c. Spong. Therid. *Verat.* Viol-tr.
As if beaten, pain, Amm-m. Arn. Creos. *Evon.* Ferr. Lact. Lyc. Mang. Merc Murex. Mur-ac. Ol-an. Ran-sc. Sil. Stann. Verat. (compare Sect. 27.)
Blood, congestion, Cocc. Lact. Nux. Ol-an. Plb. Rhod. Seneg. *Sep.* Thuj.
— congestion to chest, Acon. Aloe *Amm-c. Aur. Bell.* Brom. Carb-veg. Chin. Cocc. Cupr. Cycl. Dig. Ferr. Glon. Iod. Kali-c. Lact. Mgn-m. Merc. *Nitr-ac.* Nitr. Nux Ol-an. *Phosp.* Puls. Rat. *Rhod.* Rhus. Scill. *Seneg. Sep.* Sil. *Spong.* *Sulph.* Thuj.
— — at night, Puls.
— — after exertion and motion, *Spong.*
— — writing, Amm-c.
— — with weakness and nausea, Spong.
— to the heart, Cycl. Puls. Sulph.
— — at night, Puls.
— as if stopping, sensation, Sabad. Seneg.
— from sea-bathing, Mgn-m.
Boring, chest, Alum. *Brom.* Cina. Cupr. Ind. Kali-c. Lob. Mur-ac. Rhus. Seneg. Tar.
— heart, Seneg.
Bubbling and boiling about heart, Lachn.
Burning, chest, Amm-c. Ant. Arn. *Ars. Bism.* Bry. *Calc.* Canth. Carb-veg. Cast. Caust. *Cham.* Cic. Cina. Cocc. Colch.
Cop. Creos. Croton. *Euph.* Hyper. Iod. Kali-b. Kali-c. Lach. Lact. Lam. Laur. Led. Lob. *Lyc.* Mgn-m. Mgn-s. Mang. Merc. Merc-sulph. Murex. Mur-ac. Nux. Ol-an. Op. Phosp. Phosp-ac. Psor. Puls. Ran-b. Rat. Sabad. Sang. *Seneg.* Spig. *Spong. Sulph.* Tabac. Tart. Tereb. *Tong.* Zinc.
Burning, chest, right side, Carb-an.
— — rising even to face, Sulph.
— — in sternum, Cham. Kali-b.
— — at night, Lach.
— — when breathing, Kali-c.
— — coughing, Mgn-m. (compare Sect. 24.)
— heart, Carb-veg. Kali-c. Op. Puls. Rumex.
— sternum, Cham. Mgn-s. Mez. Tereb.
— — under, Cocc-c.
— — under lower part of, Gels.
Bursting, as if, pain, Bry. Carb-an Cham. Cina. Merc. Mur-ac. Rhus. Seneg. Sulph. Zinc.
— — from cough, Lact.
Chilliness, in chest, Bry. Ntr-c.
— — evening, Ars.
— — left side, Ntr-c. Ntr-m.
— begins in chest, Cic. Spig.
Clawing sensation in chest, Samb. Stront.
Clucking sound in chest, Cina.
Coldness, sensation of, in chest, Amm-c. Arn. Ars Berb Camph Carb an. Cor-r. Graph. Lach. Lact. Oleand. Petr. Rhus. Ruta. Spong. Sulph. Thuj. *Zinc.*
— — left side, Ntr-m.
Compression, sensation of, Acon. Agar. Arg. *Arn.* Calc. Carb-an. Cham. Cina. Coloc. Dulc. Evon. Hyosc. Kali-c. Laur. *Meny.* Merc. Oleand. Op. Plat. Rhod. Ruta. Seneg. Stann. Teucr. Verat. Zinc.
— — at night, Ruta.
— — at the heart, Arn. Ntr-m.
Contraction, constriction, *Alum.* Anac. Arn. *Ars.* Asa-f. Asar. Bell. Bism. Brom. Bufo. Cact. Caps. Carb-veg. Cham. Cinnab. *Cocc.* Con. Cop. *Cupr.* Dig. Dros. Dulc. Elaps. *Ferr.* Gels. Glon. Haematox. *Hell.* Hep. Hipp-m. Igt. Ip. Kali-chl. Lach. Lact. *Laur.* Led. Lith. Mgn-c. Mgn-m. Mang. Merc-cor. Mez. Mosch.

26. CHEST AND HEART.

Ntr-ac. Nitr. Nux-m. *Nux. Op.* Phosp. Poth. Puls. Rat. *Rhod.* Rhus. Sabad. Samb. Seneg. Sep. Spig. Spong. Staph. Stram. Sulph. Sulph-ac. Tabac. Tart. Verat. Verb. Zinc.
Contraction, constriction, upper part, Cham.
— lower part, Gels. Haematox.
— one-sided (right), Cocc.
— at heart, Ang. Cact. Calc. Kali-c. Mur-ac. Ntr-m.
— originating in epigastrium, Rhus.
— spasmodic, Asa f. Lact. Sec-c. Verat.
— — up to throat, Asa-f.
— — by deep inspiration, increase, must sit up in bed at night, Lact.
— of lower part of chest, Dros. Nux.
— — upper part of chest, Rhus.
— from bringing the arms together, Sulph.
— when ascending, Nux.
— — when bending forward, Dig.
— from cold air, Bry.
— in cold air, or temperature, worse, Sabad.
— in getting cold, Mosch.
— after drinking, Cupr.
— from exercise, Ars. Ferr. Nux.
— when stooping, Alum.
— from touch, eating and drinking, increased, Arn Cupr.
— when walking, Ferr. Nux.
Crackling in chest, Sabin.
— about heart, Ntr-c.
Cutting in chest, *Ang.* Arg. Aur. Bad. Bell. Calc. Cannab. Dulc. Ind. Kali-c. Kali-jod. Mur-ac. Ntr-c. Ntr-m. Nitr. Olean. Petr. Phosp-ac. Psor. Puls. Rat. Rhus. Sabin. Spig. Stann. Sulph. Tabac. Tar. Verat.
— — right side, Colch. Lachn.
— — left, lung, sudden, Ox-ac.
— — heart, Jac-cor. Kali-c. Kali-jod. Sabin.
— when breathing and bending forwards, Arg.
Detached, sensation as if viscera were, Bry.
Digging, Acon. Cannab. Carb-an. Cina. Dulc. Lach. Meny. Oleand. Stann.
Dilatation, of chest, sensation of, Oleand.
Distention, sensation of, Ars. Thuj.
Distend, as if lungs did not, Asa-f. Croton.
Drawing, Camph. Con. Evon. Lact. Oleand. Seneg.
— at heart, Bell. Nux-m. Rhus.
Dropsy of chest, Amm-c. Apis. *Ars.* Bry. *Carb-veg.* Chin. Colch. *Dig.* Dulc. Fluor-ac. *Hell. Kali-c.* Lact. Lyc. Merc-sulph. Op. Sang. Scill. *Seneg. Spig.* Stann.
— from organic diseases, Spig.
— with asthma, Psor.
Dryness, Ferr. Kali-chl. Merc. Osm. Puls. Zinc.

Emptiness, sensation of, *Calad. Cocc.* Croc. Croton. Graph. Kali-c. Oleand. Plat. Poth. Sep. Stann. Sulph. Zinc.
— in heart, Sulph.
— after expectoration, *Calad.* Stann.
As if something were falling forward in the chest, when turning in bed, sensation, Bar-c. Sulph.
— — drops were falling from heart. Cannab.
Fluttering in region of heart, Kali-jod. Ntr-m. Rhus.
Fulness, sensation of, Acon. Agar. Arg-n. Bar-m. Brom. Calc. Carb-veg. Cist. Croton. Ferr. Lach. Lachn. Lact. Lob. Lyc. Nitr-ac. Nux-m. Nux. *Phosp.* Puls. Rhus. Ruta. Sacch. Sep. Spong. *Sulph.* Sulph-ac. Tereb. Verat.
— in heart, Glon.
— — morning, Sulph.
Gangrene of lungs, Lach.
Gnawing, (corroding,) pain in chest, Ran-sc. Ruta.
Gurgling, when breathing, Cina. Ind. Mur-ac.
As of something hard falling down, Bar-c.
Heart affections of, in general, Acon. Aur. Hyosc. *Puls. Spig.*
— as if on right side, sensation, or would be crushed, Borax.
Heart beat, double one hard, and full, the other soft and small, Lachn. Op.
— — each beat with a bellows sound, Spong.
— fluttering, Ntr-m.
— increased, Ars. *Bar-c.* Bar-m. *Dig.* Dulc. Ferr-m. *Mur-ac.* Sabin.
— intermitting, Bry. Chin. Dig. Kali-c. *Ntr-m.* Op. Ox-ac. Phosp-ac. Samb. Sec-c. Sep. Stram. Sulph.
— irregular. Aeth. Ars. Hydroc-ac. *Laur. Ntr-m.* Zinc.
— — feeble, Hydroc-ac.
— lower, seemingly, Cannab.
— slow, Laur.
— tremulous, Ars. *Calc.* Camph. Cic. Creos. Ntr-m. Rhus. Sabin. Spig. Staph.
— twitching, Arn. Daph.
— organic diseases of, Cact. Calc. Caust. Crotal. Lach. Lyc. Naja. Puls. Spig.
Heart, palpitation of, *Acon.* Alum. *Ambr.* Amm-c. Ang. Arn. Ars. Asa-f. Aur. *Bar-c.* Bar-m. *Bell.* Berb. Bism. Bov. Brom. *Bry.* Cact. *Calc. Cannab.* Canth. Carb-an. Carb-veg. *Caust.* Chin. *Cocc. Colch.* Coloc. Con. Cop. Creos. Crotal. Cupr. *Cycl.* Daph. *Dig.* Ferr. *Graph.* Grat. Hell. Hep. Hydroc ac. Hyper. Igt. *Iod.* Ip. Kali-c. Kali chl. Kalm. Lach Lyc. *Mgn-m. Merc.* Millef. Mosch. Murex. Mur-ac. Naja. *Ntr-c. Ntr-m.* Nitr-ac. *Nitr. Nux-m.* Nux. Oleand.

26. CHEST AND HEART.

Petr. *Phosp.* Plat. Prun. Puls. Rheum.
Scill. *Sep.* Sil. Stann. Staph. Sulph. Zinc.
Par. Petr. *Ph.sp.* Phosp-ac. *Plat.* Plb.
Pod. Psor. *Puls.* Rhus. Rhus-rad.
Sabad. Sang. Sass. *Sec-c.* Seneg. *Sep.*
Sil. *Spig.* Spong. *Staph.* Stront. *Sulph.*
Sulph-ac Tabac. *Tart.* Tellur. Thuj.
Verat. Viol-od. Zinc.

Heat. palpitation of any kind, Phosp.
—— anxious, *Acon. Ars.* Aspar. Aur.
  Bar-c. Calc. Cannab. Carb-veg.
  Caust. Chelid. Chin. Cocc. Croc.
  Dig. Elaps. Graph. Kali-c. Lach.
  Lyc. Merc. Mosch. Ntr-c. *Ntr-m.*
  Nitr-ac. Nux. *Oleand.* Phosp. *Plat.*
  Plb. Psor. *Puls.* Rhus. Ruta. Sass.
  Sec-c. Sep. *Spig. Sulph. Tart.*
  Verat. Viol tr. Zinc.
—— audible, Bell. Camph. Dig. Spig. *Thuj.*
—— concussive, Seneg.
—— felt in face, Mur-ac.
—— labored, Glon.
—— nervous, Cocc.
—— palpable, externally, Cycl. Dulc.
  Mur-ac. Plb.
—— reverberating in head, Bell.
—— spasmodic, *Iod.* Sec-c.
—— vehement, *Ang.* Aur. Bell. Bry.
  Carb-veg. *Chin. Colch.* Croton.
  Dig. Hep. *Iod.* Lachn. *Ntr-c.*
  Ntr-m. *Nitr.* Oleand. *Phosp.* Puls.
  Rhus. Sec-c. Seneg. Sep. *Spig*
  Sulph. Thuj. Verat. Viol-od.
—— visible, Spig. *Sulph. Tart. Verat.*
—— in morning, Carb-an. Nux. Phosp
  Rhus. Spig. Thuj.
———— in bed, Igt. Kali-c.
———— when hungry, Kali-c.
—— evening, Ang. Carb-an. Hipp-m.
———— in bed, Ang. Lyc.
—— at night, Agar. Arg-n. *Ars.* Bar-c.
  Calc. *Dulc.* Igt. Mur-ac. Ntr-c.
  Ntr-m. Nitr-ac. Nitr. Ox-ac. Puls.
  Sulph.
—— from anger, Phosp.
—— when ascending, Bell. Sulph.
———— steps, Croton. Ntr-c. Nitr-ac. *Thuj.*
—— after drinking, Con.
———— evacuation, Caust. Grat. Tart.
—— exercising, Bad. *Graph.* Ntr-m.
  Nitr-ac. Par. *Staph.*
———— relieved, Mgn-m.
—— from physical exertion, Amm-c. Pod.
—— by exertion, increased, Iod.
—— when expanding chest, Lach.
—— from the hymn-tune in church.
  Carb-an.
—— when lying down, Nitr. Ox-ac. Viol-od.
———— on the side, Ang. Bar-c. Daph.
  Ntr-c. Ntr-m. Puls. Tabac.
  Viol-tr.
———————— left side, Ang. Brom. Cact.
  Ntr-c. Puls. Tabac.

Heat, palpitation of, when lying on back, Ars.
—— after meals, Bufo. *Calc.* Camph.
  Igt. *Lyc.* Nitr-ac. Nux. Phosp.
  Puls. Thuj
—— after mental affection, Phosp. Puls.
———— from mental exertion, Igt. Sulph.
———— music, Carb-an. Staph.
———— pain in chest, Lach.
—— when at rest, Mgn-c. Par. Phosp.
  Rhus. Spig.
—— by rising and walking about, relieved, Glon.
—— when sitting, Carb-veg. Mgn-m.
  Phosp. Rhus. Spig.
———— bent, Ant. Dig.
—— after sleep at noon, Staph.
———— speaking, Puls.
—— when standing, Agar.
—— from stooping, Ang. *Spig.* Sulph-ac.
—— when walking, Acon. Cact. Nitr-ac.
———— in open air, Ambr.
— attended by, blood, congestion of,
  Glon. *Kali-c.* Sabad.
—— chest, pain in, Nux.
—— choking from, least exertion, Lach.
—— cold feet, Kali-chl.
—— coldness, sensation of, in heart,
  Kali-chl.
—— epigastriaum, retraction of, Amm-c.
—— face hot, Acon. Glon.
—— pale, Ambr.
—— giddiness and restlessness, Bov.
—— headache, Bov.
—— pain in heart, Igt.
—— heat, Nitr-ac.
—— flushes of, Calc. Lach.
—— vital, increased, Acon.
—— loosening all clothing, Puls.
—— nausea, Arg-n. Bov. Bufo. Nux. Thuj.
—, respiration affected, Acon. Bry.
  Puls. Verat.
—— sight, obscuration of, *Puls.*
—— small of back, pain in, Lach.
—— syncope, Lach. Nux-m.
—— throbbing in whole body, followed
  by sweat, Tellur.
———— weakness in pit of stomach,
  Amm-c.

Heat in chest, Acon. Amm-c. Apis. *Ars.*
  Bar-m. Bism. Bry. Cast. Cham. Cic.
  Cocc-c. Croton. Dig. Grat. Hyosc. Iod.
  Lachn. Meny. Ntr-m. *Nux.* Op. Puls.
  Ran-sc. Rat. Rhus. Ruta. Samb. Spig.
— about heart, Glon. Lachn. Op.
— from chest to liver, Sang.
— rising in thorax, sensation of, Ol-an.
  Phosp. Plat. Thuj.

Heaviness (weight) sensation in chest,
  Acon. Alum. *Amm-c. Amm-m.* Arn,
  Bar-c. Bov. Bry. *Cast.* Cop. Creos. Gels.
  Lach. Lact. Laur. Lyc. Mgn-c. Mgn-m.
  Nicc. Nitr. *Nux-m. Nux.* Oleand. Ox-ac.

26. CHEST AND HEART.

Heaviness, weight lower part of thorax, Prun.
— morning, Sulph.
— night, Amm-m.
— when ascending, Bar-c.
— — breathing deep, Cast.
— during meals, Mgn-m.
— when sitting, Staph.
— — walking, Amm-m. Lact. Sulph.
— by walking, relieved, Staph.
— sensation of, at heart, Croc. Glon. Puls.
Hollow, as if chest were, Poth.
Hypertrophy of heart, Kalm.
Inflammation of heart, Acon. Ars. *Bry.* Cannab. Cocc. Puls. *Spig.*
— lungs, *Acon.* Ars. Bell. *Bry.* Cact. Cannab. Canth. Carb-veg. *Chin.* Cop. Crotal. Hyosc. Kali-c. Lach. Lachn. Lyc. *Merc. Nitr.* Nux. Op. *Phosp.* Phosp-ac. *Puls.* Rhus. *Sabad.* Sacch. Sang. *Scill. Seneg. Sep.* Spig. Stram. Sulph. Tart. Verat.
— — left side, Phosp.
— — lower lobe, Sulph.
— — right side, Brom.
— — lower lobe, Kali-c.
— — after abuse of aconite, Bry.
— — in aged persons, Bry.
— — after a cold, Camph.
— — neglected, Lyc. Sulph.
— — nervous, Bell. Bry. *Chin.* Con. *Hyosc.* Laur. *Lyc.* Op. Phosp. Phosp-ac. Puls. *Rhus.* Stram. *Tart.* Verat.
— — from weakness, Chin.
— pleura, *Acon. Bry.* Phosp. *Scill.*
— — rheumatic, *Arn.* Bry. Nux. Sabad.
Itching in chest, Ambr. Ars. Con. Iod. Phosp. Puls. Sep. Stann.
— — and thyroid gland, Ambr.
— under ribs of left side, Fluor-ac.
Jerks in chest, Cina. Scill. Valer.
— — when breathing, Lyc.
— — at heart, Fluor ac. Ntr-m.
Jumping sensation in chest, *Croc.*
Langor in chest, Carb-veg. Phosp.
— — evening. Ran-sc.
— from reading aloud, Cocc.
— — singing, Carb-veg.
Lightness sensation of, when breathing, Stann.
Like something living in chest, sensation, *Croc.* Led.
Looseness, sensation of, *Bry.*
Like a lump, sensation, Ambr. Cocc. Sulph.
Motion spasmodic in chest, Arn.
Oppression at heart, Cannab. *Caust.* Mgn-m. Spig. Tabac. Viol-tr.
— — with melancholy, Caust.
— of chest, (compare. Sect. 25.)
— — alternating with headache, Glon.
Pain in general chest, Coloc. Creos. Dulc. Hydroc-ac. Lachn. Lact. Lob. Ox-ac. *Phosp.* Poth. Sabad. Sep.

Pain in general, must press chest with hand, Creos. Sep.
— right side with, with aggravation from 4 to 5 p.m., Merc-sulph.
— starting from shoulder, Sabad.
— from overlifting, Sulph.
— as from a sprain, Kalm.
— after inflammation of lungs, Amm-c. Lach. Lyc. Phosp. Sulph.
— in right lung, Rumex.
— — centre of left lung, Rumex.
— through apex of both lungs, Dolich.
— dull, under sternum, on raising head and drawing breath, Jac-cor.
— about heart, Benz-ac. Hydroc-ac. Lach. Laur. *N'tr-m.* Ox-ac. Pallad. Spong. Tellur. Thuj.
— — after pains in bladder, Lith.
— extending to head, Lith.
— as if a bar were extending, to right side anxiety, palpitation of heart small pulse, hot hands and chills, Hoematox.
— in evening, Ran-sc. Verb.
— at night, Ran-sc. Tart.
— when ascending, steps, Acon.
— with anxiety, Spong.
Paralysis of lungs, Bar-c. Chin. Hydroc-ac. Lach. Laur. Seneg. Tart. (compare Sect. 25.)
— sensation of, Lob. (compare Sect. 25.
Perforation sensation of, Lob.
Phthisis pulmonalis, Calc. Creos. Dulc. Nitr-ac. Phosp. Psor. Sang. Seneg. Sep. Sil. Stann.
— acute, Ars. Bry. *Chin.* Dros. Dulc. *Ferr. Laur.* Ntr-m. Puls.
— after hæmorrhages, Chin.
— — mechanical injuries to chest, Ruta.
— mucus, Dulc. Merc. Phosp. Seneg. Stann.
— purulent, ulcerative, Ars. Brom. Bry. *Calc.* Carb-an. *Carb-veg.* Chin. Creos. Dros. Guaj. Hyosc. Iod. *Kali-c.* Led. *Lyc.* Merc. Ntr-m. *Nitr-ac.* Nitr. Nux-m. *Phosp.* Puls. Ruta. Sep. Sil. Stann. Sulph. (compare Sect. 24;—expectoration purulent.)
— tuberculous, Calc. Kali-c. Lyc. Phosp. Puls. Stann.
— with rapid emaciation, Dros.
Pinching pain chest, Agar. Alum. Bell. Carb-an. Carb-veg. Cina. Cupr. Dulc. Ip. Kali-c. Par. Phosp-ac. Ran-sc. Rhod. Seneg.
Like a plug, sensation, Anac. Aur.
Pressing sensation, Ambr. Carb-veg. Cic. Seneg.
— — during meals, Paeon.
— asunder, Euph.
Pressure, *Alum.* Ambr. Amm-c. *Anac.* Arg. Ars. *Asa-f.* Asar. Bar-c. *Bell.* Bism. Brom. *Bry.* Calc. *Carb-veg.* Cast. Caust. Chin. Cic. Cist. Cocc. Cocc-c. *Colch.*

26. CHEST AND HEART.

Croton. Cupr. Cycl. Dig Fluor-ac.
Graph. *Grat.* Hyosc. Hyper. Igt. Kali-b
Kali-c. Lach. Lact. Lam. Laur.Lith.Lyc.
Mgn-m. Merc. Mez. Mur-ac. *Ntr-c.*
Nicc. Nitr. *Nux-m.* Nux. Ol-an. Op.
Phosp. *Phosp-ac. Plat.* Plb. Psor.Ran-b.
Ran-sc. *Rhod. Ruta.* Sabad. Sabin. Samb.
Sang. Scill. *Seneg. Sep. Sil.* Spig. Stann.
Staph. Stram. Stront. *Sulph.* Sulph-ac.
Tabac. Tar. Thuj. *Verat.* Verb.Viol-od.
Zinc.
Pressure lower chest, Bism. Lact. Teucr.
Valer. (compare, Sect. 16.)
— cutting on both sides, Ang.
— about the heart, *Ambr.* Bell. Calc.
Cocc-c. Con. Cycl Hydroc-ac. Kali-b.
Ntr-m. Ol-an Pallad. Puls. Seneg.
— towards the heart, Cocc-c
— as from a load, Asa-f. Samb.
— on sternum, Agn. Arg. Ars. Asa-f. Bry.
Con. Gum-gut. Lact. Laur. Poth.
Sulph.
— in the sides, Arg. Aur. Lact. Par.
Sulph-ac.
— — — left side, Acon. Pallad.
— constant, *Lyc.*
— in morning, Sulph.
— — — in bed, Mgn-m. Phell. Seneg.
— — evening in bed. Sep.
— at night, *Alum.* Mgn-s. Seneg.
— periodical, Pallad.
— when ascending, Bar-c.
— coughing, Sil. Sulph. (compare, Sect. 24.)
— after drinking, Verat.
— during exertion, Rat.
— when gaping, Sulph.
— — laughing, Plb.
— — lying, Asa-f.
— — on affected side, better, Phell.
— after meals, Chin. Thuj. Verat.
— when respiring, Chelid. Kali-c. Scill.
— — — deeply, Agn. Plb.
— — at rest, *Seneg.*
— — sitting, Staph.
— — — bent, Dig.
— when sneezing, Sil. Sulph.
— from talking, Stram.
— when walking, better, Staph.
— with paralysis, of left arm, Pallad.
Pulsation, Amm-m Asa-f. Cinnab. Seneg.
(compare, Throbbing.)
— trembling, Ars. Calc. Creos. *Ntr-s.*
Rhus. Sabin. *Spig.* Staph.
— when standing, Amm-m.
Rasping pain in chest, *Carb-veg.*
Rawness, Anac. (compare Soreness).
Rending, tearing, Berb. *Colch.* Cycl. Elaps.
Kali-c. Phosp. Puls. Spig. Zinc.
Restlessness, in chest, Bell. Petr. Seneg.
Staph. Thuj.
— about heart, Anac.
Revolving of heart, sensation of, Tart.

Rheumatic pains, Ambr. Arn. Bry.Carb veg.
Caust. Lach. Lyc. Nux. *Ran-b.* Tart.
— — at heart, Cact. Kalm. Lach. Lith.
Sacch. Spong.
Rising up, hot in chest, Lact.Ol-an.Phosp.
Plat. Thuj.
Rolling, Cocc.
Roughness Calc. Carb-veg. Creos. Lyc.
Sep. Sulph. Zinc.
Scratching, Anac. Creos. Puls. Staph.
Shattering, Led. Lyc. Rhus.
Shocks, Alum. *Ang.* Arn. Calc. Cannab.
Clem.Con. Croc. Dulc. Hep. Lyc. Mang.
Mur-ac. Nux. Ol-an. *Plat.* Ruta. Sep.
Sulph. Tart. Zinc.
Soreness sensation of, Alum. Ambr. Anac.
Apis. Arn. Bar-c. Berb. Bruc. Bry.
Calc. Carb-an. *Carb-veg.* Caust. Chelid.
Cina. Colch. Cocc-c. Dig. Eupat. *Lvon.*
Ferr. Gels. Gum-gut. Hep. Ip. Lach.
Led. Lob. Lyc. Mgn-c. Mgn-m. Meph.
Merc. Mur-ac.Ntr-s. Nicc. Nitr-ac. Nitr.
Nux-m. Nux. Ox-ac. Phosp. Psor. Rat.
Rhus. *Seneg.* Sep. Sil. Spong. *Stann.*
Staph. Sulph. Tabac. Tart. Zinc.
— — — in middle of chest, Sep.
— — — deep in chest, four inches either
side of sternum, hurts or weakens
her to breathe or speak, Agar.
— — — presses hand against chest, Dros.
— — — when breathing, Calc. Lob.Nitr-ac.
— — — — left chest, Calc. Lac can.
Ran-b. Stann.
— — — deeply, Eupat.
— — — coughing, Nitr-ac. (compare Sect. 24.)
— — — exercising, Colch. Lob.
— — — from talking, Lyc.
— — — when touched, Ang. Calc. Colch.
Ran-b.
— — at the heart, Bar-c. Fluor-ac. Mgn-c.
Ox-ac.
— sternum, Led. Mez. Rumex. Sabin.
— under sternum, Led.
— — arms, on pressing, Mosch.
Spasms in chest, Ang. Ars. Bell. Camph.
Cina, *Cocc. Colch. Cupr. Ferr.* Graph.
Hyosc. Ip. *Kali-c.* Lach. Lact. Laur.
Led. *Merc. Mosch.* Nitr-ac. *Nux.* Op.
Phosp. Phosp-ac. Plb. Puls. Samb. Sang.
Sass. Secc-c. Sep. Spig. Spong. Staph.
Stram. Sulph. *Verat.* Zinc.
— in diaphragm, Staph.
— of heart, Lach.
— hysteric, Ars. Bell. *Cocc. Mosch. Stram.*
— of muscles of chest, Cic. Stram.
— to bend forward, compelling, Hyosc.
— when coughing, Kali-c. Merc.
— by exercise and walking, increased, Ferr.
— from the fumes of arsenic and copper,
Camph. Ip. Merc. Nux.
— with heat and congestion of the blood,
Puls.

26. CHEST AND HEART.

Sprained, sternum feels, Rumex.
— heart feels, Tart.
Squeezing, sensation in chest, Brom. Cina. Dros. Graph. Lact. Merc. *Phosp-ac. Plat.* Seneg. Teucr. Thuj. Verat.
— — heart, Iod.
Stoppage, sensation in lungs, Seneg.
Stinging, stitches in chest, *Acon.* Agar. Amm-c. Amm-m. *Ang. Ant. Arn.* Ars. Asa-f. Asar. Aur. Bad. Bar-c. Bell. Berb. Borax. Bov. *Bry.* Calc. Camph. Cannab. *Canth.* Caps. Carb-an. Carb-veg. Caust. Cham. Chelid. Chin. Cina. Cinnab. Clem. Colch. Con. Creus. Croc. Croton. Cycl. Dros. *Dulc Evon.* Ferr. Graph. *Guaj.* Hep. Ign. Iod. Ip. Kali-b. Kali-c. Kali-jod. Lach. *Laur.* Led. *Lyc.* Mang. *Merc.* Merc-cor. Merc-jod. Mez. Mosch. Mur-ac. Ntr-c. Ntr-m. Ntr-s. *Nicc. Nitr-ac.* Nitr. Nux. Oleand. Ol-an. Ox-ac. *Pœon.* Par. *Phosp.* Plat. *Plb.* Psor. *Puls. Ran-b.* Ran-sc. *Rut.* Rheum. *Rhus. Ruta.* Sabad. Sang. *Scill.* Seneg. *Sep. Sil.* Spig. *Stann. Staph. Sulph. Sulph-ac.* Tabac. Tar. Therid. *Thuj.* Tong. *Valer.* Verat. *Verb.* Viol-od. Zinc.
— — as from knives, Bell. Merc.
— to shoulders, Ox-ac.
— in sternum, Hipp-m.
— in upper part of each lung, better on walking, Elaps.
— intercostal muscles, Borax. Creos.
— at and about heart, Acon. *Anac.* Arn. Berb. Cact. Calc. *Caust.* Chin. Creos. Croton. Cycl. Gels. Glon. Hep Hydroph. Ign. Jac-cor. Kali-b. Lachn. Laur. Mgn-c. Mgn-m. Meny. Merc-jod. Mur-ac. Ntr-m. Ox-ac. *Pœon.* Psor. *Ran-sc.* Rhus. Spig. Sulph-ac. Valer Verb. Viol-tr. *Zinc.*
— — as from needles, Hipp-m.
— — from within to without, Clem.
— — which seems to beat slowly, Jac-cor.
— sides, *Acon.* Amm-c. Ang. Arg. *Bry.* Calc. *Canth.* Cham. Chin. Clem. Con. Coc. *Dulc.* Grat. Hyosc. Ign. *Meny.* Ntr-c. *Ntr-m. Ntr-s.* Nitr-ac. Nux. Op. Par. Petr *Phosp.* Phosp-ac. Plat. *Plb.* Puls *Ran-b.* Rhus. *Salad.* Samb. Sass. Scill. Sep. Sil. *Tabac. Tar.* Verat. Zinc.
— — left Amm-c. Arn Berb. Clem Elaps. Euph. Guaj Hep. Hipp. Ign. Lach. Lachn. Lact. Lyc. Mgn-c. Ntr-s. Nicc Oleand. Phosp. Psor. Rumex. Sacch. Sep. *Stann. Sulph.* Valer. Zinc. Zing.
— — upper, when sitting bent, Kali-jod.
— — right. Arg. Bufo. Creos. Evon. Gels. Kali-c. Merc. Merc-cor. Merc-jod. Mez. Nitr-ac. Pallad. Ran-b.
— — lower part, Kali-c.
— from both sides, going to each other, Gum-gut.

— outwards, *Asa-f.*
— through to back, Ambr. Anac. Bov. Caust. Croton. Ferr. Glon. Hep. Lyc. Merc. Nitr. Pallad. Rhod. Sep. Sil. Sulph. Sulph-ac Zing.
— below sternum, extending to back, Kali-b.
— middle sternum, extending to back, Kali-jod.
— chronic, Phosp.
— to bend together, compelling, Sass.
— — sit up, compelling, Bry.
— only supine position, allowing, Bry.
— in evening, Ran-sc. Verb.
— at night, Amm-c. Merc-cor. Ran-sc. Sabad.
— when raising arms, Berb. Sulph. Thuj.
— — exerting, arms, Led.
— — ascending steps, Stram. Ruta.
— — breathing, *Acon.* Amm-c. Ant. *Bry.* Cannab. Caps. Chin. Colch. Euphr. Hep. Kali-c. Lyc. Meny. Mur-ac. Nicc. *Sabad.* Scill. *Sep.* Spig. Stann. *Tabac.* Verat.
— — deeply, Acon. Arg. Arn. Berb. Borax. Bruc. *Bry.* Calc. Caust. Guaj. Mez. Mur-ac. Ntr-m. Nitr-ac. *Nitr.* Oleand. Pallad. Puls. Rhus. Spong. Sulph. Valer. Zinc.
— — inspiring, Arg. Asar. Bar-c. *Bry.* Canth. Carb-an. Clem. Grat. Mez. Ntr-s. Op. Plat. Seneg. Valer.
— — expiring, Croton.
— from cold drinks, Staph. Thuj.
— when coughing, Acon. Bell Borax. *Bry.* Merc. Ntr-m. Ntr-s. Nitr. Puls. *Sabad.* Scill. Seneg. Sep.
— — exercising, Bry. *Calc.* Cannab. Graph Meny. Mur-ac. Phosp. Puls. Rhus. Spig. Spong. Staph. Sulph.
— — better, Euph.
— from flatulent colic, Ign.
— when hiccoughing, Amm-m.
— from labor, bodily, Caust.
— — mental, Sep.
— when laughing, Nicc.
— — lying, Asa-f. *Nitr.* Psor.
— — — on side affected, Calc. Sabad.
— — — sound side, Stann.
— — singing, Amm-c.
— — sitting crooked, Rhus.
— — stooping, Amm-c.
— — talking, Cannab. Rhus.
— — touched, Phosp.
— — walking, Amm-c. Cinnab. Cocc. Hep. Kali-jod. Rhus.
— — yawning, Aur. Bell. Borax. Nitr-s. Pheil.
Suppuration of lungs, Calc. Kali-c. Led. Nitr. Psor.
— — acute, Chin. Creos. Dulc. Ferr. Laur. Puls.
— — after haemorrhages, Merc.

26. CHEST AND HEART.

Swelling sensation of, in chest, Merc.
Tearing, loose pain, Nux.
Tenderness of chest, Ang. Calc. Canth. Croton. Hep. Ntr-c. Petr. Phell. Ran-sc. Seneg. Sulph.
— — when inspiring, *Calc.*
— — — pressed upon, Ang. *Croton.*
— — touched, Calc. Seneg.
Tension of chest, Ars. Bell. Brom. Cocc. *Colch.* Dig. *Euph.* Ferr. Hydroc-ac. Lact. Lob. Lyc. Mgn-m. Merc. Ntr-c. Ntr-m. Nitr. Nux. Oleand. Op. *Phosp.* Plat. *Puls.* Rhus. Sabin. Sep. Spig. Stann. Sulph. Verb.
— — lower part, Puls.
— — upper part, Phosp. Rhus.
— about heart, Cannab.
— sternum, Mur-ac. Sabin. Zinc.
— when breathing, Puls. Ntr-c. Seneg. Tar.
— — walking, Bry.
Throbbing, Asa-f. Bell. Calad. Caps. Chelid. Cinnab. Croton. Hipp-m. Igt. Lact. Mang. Nux. Paeon. Seneg. Sulph. (compare Pulsation.)
— — in arteries, Murex.
— about heart, Croton. Graph. Lith.
— sides, Nux.
— sternum, Sil. Sulph.
Tickling, Cham. Con. Igt. Iod. Merc. Mez. Mur-ac. Phosp. Phosp-ac. Rhus Sep. Sulph-ac. Verat. Verb. Zinc.
Tingling, (crawling,) Acon. Ars. Colch. *Rhus.* Seneg. Spong. Stann.
Torn loose, as if something were, Nux.
Tremor, Ambr. Carb-an. Kali-c. Lachn. Sabin. Spig.
— at heart, Bell. Calc. Camph. Cina. Lith. Ntr-m. Nitr-ac. Nux-m. Op. Spig. Staph.
— at night, Ambr.
Turning over in chest, as if something were, Stann.
Ulcerative pain, in chest, Bry. Carb-an. Creos. Mgn-m. Merc. Psor. *Puls. Ran-b.* Spig. Staph. Sulph.
Undulating pains, Dig. Dulc. Spig.
Undulation at heart, sense of, Spig.
Velvety feeling in chest, Tart.
Warmth, sensation of, in chest, Euphr. Hell. Lact. Mang. Ol-an. Rhod.
— — about the heart, Croc. Rhod.
Weakness, Borax. Brom. Canth. Carb-veg. Cycl. Dig. Hep. Iod. Kali-c. Lact. Lam. Phosp. *Phosp-ac.* Plat. Psor. Rhus. Ruta. Stann. *Sulph.* Sulph-ac.
— impeding cough, Stann.
— — speech, Dig. Hep. Phosp-ac. Rhus. Sulph. Sulph-ac.
— in evening, Ran-sc.
— after expectoration, Stann.
— when reading aloud, Cocc.
— — singing, Carb-veg. Sulph.

Weakness after speaking, Calc. Phosp-ac. Rhus. Stann. Sulph. Sulph-ac.
— — a walk in open air, Rhus.
— sensation of, about heart, Rhus.
Whirling, sensation of, about heart, Tart.
In morning, pain in chest, Scill. Sulph.
— — in bed, Phell. Phosp. Seneg.
— evening, pain, Merc. Nitr. Nux-m. Ran-sc. Stann. Sulph.
— — in bed, Sep. Verb.
At night, Alum. Amm-c. Cact. Creos. Lach. Mgn-m. Mgn-s. Merc-cor. Nux. Puls. Ran-sc. Ruta. Sabad. Selen. Seneg.
When ascending, Bar-c. Graph. Nux.
— — steps, Rat. Ruta.
— bending to affected side, pain in chest, Calc.
— — forward, Arg. Dig.
— breathing, *Acon.* Amm-m. Ant. *Bry.* Cannab. Caps. Chin. Colch. Creos. Hep. Kali-c. Lach. Led. Lyc. Merc. Merc-sulph. Mur-ac. Ntr-c. Nitr-ac. Ox-ac. Plat. Puls. Rumex. *Sabad.* Scill. *Sep.* Spig. Stann. Sulph. Tabac.
— — deeply, Agn. Berb. Borax. *Bry.* Calc. Cast. Caust. Kobalt. Meph. Ntr-m. *Nitr.* Plb. Puls. Rhus. Sabin.
— expiring, Colch. Dulc. Oleand.
— inspiring, *Acon.* Ang. Agar. Bar-c. *Bry. Calc.* Carb-an. Chelid. Clem. Grat. Guaj. Kali-c. Laur. Mez. Op. Plat. Scill. Seneg. Valer.
From cold air, pain in chest, Bry. Carb-veg. Petr. Phosp.
— — cold drinks, Thuj.
When coughing, pain, Acon. Ars. Bell. Borax. *Bry.* Chin. Dros. Lyc. Mgn-m. Meph. Merc. Ntr-m. Ntr-s. Nitr-ac. Nitr. *Sabad.* Scill. Seneg. *Sep.* Sil. Sulph.
From drinking, pain in chest, Arn. Cupr. Thuj. Verat.
By eructation, pain relieved, Bar-c.
When exercising, pain, Arn. Ars. *Bry. Calc.* Cannab. Caps. Colch. Ferr. Graph. Mur-ac. Nux. Rhus. Seneg. Sep.
— — relieved, Euph.
— gaping, pain, Bell. Borax.
— hiccoughing, pain, Amm-m.
From labor, bodily, Caust.
— — mental, Sep.
— laughing, pain, Lyc. Nicc. Plb.
— lifting wrong, pain, *Sulph.*
When lying, pain, Asa-f. *Nitr.*
— — on side, pain, Plat. Sabad. Seneg. Sulph. Tellur.
— on affected side, pain, Borax. Cact. Calc. Lyc. Sabad. Sulph.
— — sound side, pain, Stann.
Must lie on back, Bry.
During meals, pain, Pæon.
After meals, Arn. Chin. Evon. Lach. Lam. Phosp. Thuj. Verat.

When moving in bed, Sulph.
In open air, Nux.
After pneumonia, pain in chest. *Sulph.*
By pressing upon, increasing pain, Chin. Lact. Seneg.
— — pain relieved, (must press chest with hand,) Creos. Dros. Sep.
When raising, arms. Ant. Led. Spig. Sulph.
— moving arms, Ang. Camph. Led. Spig.
— at rest, pain in chest, Euph. Rhus. *Seneg.* Tabac.
From riding on horseback, pain in chest, Graph.
When rising from seat, pain in heart, Gels.
— running, Borax.
— singing, Amm-c.
— — after, Sulph.
— sitting, pain, Staph.
— — bent, Dig. Rhus.
— sneezing, pain, Dros. Meph. Merc.

Sec-c. Sil. Sulph.
When stooping, pain, Alum. Amm-c. Meny. Mez. Oleand.
— stretching the arms, tearing pain in chest, Berb.
From talking, pain in chest, Borax. Cannab. Kali-c. Rhus. Stram. Sulph.
When thinking of the pain, Bar-c.
When touched, pain, Alum. Amm-m. Arn. Calc. Colch. Graph. Meph. Phosp. Puls. Sulph.
— throwing back the shoulders, Borax. Rat.
— turning around in bed, pain in chest, Sulph.
— walking, Amm-c. Bry. Cinnab. Hep. Ferr. Kali-jod. Led. Nux. Rhus.
— — fast, Kali-c.
— — ameliorated, Staph.
From warmth, external, pain ameliorated, Bar-c.

27 Mammae and Nipples.

Abscess on breast, *Hep.* Phosp. Sil.
Aphthae, bleeding, of nipples, Borax.
As if beaten, pain, Amor. *Ang. Arn.* Arum-trif. Bry. Calad. Rhod. Sil. (compare Sect. 26.)
— sides and sternum, Acon.
— at lower end of sternum, Cic.
Biting, on the breasts, Led.
Blood, extravasation of, on chest, Lach.
As from a blow, pain, Ant. *Cic.*
Blueness of skin, near the clavicles, Ars. Lach. Thuj.
Bluish color of ulceration of mammae, Lach. Phosp.
Bluish-red mammae, Creos.
Brown spots, Carb-veg. Lyc. Phosp. Sep. Thuj.
Burning, Bell. Calc. Iod. Led. Mez. Selen.
— in pectoral glands, Bell. Iod. Laur. Phosp.
— — nipples, Agar. Cic. Graph. Phosp. Sulph.
Cancer in breasts, Apis. Arn. *Ars.* Asterias. *Bell.* Bry. Calc. Calc-ox. Carb-an. Cham. Clem. Coloc. *Con.* Creos. Graph. *Hep.* Lach. Lyc. Merc. Nitr-ac. Phyt. Phosp. Puls. Sep. *Sil.* *Sulph.*
Caries, Con.
Chilliness, Cic. Par. Ran-b. Sp'g.
Cicatrices, old, from previous suppurations, Graph.
Contracting, sensation of, Stram. Verat.
— of left mamma, when child nurse, from right, Borax.
Cracks, nipples, Arn. Cast-eq. Caust. Graph. Sep. *Sulph.*
Cramp-pain gradually increasing and decreasing, Plat.
Darting in right mammae, Grat.
Deformed nipples, Merc.
Drawing, Carb-veg. Stront.
— in mammae, Creos.
— — left nipple, Evon. Tilia. Zinc.
Erect, nipples are, Lach.
Emaciation, Sacch.
Eruption, Grat. Hep. Led. Lyc. Staph. Tabac. Valer.
— burning after scratching, Grat.
— like chicken-pox, Led.
— hard, Valer.
— itching, Kali-c. Staph. Tabac.

Eruptions, itching, in warmth, Staph.
— mealy, Petr.
— miliary, Led. Staph. Tart.
— moist, oozing, Lyc.
— painful, Lyc.
— — to touch, Hep. Phosp-ac.
— pimples, Grat. Tabac. Valer.
— pustulous, Evon. Hep.
— red, Staph.
— scurfy, protuberances, bleeding when scurf is removed, Creos.
— sore, smarting, when touched, Hep.
— stinging, Hep.
— vesicular, Graph.
— on mammae, Graph.
— — nipples, sore, corrosive blisters, Graph.
— — yellow, scaly, itching spots, Kali-c.
Erysipelas, of pectoral glands, Arn. Calc. *Carb-an.* Carb-veg. Cham. Graph. *Phosp.* Sulph.
— in lying, in women, Carb-an.
Flatbiness, Cham. Iod.
Fulness of breast in lying, in women, *Bry.*
Furuncles, Amm-c. Chin. Mgn-c. Phosp.
Galactorrhœa, Acon. *Bell.* Borax. Bry. Calc. Chin. Con. Creos. Lach. Lyc. Nux. Phosp. Puls. *Rhus.* Staph. Stann. Tart.
Gurgling, Croton.
Hardness, *Bell.* Cham. *Clem.* Con. Merc. Phosp. Sil. Sulph. (compare Induration.)
— nipples, Agar. Sulph.
Heat, on breast, Bry. Mang. Raph.
Herpes on breast, Ars. Caust. Dulc. Petr. Psor. Staph.
Induration, pectoral glands, Bell. Bry. Calc. *Carb-an. Cham. Clem.* Coloc. *Con.* Graph. Lac-can. Lyc. Merc. Nitr-ac. Phosp. Phyt. Ruta. Sil. Sulph. (compare Hardness).
— — after contusion, Con.
Inflammation, of pectoral glands, Bell. Bry. *Carb-an. Carb-veg.* Cist. Con. Hep. Merc. Phosp. Phyt. Sil. Sulph.
— — nipples, Arn. Cham. Phosp. Sil. Sulph.
— in lying, in women, Carb-an.
Itching, Agar. Alum. Anac. Ang. Ant. Arn. Bar-c. Berb. Bov. Calc. Canth. Carb-veg. Con. Hipp. Kali-c. Led. Lyc. Mez. Ntr-m. Nicc. Nux-jug. Phell

27. MAMMAE AND NIPPLES.

Phosp. Sabad. Scill. Sep. Spong. Stann. Staph. Sulph.
Itching, pectoral glands, Alum. Con.
— nipples, Agar. Hep. Petr. Sulph.
Lancinations, Amm-c. Calc. Chin-sulph. Iod. Oleand. Sabin.
Miliary eruption, Led. Staph. Tart.
Milk, bad, Borax. Carb-an. Cham. Cina. *Merc.* Nux. Puls. Stann.
— bitter, Rheum.
— cheesy or mixed with pus, Cham.
— in mammae, Lyc. Phosp.
— disappearing, Agn. Asa-f. Bry. *Calc.* Caust. Cham. Chelid. Chin. Dulc. Lac-can. Lyc Merc. Millef. *Phell. Puls.* Rhus. Sep. Sulph. Urt-ur. Zinc.
— — after a cold, Dulc.
— — too thick and tastes badly, Borax.
— — thin and tastes saltish, Carb-an.
— thin and blue, Lach.
— — watery, Puls.
— stringy and watery, Kali-b.
— wanting, Agn. Asa-f. Urt-ur.
— yellow, Rheum.
Milk-fever, Acon. *Arn. Bell. Bry.* Cham. Coff. Igt. Merc. Op. *Rhus.*
— with delirium, Acon.
Muscles twitching, Asar. Tar.
Nodosity, hard, burning, on mammae, Lyc.
Numbness, Graph.
Pain, in general, Bell. Chin. Creos. Lact. *Ran-b. Ran-sc.* Sulph.
— — in morning, Calad.
— when exercising, Ang. Laur. Ran-b.
— — the arms, Ang. Ant.
— — — extending and stretching, *Ran-b.*
— — pressed upon, Ant.
— compelling one to press thereon, Creos.
— by rest, increased, Rhus.
— when touched, *Ran-b.*
— — as soon as child nurses, Croton.
— in mammae, Murex. Phosp. Rheum.
— intolerable pains in lactiferous tubes as soon as child nurses, Phell.
— during lactation, Borax.
— in nipples, Graph. Sulph.
Painfulness of the pectoral glands, Bry. Phosp. Rheum.
— nipples, Graph. Lach. Ocim. Sang. Sulph.
— of spot on sternum, Ruta.
Perspiration, Arg. Arn. Bov. Calc. Hep. Lyc. Nitr. Plb. Rhus. Selen. Sep.
— on chest, Chin. Cocc. Dros. Euphr. Merc. Nitr. Nitr-ac. Phosp. Phosp-ac. Tabac.
— reddish, Arn.
— in morning, Bov. Cocc. Graph. Nitr.
— at night, Agar. Bar-c. Calc. Kali-c. Lyc. Sil. Stann. Sulph.
Pores black, Dros.
Pressing sensation, Ambr. Carb-veg. Euph. Sulph.

Pressing sensation, superiorly on sternum, Ferr.
— behind left nipple, Berb.
Prickling, Calc. Ran-sc.
Red, points, Sabad.
— spots, Cocc. Led. Sabad.
— streaks on breast, Rhus.
— — — radiating from central point, Bell. Sulph.
Rending (tearing) in pectoral glands, Amm-c. Amm-m. Carb-veg. Croton. Kali-c.
— during catamenia, Calc.
Retraction of nipples, Sass.
Rheumatic pain, Ambr. Arn. Carb-veg. Nux. Ran-b. Tart.
— — in pectoral glands, Bry.
Scabs on nipples, Lyc.
Scales on mammae, Petr.
Scars hard, after mammary abscess absorbed, Graph.
Shuddering in mammae, Petr.
Smallness, excessive of mammae, Nux-m.
Smarting, Led.
Soreness, of chest, Hyosc. Lach. Mez.
— — nipples, *Arn.* Calc. *Cast-eq.* Caust. Cham. *Graph* Ham. Helianth. Hyper. Igt. Lyc. Merc. Phosp. Puls. Sang. *Sep.* Sulph.
Sore pain, mammae, *Cic.* Phyt.
— nipples, Caust. Nux. Sang. Zinc.
Spasm in pectoral muscles, Ang. Cic. Stram. Verat.
Spasmodic pain, Arg.
Stinging, stiches, Amm-c. Calc. Con. Iod. Oleand. Sabin.
— in mammae, Berb. Carb-an. Con. Creos. Graph Grat. Ind. Iod. Kali-c. Laur. Lyc. Murex. Ntr-m. Phosp. Rheum. Sang. Sep.
— below the mammae, Hyper. Laur.
— — right mammae, Bruc.
— in nipples, Bism. *Cast-eq.* Igt. Lyc. Mang. Mur-ac. Sabin. Sulph.
— momentarily by rubbing, relieved, Ind.
Suppuration of mammae, Cist. Creos. Hep. *Merc. Phosp.* Phyt. Sil.
— nipples, Cast-eq. Cham. *Merc.* Sil.
— in lying, in women, Sil.
Swelling. mammae, Bell. Bry. Calc. Cham. Clem Con. Graph. Hep. Lach. Lyc. Merc. Merc-cor. Ocim. Phosp. Phyt. Puls. Sabin. Samb. Sil. Sulph.
— hot, Bell. Bry. Calc. Merc. Phosp.
— with each attack of neuralgia uteri, Nux.
— — secretion like milk, Cycl.
— of the nipples, Lach. Lyc. Merc.
— — lower part of sternum, Sacch.
Tearing stitches in milk-breasts, Kali-c.
Tenderness, breast, Bell. Bry. Calc. Lac-can. Mosch. *Ran-sc.* Zinc-ox.
— mammae, Cham. Graph.
— nipples, Graph. Millef.
— sternum, Zinc.

Tenderness, to deep pressure, Calc. Lac-can. Merc. Mosch. Murex.
Tension, *Euph.* Iod. Lyc. Mez. Oleand. Rhus. Sass. Stann.
— as if too short when rising up, Sass.
Throbbing, Croton.
Tingling (crawling), on breast, Colch. Puls. Ran-sc.
— mammae, Sabin.
Tubercles, nodosities, *Carb-an. Coloc.* Con. Graph. Lyc. Nitr-ac. Phosp. Puls.
Ulceration of mammae, Phosp. Sil. Sulph.
Ulceration, mammae, fistulous, Phosp. Sil.
Ulcer, scirrhous, stinging, burning on edges, odor of old cheese, Hep.
— on nipple, Calc.
Vesicles, in nipples, Graph.
Wasting away, of mammae, Ars. Con. Iod. Kali-jod. Nitr-ac.
— — — nipples, Sass.
Whiteness of nipples in centre without ulceration, Nux.
Wrenching pain, *Arn.*
Yellow spots, Ars. Carb-an. Lyc. Phosp. Sep. Sulph.

28. Nape, Back and Sacral Region.

Abscess on back, *Sil.* Staph. Sulph.
Aching, in sacrum, Alum. Aur. *Calc.* Canth. Carb-an. Cham. Chin. Coff. Con. Graph. Hep. *Igt.* Kali-c. *Lach.* Lyc. Merc. Ntr-m. *Nux.* Op. *Puls. Rhus* Sep. Staph. Stram. *Sulph.* Verat.
— — and coccyx, Kali-b.
— as if flesh was detached from bones, Acon. Kali-b.
— — in nape of neck, Bar-c.
— — lumbar region, Hyper.
As from a bar in back, sensation, Ars. Lach.
— if beaten, (or broken), pain, in cervical vertebrae, Gels. Sabin.
— — neck, Ars.
— — nape, Acon. Agar. Caust. Nux. Sabin. Thuj.
— — scapulae, Creos. Hell. Merc. Merc-jod. Ran-b. Sil.
— — back, Acon. Alum. *Agar. Arn.* Asar. Bell. Berb. Chin. Clem. Dros. Kali-c. *Mgn-c.* Mgn-m. Mgn-s. *Merc.* Ntr-s *Nux-m. Nux. Phosp.* Plat. Psor. Puls. Ran-b. Rat. Rhod. *Ruta.* Sabad. Spig. Stram. Stront. Sulph. Thuj. *Verat.*
— — sacrum, *Acon. Alum.* Agar. Amm-m. Ang. Arg. *Arn.* Ars. Bry. Calad. Caust. Chin. Cina. Cinnab. Cor-r. Creos. Dig. *Graph.* Gum-gut. *Hep.* Hyper. Kali-jod. Lact. Lam. Mgn-c. Mgn-m. Meny. Merc. Ntr-c. Ntr-m. Ntr-s. *Nux-m. Nux.* Ox-ac. Phell. Phosp. *Plat.* Ran-b. Ran-sc. Rhod. *Rhus. Ruta.* Sabad. Sass. Staph. Stront. Sulph. Thuj. *Verat.*
— — os coccygis, Cist.
Blisters, on back, Calc.
Boils on neck, Graph. Hep.
— painful to touch, *Hep.*
Bones, pain in, neck, Bar-c. Bell.
— as if the flesh was loose, Acon. Kali-b.
Boring, back, Acon. Agar. Bar-c. Bism. Cocc. Laur. Ntr-c. Thuj.
— scapulae, Acon. Meny.
— sacral region, Acon.
Break, as if spinal column would, from within, Kalm.
Breath, obstructing, pain, back, Berb. *Cannab.* Led. Ruta. Sulph. Tart.

— scapulae, Calc. *Cannab.* Nitr. Sulph.
— sacral region, Berb. Ruta. Sulph. Tar.
Broken as if sacrum were, Phosp.
Brown spots, arm-pits, Thuj.
— back, Sep.
— greasy skin of neck, Apis. Lyc. Thuj.
Bubbling sensation, back, Petros. Tar.
Burning, neck, Bar-c. Merc.
— scapulae, Lachn. Sil. Sulph.
— — between, Glon. Lyc. Nux.
— left scapula, Ambr. Bar-c. Ntr-m. Sil. Teucr. Zinc.
— right scapula, Bar-c. Cannab. Caust. Iod. Laur. Seneg. Sulph. Verat.
— supra-sternal fossa, Ars.
— back, *Ars.* Asa-f. Bar-c. Berb. Borax. Bry. Cannab. Carb-an. Coloc. Dulc. Lach. Lachn. Lob. Mgn-c. Mgn-m. Merc. Nux-m. Nux. Oleand. *Phosp.* Selen. Seneg. Sep. Zinc.
— — in whole spinal column, Glon.
— — from small of back to between scapulae, Phosp. Sep. Thuj.
— — as if a hot iron was pierced through, Alum.
— sacral region, Borax. Murex. Phosp. Phosp-ac. Sep.
Bursting pain, under right scapula, Seneg.
Chills in back, All-cep. Bell. Bov. Caps. ¯[Cocc. Coff. Colch. Croton. Guaj. ¶!Gum-gut. Hipp. Igt. Lach. Mgn-c. Phosp. Rumex. Ruta. Sang. Sep. Spong.
₂ Stann. Staph. Stram.
— running through back, Ars. Puls. Rhus. Thuj.
— as from a piece of ice between the shoulders, Lachn.
Coldness, sensation of, in neck, chronic, Calc.
— back, Amm-m. Berb. Calc. Carb-veg. Croc. Elaps. Hyosc. Laur. Ox-ac. Phosp. Rhus. Sec-c. Spong.
— in whole spinal column, Glon.
— between shoulders, Haematox.
— cold spot between shoulders, Amm-c.
— — — — like ice, Lachn.
— sacral region, Hyosc. Laur. Stront.
Compressing pain, back, Con.
Concussions in neck, Mez.
Congestion of blood to neck, it seems larger and neck cloth too tight, Glon.

28 NAPE, BACK AND SACRAL REGION.

Constringing pain, back, Canth. Nux. Sabad.
— supra-sternal, fossa, Rhus. Staph.
Contracting pain, neck, Amm-c. Asar. Cinnab. Lyc.
— — right side, Gels.
— supra-sternal fossa, Phosp-ac.
— back, Bry. Graph. Guaj. Mez. Viol-tr.
— lumbar region, Lach.
— sacral region, Hell. Mgn-m. Tabac.
— muscles generally, Con. Nux.
Cracking sound in cervical vertebrae when moved, Cocc. Ntr-c. Nicc. Ol-an. Puls. Stann.
Cramping pain, nape, Arn. *Asar.*
— neck, Arn. *Asar.* Scill.
— between scapulae, on motion. Ip.
— back, Bell. Bry. Chin. Con. Euph. *Euphr.* Sep. Viol-tr.
— — in small of back, and os coccygis, can sit for but a short time, Bell. Mgn-m. Sil.
— sacrum, Sil.
Curvature (distortion), cervical vertebrae, *Calc.*
— dorsal vertebrae, *Calc.* Lyc. Plb. *Puls.* Rhus. *Sil. Sulph.*
— — upper part, Puls.
Cutting, in whole spine, from occiput to sacrum, Elaps.
— nape, Grat.
— neck, Samb.
— — left side, Elaps.
— between shoulders (stabbing) Ntr-s.
— back, Arg-n. Graph. Igt. Ntr-s. Seneg.
— sacral region, Lob. Ntr-m. Samb.
Digging in back, Acon. Dulc. Sep.
Drawing pain, nape, Ambr. *Amm-c.* Ant. Berb. *Carb-veg* Cast. *Chin.* Lact. Lyc. Merc. Mosch. Ntr-c. Nitr. Nux-m. Nux. *Puls.* Rat. *Rhod.* Ruta. Sep. *Staph.* Sulph. Tereb.
— neck, Ant. *Carb-veg.* Cycl. Hep. Kalm. Lact. Phosp-ac. Puls. *Rhod.* Scill.
— scapulae, Ars. Berb. Borax. Calc. Camph. Caust. *Chin.* Hep. Rhod. Ruta. Seneg. Sil.
— between scapulae, Bell. Borax. Ntr-c.
— back, Ambr. Amm-c. *Ars.* Bell. Brom. Bry. *Canth.* Caps. Carb-veg. *Cham. Chin.* Cina. Cocc. Con. Cycl. Dig. Hep. Kali b. *Kali-c.* Kalm. *Lyc.* Merc. Mosch. Ntr-m. Nux-m. Nux. Puls. Rat. Rhod. Rhus. Rhus-rad. Seneg. Stront. *Sulph.* Sulph-ac. Tart. Teucr. Thuj. Valer. Verat.
— — spine, Berb. Daph.
— sacral region, *Amm-c.* Arg. *Chin.* Cocc. Colch. Croc. Dig. Dulc. Igt. Kali-c. Lyc. Ntr-m. Nux. Sabin. Samb. Sil. Spong. Stram. *Sulph.* Sulph-ac. Tereb. Thuj. Valer. Verat.
Emaciation, back, Tabac.

Emaciation, neck, Ntr-m.
Emprosthotmos, *Canth. Ip.*
Eruption on the nape, Ant. Bell. Berb. Caust. Hep. Petr. Sec-c. Sil. Staph. Tart.
— neck, Bry. Clem. Gels. Lyc. Phosp-ac. Puls. Scill. Spig. Verb.
— — brown spots on throat, like freckles, Kali-b.
— scapulae, Ant. Caust. Lach. Phosp-ac.
— back, Alum. Ant. Ars. Bar-c. Bell. Berb. Carb-veg. Caust. Cina. Cist. Clem. Evon. Lach. Led. Merc. Ntr-m. Nitr-ac. Petr. Phosp-ac. Scill. Sep. Staph. Tabac. Tart.
— biting, Bry.
— burning, Cist.
— in groups, Berb.
— hepatic, Lach.
— itching, Bry. Carb-veg. Caust. Cham. Lyc. Puls. Scill. Sep. Staph. Tabac.
— lumps, Verb.
— miliary, Ant. Bry. Caust. Phosp-ac. Psor. Sec-c. Tart.
— moist, extending to neck, Clem.
— oozing, Clem. Ntr-m.
— painful, Lyc. Spig.
— — to touch, Cist. Hep. Phosp-ac. Psor. Scill. Spig. Verb.
— pimples, Carb-veg. Lach. Lyc. Nicc. Puls. Scill. Sil. Spig. Staph
— pustular, Bell. Berb. Clem. Evon.
— red, Bell. Bry. Spig. Tabac. Verb.
— smarting, Bry.
— sore smarting, Spig.
— vesicular, Lach.
Erysipelas, from nape to face, Graph.
— around the waist, *Merc.* Rhus.
Excoriation, axilla, Carb-veg.
— — pain as from, under, Mez.
Exostosis, painful, on sacrum, Rhus.
Foreign body, in lumbar region, pain as from, Nux.
Furuncles, nape, Nitr-ac Phosp. Sil.
— neck, Mgn-c. Ntr-m. Sep.
— blood-boils on shoulder and region of liver, Nux-jug.
— arm-pit, Borax. Lyc. Phosp-ac.
— scapulae, Amm-c. Bell. Led. Lyc. Nitr-ac. Zinc.
— back, Caust. Mur-ac. Sulph-ac. *Thuj.* Zinc.
— sacrum, Aeth. Thuj.
— back, blood-boils, Caust. Graph. Hep. Thuj.
— — small, on back, Iris.
— blood-boils on right side of spine, painful on motion, Kali-b.
— — under axilla, Borax. Lyc.
Glandular affections of the nape:
— induration, Bar-c. Dulc.
— inflammation, Sulph.
— swelling, *Bar-c.* Cist. Dulc. *Iod.* Petr. Sil. *Staph.* Sulph.

28. NAPE, BACK AND SACRAL REGION.

Glandular affections of the neck, drawing, (compare, Sect. 18.)
— drawing sensation, Bov.
— induration, Bar-c. Carb-veg. Dulc. Kali-c. Spig.
— inflammation, Bell. *Cham.* Kali-c. Merc. Nitr-ac. *Sulph-ac.*
— — right side, Bar-c.
— pain, Alum. Amm-m. Arn. Bell. Calc. Caust. Hell. Kali-c Lyc. Merc. Ntr-m. Nitr-ac. Phosp-ac. Puls. Selen Sep. Spig.
— pressing pain, Bell. Igt. Merc.
— rending, tearing, Graph.
— stinging, stitches, Bell. Carb-an. Lyc. *Merc.*
— suppuration, Bell. Cist. Sil.
— swelling, Alum. Amm-c. Arn. Bar-c. *Bell. Bov.* Brom. *Calc. Carb an.* Carb-veg. Caust. *Cham* Cina. Cist. Creos. Cupr. *Dulc.*Ferr. Graph. Hell. Hep. *Iod. Kali-c.* Lach. *Lyc.* Mgn-c. Mgn-m. *Merc.* Ntr-c. *Nitr-ac.* Phosp. Puls. Rhus. Sil. Spig. Spong. Staph. *Sulph.* Thuj. Viol-tr.
— — painless, Igt.
— — and tickling, relieved by pressure with the cold hand, Kali-c.
— lancinations, Lyc.
— tension, Bov. Graph.
— of axilla, from contusion of little finger Bufo.
— — induration, Amm-c. Bufo. Calc. Carb-an. Clem. Iod. Kali-c. Lac-can. Sil.
— — heaviness, sensation of, Caps.
— — pain, Amm-c. Bar-c. Kali-c. Prun. Rhus. Sulph-ac.
— — stinging, Lyc.
— — suppuration, Amm-c. Ars. Bell. Bufo. Calc. Coloc. *Hep* Kali-c. Lac-can. Merc. Ntr-m.*Nitr-ac.* Petr. Phosp-ac. Prun. Sil. *Sulph.*
— — swelling, Amm-m. Bell. Brom. Calc. Carb-an. Clem. Coloc. *Iod.* Kali-c. Lyc. Merc. Ntr-m. *Nitr ac.* Petr. Phosp. Rhus. Sep. Sil. *Staph. Sulph.* Sulph-ac.
Gnawing, sensation, Hell. Ntr-s.
— vertebrae, Bell.
— small of back. Canth. Mgn-m. Nicc. Phosp. Stront. Sulph.
— os coccygis, Gum-gut.
Goitre, (struma,) Ambr. *Brom. Calc.*Canth. Carb-an. Caust. *Iod. Kali-c.* Lyc. *Ntr-c.* Ntr-m. *Spong.* Staph.
— hard, *Iod. Ntr-c.* Spong.
— itching, Ambr. Mgn-c.
— — and stinging, Spong.
— large, *Iod.* Ntr-m. Spong.
— pressing pain in, Ntr-c.
— — constrictive pain in, Iod. Spong.
— sensitive to contact, Kali-jod.

Goitre stitching, piercing pain, Scill.
— swelling, Iod. Spong.
— ulcerative pain, Carb-veg. Iod.
Greasy, brown skin of neck, Apis. Lyc. Thuj.
Griping, back, Paeon. Sil. Viol-tr.
Heat in lumbar region, Berb.
Heaviness, sensation of, nape, Meny.Nux. Par. Samb.
— neck, Meny. Nux.
— arm-pit, Berb.
— back, Ambr. Par.
— sacral region, Berb. Mgn-s.
Herpes, nape, Carb-an. Caust. Clem. Lyc. Ntr-m. Nitr. Petr. Sep. Sulph.
— axilla, Carb-an. Elaps. Lyc. Ntr-m.
— back, Ars. Lach. Zinc.
— itching, Caust.
— moist, Carb-an. Caust. Ntr-m. Sep.
Herpetic spots, nape, Hyosc.
— neck and back, Sep.
Itching, axilla, Carb-veg. Elaps. Phosp.
— back, Caust. Cist. Daph. Guaj. Nicc. Nitr-ac. Raph. Seneg.
— — burning, Daph.
— os coccygis, Borax. Bov.
Jerking pain, nape, Aeth. *Chin.* Tar.
— neck, Tar.
— back, Ang. *Chin.* Cinnab.
— sacral region, Chin.
Labor-like pains, sacral region, Cinnab. Creos. Croc. Kali-c. Kali-jod. Puls.
— back, Sep.
As from lifting, overstraining back, Calc. Lyc. Mur ac. Oleand. Rhus. Valer.
— sacral region, Rhus. Staph.
Livid spots, nape, Lyc.
To lie down, necessity from pain in sacral region, Sil.
— — from pain in back, *Ars.*
Lump in back, sensation of, Arn.
Lumps in neck, Graph. Hep.
— — painful, Hep.
— between scapulae, Calc.
Moisture, axilla, Carb-an. Carb-veg.
Motion, pain, impeding, back, Petr.
— sacral region, Caust. Phosp.
Muscles, twitching, neck, Ang.
— back. Sol-m.
Nocturnal pain back, Calc.Carb-an.Cham. Cinnab. Dulc. *Ferr.* Hell. Kali-b. Lyc. Mgn-c. Mgn-s. Ntr-m. Nitr.
— sacral region, *Amm-c.* Ang. Cham. Chin. Lach. Lyc. *Mgn-c.* Mgn-s. Ntr-s. Nux. *Staph.*
— — in nape of neck, Oleand.
— — at 1 A.M., Staph.
Numbness, sensation of, nape and os coccygis, Berb. Plat.
— sacral region, Berb. Ox-ac. Spong.
Opisthotonos, Ang. Bell. *Canth. Cham.Cic. Igt. Ip.* Led. *Op. Rhus.* Stann. *Stram.*
Oversensitiveness of spine, Ntr-m.

28. NAPE, BACK AND SACRAL REGION.

Pain in general, nape, Amm-c. Daph. Graph. Igt. Lact. Pod.
— supra-sternal fossa, Nux. Tart.
— neck, Bell. Brom. Coloc. Cycl. Hell. Meph.
— scapulae, Bell. Cist. Coloc. Graph. Lob. Nitr-ac.
— below left scapula. Chenop. Gels.
— shoulder, as if inflamed, Hæmatox.
— back, Actea-r. Ars. Asa-f. *Aur. Bov.* Calc. Cannab. Caust. Cham. Coloc. Hyosc. Kali-b. Kali-c. Kobalt. Lact. *Led* Lyc. Nitr-ac. Nitr. *Petr.* Phosp. Puls. *Rhod.* Rhus-rad. *Sep. Tart. Zinc.*
— — to pubis, Sabin.
— — in whole spinal column, Glon.
— — — spinal marrow, Lact.
— — after a fall, Kali-c.
— — one-sided, Guaj.
— — under scapulæ between shoulders, to loins, Ox-ac.
— lumbar region, Asa-f. Calc. Con. Cycl. Dulc. Hyosc. Kobalt. *Led.* Murex. Ntr-m. *Puls.* Sil. Stront. *Valer.*
— sacral region, Amm-m. Ant. *Bar-c.* Berb. Borax. *Bry.* Calc. Calc-phosp. Cannab. Caust. Cham. Chin. Cimex. Con. Creos. Ferr-ac. *Graph.* Igt. Kali-b. *Kali-c.* Kobalt. Lach. Led. Lith. *Lyc.* Mgn-s. Merc. Mez. Murex. Nitr ac. Nitr. Ol-an. Petr. *Phosp.* Pod. Psor. *Puls.* Rhod. Rhus. Rhus-rad. Sang. *Sep. Sil.* Staph. *Sulph.* Tong. *Zinc.*
— — in sacrum, on retaining urine, Ntr-s.
— — — to right thigh, worse by pressing at stool and coughing, Tellur.
— os coccygis, when touched, Carb-an. Kali-b. Lact.
— — as from a fall, Kali-jod.
— — as if sitting on something sharp, Lach.
— — after micturition, Graph.
— pelvis, Murex.
— with coldness of limbs, Pallad.
— — cold feet and strangury, Elaps.
Palsy, of neck, Lyc.
— back, Cocc. Sil.
— sacral region, *Cocc. Ntr-m.*
Paralytic pain, nape, Sil. Verat.
— neck, Cycl. Lachn.
— back, Agar. Asar. Berb. Meph. Pallad. Sil. Zinc.
— sacral region, Acon. *Cocc. Ntr-m.* Nitr. Nux. Ran-c. Selen. Sil. Zinc.
Perspiration, nape, Calc. Chin. Phosp-ac.
— neck, Bell. Clem. Euph.
— — sour, Ars. Bell. Mgn-c. Nux. Sulph.
— — at night, Mang.
— axilla, Asar. *Bov.* Bry. Gymnoc. Kali-c. Ntr-m. Scill. Selen. Sep. Sil. *Sulph. Thuj.*
— — fetid, Dulc. Hep. Lac-can. Nitr-ac. Phosp. Rhod. Selen. Sep. Sulph.

Tellur. Thuj.
Perspiration, axilla, greasy, oily, Merc.
— — with smell of onions Bov. Osm.
— back, Anac. *Chin.* Chin-sulph. Dulc. Guaj. Hep. Lyc. Mur ac. Ntr-c. Nux. Petr. Phosp. Phosp-ac. Puls. Rhus. Sep. Stram. Sulph.
— — at night, Anac. Lyc.
— — from a little exercise, *Chin.*
— — when walking, Lac-can. Lach. Petr. Phosp. Rhus. Sep.
Pimples on neck, painful to touch, Hep.
Pinching, sacral region, Graph. Sulph.
— under right scapulæ, preventing motion, Chelid.
Like a plug, in back, sensation, Lach.
Pressing, pain in sacral region, Carb-an.
— outwards, in sacral region, Cannab.
Pressure, in nape, Ambr. Bar-c. Croton. Cupr. Laur. Ntr-m. Ol-an. Samb. Sass. Staph. Tar.
— neck, Calc. Cycl. Elaps. Ferr. Guaj. Tar.
— scapulae, Anac. Bell. Calc. Chin. Cor-r. Elaps. Graph. Kali-c. Kalm. Lach. Laur. Nitr-ac. Nux. Ran-sc. Seneg. Sep.
— — as from a stone between shoulders, Chin.
— back, Ambr. Anac. Aur. Berb. Calc. Caps. Carb-veg. Caust. *Chelid.* Cocc. Con. Cycl. Dulc. Euph. Euphr. Graph. Kali-c. Led. Lyc. Mgn-m. *Mur-ac.* Ntr-m. Nitr. Ol-an. Petr. Phosp. Plat. Puls. Rhod. Sabin. *Samb.* Sass. Seneg. Sep. Sil. Spong. Stann. Staph. Tar. Thuj. Verat.
— sacral region, Berb. Borax. Caust. Meny. Sabin. Samb. Spong. Tar. Verat.
— os coccygis, Cannab.
Prickling, back, Acon. Lact. Ox-ac. Ran-sc.
Pulsation, neck, Acon. Hipp. Glon. Op.
— carotids, Hep. Oleand.
— — during pregnancy, Gels.
— between scapulae, Merc-jod.
— back, *Bar-c.* Thuj.
— sacral region, Caust. Graph. Kali-c. Lach. Ntr-m. Nitr-ac. Nux. Ol-an. Sep. Tabac.
Rasping pain, nape, Cycl. Graph.
— back, Graph.
Red spots, neck, Bry. Cocc. Iod. Lach. Sep.
— under axilla, Bell.
— — scapulae, Cist.
Red, swollen streak on left side neck, Mang.
Rending (tearing), nape, Aeth. Berb. Carb-veg. *Chin.* Mgn-c. Oleand. Rat. Sulph. *Zinc.*
— neck, *Amm-m.* Berb. *Carb-veg.* Mez. Ntr-s. *Zinc.*

28. NAPE, BACK AND SACRAL REGION.

Rending, tearing, scapulae, *Anac.* Arg. Ars. Berb. Borax. Caust. *Chin. Ferr.* Guaj. Phosp. Plb. Rhod. Rhus. Sil.
— back, Anac. Ars. Aur. *Canth. Caps. Carb-veg. Chelid. Chin.* Cina. Cocc. Colch. Led. Lyc. Mgn-m. Mgn-s. Mang. Meph. Ntr-s. *Nux.* Plb. Rhod. Sabin. *Sep.* Sil. Sulph.
— — spine, Berb.
— — one-sided, Guaj.
— from small of back through right leg, Ambr.
— in loins, sensation of, Berb.
— sacral region, Alum. As-i-t. Berb. Calc-ph. Canth. Carb-veg. Caust. *Chin.* Croc. Dig. Lach. Led. Lyc. Mgn-m. Mez. Phosp-ac. Plb. Raph. Rhod. Sep. Spong. Stram. Stront. Sulph. Zinc.
Restlessness, in nape and neck, Thuj.
Rheumatic pain, nape, Acon. Ambr. *Ant.* Berb. *Bry.* Merc. Puls. Rhod. Rhus. Sang. Staph. Sulph. Verat.
— neck, *Bry.* Cycl. Merc. Puls. Rhod. Rhus. Scill.
— scapulae, Ferr-m. Mgn-s. Mez. Ran-b. Rhod. Rhus. Valer.
— back, Acon. Ambr. Anac. Asar. Bell. Calend. Carb-veg. Cham. Cycl. Dros. Graph. Hep. Kali-b. Lach. Lyc. Mcz. Nux. Ol-an. Puls. Ran-b. Rhod. Rhus. Scill. Stram. Sulph. Tart. Teucr. Valer. Verat. Zinc.
— sacral region, Sulph.
Rising up, pain, impeding, back and sacral region, Phosp. Sil.
Scabs, axilla, Ntr-m.
Sciatica, Curare. Graph. Iris. Kali-c. Lach. Lyc. Phyt. Plantago.
As if screwed together, pain, sacral region, Aeth. Alum. Puls. Stront. Zinc.
Seizing, catching pain, in lumbar region, Igt.
Sensitiveness, Ant. Kali-c. Kali-jod. Lach. Nicc. Phosp. Scill.
— from last cervical to fifth dorsal vertebrae, Tellur.
Senselessness, back, Sec-c.
Shingles, *Merc.*
Shivering in back, Bell. Bov. Caps. Igt. Senna. Sep. Spong. Zinc.
Solidity, sensation of, sacrum, Sep.
Sore pain, nape, Cycl. Sang.
— neck, Cic. Lyc.
— under axilla, Mez.
— cervical vertebrae, Con.
— back, Cast. Kalm. Sulph-ac.
— sacral region, Cast. Colch. Ntr-s. Sulph-ac.
Spasms neck, Asar. Cic. Spong.
— — after drinking, Amm-c.
— back, Cham. Iod. Lach.
— — bending, forwards, *Canth. Ip.*
— — — backwards, Ang. Bell. *Canth. Cham.*

Cic. *Igt. Ip.* Op. Rhus. Stann. *Stram.*
Spasmodic pain, nape, Ant. Arn. Asar. Ntr-c.
— neck, Ant. Arn. Asar. Lach. Phosp-ac. Scill.
— back, Bry. Con. Euph. Euphr. Lach. Ntr-s. Sep. Viol-tr.
— sacral region, Bell. Lob. Mgn-m. Plat. Sil.
Sprain, as from, left side back and neck, Con.
Squeezing pain, nape, Lyc.
— between scapulae, Verat.
— lumbar, Aeth. Graph. Lob.
Standing impeded by pain in sacral region, Petr.
Steatoma, nape, Bar-c.
Stiffness, nape, Agar. Amm-m. Anac. *Ang.* Ars. *Bar-c. Bell.* Berb. *Bry.* Calc Camph. Canth. Caps. *Caust.* Cor r. Dig. Dros. *Dulc.* Glon. Graph. Guaj. *Hell.* Igt. *Kali-c.* Lach. *Lyc. Mgn-c.* Mang. Meny. Merc. Mez. Ntr-c. Ntr-m. *Nitr-ac.* Nux. Ol-an. Phosp. *Plat.* Psor. Rat. *Rhod. Rhus. Scill.* Sec-c. Selen. *Sep.* Sil. *Spong.* - Staph. *Sulph.* Thuj. Verat. Zinc. Zing.
— — rheumatic, Lach. Merc.
— — in morning, Ang.
— — after a strain by lifting, Calc. Lyc.
— neck, Amm-m. *Bell. Bry.* Chelid. Croc. Cycl. Dig. Ferr. Glon. Hell. Lach. Lachn. Merc. Mez. Nitr-ac. Rhus. *Scill.* Selen. Spig. *Spong.* Tabac. Zinc.
— — one sided, left, Brom. Laur. Lyc.
— — right, Elaps.
— — of both sides, Chelid.
— — when bending head forward, Kali-b.
— — with headache and nausea, Zing.
— — elongation of uvula, Kali-c.
— — sensation of, and swollen on turning it, Par.
— back, *Ang. Caust.* Kali-b. *Kali-c. Led. Ol-an.* Petr. Prun. Puls. *Sep.* Sil. *Sulph.* Sulph-ac. Thuj.
— — spine, Carb-veg.
— — as from a strain in loins, Prun.
— — one sided, Cinnab. Guaj.
— — — on moving, from ncek, extending to small of back. Guaj.
— — in morning, Ang. Carb-veg. Hipp-m. Sulph-ac.
— — sitting, Caust. Led.
— — after stooping, Bov.
— sacral region, Acon. Amm-m. *Bar-c.* Berb. *Bry.* Hipp-m. Lach. Laur. Led. Lyc. Meph. Prun. Puls. Rheum. *Rhus.* Sil. *Sulph.* Thuj.
— — morning, Thuj.
— — evening, increased, Bar-c.
— — after sitting, Ambr.

Stinging, stiches, nape, Aeth. Bar-c. Bry. Carb-veg Mgn-s. Ntr-m. Ntr-s. Sass. Sep. Stann. Tar Zinc.
— under axilla, Arn. Lact. Ntr-s. Phosp. Staph.
— supra-sternal fossa, Cham.
— neck, Bell. Carb-veg. Cocc. Hep. Merc. Ntr-c. Puls. Samb. Sass. Tar. Zinc.
— scapulae, *Amm-m. Anac.* Berb. Bry. Calc. Camph. Cannab. Chin. Cocc. Colch. Creos. Ferr. Ferr-m. Guaj. Hep. Hyosc. Hyper. Kali-b. Kalm. Lach. Meny. Mur-ac. *Nitr-ac. Nitr.* Nux. *Par. Phosp.* Plb. Prun Puls. Samb. Sass. Sep. Sil. Stram. *Sulph.* Verb. Zinc.
— left scapula, Meny.
— between scapulae. Ind.
— below scapulae, Bad.
— lower angle of left scapulae, Kali-b. Kalm.
— left shonlder and left breast, at intervals, Hipp-m.
— from left scapulae to shoulder and mammae, Grat.
— back, Acon. *Alum.* Anac. Asa-f. Berb. *Bry.* Calc. Carb-an. Carb-veg. Cham. Chin. Coloc. Con. Cycl. Dulc. Evon. Guaj. Hell. *Hep.* Hyosc. Hyper. Igt. Kali-b. Kalm. Lach. *Lyc.* Mgn-c. Mgn-m. Merc. Mez. *Nitr-ac.* Oleand. Pæon. *Par.* Phosp. Plb. Puls. Rhus. Sabin. *Sass.* Sep. Sil *Spig.* Staph. *Sulph.* Thuj. Tar. Verb Zinc.
— — spinal column, Bell. Kali-b.
— — one-sided, Guaj.
— sacral region, Acon. Ambr. Arn. Bell. Berb. *Bry.* Calc. *Carb-an.* Carb-veg. Cocc. Dulc. Hyper. Igt. Kali-b. Kali-c. Kali-jod. Lith. Lyc. Mgn-c. Merc. Ntr-c. Ntr-m. Ntr-s. Nicc. Nitr-ac. Nitr. Nux-jug. Ox-ac. Plb. *Puls.* Ruta. *Sulph.* Tar.
— — after stool, relieved, Ind.
— piercing pain, Scill.
Suppuration at throat-pit, Ip. (compare Sect. 23.)
Swelling, nape, *Bell.* Merc. Puls.
— neck, Ars. *Bell.* Caust. Cic. Con. Croc. *Iod.* Lyc. Merc. Merc-cor. Nux. Phosp. Puls.
— — oedematous. Bell.
— — rheumatic, Con. Merc.
— — from wound in oesophagus with a splinter, bone or other sharp body, Cic.
— — one-sided, Lyc. Ntr-c. Puls. Sass.
— cervical vertebrae, *Calc.*
— dorsal vertebrae. Calc. Sil.
— draws head to one side, Cist.
— when talking, Iod.
— tumor of neck, Graph. Hep.
Tabes dorsalis, Nux-m. Phosp. Tabac.

Talking, impeded by pain in back, Cannab. Tension, nape. Bar-c. *Bry.* Camph. *Caust.* Con. Dig. *Mgn-s.* Mosch. Ntr-s. *Ol-an.* Par. *Plat.* Plb. *Puls.* Rat. Rhod. Rhus. Sass. *Spong. Sulph.* Zinc.
— neck, Bar-c. Berb. *Bry.* Chin. Cic. Coloc. Dig. Glon. Iod. Lach. Meph. Ntr-s. Par. Phosp-ac. Puls. *Rhod.* Rhus. *Spong. Thuj.* Viol-od. Zinc.
— if he turns his head, cannot easily turn it back, Cic.
— scapulae, Bar-c. Cic. Colch. Coloc. Nux. Sil. Zinc.
— back, Amm-c. Berb. Coloc. Hep. **Mez.** Mosch. Ntr-c. Ntr-m. Oleand. *Ol-an.* Puls. Rat. Sass. *Sulph.* Tar. Teucr.
— sacrum, Amm-c. *Bar-c.* Berb. Puls. Sass. *Sulph.* Tar.
Thick, growing, the neck, Con. *Iod. Phosp.*
— when talking, Iod.
Throbbing, back, *Bar-c.* Chin. Lyc. Phosp. Sep. Thuj.
— — lumbar region, Sep.
— from sacrum to pubes, Sabin.
— stitch in os-coccyx when sitting. Par.
Tickling, supra-sternal fossa, Cham.
— thyroid cartilage, Puls.
Tingling (crawling), back, Acon. **Anac.** *Arn.* Caust. Evon. Graph. Ntr-c. *Phosp-ac.* Ran-sc. Sass. Sec-c.
— — as from ants, Evon. Graph. Ntr-c. *Phosp-ac.* Ran-sc. Sass.
— sacral region, Borax. Croton. *Phosp-ac.* Sass.
Torpor, in nape, Calc. Ntr-m.
Tremor, back, Cocc.
Tumors in neck, Cist.
— under axille, encysted, Bar-c.
— in vertebrae, small, Lach.
Twisting pain, sacral region, Graph.
Ulcerative pain, nape, Puls.
— neck, Puls.
— back, Cic. Creos.
— sacral region, Ntr-s. Prun.
Ulcers, nape, Sil.
Venis distension of, neck, Bell. Op. *Thuj.*
Walking, impeded by pain in back, or sacral region, Phosp.
To walk about, necessity, from pain in back, Mgn-s.
Weakness, cervical muscles, Arn. Cocc. Glon. Kali-c. Lyc. Par. Staph. Sulph. Tart. Verat.
— nape, Acon. Kali-c. Par. Plat. Sil. Stann. Staph. Verat.
— back, *Agar.* Coloc. Lach. Nux. Ox-ac. S.l. Zinc.
— sacral region, Ars. Coloc. Merc. Ntr-m. Nux-m. Petr. Sep. Sil. Sulph. Zinc.
Wrenching, spraining pain, nape, *Agar.* *Calc.* Cinnab. Nicc.
— neck, Cinnab.
— between scapulae, Bell. Nux.

28. NAPE, BACK AND SACRAL REGION.

Wrenching, spraining pain, back, Agar. Arg-n. Bell. *Calc.* Nux. Petr. *Puls.* Rhod Sep. Sulph.
— sacral region, *Agar. Calc.* Lach. Ol-an. Rhod. Sulph.
Yellow spots, neck, Iod.
Zona, *Merc.*
In morning, pain, nape, Thuj.
— back, Berb. Euph. Mgn-s. Phyt. Thuj.
— sacral region, Ang. Calad. Ntr-m. Nitr. Selen. *Staph.* Thuj.
— morning in bed, pain, Ang. Berb. Euph. Mgn-s. Nitr.
— evening, pain, nape, Oleand.
— — back, Cist. Led. Nux. Tereb.
— — sacral region, Led. Tereb.
Arms, moving, pain, back. Camph. Ferr.
With desire to evacuate, Creos.
When bending forward, pain, back, Chelid.
— backwards, pain, nape, Con.
— — back, Chelid. Mang. Plat.
— — sacral region, Con. Plat.
— — — relieved, Sang.
— pain in nape of neck, Graph.
— blowing nose, pain, sacral region, Dig.
— breathing pain, back, Acon. *Amm-m.* Calc. Carb-an. Cinnab. Prun. Sass. Spig. Sulph.
— — sacral region, Carb-an. Sulph.
From a cold, pain, back and sacral region, Dulc. Nitr-ac.
— cold air, pain in nape, back and sacral region, Bar-c.
By coldness increased, pain, Rhus. Sabad.
When coughing, pain, back, Bry. Cocc. Nitr.
With dyspnœa, Sulph.
In damp weather, pain, nape and back, Nux-m. Rhod.
From exertion, pain in back, Calc. Calc-ph. Sulph.
When exercising (moving), pain, neck, Ferr. Hell. Phosp-ac. Puls. Rhus. Thuj.
— nape, Acon. Amm-m. Camph. Chin. Dros. Hell. Plb. Rhus. Sass.
— scapulae, Calc. Petr.
— back, Chin. Cinnab. Mang. Meph. Petr. Samb. *Sass.* Stram.
— sacral region, Chin. Kali-b. Psor. Sass.
From exercise, pain increased, Cham. Caust.
— falling, pain, sacral region, Kali-c.
By emission of flatus, relieved, Berb.
When lifting, Lyc.
— lying, pain, nape, Agar.
— — back, Agar Berb. Creos. Euph. Nitr. Sil. Staph. Tar.
— — sacral region, Agar. Berb. Chin. Tar.
— — on back, pain in back, Chin. Euph. Igt. Nitr. Staph.
— — — — relieved, Ruta.
— — side, increased, Staph.
— — — relieved, Nitr.

— — something hard, relieved, Ntr-m. Rhus.
After manual labor, pain, back, Sulph.
— mental affection, pain, back, Bar-c.
When nursing child, pain through scapula, Croton.
Pressure, pains, neck and nape, Lach.
— — relieved by, Dulc. Ruta.
When raising head, pain, nape, Senna.
— — arms, pains, neck and back, Graph.
— at rest, pain, back, Creos. Dulc. Kali-c. Mang. Nitr. Samb. Spig.
— riding in a vehicle, pain, back, Calc. Nux-m.
With rigidity of body, Cham.
When rising from sitting, pain, back, Canth. Led. Sulph.
— — sacrum, Ant. Calc. Cannab. Con. Ferr ac. Petr. Rhod. Staph. Sulph.
— from stooping, pain, nape, Nicc.
— — back, Phosp. Sil. Sulph. Verat.
— — sacrum, Lyc. Phosp. Sass. Verat.
In room, pain nape, relieved in open air, Psor.
When sitting down, pain in back and sacrum, Aloe. Kobalt. Meny. Zinc.
— — —, back, Agar. Berb. Cimex. Lyc. Rhus. Sabad. Sil. *Tart.* Tereb. Thuj.
— — with dyspnœa, Lyc.
— — relieved, Staph.
— sacral region. Agar. Bar-c. Borax. Caust. Cist. Kobalt. Lyc. *Meny.* Ntr-c. Ntr-s. Ol-an. Phell. Prun. Ruta. Sabad. *Tart.* Tereb. Thuj.
— pain in os coccygis, Par.
— bent, Kali-jod.
After sitting, pain back, Led.
— sacral region, Berb. Phosp.
When sneezing, pain neck and nape, Arn.
— speaking, pain, back, Cocc.
By standing, pain increased, Agn. Cocc. Kali-b. Kali-c. Lith. Petr. Phosp. Sulph.
— — relieved, Arg-n.
After stool, pain sacral region, Tabac.
— — relieved, Berb.
When stooping, pain in nape, Kali-b. Par.
— — — back, Clem. Con. Lyc. Meny. Nitr. Par. Rhus. Verat.
— sacral region, Borax. Lyc. Meny. Ol-an. Ruta Sass. Verat.
Stoop, inability to, Borax.
On throwing the head back, pain in neck, Cic.
When touched pain in back, Glon. Lach. Puls. Sass.
— nape, Lach. Puls. Sang.
— back, increased, Ars.
— sacrum, Amm-m. *Colch.* Kali-b. Rhus. Sil. Tong.
When turning in bed, pain back, Hep.
— sacral region, Nux. Staph.
To urinate, with desire to, pain in loins, Creos.

28. NAPE, BACK AND SACRAL REGION.

When walking, pain in back, Agar. Cocc. Sulph.
— — relieved, Arg-n. Bar-c. Kobalt. Mgn-s. Phosp. Rhus. Ruta. Stront.
— sacral region, Kali-c. Ruta. Sulph. Zinc.
By warmth, external, pain relieved, nape, Rhus.
— — — — back, Cinnab.

29. Upper Extremities.

Aching pains, Asa-f. Benz-ac. Chin-sulph. Dros. Lach. Phosp-ac. Raph. Staph.
Agility, nimbleness, want of in hands, Graph. Ntr. Plb. Sil.
— — — in fingers, Sep.
Arthritic complaints, *Bry*. *Hep*. Lach. *Lyc*. *Merc*. Petr. Phosp. *Rhod*. Rhus. Sabin. *Sis*. Spig. (compare Rheumatic.)
— left shoulder, Guaj. Merc-cor. Sulph.
— right shoulder, Iris. Lob. Lyc. Pallad. Sang.
— elbow and wrist, Grat. Mgn-s.
— forearm, *Merc*. Nitr-ac.
— — right, Nitr-ac.
— wrist, left, Guaj. Mgn-s.
— hand and wrist, Bell. Cocc. Kali-b. *Hep*. Lyc. *Sabin*.
— fingers and fingers-joints, Ant. Bry. *Cero-an*. Clem. Grat. *Hep*. Lyc. Mang. Ncc. Nitr-ac. Ox-ac. Petr. Rhod. Rhus. Sass. Sep. Spig.
Arthritic nodes, wrist, *Calc*. *Led*. Rhod.
— hands and finger joints, Ant. Benz-ac. C. lc. Hep.
— finger-joints, Agn. *Calc*. Clem. *Dig*. *Graph*. *Led*. Lyc. Rhod. Staph.
— stiffness, elbow, Lyc.
— wrist, Lyc.
— stiffness finger-joints, *Carb-a*. Graph. Lyc.
Atrophy of arms. Chin. Graph. Selen.
As if beaten, pain in arms, *Acon*. Ang. *Arn*. Berb. Cannab. Chenop. Cocc. Creos. *Croc*. Croton. Hep. Ntr-m. Nitr-ac. *Verat*. Zinc-ox.
— shoulder-joint, *Dros*.
— under shoulder-joint, right, Kali-c.
— — left, Kali-jod.
— shoulder, Acon. Cannab. Coloc. Con. Ntr-m. Verat.
— upper arm, *Cocc*. *Hep*. Nitr-ac.
— — right, Cinnab.
— fore-arm, *Croc*. Croton. *Ruta*.
— bones of left fore-arm, radius as if crushed or broken, Gymnoc.
— hands, Arn. Ntr-m. Nicc. *Ruta*.
— wrist, *Dros*. Ruta.
Bending over easily of finger joints, Bell. Hep. Nux. Teucr.
Bloatedness hands, Cham.
— fingers when the arms hang down, Amm-c. Phosp.

— dark blue of forearms. and hands, Samb.
Blood, congestion of in arms, Nux.
— as if stopped, sensation, arms. Rhod.
— — — — fingers, Croc.
Blue spots, like sugillations, forearm, Sulph-ac.
Blueness of hands, Amm-c. Apis. Bar-c. Elaps. Verat.
— after washing with cold water, Amm-c.
— marbled of hands, Cupr.
Boring, sensation shoulder-joint, Rhod.
— humerus. Mang.
— fore-arm, Ran-sc.
— wrist, *Hell*.
— carpal bones, Daph. Ntr-c. Ran-sc.
— fingers, Ran-sc.
— finger-joints, Daph. Hell.
— finger-tips, Sulph.
Brown spots, elbow, Sep.
— wrist, Petr.
— hands, Ntr-m.
— palmar surface of hand, Iod. Ntr-c. Thuj.
Bruising pain, Acon. *Arn*. Dulc. Oleand, *Plat*. *Ruta*.
— shoulder, Acon. *Cic*. Cocc. Hep. Sulph.
— upper-arm, Cycl.
— elbow-joint, Carb-veg. *Ruta*.
— fore-arm. Acon. *Cic*. Oleand.
— — middle of, to wrist, Kali-b.
— hands and fingers, Bism. Oleand.
— thumb, left, Creos.
Bubbling sensation, upper arm, Colch. Petros.
— elbow, Rheum.
Burning, arms, Agar. Alum. Berb. Bry. Phosp. Plat. Puls. Rhus. Rhus-rad.
— humeri, Rhus.
— shoulder, Carb-veg. Graph. Rhus. Stront. Tabac.
— upper-arm, *Agar*. Berb. Sulph.
— elbow, Alum.
— fore-arm, *Agar*. Sulph,
— hand, Bry. Carb-veg. Lam. Led. Ntr-s. Phosp. Plat. Rhus. Sec-c. Sep. *Stann*. Tart.
— wrist, Ntr-c.
— palm of hand, Canth. Lach. Lyc. Petr. *Phosp*. Sang. Sep. Stann. Sulph.
— fingers, *Agar*. Alum. Borax. Croc.

29. UPPER EXTREMITIES.

Kali-c. Mosch. Ntr-c. Oleand. Plat.
Sil. Teucr.
Burning finger-tips, Mur-ac.
Callosities, horny, on hands, Graph.
Chilblains, pain as from, Nux.
Chilliness, arms, Bell. Igt.
— fingers, Meny.
Chill begins and spreads from arms, Hell.
— — in right arm, Merc.
— — — left hand, Carb-veg.
— during the pain in hand and fingers, Nux.
Cicatrices, deep, stinging, in hands, Kali-b.
Clenched thumbs, Aeth. Bell. *Cham.* Cocc. Hyosc. Igt. Merc. Stann. Stram. Viol-tr.
Cobweb, sensation of, on hands, Borax.
Coldness, arms, *Bell.* Cic. Dulc. Ip. Kali-c. Kali-chl. *Led.* Merc-cor. *Op.* *Plb.* Rhus. Sec-c. Sep. Thuj. Verat.
— wrist, Gels.
— hands, Acon. Ambr. Apis. Ars. Aur. Bar-c. Bell. Benz-ac. Carb-veg. Caust. Cham. Chin. Cocc. Cupr. Dig. Dros. Elaps. Gels. Hell. Hep. Hipp m. Hyosc. Iod. *Ip.* Kali-c. Lach. Lyc. Merc. Mez Ntr-c. Ntr-m. Nitr-ac. Nitr.Nux-m.Nux. Ox-ac. Petr. Phosp. Ran-b. Rhus. Rumex. Scill. Sep. Sulph. Tabac. Tart. Thuj. Verat. Zinc.
— — evening in bed, Carb-an.
— — at night, Phosp. Thuj.
— — icy, Camph. Carb-veg. Lach. Nux-m. Verat.
— — — one hand, Chin. Dig. Ip.
— — — — on one side, the other hot and red, Puls.
— — of right, warmth of left, Mez.
— — one hand, sweat of the other, Ip. Mosch.
— — alternately with heat, Cocc. Par.
— — feet warm, Aloe.
— fingers, Ang. Chelid. Cic. Colch. Hell Lac-can. Mosch. Mur-ac. Par. Rhod Sulph. Tar. Tart. Thuj.
— — tip, Meny. Phosp-ac.
Contraction of arms, Lyc. Sec-c.
— — upper arms, Stram. Sulph.
— bend of elbow, Elaps.
— hands, Bism. Carb-veg. Cina. Cinnab. Colch. Mgn-s. Merc.Nux. *Sol-nig.* Sulph.
— — and fingers, Phosp-ac.
— — — tendons of, Caust. Sulph.
— right hand when writing, Euph.
— metacarpal bones, Eupur.
— — right hand, Cannab.
— right thumb and index, Cycl.
— fingers, Ambr. Arg. Calc Carb-veg. Caust. Chin. Cina. Cocc. Coff. Colch. Cycl. *Graph.* Kali-jod. *Lyc.* Mgn-s. Mang. Merc. Ntr-c. Nux. Ox-ac. Phosp. Phosp-ac. Plat. Rhus. Ruta. Sabad. Sabin. Sec-c. Selen. Spig. Stann. Tart.

— — when gaping, Nux.
— of tendons, sensation of, Aeth. Lach. Sep.
— — — when bending them, Aeth.
— — — of shoulders, Bov.
— — — — elbows, Caust. Lach. Mang. Sep.
— — — — wrist, Carb-veg. Igt. Lach.
— — — — hands, Nux.
— — — — fingers, Aeth. Carb-an. Croc. Dros. Lach. Nux. Sep. Spong.
Convulsions, arms, *Bell.* Bry. Camph. Caust. *Cham.* Cocc. Igt. *Iod.* *Op.* Plb. Sabad. Scill. (compare Twitching.)
— hands, *Bell. Iod.* Mosch. Plb.
— fingers, Cham. Cupr. *Igt.* Iod. Mosch. Staph.
Convulsive rotation of arms, Camph.
Copper-colored spots on hands, Nitr-ac.
Corroding pain, Lyc. Plat.
— fingers Bar-c. Plat.
Cracked skin of hands, Creos. (compare Rhagades.)
Cracking in joints of arms, Chin-sulph. Croc. Kali-b. Merc. Tart. Thuj.
— when leaning on the arms, Thuj.
— in shoulder-joint, Ferr. Kali-c.
— — elbow-joint, Kalm.
— — wrist-joints, Con.
— — finger-joints, Merc.
Cramping pain, back of the hand, Bruc.
Cutting pain, arms, Anac.
— shoulder-joint, in bending arm forward, Igt.
— elbow, wrist and finger-joints, Phosp-ac.
— fore-arm and fingers, Mur-ac.
— hands, Mur-ac. Ntr-c.
Deadness, arms, Amm-c. Thuj.
— hands, Acon. *Calc.* Con. Lyc. Nux. *Thuj.* Zinc.
— fingers, *Amm-c. Amm-m. Calc.* Caust. *Chelid.* Cic. Creos. Hep. Lyc. Merc. Mur-ac. Nitr-ac. Par. Phosp. Phosp-ac. Sec-c. *Sulph.* Tart. Thuj. Verat. Zinc.
— — one-sided, Phosp-ac.
— in morning, Amm-c.
— at night, Amm-c. Mur-ac.
— in cold air, Nitr-ac.
— when taking hold of something, Amm-c. Calc.
— in warm temperature, Calc.
Desquamation, of the cuticle, arms, Agar.
— — — hands, Alum. Amm-c. Amm-m. Bar-c. Ferr. Laur. Sulph.
— — — — palms, Amm-c.
— — — — between fingers, Amm-m.
— — — fingers, Agar. Bar-c. Elaps. Merc. Sulph.
— — — — about the nails, Eugen. Merc. Sabad.
Detached from bones, sensation as if the flesh were, Bry. Igt. Rhus. Sulph. Thuj.

29. UPPER EXTREMITIES.

Digging pain, Croc. Diad. Ntr-m. Rhod. Rhus. Ruta.
— — arms, Carb-an. Croc. Mang. Rhus. Thuj.
Dislocation of wrist, *Amm-c.* Arn. Bov. Bry. Carb-an. *Ruta.*
— — fingers, easy, Hep.
Distortion of fingers, Graph.
Doubling the fist, Hyosc. Merc. Stram.
— with clenched thumb, Merc.
Drawing pain, arms, Arg. Bell. Berb. Bry. Calc. Caust. Cina. Cinnab. Clem. Coloc. Cycl. *Ferr.* Ind. Kali-c. Lam. Lyc. Mgn-c. *Mang.* Meny. Merc. Mez. *Nitr-ac.* Nitr. *Nux.Ol.* and *Ol-an.* Par Petr. Phosp-ac. *Plat.* Plb. Puls. *Rhod.* Sec-c. *Sep.* Sil. *Staph.* Sulph. Tabac. *Thuj.* Zinc.
— shoulder-joint, Clem. Kali-c. Lact. Puls. Rhod. *Sulph.* Teucr.
— humerus, Rhod. Tereb. Teucr. Thuj. Valer.
— shoulders, Ambr. Aur-m. Dulc. Kali-c. Mang. Ntr-c. Nux. Puls. Sep. Staph. *Sulph.* Zinc.
— upper-arm, Acon. Aur-m. Ars. Dulc. Ferr-m. Lact. Mosch. *Mur ac.* Oleand. Plb. *Staph.* Tereb. Valer.
— elbow-joint, Ambr. Lact. Mur-ac. Ntr-c. Phosp-ac. *Sulph.* Viol-od. Zinc.
— fore-arm, Ambr. *Ang.* Ant. *Carb-veg.* Croc. Croton. Cycl. Ferr-m. Mosch. Ntr-c. *Nitr-ac.* *Rhod.* Ruta. Samb. Seneg. Spong. *Staph.* Tar.
— hands, Ambr. Ang. Arg. *Caust.* Cina. Clem. Croton. Cycl. Ferr-m. Kali-c. Lact. Mgn-c. Mang. Meny. Ntr-c. *Nitr-ac. Ol-an.* Rhod. Ruta. Sil. Staph. *Sulph.* Viol-od. Zinc Zing.
— wrist, Anac. Ars. *Asar.* Bov. Carb-veg. Caust. Cist. Ferr-m. Fluor-ac. Kali-c. Mosch. Phosp-ac. Spong. Sulph. Tar. Zinc.
— carpal bones, Anac. Sabin. Samb. Spig. Teucr.
— fingers, Ambr. Aug. Ant. *Asar* Carb-veg. Coloc. Croton. Kali-c. Lam. Mang. Nux. Oleand. *Ol-an.* Petr. Phosp-ac. Puls. Ruta. Sil. Sol-nig. Staph. Sulph. Teucr. Zinc.
— finger-joints, Anac. Ant. Caust. Kali-c. Phosp-ac. Sep. *Sulph.* Teucr.
Dry skin, of the hands, Anac. Bar-c. Bell. Clem. Ferr-m. Gels. Hep. Lach. Lyc. Ntr-c. Ntr-m. Phosp-ac. Sabad. Sulph. Thuj. Zinc.
— palm of hand, Bism. Gels.
— fingers, Anac. Phosp-ac. Puls.
— — at night, Puls.
Emaciation, arms, Nitr-ac.
— hands, Chin. Graph. Selen.
Enlargement, sensation of, arms and hands, at night, Clem. *Diad.* Nitr.

Eruption, arms, Agar. Alum. Ant. Caust. Merc. Nux. Phosp-ac. Rhus. Sulph. Tart. Valer.
— upper-arms, Led. Merc. Nux. Sep. Tart.
— elbow, Berb. Sep. Sulph.
— — red papulous, not itching, Cinnab.
— fore-arms, Alum. Bry. Selen. Spong.
— wrist, Amm-m. Caust. Hep. Led. Rhus. Tart.
— hands, Amm-m. Carb-veg. Creos. Dulc. Hep. Kalm. *Lach.* Merc. *Mur-ac.* Rhus. Rhus-v. Selen. Sep. Sulph. Sulph-ac.
— — back of, Berb. Creos. Kali-chl. Mur-ac.
— palms, Kali-c. Sep.
— fingers, Borax. Caust. Graph. Hep. *Lach.* Mur-ac. Ntr-c. Ran-b. Rhus. Sass. Sep. Sil. Spig. Tabac. Tar.
— finger-joints, Cycl.
— between fingers, Lyc. Puls. Sep. Sulph-ac.
— between thumb and fore-finger, Bruc.
— blisters, on wrist, forming scabs, Amm-m.
— large, on palms of hands, Bufo.
— — spreading, on swollen hands and fingers, worse from cold water, Clem.
— itching, on hands, first pale, then red, Gum-gut.
— blue, on fingers, Ran-b.
— blotches, red, Lach.
— burning, *Ntr-c.* Rhus. Spig.
— like chicken-pox, Led.
— clustering, Rhus.
— desquamating, Agar.
— erysipelatous, Kalm.
— excresences, Lach.
— hard, Caust.
— granulated, Carb-veg. Graph. Hep.
— humid, on back of hands and fingers, and in palms, elbows, knuckles, Creos.
— itching, Ant. Carb-veg. Caust. Creos. Kali-c. Kali-chl. Lach. Led. Lyc. Merc. Nux. Rhus. Sep. Spig. Sulph. Tabac. Tart.
— itch-like, Alum. Berb. Graph. *Lach.* Merc. Nitr-ac. Phosp. Rhus. Sass. Selen. *Sep.* Sulph.
— miliary, Alum. Bry. Led. Merc. Nux. Selen. Sulph. Tart.
— nettle-rash, Berb. Hep. Hyper. *Ntr-c.* Ntr-s.
— pimples, Agar. Berb. Creos. Kali-chl. Lyc. Phosp-ac. Spig. Sulph. Tabac. Tar. Tart. Valer.
— — red, on finger-tips, Elaps.
— pustules, Ars. Borax. Rhus. Sass. Sec-c. Sep. Sil. Spig. Sulph.
— — black, Anthrax. *Ars.* Lach. Sec-c.
— — large, surrounded by inflamed base, Sep.
— rash, hot, on right wrist, Elaps.

29. UPPER EXTREMITIES.

Eruption, red, Ant. Cycl.
— scabs, Alum. Amm-m. Mur-ac. Sep.
— — itching, Sep.
— — moist, Alum.
— scaly, Agar.
— smarting, like nettle-rash, on hands, Hyper.
— smooth spots on palms and fingers, first coral-color, then dark-red, last copper-colored, Cor-r.
— stinging, Mgn-c. Puls.
— tubercles, hard, Rhus.
— vesiculous, Amm-m. Ant. Bruc. Cycl. Kali-c. Kali-chl. Lach. Mgn-c. Merc-cor. *Ntr-c.* Puls. *Ran-b.* Rhus. *Sep.* Spong. Sulph.
— — comes out in cold air, Dulc.
— — gnawing, on hands and fingers, Clem. Graph. Kali-c. Mgn-c. Nitr-ac. Sil.
— — humid, painless, between fingers, Hell.
— — itching on arms and hands, Daph.
— — suppurating on elbow, Sulph.
— — worse from washing in cold water, Clem.
— — with shooting pain, Mgn-c.
— warts, Lach. Sulph.
— white, Agar.
Erysipelas, Amm-c. Bell. Kalm. Petr. *Rhus.*
— upper arms, Bell.
— fore-arms, Ant. Lach. Merc.
— hands, Graph. Hep. Hydrast. Rhus.
— fingers, Rhus. Sulph.
Excoriation, pain as from, in fore-arm, Cic.
— — in shoulder, Cic. Con.
Excrescences on hand, Lach.
Exertion, pain in elbows impedes, Tabac.
Exostosis, Dulc. Mez. Rhus. Sil. Sulph.
To extend the arms, inclination, Amm-c. Bell. Sabad. Tabac. Verb.
Firmness, want of, in shoulder, Croc.
Fore-arm, complaints in, Acon.
From freezing, disorders, (boils, blisters, chilblains), Agar. Carb-an. *Croc.* Lyc. *Nitr-ac.* Nux. Op. Petr. *Phosp. Puls.* Rhus. Stann. Staph. Sulph. Sulph-ac.
— itching, Puls.
Fulness, sensation of, arms, Verat.
— hands. Caust. Ntr-s.
— — palms, at night, Ars.
— — when taking hold of something, Caust.
Furuncles, boils arms, Amm-c. *Calc.* Carb-an. Carb-veg. Lyc. Mgn-m. *Mez.* Nitr. Petr. Phosp-ac. *Sil.* Zinc.
— shoulders, Amm-c. Bell. *Nitr.* Phosp-ac.
— — large blood-boils on, Nux-jug.
— upper-arms, Carb-veg. Zinc.
— fore-arms, Calc. Lyc. Mgn-m. Petr.
— hands, Calc. Lyc.
— — small blood-boils on, Iris.
— fingers, Calc. Lach.
— thumb, Nitr.

Ganglion, back of head, Amm-c. Phosp-ac. Plb. *Sil.*
Gangrene of fingers, Sec-c.
Gnawing pain, hands and fingers, Ran-sc.
— — under nails, Alum.
Grasping, involuntarily, Sulph.
Hang-nails, *Ntr-m.* Rhus. Stann. Sulph.
Hard skin of hands, Amm-c. Sulph.
Heat in the hands, Acon. Anac. Borax. Carb-veg. Cast. Clem. Corc. Cub. Eupat. Ferr. Hep. Iod. Lach. Lact. Led. Lyc. Millef. Murex. Nitr-ac. Nux-m. Nux. Petr. Phosp. Rheum. Rhus. Stann. Staph.
— — alternating with coldness, Cocc.
— — sudden, when stretching out the arm, Ferr-m.
— — in the evening, Led.
— — at night, Staph.
— — with cold feet, Acon.
— of one hand, coldness of the other, Dig. Ip. Puls.
— and redness of one hand, the other pale and cold, Mosch.
— of palms, Asar. Colch. Gels. Nux. Sep. Zinc. Zing.
— — fingers, Borax. Lact. Mgn-c. Par.
Heaviness, arms, Acon. *Alum.* Amm-m. Ang. Bell. Berb. Cact. Calc. Caust. Cic. *Ferr.* Hipp-m. Mur-ac. Ntr-c. Ntr-m. Nux. Par. Plat. *Puls.* Rhod. *Sil.* Spig. Stann. Sulph-ac. Tart. Teucr.
— — from shoulder to fingers, with numbness, Ambr. Cham. Croc. Graph. Kali-c. Lyc. Mgn-m. Nux. Puls. Sep. Sil.
— — when at rest, Rhod.
— right arm, Amm-m.
— — and loss of power, Amm-c.
— left arm, Dig. Merc-jod.
— shoulder, *Puls.* Sulph. Thuj.
— — as from a burden, Sulph.
— upper arms, Teucr.
— elbow-joint, Samb.
— fore-arms, Anac. *Croc.* Mur-ac. Spong. Thuj.
— hands, Bry. Nicc. Nitr. Ox-ac. Puls.
— — at night, Nitr.
— fingers, Par.
Herpes arms, Alum. Bov. Con. Dulc. Graph. Lyc. Mang. Merc. Ntr-m. Phosp. Psor. Sec-c. Sil.
— elbow, Caust. Creos. Cupr. Hep. Phosp. Psor. Staph. Thuj.
— fore-arm, Alum. Con. Mang. Merc.
— wrist, Merc. Psor.
— hands, Bov. Cist. Creos. Dulc. Merc. *Ntr-c. Ran-b.* Sass. Staph. Verat. Zinc.
— — back of, Lyc. Sep.
— — like moist itch, itching at night, Merc.
— fingers, Caust. Creos. Ran-b. Psor. Thuj. Zinc.

29. UPPER EXTREMITIES. 213

Herpes between fingers, Ambr. Graph. Nitr-ac.
— burning, Con. Merc.
— crusty, Con. Thuj.
— dry, Verat.
— furfuraceous, mealy, Merc. Phosp.
— itching, Caust. Cupr. Mgn-s. Mang. Zinc.
— moist, Bov. Con.
— red, Mgn-s.
— scaly, Cupr. Merc.
Herpetic spots on arms and hands, Ntr-m. Zinc.
— elbows, *Sep*.
Horn-like, calli, hands, Graph.
Indolence, inactivity of arms, Nux.
Induration of cellular tissue of forearm, Sil.
— tendons of fingers, Caust.
Inflammation arm, Cupr. Petr. *Rhus*. Sep.
— forearm, Lyc.
— elbow, Ant. Lach.
— — erysipelatous, Lach.
— palmar surface of hand, Bry.
— fingers, Con. Kali-c. Lyc. *Mgn-c*. Mang. Ntr-m. Nitr-ac. Puls.
Itching, arms, Bov. Caust. Fluor-ac. Lach. Lyc. Phosp. Plat. Puls. Rhus-rad. Selen. Sulph. Zinc.
— shoulders, Gels. Kobalt. Nicc.
— hands, Anac. Berb. Carb-veg. Caust. Colch. Gran. Lach. Lyc. Merc. Mur-ac. Nitr-ac. Plat. Ran-b. Rhus. Sass. Selen. Sep. Sil. Stann. Sulph.
— spots on hands, Berb. Zinc.
— palms, Ambr. Anac. Berb. Carb-veg. Hep. Kali-c. Ntr-m. Ran-b. Sil. Spig. Sulph.
— — palms, Grat.
— fingers, Agar. Con. Lach. Lact. Ntr-c. Nux. Ox-ac. Plat. Prun. Puls. Ran-b. Selen. Sulph.
— between fingers, Cycl.
— as from chilblains, Prun.
Jerks, shocks, arms, Nux. Op.
— — left, Cic.
— upper arms, Ruta.
— elbow-joint, Ntr-m. Verat.
— hand, Sulph-ac. Valer.
Jerking pain, arms, Arn. *Chin*. Ind. Meny. Mez. Ntr-c. *Phosp-ac*. Puls. Ran-b. Rheum.
— humerus, *Chin*.
— shoulder, Mez. *Puls*. Tar.
— scapula joint, Puls.
— upper arms, Lact. Puls. Rhus. Tar. Valer.
— elbow joint, Rhus.
— hands, Chin. Mez. Ntr-m. Puls.
— wrist, Anac. Rhus.
— carpal bones, Anac. Chin.
— fingers, *Amm-c. Chin*. Meny. Mez. Ntr-c. Phosp-ac. Ran-sc. Rheum. Staph.
— finger-joints, Anac. Ntr-m. Rhus.

Joint, sensation as if shoulder were put out of, Croc. Mez.
Lameness, paralytic, arms, Alum. (compare, Paralysis, sensation of.)
— right arm, Fluor-ac.
— left arm and right foot, Hyper.
— languor, arms, Anac *Ang*. Berb. Bry. *Calc*. Hœmatox. Lach. *Ntr-c. Ntr-m*. Phosp. Sass. Seneg. Sil.
— — in morning, in bed, Iod.
— — during movement, Berb.
— shoulder and elbow, Ntr-c.
— hands, Phosp.
Laxity, relaxation, arms, Guaj. Plat.
Livid spots, arms, Lyc.
Living, as if, something, were running in arms, Igt.
Looseness, sense of in shoulder, *Croc*.
Moisture on bend of elbow, Sep.
Motion impeded by pain, arm, Mgn-c. Ntr-m.
— — — elbow, Tabac.
Muscles, twitching arms, *Asa-f*. Cupr. Mez. Ntr-m. Oleand. Sil. Tar. Tart. Teucr.
— shoulder, Spong.
— upper arm, Cocc. Hell. Nitr-ac. Spig.
— forearm, Spig.
— hands, *Asa-f*. Tart.
Nails, blueness, Chin. *Dig*. Hipp-m. Merc-sulph. Sil.
— — beginning, Chelid.
— crippled, Graph. Nitr-ac. Sep. Sil. Thuj.
— discolored, Ars. Thuj.
— dark, Ox-ac.
— gray color, Merc-cor.
— grow more rapidly, Fluor-ac.
— — too slowly, Ant.
— hang nails, Ntr-m. Rhus.
— painful Ant.
— — sore pain, margin of, red, Lith.
— — ulcerative pain, Ntr-s.
— peeling off, Merc.
— suppuration, around, Eugen.
— thickness, Graph.
— white spotted, Nitr-ac.
— yellow, Con. Sil.
— — under the nails pain, Berb.
Numbness, arms, Ambr. Bar-c. Berb. Bufo. *Cham*. Creos. *Croc*. Euphr. Graph. Kali-c. Lach. Led. *Lyc. Mgn-m*. Nitr. *Nux*. Petr. Phosp. Rhus-rad. Sep. *Sil*. Spig. Sulph. Thuj. Verat.
— — left, Acon. Cinnab. Glon. Millef. Pallad.
— — right, Kali-b. Merc-jod.
— forearms, Nux.
— left forearm and hand in morning, Fluor-ac.
— hands, Ambr. Ars. Carb-an. Cocc-c. Con. *Croc*. Euphr. Hyosc. Lam. Lyc. Mez. Nitr-ac. Nux. Phosp. Sil. Spig.
— — left, Merc-sulph.

29. UPPER EXTREMITIES.

Numbness, hand, right, Cycl.
— palm of hand, Bry.
— fingers, Acon. Amm-c. Bar-c. Calc. Carb-an. Caust. Cham. Cimex. Creos. Dig. Euphr. Ferr. Iod. Kali-c. Lam. Lyc. Mur-ac. Ntr-m. Nitr-ac. Nitr. Nux Par. Phosp. Puls. Sass. Stram. Sulph. Verat. Zinc.
— — single, Ol-an.
— — ring and little finger, Diad.
— — tips, Kali-c. Lach. Phosp. Spong. Staph.
— in morning, Nux. Puls. Zinc.
— — in bed, Mgn-m. Nitr-ac.
— — on waking, Hipp-m.
— at night, *Ambr. Croc.* Igt. *Lyc. Nux.* Puls. Sil.
— when carrying something, Ambr.
— with torpor, Nux.
— in cold weather, Kali-c.
— when lain upon, Ambr. Bar-c. Sil.
— — leaning upon the part, Sil.
— after motion or exercise, Kali-c. Ruta.
— when taking hold of anything, Cocc. Cham.
Outward pressure, shoulder joint, Cor-r.
Pain, simple, arm, Bar-c. Calc. Hæmatox. Rhus-rad.
— in upper three vertebrae, through shoulders, Kalm.
— shoulder, Dig. Gels. Igt.
— — right, Cimex. Fluor-ac. Kalm. Lact.
— — left, Cinnab.
— shoulder-joint, Amm-c. Cist. Igt. Plb.
— humeri, Diad. Igt. Iod. Lyc. Murex.
— first in left then right deltoid, with inclination to move, Ox-ac.
— elbow left, from draft of air, Gels.
— wrist, Amm-c. Calc-ph. Cor-r. Kalm. Kobalt. Lach. Plb. Ruta.
— — joint which had been sprained, Amm-c.
— — right, Lac-can. Ox-ac. Petr.
— — left, Kalm.
— hands, Cist. Kalm.
— fingers, Benz-ac. Calc-ph. Iris. Kalm.
— thumb, Calc-ph.
— — on lifting, Ruta.
Pain in bones in general, *Asa-f.* Lyc. Phosp-ac. Staph.
Panaritia, paronychia, All-cep. Alum. Apis. Bar-c. Berb. Bov. Bufo. Calc. Caust. Con. Diosc. Ferr-m. Fluor-ac. Gins. *Hep.* Iod. Kali-c. Lach. Led. Lyc. Merc. Ntr-m. Ntr-s. Puls. Sacch. Sep. *Sil. Sulph.* Teucr.
— blue black, around nail of thumb, Bufo.
— left index, (as if forming), Gymnoc.
— pain as from, Puls.
Paralysis, arms, Bar-c. *Bell. Calc.* Calc-ph. Caust. Chelid. *Corc.* Cupr. Dulc. Ferr. Lyc. Nitr. *Nux.* Op. Plb. Rhus. Sec-c. Sil. *Stann.* Verat.

— — left, Dig. Hipp. Pallad.
— — — with pain in heart, Pallad.
— upper arm, Agar. Calc-ph. Chelid. Nux.
— fore arm, *Sil.*
— wrist, right, in morning, Hipp.
— hand, Agar. Cannab. Cupr. Kali-c. Lach. Plb. *Sil. Zinc.*
— — right, Caust. Elaps.
— fingers, Calc. Calc-ph. Phosp.
— with coldness and insensibility, Plb. Rhus. Zinc.
— sensation of, paralytic pains, arms, Acon. Alum. Amm-m. Ang. Bell. Berb. *Calc.* Cham. *Chin.* Cina. *Colch. Cycl.* Dig. Dulc. *Ferr. Igt.* Lach. Meny. Mez. Ntr-m. Par. *Plat.* Plb. Prun. *Sep. Sil.* Stann. Sulph-ac. *Tabac. Verat.* Zinc. (compare Weakness.)
— — left arm and right foot, Hyper.
— — right arm, Fluor-ac.
— shoulder, Ambr. Euph. Mgn-s. Mang. Mur-ac. Ntr-m. Nux. Puls. Sep. Stann. Staph. Sulph. Valer. Verat.
— — right, Laur. Merc-cor. Pallad. Psor.
— — top, Mez.
— upper arm, Ferr-m.
— elbow joint, Ambr. Ang. Samb. Valer.
— fore arm, Acon. Ambr. Bism. Bov. Creos. Prun. Seneg. Staph Stront.
— wrist, Asar. Bism. Bov. Carb-veg. Kali-c. Merc. Petr.
— — right, Laur. Lyc. Ox-ac.
— hand, Acon. Ambr. Ang. *Chin.* Meny. Merc. Nux. Prun. Staph. Stront. Sulph. *Tabac.*
— fingers, Acon. Asar. Aur. *Carb-veg. Chin.* Creos. Cycl. Dig. Evon. Lact. Meny. Staph.
— — thumb and index, Lachn.
— — right, Prun.
— — joints, *Aur.* Par. Verb.
Perspiration, upper arms, Petr.
— in axilla, smelling like onions, Osm.
— hands, Acon. Anac. Ars. Bell. *Calc.* Canth. Carb-veg. Cham. Con. Hell. Hep. Igt. Iod. Merc. Ntr-c. *Ntr-m.* Nitr-ac. *Nux.* Petr. Phosp. Puls. Sass. Sep. Sil. *Sulph.* Tabac. *Thuj.* Zinc.
— — only, Agn.
— — clammy, Anac. Phosp. Spig.
— — cold, Acon. Bell. Canth. Caps. Cham. Cina. Cocc. Hep. Iod. Ip. Kali-b. Nux. Rheum. Sass. Sep. Spig. Tabac.
— — fetid, Hep.
— — itching, Sulph.
— — warm, Igt.
— — at night, Coloc.
— — palms, *Acon.* Amm-m. Anac. Bar-c. Cadm. *Calc.* Carb-veg. *Con.* Creos. *Dulc.* Gymnoc. Hell. Hep. Igt. Led. Lyc. Merc. Ntr-m. Nitr-ac. Nux.

29. UPPER EXTREMITIES.

Petr. Phosp. Psor. Rheum. Sil. Sulph.
Perspiration, hands, back, Lith.
— finger tips, Carb-an. Carb-veg.
— between fingers, Sulph.
Petechiae, like, or fore-arm and back of hand, Berb.
Phagedenic blisters, on hands and fingers. Graph. Kali-c. *Mgn-c. Nitr-ac.* Sil.
— — with a pungent pain, Mgn-s.
Pressing pain, arms, Anac. *Arg.* Bell. Berb. Clem. Coloc. *Cycl.* Dulc. Led. Puls. *Sass.* Sulph.
— shoulder joint, Anac. *Bell.* Bry. Carb-an. Caust. Croton. Kali-c. Ntr-c. Phosp. Puls. Staph. Sulph.
— — right, Laur. Prun.
— shoulder joint, Cor-r. *Led.* Nitr-ac. Stann.
— upper arm, Aur. Camph. Chelid. Cycl. Mur-ac. *Phosp-ac.* Sabin. Sass. Stann. *Staph.*
— — and axilla, Agn.
— elbow, Camph. *Led.*
— fore-arm, Aur. Berb. Bism. Camph. Croton. Cycl. Ferr-m. *Oleand. Phosp-ac.* Plat. Ruta. Sabin. *Sass.* Staph. Verb.
— wrist, Arg. Bell. Berb. *Bism. Sass.* Stann. Viol-od.
— carpal bones, Arg. Bell. Cupr. *Oleand.* Plat. Puls.
— hands, Arg. Clem. *Phosp-ac.* Puls. Ruta. Stann. Staph. Verb.
— — back of, Berb.
— fingers, *Arg.* Cycl. Oleand. *Phosp-ac.* Plat. Ruta. Sabin. Stann. Staph. Verb.
— finger joints, Arg. *Sass.* Stann.
Prickling, arms, hands, fingers, Dig. Fluor-ac. Mez. Plat. Rhus-rad.
— left upper arm, Elaps.
— finger tips, Lach.
Pulsation, shoulder and upper arm, Tar.
— fingers, Glon. Sulph. Teucr.
— — left index, Gymnoc.
Pustules at root of nails, sperading over hands to wrists arms and axillary glands get red, pustules secrete a watery fluid if broken, if not broken, fluid thickens to a yellow tough mass, Kali-b.
To raise the arms, inability from pain, arm, Ntr-c. Ntr-m.
— — shoulder, Ferr. Ntr-m.
— — upper arm, Ferr. Nitr-ac.
Red spots, arms. Rhus. Sabad. Sulph.
— — with yellowish pellicle, wrist, Jac-cor.
— shoulder, Tabac.
— fore-arm, Berb. Euph. Thuj.
— hands, Cor-r. Elaps. Hipp-m. Lach. Ntr-c. Sabad. Stann. Tabac.
— fingers, Cor-r. Lach. Plb.
— burning, Berb Sulph. Tabac.
— itching, when touched, Berb. Euph. Zinc.

— marbled, Berb. Thuj.
— swollen, Plb.
— after washing, Sulph.
— with vesicles, Lach.
Redness, arms, Ant.
— — scarlet, Ars. Bell. Bry. Merc. Rhus. Sulph.
— hands, Bar-c. Berb. Carb-an. Fluor-ac. Hep. Ntr-s. Nux. Phosp. Puls. Staph. Sulph.
— — scarlet, Bell. Bry. Hep. Mez. Rhus. Stram.
— fingers, Agar. Borax. *Lyc.* Nux.
— — knuckles, Cannab. Pallad.
— — points and backs of fingers, Berb. Calc.
Relaxation of arms, Guaj. Plat.
— — — when laughing, Carb-veg.
Rending (tearing) arms, *Ambr.* Amm-m. *Arg.* Ars. Bell. Berb. Calc. *Canth. Caust.* China *Cina.* Cinnab. *Cocc. Colch.* Creos. Crotal. Dig. Ign. Ind. Iod. Kalm. *Led.* Mgn-m. Mgn-s. Mang. Meny. *Ntr-c.* Ntr-s. *Nitr. Ol-an.* Par. Phell. Phosp. *Phosp-ac.* Puls. Ran-b. *Sass.* Sil. Stront. Sulph. Tart. *Thuj.* Zinc.
— arm joints, Amm-c. Bov. Chin. Graph. Kali-c. Lact. Lyc. Nitr. Phosp-ac. Puls. Stront *Sulph. Teucr.* Zinc.
— brachial bones, Berb. *Chin.* Hell. *Ntr-s.* Rhod. Ruta. *Teucr.*
— shoulder, Acon. *Alum.* Ambr. *Amm-m.* Bell. Bry. Carb-veg. *Cast.* Chenop. Croton. *Evon.* Ferr. Graph. Kali-b. Kali-c. Kali-jod. Lachn. Laur. Lyc. Mgn-m. Mgn-s. *Mang. Merc.* Ntr-c. Nitr. Phell. Phosp. Puls. *Rat. Rhus.* Sep. Stann. Staph. *Sulph. Thuj.* Verb. *Zinc.*
— — right, Colch.
— — left, Ferr.
— upper arm, Ars. Berb. Bry. Camph. Cast. Chenop. Croton. Ferr. Hyper. Kali-b. Kalm. Laur. *Merc.* Mur-ac. Oleand. Plb. Puls. Rat. Rheum. Sabin. Stann. *Staph.* Valer.
— elbow joint, Ambr. Kalm. Lachn. Lyc. Ntr-c. Rhus. Ruta. Verb. Zinc.
— fore-arm, Aeth. *Ambr.* Asa-f. Berb. *Bism. Calc.* Camph. *Carb-veg.* Croton. Guaj. Ind. Kali-c. Kali-chl. Lact. Mgn-c. Mez. Mur-ac. Ntr-s. *Nitr-ac.* Phosp. Ran-b. Rat. Rheum. *Rhod.* Ruta. Sabin. *Sass.* Staph. Tar. Tilia. Verb.
— hands, *Ambr.* Amm-m. Arg. Arn. Ars. *Caust.* Chin. Chin-sulph. *Cina. Colch.* Graph. Kali-c. Kalm. Led. Mgn-s. *Mang.* Meny. Mur-ac Ntr-s. *Nitr-ac. Ol-an.* Petr. Phosp. *Rhod.* Rhus. Ruta. Selen. Sil. Stann. Staph. Stront. *Sulph.* Verb. Zinc.
— wrist, Amm-c. Amm-m. Arg. Ars. Aur.

29. UPPER EXTREMITIES.

Bell. Berb. *Bism.* Carb-veg. Kali c. Kali-jod. Lact. Nitr. Rat. Rhus. Sabin. *Sass.* Stann. Stront. *Sulph.* Tar. Teucr. Zinc.
Rending (tearing) wrist, right, Caust.
— carpal bones, *Arg. Aur.* Bell. Chin. Cupr. Lachn. Lact. Ntr-c. Sabin. Spig. Teucr.
— fingers, Agar. *Ambr. Amm-m. Arg.* Aur. Carb-veg. *Chin. Colch.* Creos. Croton. Daph. Hell. Iod. Kali-c. Lam. Led. *Mgn-s Mang.* Meny. Mur-ac. Ntr-s. Oleand. *Ol-an.* Phosp-ac. Plb. Puls. Ruta. Sabin. Sil. Stann. Staph. Stront. Sulph. Teucr. Verb. Zinc.
— — back of, Berb.
— — joints, Amm-c. Arg. *Aur.* Berb. Carb-veg. Dig. Hell. Kali-c. Lachn. *Lyc.* Nitr. Rheum. Rhus. Samb. *Sass.* Stann. Stront. *Sulph.* Teucr. Zinc.
— — tips, Berb.
— — right hand, Chelid.
— between fingers, Cycl.
— under nails, Bism.
Restlessness, arms, Fert. Glon.
— — left, Meph.
Rhagades, arms, Sil.
— hands, *Alum.* Arn. *Aur.* Bar-c. *Calc.* Creos. Cycl. Graph. *Hep.* Kali-c. Lach. Mgn-c. Merc. Ntr-c. *Ntr-m. Petr. Rhus.* Ruta. Sil. *Sulph.* Zinc.
— — deep and bleeding, *Merc.* Petr. Sass.
— — in winter, Petr.
— — on back of hands, Ntr-c. Rhus. Sep.
— — palms, Sulph.
— — on ball of hand, Hep.
— fingers, Mgn-c Merc. *Petr. Sass.*
— finger-joints, Mang. Phosp. Sulph.
— between fingers, Ars. Graph. Sulph. Zinc.
— on the nails, *Ntr-m.*
Rheumatic pain, *Ant.* Ars. Bell. Bry. Calc-ph. Chenop. Colch. Dros. Dulc. Fluor-ac. Grat. Igt. Kali-b. Lach. Led. *Merc.* Mez. Ntr-c. Nux. Phosp. Pod. Puls. *Rhod. Rhus.* Rhus-rad. Scill. *Sulph Tart.* Teucr. Thuj. *Valer. Verat.*
— — right side, Kalm. Sang.
— shoulder, Kali-b. Mgn-c. Mgn-m. Mang. Ntr-c. Nitr.
— left arm, Fluor-ac. Jac-cor.
— elbows, Grat. Mgn-s. Prun.
— wrist, Kali-b. Lach.
— hands, Lach. Zinc.
— small bones of hand, Cauloph.
— finger joints, Colch. Kali-b. Lach. Teucr.
Rigidity, stiffness, arms, Agar. Amm-c. Amm-m. Canth. Caps. *Cham.* Kali-c. Lyc. Meny. Merc-sulph. Ntr-c. *Nux.* Petr. Plat. Rhus. Sass. Sep.
— — at night, *Nux.*
— — when taking hold of something.

Cham.
— — after movement and in cold air, Kali-c.
— of right arm, Amm-m. Kali-b.
— shoulders, Kali-b.
— — in morning, Staph.
— elbow-joints, Alum. Ang. Asa-f. Bell. Bry. Kali-c. Lach. Phosp. Puls. Sep. Spig. Sulph. Zinc.
— wrist, *Bell.* Chelid. Kali-c. Lyc. Merc. Ntr-s. Rhus. Sabin. Sep. Staph. Sulph.
— — right, Merc.
— — paralytic, Ruta.
— hands, Asa-f. Cham. Creos. Hyosc. Merc.
— — paralytic, Cham.
— rheumatic, of metacarpal bones, Bell. Chelid. Kali-c. Lyc. Merc. Ntr-c. Phosp-ac. Puls. Rhus. Ruta. Sabin. Sep. Staph. Sulph. Thuj. Viol-od.
— fingers, Amm-c. Ars. *Carb-an.* Chin. Coloc. Dig. Dros. Graph. Hell. Hipp-m. Lyc. Ntr-m. Nitr. Oleand. Pe,r. Puls. Rhus. Sang. Sil. Spong. Sulph.
— — when taking hold of something, Dros.
— — during labor, Lyc.
Rigor of hands, Hyosc.
Rough skin of hands, Graph. Hep. Kali-c. Laur. Ntr-c. Nitr-ac. Phosp-ac,
— in spots, Zinc.
— fingers, Phosp-ac.
Scabs, elbows. *Sep.* Staph.
— forearm, Alum.
— hand, Mur-ac. Sass. Sep.
— wrist, Amm-m.
— fingers, Kali-b. Mur-ac.
— itching. *Sep.*
— moist, Alum.
Scarlet redness of forearm, *Euph.*
— — hands, *Bell.* (compare Redness).
Senselessness, insensibility arms, *Alum.* Ambr. Bell. Nitr. Plat. *Puls. Rhus.* Stront.
— shoulder, *Puls.*
— hands, Acon. Asa-f. Bry. Carb-an. Cocc. Hyosc Lam. Lyc. Ntr-m. Nitr. *Puls.* Stront.
— fingers, Anac. Bell. Calc. Carb-an. Caust. Colch. Con. Cupr. Dig. Ferr. Kali-c. Lam. Lyc. Mur-ac. Oleand. Ol-an. Phosp. Plat. Rhus. Sec-c. Spong. Staph. Sulph.
— — at night. Mur-ac.
Shaking, arms, Bry.
Shivering on the arms, Bell. Igt.
— — fingers, Meny.
Shrivelled skin, of hands, Ang.
— — fingers, Ambr. Cupr. Phosp-ac.
Sore pain. shoulder, *Cic. Con.* Nux.
— — right, Psor.
— fore-arm, *Cic.*
— right arm, Merc-jod.

29. UPPER EXTREMITIES.

Soreness between fingers, Ars. Graph.
— of flesh, Bad.
Spasm and distortion of the arms, *Bell.* Bry. Cupr. Jatr. Lyc. Meny. Ntr-m. Phosp. Plat. *Sec-c.* Sil. Sulph. Verat.
— hands, Ambr. *Bell.* Calc. Cannab. Coloc. Graph. Kali-b. Ntr-m. Pæon. Plat. Sec-c. Stram. Sulph-ac.
— fingers, Amm-c. Arn. Ars. *Calc.* Cannab. Cocc. Coff. Dros. Ferr. Hell. *Lyc.* Ntr-m. Nitr. Nux. Phosp. Sec-c. Stann. Staph. Sulph. Tabac. Verat.
— thumb, Ntr-m.
— at night, Nux. Sulph.
— when taking hold of something, Ambr. Dros.
Spasmodic pain, Arg. *Cina.* Ran-b. Sulph-ac.
— left side, *Meny.*
— upper arm, Lact. Mosch. Oleand. Valer.
— elbow-joint, Creos. Rat.
— fore-arm, Ang. Berb. Calc. Creos. Ferr-m. Mosch. Mur-ac. *Phosp-ac.* Plat. Ruta. Verb.
— hands, Ang. Arg. Calc. Cina. Coloc. Euph. *Euphr.* Ferr-m. Mang. *Meny.* Merc. Phosp-ac. Plat. Ruta. Sil. Verb.
— wrist, *Anac. Aur.* Bov.
— carpal bones, *Anac. Aur.* Spig.
— fingers, Agar. Ang. Calc. *Euphr. Meny.* Mur-ac. *Oleand.* Phosp-ac. Plat. Rat. Ruta. Sil. Verb.
— finger-joints, Anac. Mgn-c. Nitr.
Splinter of glass, like a, under the finger-nails, Cocc-c.
Sprained, as if in arm-joints and wrists, Arn.
— wrists, Cina. Cist. Hipp. Lach.
— — right, Gels.
— hands, Kalm.
Spraining, easily, the upper arm, right, Euphr.
— elbow, right. Gels.
— fingers, Bell. Hep. Nux.
Stinging, stitches, arms, Cinnab. *Cocc.* Dros. Dulc. Guaj. Ind. Kali-b. Ol-an. Phosp. Puls. Ran-b. Rheum. Sacch. Sabin. *Sass.* Sep. Sulph. Tart. *Thuj.* Viol-tr. Zinc.
— brachial bones, Dros.
— arm-joints, Bry. Dros. Ferr. Graph. Laur. Led. Lyc. Nitr. Phosp. Puls. Sep. Staph. *Sulph.* Sulph-ac. Tabac. *Thuj.* Viol-tr.
— shoulder, *Bry.* Chin. Croton. Dulc. Ferr. Graph. Gum-gut. Laur. Led. Lvc. Ox-ac. Phosp. Puls. Staph. Sulph. Sulph-ac. Tabac. Verb. Viol-tr. Zinc.
— — right. Pallad.
— — top of shoulder, at every inspiration, Hyper.
— upper arm, Berb. *Bry.* Dulc. Ferr. Lact. Laur. Rhus. Sabin. *Sass.* Staph.
— elbow-joint, Bry. Lam. Lyc. Nitr. *Spig.* Tabac. Tar. Viol-tr. Zinc.

— — left, Kali-b.
— fore arm, Anac. Ant. Caust. Guaj. *Ran-sc.* Sabad. Sabin. Sass. Staph. Stram. Viol-tr.
— (shootings) wrists, Alum. Ars. Aur-mur. Bov. Bry. Hell. Kali-c Ntr-m. Nitr. Ox-ac. Ruta. Sabin. Samb. Sass. Scill. Sep. Sil. Spig. Sulph. Zinc.
— wrist joints, Kobalt.
— hands, Ars. Bar-c. Berb. Bry. Hell. Kali-c. Kalm. Led. Mgn-s. Mur-ac. Ntr-m. *Ntr-s.* Ol-an. Phosp. Sass. Sep. Staph. *Sulph.* Verb. Zinc.
— metacarpus, Berb. Lach.
— fingers, *Amm-m.* Bry. Carb-an. Con. Daph. Kalm. Mgn-s. Mang. Ntr-m. *Ntr-s.* Nitr-ac. Par. Phosp-ac. Ran-sc. Sabin. Sep. Stann. Staph. Sulph. Sulph-ac. Thuj. Verb. Viol-tr. Zinc.
— — joints, Ferr-m. *Hell.* Ntr-m. Nitr-ac. Pæon. Phosp-ac. Sass. *Sep.* Spig. *Sulph.* Sulph-ac.
— — tips, Lach.
— thumb, right, Guaj.
— — left, Lith.
— under the nails, Ntr-s.
Stitches, sudden, penetrating into the bone, Berb. Pallad.
Straining, as if too short, arms, Aeth. *Sep.*
— when bent, Aeth.
— shoulder, Berb. Bov.
— elbow-joint, Caust. Mang. *Sep.*
— when stretched out, Caust.
— wrist, Carb-veg. Ign.
— fingers, Aeth. Carb-an. Croc. *Sep.* Spong.
Stretching, spasmodic arms, Chin.
— out, impeded by pain, Tabac.
Suppleness, want of, hands, Sep. (compare Unwieldiness.)
— — fingers, Graph. Ntr-m. Plb.
Suppuration on the fore arm, Lyc.
— — — fingers, Borax. Mang.
— — — nails, Eugen.
Swelling, arms, Acon. Alum. *Ars.* Bar-c. *Bell. Bry.* Crotal. Dulc. Elaps. Lyc. Merc. Merc-cor. Mez. *Rhus.* Sep. Sil. *Sulph.*
— brachial bones, Aur. Bry. Dig. Dulc. Mez. Rhus. Sil. Sulph.
— shoulder, Acon. Bry. Calc-ph. Kali-c. Kali-chl.
— upper arm, Acon. Bry. Calc-ph. Sep. Sulph.
— elbow joint, Acon. Bry. Merc. Puls.
— fore-arm, *Ant.* Berb. Lach. *Merc.* Nux. Sulph.
— wrist, Amm-c. Euphr. Merc. *Sabin.* Sec-c.
— hands, Acon. Ars. Bar-m. *Bell. Bry.* Calc. Cham. Clem. *Cocc.* Cupr. Dig. Elaps. Euphr. Ferr. *Hep.* Hyosc. Lach. Lyc. Mez. Mosch. Nux. Phosp. Rhus. Samb. Sec-c. Spong. *Stann.* Sulph.

29. UPPER EXTREMITIES.

Swelling, hands, right, Ntr-m.
— — dorsum, left, Chin.
— — palms, Cham.
— — — at night, Ars.
— fingers, Alum. Amm-c. Ant. Ars. Borax. Dig. Euphr. Graph. Hep. *Lyc. Mgn-c.* Merc. Mur-ac. Ntr-c. Nitr. Nitr-ac. Nux. Oleand. Phosp. Ran-sc. *Rhus.* Spong. Sulph. Tabac. *Thuj.*
— — on letting arms hang down, Amm-c. Phosp.
— finger-joints, Agn. Amm-c. Berb. Bry. Chin. Euphr. Hep. Lyc. Merc. Nitr-ac. Spong.
— finger-tips, Mur-ac. Rhus. Thuj.
— thumb, Nux.
— — joints of, Nux. Sulph.
— bluish, Lach. Samb.
— burning, Mur-ac. Oleand. Sulph.
— burn, with pain as from a, Nux.
— cold, Lach.
— dropsical, lymphatic, soft, Berb. Sec-c.
— erysipelatous. Bell. Petr. Rhus.
— hard, Ars. Lach. Sulph.
— — of axillary glands, Amm-m.
— hot, Ant. Bry. *Cocc.* Hep. *Merc.* Mez. Rhus. Sulph.
— lancinating, Mosch. Sulph.
— large, Sulph.
— lymphatic, Berb.
— painful, Ant. Chin. Hep. Kali-c. Lach. Nux. Sep. Sulph. *Thuj.*
— painless, Euphr. Lyc.
— pale, Bry. Nux.
— red, Ant. Bry. Hep. Lyc. Mgn-c. *Merc.* Sep. Spong. *Thuj.*
— scarlet-red, Bell.
— shining, Bry. Sulph.
— ending in suppuration, Nux.
— in afternoon, Ntr-c.
— — evening, Rhus. Stann.
— at night, Dig. Nitr. Phosp.
— on moving the parts, Euphr.
— after paralysis, Sulph.
— with putrid-smelling black blisters, Ars.
— — rigidity, Sulph.
— sensation of arms, Verat.
— — at night as if hands were swollen and heavy, Diad. Nitr.
— — shoulder, Kali-jod.
— with heaviness, in arms, and hands, at night, Diad. Nitr.
— hands, when entering in room, Aeth.
— veins on forearms and hands, Puls.
Tenderness of arms to cold, Agar. Calc-ph.
— — fingers, Agar.
— — finger-tips, Lach.
— — skin at nails, Ant.
Tendons, twitching of, fingers, Iod.
Tension, arms, Anac. Arg. Chin. Hyper. Kali-c. Lach. Mang. Meny. Mez. Prun. Rhus. *Sep.* Tabac.

— arm-joint, Kali-c. Mang. *Sep.*
— shoulder, *Bry.* Eup-a. Kali-c. Kali-jod.
— upper arm, Bry. Croton. Prun.
— elbow joint, Acon. Dros. Kali-c. Lach. Laur. Mang. Mur-ac. Nitr. Puls. Rhus. *Sep.* Stann. Sulph-ac. Tabac.
— forearm, Ant. Croton. Lach. Ntr-c.
— wrist Amm-m. Carb-veg. Kali-c. Lach. *Mang.* Phosp. Puls. Verb.
— hands, Arg. Chin. Ferr-m. Hyper. Kali-c. Lach. Mang. Ntr-c. Prun.
— fingers, Aeth. Kali-c. Lach.
— finger-joints, Caust. Croc. Kali-c. Mgn-c. Nitr-ac. Nitr. Phosp. Puls. *Sep.* Spong.
Throbbing, arms, Berb. Sil. Thuj.
— shoulder, Sil. Tar. Thuj.
— upper arm, Tar.
— finger, *Amm-m.* Borax. Ferr-m. Lith. Plat.
— thumb, Borax.
Thumbs clenched convulsively, Merc.
Tingling (crawling), arms, Arn. Bell. Cannab. Caps. Igt. Mgn c. Nitr. Ol-an. Pæon. Rhod. Sabad. Sec-c Sulph.
— hands, Arn. Bar-c. Lam. Mur-ac. Ntr-m. Nitr. Ruta. Stram. Verat.
— — left, Lach.
— fingers, *Acon. Amm-m.* Calc. Croc. Lact. Lam. Mgn-c. Mgn-s. Ntr-m. Ol-an. Pæon. Rut. Rhod. Rhus. Sec-c. Sil. Spig. Sulph. Tabac. Thuj. Verat.
— finger-tips, Coloc. Hep. Ntr-s.
Tired, as if, pain, arms, Lach. Nux. Verat.
Tophi, (arthritic Nodes), wrists, *Calc.* Led. Rhod.
— finger joints, Agn. *Calc. Dig. Graph. Led.* Lyc. Rhod. *Staph.*
Torpor, rigidity, arms, *Amm-c.* Amm-m. Kali-c. Petr. Plat.
— — after exercise and in cold, Kali-c.
— hands, Asa-f. Hyosc.
— wrist, Puls. Sep.
— fingers, Amm-c. Hell. Petr.
Torpor, sensation of, arms, Arg. Caust. Petr. Plat.
— hand, Asa-f.
Tremor, arms, Ambr. Anac. Bry. Colch. Hipp-m. Hyosc. *Iod.* Lyc. Murex. Nitr-ac. *Op. Phosp.* Phosp-ac. Rhus. Sabad. *Sil.* Spig. Spong. Thuj. Verat.
— left, Hyper.
— biceps, and triceps of right arm, Fluor-ac.
— hands, *Agar.* Amm-c. *Anac.* Ars. Bell. Bism. Bov. Calc. Caust. Chin. Cic. Cocc. Coff. Colch. Gels. Hipp-m. *Hyosc. Iod.* Kali-c. *Lach.* Lact. Laur. Led. Mgn-s. Merc. Ntr-c. Ntr-m. Ntr-s. Nicc. Nitr-ac. *Nux.* Op. Par. *Phosp.* Phosp-ac. Plat. Plb. Puls. Rhus. Sabad. Samb. Sass. Sep. Spig. Stann. Stram. *Sulph.* Tabac. *Tart.* Thuj. Valer. Zinc.

29. UPPER EXTREMITIES.

Tremor, hands, right, All-cep. Anac. Mez
— — when taking hold of anything, Led. Verat.
— fingers, Bry. Glon. Iod. Nitr-ac. Oleand. Rhus.
— in evening, Hyosc.
— after slight exertion, Rhus. Sil.
— — meals, Bism.
— — when moving, Led.
— after moving, Hyosc.
— with fine work, Sulph.
— when holding anything, Coff. Led. Lyc. Phosp.
— — writing, Bar-c. Caust. Chin. Colch. Hep. Kali-c. Ntr-m. Ntr-s Oleand. Phosp-ac. Sabad. Samb. Sep. Sulph. Thuj. Valer. Zinc.
Tumor, steatoma, on point of elbow, Hep.
Twitching, arms, Asa-f. Bar-m. Bell. Bry. Caust. Cic. Cina. Cupr. Hyosc. Igt. Kali-c. Lact. Lyc. Mgn-s. Meny. Merc. Ntr-c. Op. Rheum. Scill. *Thuj.* Verat.
— — in sleep, at noon, Lyc.
— — at night, Bar-m.
— shoulders, Fluor-ac. Lyc. Sulph.
— deltoid muscle, Igt.
— hands, Bell. Cupr. Lact. Meph. Ntr-c. Ntr-s. Rheum. Stann. Sulph.
— — in morning, Cupr.
— — when taking hold of something, Ntr-c.
— fingers, Bry. Cham. *Cic.* Cina. Croton. Cupr. Igt. Kali-c. Lyc. Merc. Ntr-c. Ox-ac. Phosp. Rhus. Sulph.
— — when moved, Bry.
— — — sewing, Kali-c.
Ulcers, arm, burning and sanious, Rhus.
— — malignant, Lach.
— — painless, Carb-veg. Plat. *Ran-b.* Sep.
— right forearm, fistulous, yellowish thin pus, Sacch.
— hands, Ars. Sep. Sil.
— fingers, Carb-an. Kali-b. *Plat. Ran-b.* Sep. Sil.
— finger joints, Sep.
— knuckles, Sep.
— finger tips, Ars. Fluor-ac.
— at nails, (panaritia,) Alum. Bar-c. Caust. Con. *Hep.* Iod. Merc. Ntr-m. Puls. Sang. Sep. *Sil. Sulph.*
— around nails, Hell.
Ulcerative pain, arm, shoulder, Berb.Thuj.
— finger, Amm-m. Berb. Sass. Sulph.
— right thumb, Ol-an.
— nails, Ntr-s.
Unwieldiness, clumsiness of hand, Sep.
— fingers, Calc. Graph. Ntr-m. Plb. Sil.
Veins distended, hand, Amm-c. Arn. Bar-c. Calc. Cast. Chelid. Chin. Cic. Ind. Laur. Nux. Oleand. Op. Phosp. Puls. Rheum. Rhus. Ruta. *Thuj.*
— — after washing with cold water, Amm-c.

Vibrating pains and sensation, Berb.
Warts, arm, Ars *Calc.* Caust. Dulc. Ntr-c. Nitr-ac. Rhus. *Sep.* Sil. Sulph.
— hand, Berb. Borax. Calc. *Dulc.* Ferr-m. Lach. Lyc. *Ntr-c. Ntr-m.* Nitr-ac. Rhus. Sep. Thuj.
— — palm, Ntr-m.
— knuckles, Pallad.
— fingers, Berb. Lach. Lyc. Petr. Rhus. Sulph.
— — flat, Berb.
— finger tips, Caust.
Weakness, arms, Acon. Agar. Amm-c. *Anac.* Ars. Berb. Bism. Caust. Cham. Cic. Chin. Glon. Guaj. Kali-c. Kalm. Lact. Lyc. Ntr-c. Ntr-m. Nitr. Nux. Ol-an. Par. Petr. Phosp-ac. Plat. Plb. Psor. Rhod. Rhus. Ruta. Sec-c. Sep. Sulph. Tabac. Tilia.
— — left, Calc. Ntr-s.
— shoulder, Acon. Nux.
— elbow joint, Ang. Sulph.
— fore-arms, Nitr-ac. Rhus.
— hands, Acon. Ang. Arn. *Bov.* Canth. *Carb-veg.* Caust. Chin. Cina. Cupr. Fluor-ac. Hell. Hipp. Kali-b. Kali-c. Merc. Ntr-s. Nitr-ac. Nitr. Nux. Plb. Rhus. Sabin. Sil. Stann. Sulph. Tabac. Zinc.
— fingers, Ambr. *Carb-veg.* Hipp. Lact. Nitr. Par. Rhus. Sil.
— sudden, as from paralysis, Calc.
— in morning, Nux. Sulph.
— — — in bed, Kali-c.
— at night, Ambr.
— when at rest, Acon. Rhod.
— with swelling, Acon.
— when taking hold of something, Arn. Bov. Carb-veg. Cina. Colch. Ntr-m. Sil.
— when writing. Acon. Agar. Cocc. Sabin.
Wen on hand, Plb.
— between metacarpal bones, Phosp-ac.
Withering of skin of hands, Bism.
Wrenching, (spraining.) pain, arms, *Ambr.* Arn. Bov. *Igt.* Lach. Lact. Oleand. Prun. Tereb. Thuj.
— shoulder, *Ambr.* Asar. Bry. Caust. Croc. Igt. Mgn-c. Mur-ac. Ntr-m. Nicc. Petr. Puls. Rhod. Ruta. Sabin. Sep. Staph. Sulph. Tereb. Thuj.
— elbow, *Ambr.* Ferr-m. Nicc. Puls.
— wrist, Ambr. Amm-c. *Arn. Bov. Bry.* Calc. Caust. Cist. Hep. Nux. Puls. *Rhod.* Ruta. Su'ph. *Verb.*
— — when bent, Ferr-m.
— hand, *Ambr. Amm-c.* Arn. Bov. *Bry.* Calc. Carb-an. Caust. Hep. Nitr. Phosp. Prun. Puls. Rhod. *Ruta.* Sabin. Seneg. Sulph. Verb.
— fingers, Graph. Ntr-m. Nitr. Phosp. Puls. Sulph.
— thumb, Creos.

29. UPPER EXTREMITIES.

Wrenching, dislocation. of wrist, *Amm-c.* Arn. Bov. Bry. Carb-an. *Ruta.*
Wrinkled fingers, Ambr. Cupr. Phosp-ac.
Wrist joint which had been sprained, pain in, Amm-c.
Yellowness of hands, Sil. Spig.
— fingers, Chelid. Phosp-ac.
— joints of fingers, right hand, cold and dead, Chelid.
Yellow spots, arm, Petr.
— fingers, Con. Elaps. Sabad. Tart.
Yellow rings on hands, fingers, elbows and around nails, Ntr-c.
In morning, aggravation of pain, carpal bones, Amm-c. Cupr. Iod. Kali-c Mgn-m. Nux. Puls. Staph. Sulph. Zinc.
— — in bed, Ntr-c.
— afternoon, Nux.
— evening, pain arm, Hyosc. Led. Puls. Rhus. Stann.
— — in bed, Carb-veg. Creos. Mgn-m.
— pain in hand, Ntr-c
At night, pain, arm, Ambr. Amm-m. Bry. *Calc.* Caust. Cham. Coloc. Croc. Diad. Dig. Dros. Dulc. Igt. Iod. *Lyc.* Mgn-c. Merc. Mur-ac. Nitr. *Nux.* Phosp. Puls. Sang. Sil. Staph. Sulph.
— — in bed, Igt. Sulph.
— brachial bones, Amm-m. Lyc.
— shoulder, Bell. Cast. Mgn-c. *Merc. Nitr.* Phosp. Sulph.
— upper arm, Ars. *Cast.* Cham. *Merc.* Nux. Puls. Sulph.
— elbow joint, Nitr.
— wrist, Nitr. Sil.
— hands, Phosp. Selen. Sulph.
— fingers, Borax. *Mgn-s.* Puls. Sulph.
— finger joints, Nitr. Sulph.
— after midnight, pain, arms, Nux.
— day and night, pain, arm, Borax.
In autumn, arm, pain, *Rhus.*
On bending arms, Aeth.
When carrying something, Ambr.
During chills, pain in hands and fingers, Nux.
In cold weather, Agar. Kali-c.
— — pain relieved, Thuj.
From cold air, pain, arm, Igt. Nitr-ac. *Rhod.*
In damp weather, pain, arm, *Rhod.* Rhus.
From exertion, pain arms, hands, *Sep.* Sil.
During exertion, Alum. Iod. Merc. Sulph.
After exertion, Ruta.
When hanging down, pain arms, Alum. Berb. Sabin. Thuj.
— — — shoulder, Ruta.
When taking hold of anything, pain arms and hands, Amm-c. Arn. Calc. Carb-veg. Caust. Cham. Dros. Led. Plat. Verat.
— — — relieved, Lith.
— — wrist, Bov.
— tips of fingers, powerless, can't hold, Mez.

— holding anything in hands, pain, Coff. Guaj. Phosp. Sep. Sil.
— lain upon, pain, arm, increased, Ars. Iod.
— laughing, pain, Carb-veg.
— leaning upon part, pain, Ruta. Sil. Thuj.
— lifting a load, Ruta. Sep.
— moved, pain, arm, Berb. Bry. Cannab. Chelid. Hyosc. Kali-c. Led. Mgn-m. Nux. Staph.
— shoulder, Asar. Bell. Cannab. Led. Mgn-c. Merc. Puls. Sang.
— scapula, Puls.
— upper arm, *Cocc.* Fluor-ac. Lac-can. *Merc.*
— fore arm, Croc.
— hand, Laur. Puls. Sep.
— wrist, *Bry.* Hep. Kali-c. Merc.
— fingers, Hep. Kali-c. Lam.
By moving, pain increased, Berb. Iris. *Led.* Mgr-c. Mgn-c. Nux.
— — relieved, Meph. Thuj.
Passion, after being in a, Coloc.
After perspiration, pain in arms relieved, Thuj.
When pressing the parts, pain, Berb. Sil.
— raising arms, pain, Cocc. Oleand. Sang.
— — shoulder, Ferr. Led. Ntr-m. Prun. Puls. Sulph-ac.
— — scapula joint, Puls.
— — upper arm, Bar-c.
During rest, pain, arms, Acon. Dulc. Rhod.
— shoulder, Cocc. Euph. Rhus.
— upper arm, Cocc.
— fingers, Lith.
By rest, pain increased, *Rhod.*
On entering a room, pain, arm, Aeth.
From rubbing, pain, arm, Berb.
— scratching, pain, arm, Berb. Lach.
— sewing, pain carpal bones, Kali-c. Lach.
During the siesta, Lyc.
When stretching out the arm, pain in arm, Alum. Caust.
— — sudden heat, Ferr-m.
— touched, pain, arm, Agar. *Chin.* Euph. Lam.
— shoulder, Acon.
— upper arm, Agn.
— elbow, Ambr.
— wrist, Merc.
By touch, pain increased, Agar. Berb. *Chin* Cocc. Lam.
After vexation, pain shoulder, Coloc.
— a walk, pain shoulder and elbow, Valer.
— — — fingers, Croc.
By walking relieved, Daph.
— warmth, pain increased, Calc. Sulph. Thuj.
— relieved, Cinnab.
From warmth of bed, pain, shoulder, Rhus.
— — pain relieved, Amm-c.

From washing, Amm-c. Sulph.
— — in cold water, Amm-c.
— cold water, Clem.
In winter, Petr.
When working, pain, hands, Alum. Iod. Merc. Sulph.
From writing, pain, fore arms, Acon.

— — hands, Acon. Agar Bar-c. Cinnab. Euph. Fluor-ac. Kali-c Merc-jod. Sabin. Samb. Sulph-ac. Thuj. Valer. Zinc.
— — fingers, Acon. Bry. Cist. Iris. Mur-ac.
— yawning, pain, Nux.

30. Lower Extremities.

Abscess on buttock, Sulph.
— — calf of leg, Chin.
— — ankle joint, Ang.
— — heel, Lach.
Aching of toes, Mosch.
Arthritic complaints, lower extremities, Ambr. Arn. Led. *Puls. Rhod. Rhus.* Sabin.
— hips, (coxalgia.) *Ang. Ars. Asa-f. Aur. Bell.* Bry. *Calc. Canth. Cham. Coloc.* Dig. Graph. *Hep. Merc. Nux. Puls. Rhus.* Sep. Staph.
— — with commencing suppuration, (throbbing), *Hep. Merc. Staph.*
— knees, Chin. Con.
— feet, Ambr. *Bry.* Graph. Verat.
— toes, (gout), Ambr. *Arn.* Colch. Con. Graph. *Led. Sabin. Sulph.* Verat.
Atrophy of legs, Chin.
As if bandaged, pain, *Anac.*
— — knees, *Anac.* Aur.
As if beaten, *Ang. Arn.* Berb. Bruc. Carb-veg. Croton. Cupr. Merc. Phosp. Sil. Spig. Spong. Tart. Valer. *Verat.*
— — joints, Arg.
— — bones, *Led.* Puls. *Ruta.*
— — buttocks, Puls.
— — hips, *Acon.* All-cep. *Amm-c.* Arn. Phosp-ac. *Ruta.* Sulph.
— — — right, Sep.
— — thighs, *Acon. Amm-c.* Ang. Camph. Caust. Cocc. Creos. Grat. Guaj. Hep. Led. Meny. Merc. Murex. Nux. *Phosp-ac. Plat.* Puls. Sang. Spig. Staph. Tabac. Viol-tr.
— — knees, Ars. Berb. Camph. Cupr. Hep. Led. Meph. Phosp. *Plat.* Staph. Verat.
— — legs, Ang. Caust. Croc. Gels. Merc. Puls. Valer.
— — tibia, Puls.
— — tarsal joint, when walking and touching it, Ntr-m.
— — feet, Arg. *Arn.* Bry.
— — soles, Ambr. Arum-trif. Calc. Graph. Igt. Lac-can. Phosp. Puls. Xiphos.
— — instep, left, Kali-jod.
— — os calcis. Cocc.
— — toes, Daph.
Black and painful spots, Nux.

Blister on thighs and legs, after scratching, Lach.
— — heel, from rubbing of shoes, then smarting ulcer, Lam.
Bloatedness, Dulc.
Blood, congestion to feet when standing, Graph.
— as if stagnating, sensation in, knees, Lact. Phell.
— — legs, Lact. Zinc.
Blood-specks, legs, Phosp.
Blueness, of feet, Arn. Elaps.
Bluish spots, Creos. Sulph.
Boring pain, Canth. Merc. Ran-b. Ran-sc.
— thighs, Ran-b.
— knee joint and ankle joint, *Hell.*
— feet and toes. *Ran-sc.*
— heels. Puls.
— os calcis, relieved by continued motion, Diad.
Brown skin of legs (inside thigh), Thuj.
Burning, pain, in general, Kali-c. Led. Lyc. Phosp. Prun.
— — bones, Euph.
— hips, Bell. Carb-veg. Euph. Hell. Rhus. Valer.
— thighs, Bov. Croton. Rat. Rhus.
— knees, Lyc. Tabac. Tar.
— legs, Agar. Anac. Borax. Lyc. Prun. Tar.
— calf of leg, Dig.
— tibia, Mgn-c. Phosp-ac.
— ankle-joint, Euph. Ntr-c. *Puls.*
— — top of, *Puls.*
— tarsal bones, Ruta.
— feet, Amm-c. Ars. Berb. Borax. Calc. Cham. Cocc. Dulc. Graph. Hep. *Kali-c.* Led. Lyc. Ntr-m. Phosp. *Phosp-ac.* Scill. Sec-c. *Sep.* Sil. *Stann.* Zinc.
— instep, *Puls.*
— soles, *Ambr.* Anac. Ars. Berb. Calc. Canth. Carb-veg. Cham. Creos. Croc. Crotal. Cupr. Eupat. *Graph.* Kali-c. Lach. Lachn. Lyc. Mgn-m. Mang. Mur-ac. *Ntr-c.* Ntr-m. Nux. Petr. *Phosp-ac.* Puls. *Sang.* Scill. Sil. Sulph. Tabac.
— heels, Igt.
— toes, *Agar.* Alum. Ant. Arn. Berb. Borax. Carb-an. Dulc. Kali-c. Lith. Nux. Pæon. Phosp-ac. Sabin. *Staph.* Tar.

30. LOWER EXTREMITIES.

Burning toes, tips, Mur-ac.
Burning spots, Lyc. Mgn-c. Phosp-ac.
Buzzing and humming in, Creos.
Buzzing, sensation of, Ambr.
— in legs, Puls.
— especially in soles, Oleand.
Caries, ankle-joint, Asa-f.
Chafed, between thighs, Bar-c. Caust. Chin. Graph. *Hep.* Kali-c. Lyc. Merc. Ntr-c. Ntr-m. Nitr-ac. *Petr.* Rhod. *Sep. Sulph.*
— bend of knee, Ambr.
— legs, Lach.
— heel, skin rubbed from, by shoes, All-cep.
— between toes, *Graph.* Lyc. Mang. Ntr-c. Phosp-ac.
Chilblains, *Agar.* Amm-c. Carb-an. Carb-veg. *Croc. Nitr-ac.* Nux. Op. Petr. *Phosp.* Phosp-ac. *Puls.* Rhus. Stann. Staph. *Sulph. Thuj.* Zinc.
— large, Nitr-ac.
— looking red, Cycl.
— heel, swelling and red, Petr.
— toes, Croc. Kali-c. Nitr-ac. Phosp.
— pain, as from, Berb. Borax. Cham. Nux.
Chilliness, Cocc. Par. Sep.
Coldness, Apis. Ars. *Bell.* Calc. Cic. Ip. Lac-can. Led. *Nitr-ac.* Nux. Op. Ox-ac. Plb. Rhod. Rhus-rad. Sec-c. Sep. Sil.
— in evening, when lying down in bed, Sass.
— at night, Phosp.
— hip-joint, Merc.
— thighs, Merc. Nux.
— knees, Ars. Benz-ac. Cimex. Coloc. Daph. Merc. Raph. Puls.
— — up to, Chenop. Igt.
— legs, Ambr. Chenop. Mosch. Nux. Sil.
— — right, Elaps. Sabin.
— — left, Ol-an.
— — from knees to toes, Tabac.
— — middle of right tibia, Samb.
— — ankle-joint, Berb.
— feet, Acon. Alum. Ambr. *Anac.* Ars. Aur. Bell. Bufo. *Calc. Carb-an. Caust.* Chenop. Chin. Cinnab. Cist. Cocc. *Con.* Creos. Daph. Dig. Dros. Ferr. Gels. *Graph.* Hipp. Hipp-m. Hyosc. Iod. *Ip. Kali-c.* Kali-chl. Lach. Lact. Laur. Lyc. Mgn-s. Mang. Merc. Merc-cor. Mez. Mur-ac. *Ntr-c.* Ntr-m. *Nitr-ac.* Oleand. Petr. Phosp. Plat. Plb. *Rhod.* Samb. Sass. Scill. *Sep. Sil.* Stann. Staph. Stront. Sulph. Sulph-ac. Tart. Verat. Zinc.
— — on one side, the other red and hot, Puls.
— — in morning, Anac.
— — evening, *Calc.*
— — — in bed, Amm-c. Carb-an. Graph. Kali-c. Nux. Par. Sulph.
— — when walking, Anac.

— — after foot-sweat suppressed, Sil.
— soles, Coloc. Merc. Sulph.
— toes, Acon. Meny. Sulph.
— — begins in, Sulph.
— in joints, Cinnab.
— sensation of, Berb. Merc. Rhod.
— icy, on single spots, Berb.
To take cold, liability, feet, Con. *Sil.*
Contraction of tendons, *Mez.* Sulph.
— left hip, Amm-m.
— bend of knee, *Amm-m.* Ars. Carb-an. Graph. *Ntr-c. Ntr-m.* Ruta. Sulph.
— instep, Caust.
— toes, Nitr. (compare Shortening.)
Contracting pain, Amm-c. *Caust.* Lyc. Rat.
— — right leg, leg seems shortened, Ambr.
— — — on walking, Coloc.
— — calf of leg, Lyc.
— — instep, *Caust.*
Convulsions, Cupr. Hyosc. *Igt. Ip.* Mosch. Nux. *Op.* Plb. *Scill. Sec-c.* Spong.
— toes, Cupr.
Corns, *Amm-c. Ant.* Bar-c. Bov. Bry. *Calc.* Caust. *Lyc.* Ntr-c. *Ntr-m.* Nitr-ac. *Petr. Phosp. Phosp-ac.* Rhod. Sep. Sil. Staph. Sulph.
— on soles of feet, horny, Ant.
— boring, Ntr-c. Ntr-m.
— burning, Amm-c. Bar-c. Bruc. Bry. Calc. Chenop. Igt. Lith. Meph. Phosp-ac. Ran-sc. Rhus. Thuj.
— inflamed, *Sep.*
— painful, in general, Bry. Calc. Caust. Iod. Kali-c. Lith. Ntr-m. Nitr-ac. Phosp. Sulph.
— — when touched, Bry. Kali-c.
— pinching, Bar-c.
— pressing, Ant. Bry. Sulph.
— rending, Amm-c. Sulph-ac.
— sore, smarting, Ambr. Bry. Calc. Fluor-ac. Graph. Lyc. Rhus. Verat.
— stinging, stitches, Amm-c. Bar-c. Bov. Borax. Bry. Caust. Chenop. Hep. Kali-c. Mgn-m. Ntr-c. *Ntr-m.* Petr. Phosp. Phosp-ac. Ran-sc. Rhod. Rumex. Sep. Sil. Sulph. Sulph-ac. Verat.
Coxalgia. *Arg.* Ars. Asa-f. Aur. *Bell.* Bry. *Calc.* Canth. *Cham.* Colch. *Coloc.* Dig. Graph. Hep. *Merc. Nux. Puls. Rhus.* Sep. Staph. Sulph.
— hip becomes elongated, Coloc. Rhus. Thuj.
— with spasmodic pains in bladder and strangury, Canth.
Cracking, in the joints, Benz-ac. Bry. Camph. Cocc. Con. Led. Nux. Petr. Puls. Ran-b. Selen. Tabac. Thuj.
— knee, Cham. Cocc. Igt.
— — right, Mez.
— when bending, Selen.
— moving, Cham. Cocc. Nux.
— stepping, Euphr. Mgn-s.

30. LOWER EXTREMITIES.

Cracking, when stooping, Croc.
— — stretching out, Thuj.
— — walking, Bry. Led. Nux. Tabac.
Cramp, Actea-r. Ambr. Ars. *Calc.* Graph. Hyosc. Phosp. Plb. Sec-c. Sep. Sil.
— buttocks, Graph.
— hips, *Coloc.* Phosp-ac.
— thighs, *Asar. Cannab. Hyosc.* Ip. Petr. Rhus. Sep.
— bend of knee, *Calc. Cannab.* Caust.Nitr. Pæon. Petr. Phosp. Sulph.
— legs, Bufo. Carb-an. Carb-veg. Coloc. Cupr. Hipp-m. Jatr. Ntr-m. Pod. Sass. Sec-c. Tabac. Verat.
— tibia, Amm-c.
— calves, Alum. Ambr. Amm-c. *Anac.* Arg. *Ars.* Bar-c. Bov. Bry. *Calc. Camph. Cannab.* Carb-an. Carb-veg. *Cham.* Coff. Coloc. Con. Cupr. Elaps. Ferr. Ferr-m. Graph. Gum-gut. Hep. Hyosc. Jatr. Lach. Lact. Lob. Lyc. Mgn-c. Mgn-m. Merc. Merc-cor. Ntr-c. Ntr-m. *Nitr-ac. Nux.* Oleand. Petr. Rhus. Sacch. Sass. *Sec-c.* Selen. *Sep.* Sil. *Sol-nig.* Staph. Sulph. *Tart.* Verat.
— feet, Amm-c. Berb. Camph. Caust. Graph. Hipp-m. Lac-can. Lachn. Lyc. Meph. Ntr-c. Nux. Petr. Ran-b. Rhus. Sec-c. Sil. Stram. Sulph.
— soles, *Amm-c.* Ang. Berb. Calad. *Calc.* Carb-veg. Chelid. Coff. Eugen. Ferr. Hep. Hipp. Petr. *Phosp.* Plb. Sec-c. Selen. Sil. Staph. *Sulph.*
— — at every step, Petr. Sil. Sulph.
— toes, *Amm-c.* Bar-c. *Bar-m. Calc.* Carb-an. Caust. Ferr. Gels. Gum-gut. Hep. *Lyc.* Nicc. Nux. Ol-an. Plat. Sec-c. Sil. Sulph.
— in morning, in bed, Bov. Bry. Nitr-ac.
— evening, Hipp. Sil.
— at night, *Ambr.* Ars. Bry. Carb-veg. Cham. Eugen. Iod. Ip. Lachn. Lyc. Mgn-c. Mgn-m. Nitr-ac. Nux. *Rhus.* Sec c. Sep. Staph. *Sulph.*
— when bending the foot forwards, Coff.
— — crossing the legs, Alum.
— — extending the leg, Bar-c. Calc.
— — going down stairs, Arg.
— — lifting the legs, Coff.
— — pulling on boots, Calc.
— — sitting, Oleand. Pæon. *Rhus.*
— after sitting, Nitr-ac.
— when standing, Euphr.
— — stepping out, Alum.
— — walking, Amm-c. *Lyc. Nitr-ac.* Sep.
— after a walk, when sitting, *Rhus.*
— with colic, Coloc.
Cramping pain, *Cina.* Iod. *Phosp-ac.*
— hips, Ang. *Arg.* Aur. Cannab.Carb-veg. Caust. *Coloc.* Ntr-m. Ruta.Sep.Sulph-ac. Valer.
— thighs, Carb-veg. Cycl. Mang. Mur-ac. Ol-an. Phosp-ac. Plat. Ran-b. Ruta.

Sabin. Valer. Verb.
— knees, Arg. Bry. Carb-veg. Led. Ol-an.
— legs, Anac. Ang. Bry. Camph. Caust. Ntr-c. Oleand. Phosp-ac. Plat. Verb.
— tibia, Eugen.
— calves, *Anac.* Berb. Caust. *Euphr.* Led. *Lyc.*
— heel, Eugen. Led.
— feet, *Ang.* Arg. Camph. Oleand. Phosp-ac. Plat. Verb.
— toes, Phosp-ac. Plat.
Crawling, Bov. Caps. Euphr. Lachn. Ol-an. *Plat.* Rhod. Sabad. *Sec-c.* Sulph.
— bones, *Guaj.*
— thighs, *Guaj.*
— legs, Kali-c. Sec-c. Sulph. Tabac.
— calves, Sulph. Zinc.
— feet, Arn. Bell. Caps. Caust. Croc. Dulc. Hipp-m. Kali-c. Ntr-m. Par. Sep. Tar. Zinc.
— soles, Raph.
— — one spot in middle of, Ol-an.
— toes, *Amm-m.* Hep. Jatr. Lach. Lact. Ntr-m. Ran-sc. *Sec-c.* Sulph.
— — tips, *Colch.*
Crooking of the knees, Lyc. Sulph.
To cry out, pain in legs, *Sep.*
Cutting pain, Bell. Dros. Graph. Igt Ntr-c.
— — hips, Calc. Igt.
— — — left, Kali-jod.
— — — — after a fall, Ntr-s.
— — thighs, Dig. Gels.
— — knees, Arg.
— — ankle-joint, Arg.
— — feet, Ambr. Ntr-c.
— — heel, Ntr-s. Puls.
— — sole, Ol-an.
— — toes, Aur-m Led. Pæon. Phosp-ac.
Deadness, in open air, paleness and torper, Graph.
— legs, Amm-m. Nux.
— middle of right tibia, Samb.
— feet, *Calc.* Iod. Nux. Rhus. Sep.
— — — — in evening, Calc.
— toes, Calc. Chelid. Cycl. Sec-c.
— — after walking, Cycl.
Digging, Diad. *Rhod.*
— — knees, Croton.
Dragging, from hip to groin, as if everything would be pressed out, Ox-ac.
Drawing up of knees, involuntary, when walking, Igt.
Drawing pain, Acon. Amm-m. *Ang. Ant. Bar-c.* Berb. *Bry. Carb-veg. Cham.* Chelid. Chenop. Cina. Con. Creos. Dulc. *Graph.* Iod. Kali-c. Lach. Led. Lyc. Mgn-c. *Merc.* Ntr-m. *Nux.* Par. Puls. Rhus-rad. Sep. *Sil.* Stann. Stront. *Sulph.* Thuj. Verat. *Zinc.*
— buttocks, Croton.
— joints, Chelid. Rhod. Stront.
— bones, *Chin.* Con. Kali-c. *Rhod.* Valer.

30. LOWER EXTREMITIES.

Drawing pain, hips, Ant. Benz-ac. Bry. Calc. Carb-veg. Chelid. Con. Evon. Ntr-m. Par. Plb. Rhus. Ruta. Stann. Tereb.
— thighs, Anac. *Arn.* Bar-m. Berb. Caust. Cham. Cinnab. Colch. Creos. Cupr. Dulc. Iod. Mang. Mez. Mur-ac. *Ntr-m.* Nux. *Ol-an.* Puls. Rat. *Ran-b.* Rhus. Ruta. Sabin. Samb. Scill. Sep. Stram. Tereb. Valer. Zinc.
— knees, Acon. Alum. *Anac.* Asar. Bry. Caust. Cham. Chenop. Cocc. Cupr. Iod. Mgn-m. *Ntr-m. Phosp.* Puls. Rat. Sabin. Sep. Stann. Staph. Zinc.
— legs, Acon. Agar. Amm-c. Anac. Borax. Bry. Calc. Carb-an. Caust. Cham. Chenop. *Ferr.* Kali-c. Lact. Led. Mgn-c. Mez. Mur-ac. Ntr-c. *Ntr-m. Ntr-s.* Oleand. Ol-an. Phosp. Puls. Rat. *Rhod.* Rhus. Scill. Sep. Sil. Spong. Staph. Viol-tr. Zinc.
— tibia, Chenop.
— calves, Puls.
— tendo achillis, Benz-ac. Mur-ac. Ntr-s.
— ankle-joint, Cannab. Stront. Valer. Zinc.
— tarsal bones, Cupr. Rhod. Staph.
— feet, Borax. Cannab. Caust. Cocc. Ferr. Mgn-c. Mez. Oleand. *Ol-an.* Puls. Rat. *Rhod.* Spong. Stront. Verat. Zinc.
— soles, Chenop.
-- heel, Sep.
— toes, Aur. Berb. Cocc. Mez. Ol-an. Rat. Sep. Sil. Stront.
Dryness, knee-joint, Nux.
— feet, Hipp. Phosp. Sep. Sil.
Emaciation, wasting, Berb. Chin. Selen.
— of ham and thighs, Sacch.
— legs, Nitr-ac.
— feet, Caust.
Eruption, Ant. Clem. Dulc. Merc. Rhus-rad. Sulph.
— buttocks, Ant. Nux. Selen. Thuj.
— thighs, Merc. Nitr-ac. Nux. Osm. Petr. Thuj.
— between the thighs, Petr. Selen.
— knees, Anac. Ant. Lach. Merc. Nux. Phosp-ac. Thuj.
— bend of knees, Ntr-m.
— legs, Alum. Bov. Daph. Lach. Merc. Mez. Phosp-ac. Sep. Sulph.
— calves, Petr. Sil. Thuj.
— ankle, Osm.
— feet, Con. Lach. Rhus. Sep.
— toes, Ntr-c. Sulph.
— blisters, large, on soles, Bufo.
— — full of serum on sole of right foot, Kali-b.
— blisters spreading on toes, Graph.
— blotches, Ant. Lach. Ntr-c. Sulph.
— burning, Nux.
— confluent, Phosp-ac.
— gangrenous, Hyosc.
— gnawing, corroding, Nux. Sulph.
— humid, on malleoli, Creos.

— itching, Anac. Daph. Dulc. Lach. Merc. Nux. Petr. Rhus. Selen. Sep. Sil. Sulph.
— lumpy, Petr. Therid. Thuj.
— miliary, Alum. Bov. Daph. Merc. Nux. Sil. Sulph.
— papular, Lach. Lachn. Merc. Nux. Phosp-ac. Rhus. Selen. Sep. Thuj.
— phagedenic, Sulph.
— pustular, Clem. Dulc. Rhus. Thuj.
— — black, *Ars.* Ntr-c. Sec-c.
— — — ulcerated, on heel, Ntr-c.
— — suppurating, Con. Thuj.
— — with a red areola, Ant.
— scabby, Lach.
— elevated, white scabs, Mez.
— spots, like a burn, Lach.
— ulcerating, Phosp-ac.
— vesicular, Hyosc. Ntr-c. Sulph.
— — comes out in cold air, Dulc.
— — corroding, gnawing, Borax. Caust. Graph. Sep. Sil. Sulph.
— — humid, painless, between toes, Hell.
— white, Mez. Thuj.
Erysipelas, legs, Ars. Borax. *Hep.* Ntr-c. Sil. Sulph. Zinc.
— knee, Nux. Sulph.
— feet, *Arn.* Borax. Bry. Dulc. Nux. Puls. Rhus. Rhus-rad. Sulph.
Erysipelatous, desquamation of feet, Dulc.
Extend the limb, need to, Sulph-ac.
Extention, spasmodic of legs, Cina.
Fall to readily, liability, *Caust.* Mgn-c. Nux. Phosp. Phosp-ac.
Fatigue, sensation of, legs, Arg-n. Chenop. Creos. Lact. Mgn-m. Merc-jod. Mosch. Murex. Ntr-s. Psor. Puls. Ruta. Sulph.
— hips, Creos.
— knees, Anac. Cor-r. Croc. Kobalt. Ox-ac. Puls. Stann.
— feet, Alum. *Cannab.* Cor-r. Croc.
— after walking, Murex. Ruta.
To fall liability, Caust. Mgn-c. Nux. Phosp. Phosp-ac.
— in children, Caust. Nux.
— on making a false step, Phosp-ac.
Flaccidity, Ang. Camph. Canth. Cic. Hell. Lach. Lyc. Ntr-c. Nitr-ac. Nux-m. Op. Plb. Puls. Stram. Verat.
Flexibility, hips, Chin.
— knees, Acon. Arn. Bry. Cannab. Chin. Lach. Nitr-ac. *Nux.* Puls. *Ruta.* Stann. Stram. Sulph. Viol-tr.
— — when ascending stairs, *Cannab.*
— — going down stairs, Ruta.
— — walking, Stann. Stram. Viol-tr.
— legs, Murex.
— feet, Bell. Chin. Cic. Nitr-ac.
— easily, Carb-an. Sulph.
— toes, Carb-an. Lyc.
Flexion of knees, Lyc. Sulph.
Fungus, articulorum, white swelling on knee, Arn. Ant. Sil. Sulph.

30. LOWER EXTREMITIES.

Furcunles, buttocks, Agar. Alum. Amm-c. Bar-c. Graph. *Hep.* Lyc. Nitr-ac. *Phosp-ac. Rat.* Sabin.
— thighs, Calc. *Cocc. Clem. Hyosc. Igt.* Lach. *Lyc* Mgn-c. *Nitr-ac.* Nux. Petr. Phosp. Sep. *Sil.*
— on right thigh, painful on motion, Calc. Hell. Kali-c.
— knees, Ntr-m. Nux.
— bend of knees, Sep.
— legs, Calc. Mgn-c. Nitr-ac. Petr.
— — small blood boils, Mgn-c.
— calves, *Sil.*
— ankle, Merc.
— feet, Calc.
— soles, Rat.
Ganglion on instep, Ferr.
Gangrenous spots, legs, Hyosc.
Gangrena, senilis, Carb-veg.
Gangrene of toes, Sec-c.
Gnawing (corroding) pain, Lyc. Plat. Ran-sc. Ruta.
— hip, Kali-jod.
Greenish, yellow spots, as from a bruise, Con.
Hard, callous, skin of soles, Ant. Sil.
— toes, Graph.
Heat, hip, Phosp.
— thighs, Murex.
— knee, Igt. Phosp.
— — as if hot air blowing through knee-joint, Lach.
— legs, Acon. Ntr-s.
— — flushes, Kobalt.
— — in morning and evening, Ntr-s.
— tibia, Croton.
— feet, Acon. Cub. Led. Millex. Petr. Phosp. Psor. Puls. Stann. Staph.
— — in the evening, Led.
— — at night, Staph.
— of one foot, coldness of the other, Lyc.
— soles, in morning, Eupat.
— heels, cold to touch, Igt.
— toes, Borax. Zinc.
Heaviness, Acon. *Agar.* Alum. Ambr. Ang. Arg-n. Ars. Bar-c. *Bell.* Berb. *Calc.* Camph. Carb-an. Carb-veg. Chin. Creos. Graph. *Igt.* Iod Kali-b. Lach. Lyc. Mgn-m. Merc. *Ntr-c. Ntr-m.* Nitr-ac. Nux-m. *Nux.* Op. Osm. *Phosp.* Plb. Puls. *Rhus.* Sec-c. Sep. Sil. Spig. *Stann. Sulph.* Sulph-ac. Tart. Thuj. Verat. Verb.
— — at night, Sulph.
— — when ascending steps, Thuj.
— — in open air, Graph.
— — when walking, Thuj.
— hip, Mgn-s. Tart.
— thighs, Agar. Ang. Lach. Merc. Nux. Stann. Thuj.
— knees, Lach. Puls. Rhus. Ruta. Stann. Verat.
— legs, Ang. Cannab. Coloc. *Ferr.* Merc.

Ntr-m. Puls. Ruta. Stann. Verat.
— calves, Euphr. Rhus.
— feet, Acon. Agn. *Bell.* Bry. Colch. Creos. Igt. Kali-c. Lach. *Ntr-c. Ntr-m.* Ntr-s. Nicc. Nitr-ac. Op. Plb. Puls. Sabad. Tart. Verat. Verb.
Herpes, Alum. Bov. Graph. Lyc. Merc. Petr. Staph. Zinc.
— between thighs, Ntr-m. Petr.
— on buttocks, Ntr-c.
— hip, Nicc.
— thighs, *Clem. Graph.* Merc. Ntr-m. Petr. Staph. Zinc.
— knees, Carb-veg. Dulc. Petr. Phosp.
— bend of knee, Ars. Graph. Led. Ntr-c. Ntr-m. Petr. Phosp. Sulph.
— legs, Merc.
— calves, Cycl. Lyc.
— ankle, Cact. Creos. Cycl. Ntr-c. Ntr-m. Petr. Sulph.
— between toes, Alum. Graph.
— chronic, Led.
— itching, Mur-ac. Nicc. Staph.
— scaly, Clem.
Herpetic spots, on hams, Creos.
— thighs, Mur-ac.
— calves, Sass.
Horn like spots on the soles, Ant. Sil.
— toes, Ant. Graph.
Inflammation, thigh, Ntr-c. Sil.
— knees, Bry. *Cocc.* Led. Nux. *Puls.* Rhus. Sulph.
— legs, *Acon.* Borax. *Calc.* Ntr-c.
— tendo achillis, Zinc.
— ankle joint, Mang.
— feet, Acon. *Aru.* Borax. Bry. *Carb-an.* Kali-b. Zinc.
— instep, Mgn-c. Puls. Thuj.
— toes, *Carb-an.* Phosp. Puls. Thuj. Zinc.
Itching, Bar-c. Calc. Euph. Lyc. Spig. Zinc.
— buttocks, Mgn-c. Therid.
— hips, Alum. Dig. Puls. Sep.
— thighs, Bar-c. Calc. Croton. Nitr-ac. Petr. Ran-b. Thuj.
— between thighs, Carb-veg. Cinnab. Kali-c. Ntr-m. *Petr.*
— knees, Kobalt. Lyc.
— bend of knee, Ars. Ntr-m.
— legs, Bism. Calc. Caust. Lach. Rhus.
— tibia, Croton. Grat. Kali-c.
— calves, Ip.
— ankle, Berb. Borax. Calc. Kali-c. Lyc. Ran-b. Selen.
— feet, Bell. Berb. Bism. Bov. Calc. Caust. Cham. Dulc. Igt. Lach. Rhus. *Selen.* Sep. Zinc.
— soles, Ambr. Creos. Psor. *Sil.*
— heel, left, Nicc.
— toes, *Agar.* Clem. Graph. Jatr. Lact. Ntr-s. Nux. Pæon. *Staph.* Zinc.
— — which have been frozen, Ntr-c. Nux. Pæon. Staph. Sulph. Zinc.
— — when undressing, in evening, Ntr-s.

30. LOWER EXTREMITIES.

Jerking, of legs, Ambr. Amm-c. Asa-f. Bar-c. Berb. Carb-veg. Cic. Cina.*Igt.Ip.* Kali-c. Lyc. Ntr-c. Ntr-m. Op. Plat. Puls. Scill. Sep. Sil. Stram. Stront. Sulph.
— right leg, Mez.
— hips, Ars.
— hip-joint, Nux. Puls.
— thighs, Kali-b. Lact.
— right thigh, relieved by standing or drawing leg up, Meny.
— feet, *Cic.* Cina. *Ip.* Lyc. Ntr-s. *Sep.*
— — in sleep, Sep.
— soles, Croton. Ferr-m.
— spasmodic, of limbs on stepping out, Coff. Rhus.
Jerking pain, hips, Mgn-m. Mez. Puls.
— thighs, Ang. Cinnab. Mang. Mez.Ntr-c. Puls. Rat. Rhus. Valer.
— knees, *Amm-c. Anac.* Chin.
— legs, Amm-c. Anac. Cinnab. Mez. Nitr-ac. Phosp. Rat. Rhus.
— feet, Nitr. Rat.
— toes, *Amm-m.* Mez. Par. Ran-sc.
Knocking, feet, *Cannab.*
— toes, *Asa-f.* Plat.
Lameness, left hip, Fluor-ac.
Languor, lassitude, *Agar.*Amm-c.Amm-m. Ang. Bell. Berb. Bry. Cast. Con. Gum-gut. Hep. Ind. Lob. Mgn-m. Nitr-ac. Nitr. Nux-m. Nux. Phosp. Plat. Sec-c. *Senna. Stann.* Sulph. *Thuj.* Verb.
— thighs, Agar. Ang. *Arn.* Ars. Bry. Croc. Rheum. Sass.
— knees, Anac. Asar. Berb. Cannab. Con. Hyosc. Merc. Ntr-m. Nitr-ac. Nux-m. Puls. Sass. Staph. Sulph.
— legs, Ang. Asar. Bry. Croton. Ferr. Lact. Ntr-m. Nitr. Plat. *Puls.* Valer.
— feet, Bell. Croc. Gum-gut. Lyc. Merc. Ntr-s. Nitr-ac. Plb. Sass. Verb.
— in evening, in bed, Ind.
— when ascending steps, Bry. Thuj. Verb.
— in open air, Graph.
— when sitting, Croc. Mgn-m. Plat.
— — standing, Bry.
— while walking, Arn. Bry. Hep.
— after walking, Nitr.
Laxity of legs, Amm-c.
Limbs, inability to bend the, Ang.
Limping involuntary, Bell. Calc. Coloc. Kali-jod. Lyc. Puls. Rhus. Zinc.
Luxation, dislocation, spontaneous, of the hip, Bell. Bry. Calc. Caust. *Coloc.* Lyc. Puls. *Rhus.* Sulph. Zinc.
— — from pain, Carb-an. Dros. Kali-jod. Nitr-ac.
— — on sitting down, Ip.
— of patella, Gels.
— — when going up stairs, Cannab.
— ankle, Bry. Ntr-c. Nux. Ruta. Sulph.
— — left, Kali-b.

Marbled skin, legs, Caust.
— instep, Thuj.
Milk leg, phlegmasia alba dolens, Ant. Apis. Arn. Ars. Bell. Bry. *Calc.* Cham. *Chin.* Graph. Ham. Hep. *Iod.* Kali-c. Lach. *Led.* Lyc. Merc. Nux. Puls. Rhod. Rhus. *Sep.* Sil. Sulph: Verat.
Mobility, Alum. *Anac.* Calc. Caust. *Chin.* Cina. Coff. *Creos.* Cupr. Hell. Hyosc. *Lach.* Ntr-m. *Op. Rhus.* Sec-c. *Stram.* Tart. Zinc.
— knees, Acon. Arn. Bry. Cannab. Chin. Lach. Nitr-ac. *Nux.* Puls. *Ruta.* Stann. Stram. Sulph. Viol-tr.
— — when ascending stairs, *Cannab.*
— — — descending stairs, Ruta.
— — — walking, Stann. Stram. Viol-tr.
— legs, Murex.
— — feet, Bell. Cic. Chin. Nitr-ac.
— — easily, Carb-an. Sulph.
— toes, Carb-an. Lyc.
— hips, Chin.
Moisture, between scrotum and thighs, *Bar-c.* Carb-veg. *Hep.* Lyc. Merc. Ntr-c. Petr. Rhod. Sulph.
— on thigh, Sulph.
— water, oozes from legs, Sacch.
Motion, voluntary, loss of, Gels.
Mouse, running over legs, sensation of, Sep.
Muscles, twitching, Arg. Asa-f. Asar. Cupr. Graph. Kali-c. Mang. Ntr-m. Rheum. Spong. Teucr. Viol-tr.
— when exercising, Mang.
Nails, blue, Dig. Graph.
— crippled, Ars. *Graph.* Sabad. Sep. Thuj.
— discolored, Ars.
— painful, Merc-sulph. Teucr.
— thick, Graph.
Nail, as if, of big toe, would grow into flesh, Kali-c. Teucr.
Numbness, Alum. *Ambr.* Ant. Berb. Bov.)Calc. Carb-an. Carb-veg. *Chin.* Cocc. Croc. Euphr. *Graph.* Kali-c. Lact.' Led. Lyc. Merc. Merc-cor. Mez!Nux.Oleand.)Op.'Ox-ac. *Petr.* Plat.'Plb. Psor. *Puls.* Rheum.*Rhus*,\\Sep.\\Sil. Sulph.Sulph-ac. Thuj. Verat.
— — in evening, Sil.
— — at night, Alum.
— — when crossing the legs, Laur.Rheum.
— — after meals, Kali-c.
— — when sitting, Calc. Chin. Euphr. Sil. Tart.
— thighs, Ferr. Lach. Ocim.
— knees, Carb-veg. Lach.
— in middle of right tibia, Samb.
— feet, Cocc. Con. Kali-c. Lach. Laur. Millef. Ntr-m. Nitr. Nux. Oleand. Plb. Sep. Sil. Tart.
— — first right, then left. Coloc.
— — — left then right, Millef.
— soles, Bry. Oleand. Sep.

30. LOWER EXTREMITIES.

Numbness, toes, Cham. Phosp.
Offensive smell of feet, Sil.
Pain, simple, Ant. Ars. Calc. Cupr-carb.
  Kalm. Lyc. Nitr-ac. Psor. Sec-c. Sulph.
— buttocks, *Sulph.*
— joints, Phosp. Sulph.
— bones, Diad Merc. Mez. Oleand. Sulph.
— in periosteum of long bones, worse by least touch, Mez.
— hips, *Acon.* Agar. Ars. *Bar-c. Bell.* Calc-ph. Carb-an. Caust. Coloc. Dig. Evon. Kali-b. Kali-jod. Lyc. Mez.Ntr-s. Nux-jug. Phosp. Phyt. Prun. *Rhus.* Verat.
— — right, to knee, Kali-b.
— — — to left, Lith.
— thighs, Ars. Merc. Mez. Murex. Nitr-ac. Pareria. Phyt.
— — right, Cist.
— knees, Calc-ph. Cannab. Caps. Cist. Evon. Kali-chl. Kalm. Lac-can. Nitr-ac. Nux-jug. Ruta. Zinc.
— — right, Fluor-ac.
— — left, Kalm.
— patella, Nitr-ac,
— — right, Cocc.
— legs, Anac. Bell. Caps. Diosc. Mez. Rhus.
— — middle of left, Ntr-c.
— tibia, like labor-pains, Carb-veg.
— — rightly, Phyt.
— — middle of, Kali-b.
— calves, Lach. Sulph.
— ankle joint, Acon. Kalm. Lith. Phosp. Ran-b.
— — inner side of, limbs, Ang.
— heel, Agar. Calc. Cinnab. Diad. Eupat.
— — as if from a knife-thrust, Eupat.
— soles and toes, Pareira.
— soles, Ars. Croc. Lith. Lyc. Merc-jod.
— toes, Amm-m. Calc. Lact. Lith.
— big toe, as if being pinched off, Meph.
— — first joint of, as if pulled out, Prun.
Painful spots, on tibia, Ambr.
— on foot, when touched, Ferr-m.
Paralysis, Anac. Ang. Ars. *Bell.* Bry. Chin-sulph. *Cocc.* Iod. Lach. Lyc.Ntr-m. *Nux. Oleand. Op.* Ox-ac. *Plb.* Rhus. Ruta. Sec-c. Sep. *Sil. Stann.* Stront. *Sulph.* Zinc.
— hips, Verat.
— thighs and knees, left, *Chelid.*
— feet, Ang. Ars. *Bell. Chin.* Cocc. *Nux. Oleand.* Phosp. *Plb.* Rhus. Sulph. Zinc.
— painless, Oleand.
As if paralyzed, sensation of, Acon. Berb. Lach. Hyper. Rheum.
— — especially in ankles, Ntr-m.
— thighs, Berb. Croton. Lach. Nux.
— knees, after walking, Berb. Hyper. Lach.
Paralytic, paralyzing pain, *Amm-m.* Carb-veg. Cham. Chelid. Chin. Cina.
Dig. *Ntr-m.* Pod. *Seneg. Sep. Sil. Stann.* Stront. *Sulph.* Verat.
Paralytic pain after vexation, Sep.
— hips, Acon. Arg. Cham. Chelid. Dros. Evon. Led. Lyc. Plb. Sol-m.
— right, Mez.
— — left, Laur.
— thighs, Ars. Carb-veg. Cham. *Chin.* Colch. Dros. Ferr. Guaj.
— knees, Anac. Arg. Berb. *Chin. Evon.* Hipp. Mgn-m. Mosch. Plb. Ruta. Sulph. Valer.
— — left, Lach.
— legs, Cham. Chin. Eugen. Mosch. Nitr. Ruta.
— feet, Ang. Cham. *Chin.* Eugen. Kalm. Ntr-m. Oleand. Ol-an. Par. *Plb.* Tabac.
— — left, Hyper.
— toes, Aur. *Chin.*
Periodical pain, Lyc.
Perspiration, Cocc-c. Coloc. Phosp. Sep.
— at night, Coloc. Mang. Tereb.
— thighs, Ambr. Carb-an. Nux. Thuj.
— — between the, Cinnab.
— — when walking, Ambr.
— — at night or in morning, Carb-an.
— legs, Calc. Hyosc. Petr. Rhod. Sep.
— feet, Acon. Amm-c. Ang. *Bar-c. Calc.* Cannab. Canth. *Carb-veg.* Cocc. Creos. Cupr. Cycl. Graph. *Hell.* Hep. Iod. *Kali-c.* Lact. *Lyc. Mgn-m.* Merc. Ntr-m. Nitr-ac. Petr Phosp. Phosp-ac. Plb. Puls. Sabad. Scill. *Sep. Sil.* Staph. *Sulph.* Thuj. Zinc.
— — at night, Coloc.
— — cold, Ars. Canth. Cocc. Dros. Euph. Hep. Ip. *Lyc.* Merc. Scill. Staph. Stram. *Sulph.*
— — excoriating, Iod. Lyc. Nitr-ac. Sil. Zinc.
— — fetid, Amm-c. Amm-m. *Bar-c.* Cycl. Graph. *Kali-c.* Kobalt. Nitr-ac. Phosp. Plb. Puls. Sep. *Sil. Thuj.* Zinc.
— — like sole leather, Kobalt.
— — suppressed, Apis. Cupr. Hæmatox. Kali-c. Ntr-m. Nitr-ac. Rhus. Sep. Sil. Thuj.
— soles, Acon. Amm-m. Nitr-ac.
— between toes, Acon. Clem. Cycl. Ferr. Kali-c. Kobalt. Scill. Sil. Tar. Thuj.
Petechiæ on legs, Phosp.
Phagedenic blisters, Caust. *Graph.* Sep. Sil. Sulph.
Pimples, blisters, on thigh and leg, after scratching, Lach.
Podagra, Ambr. *Arn.* Con. Graph. *Led. Sabin.* Sacch. *Sulph.* Verat.
Pressing pain, *Arg.* Cycl. Kalm. Led. Ntr-m. *Oleand. Phosp-ac.* Ruta. *Sass. Stann.* Staph. Verat.
— bones, Guaj.
— hips, Arg. Asar. Ferr-m. Hell. Led. Stann.

30. LOWER EXTREMITIES.

Pressing, pain thighs, Agar. *Anac.* Asar. Cupr. *Guaj.* Kali-c. Led. *Oleand.* Phosp-ac. Sass. Sil. Verb.
— knees, Cupr. Led. Mgn-m. Sass.
— legs, Anac. Kali-c. Kalm. Ntr-c. Phosp-ac. Sass. Verb.
— tibia, Mez. Staph.
— calves, *Anac.*
— ankle-joint, Agar. Cron.
— tarsal bones, *Bism.* Cupr. Sabin. Staph.
— feet, *Oleand.* Phosp-ac. Verb.
— toes, Oleand. Phosp-ac.
Pricking, in nates, as if sitting on needles, Guaj.
— knee, Puls.
— feet, as if from needles, Hyper. Nitr-ac.
Prickling in feet, Dig. Sep. Thuj.
— under toe-nails, Elaps.
Pulsation, heels, Ran-b.
— toes, Zinc.
— big-toe, Asa-f.
Rasping, (smarting) pain, in hams, Creos.
— ankle joint, Plat.
— heels, Raph.
— toes, between the, Ntr-c.
Redness, one side, Puls.
— inflammatory, of heel, Ant.
— toes, *Agar.* Amm-c. Berb. Borax. *Carb-veg.* Ntr-m. Phosp.
— — tips, Mur-ac.
Red spots, Sulph.
— buttocks, Mgn-c.
— thighs, Cycl. Sulph.
— legs, Calc. *Con.* Lyc. Sass. Sil. Sulph-ac.
— foot, Elaps.
— — instep, Thuj.
— burning, Lyc. Phosp-ac.
— itching, Sulph-ac.
— turning livid, as after a bruise, Con.
— marbled, Thuj.
— oozing, Sulph.
— painful, Lyc. Sulph.
— smarting, Sil.
— as if scalded, Cycl.
— after scratching, Mgn-c.
Relaxation of legs, Amm-c. Guaj.
Relaxed, as if, muscles of thigh and calf, Merc-cor,
— hip-joint feels, Apis. Calc. Staph. Thuj.
Rending, tearing, Acon. *Agar.* Alum. *Ambr.* Ant. Arn. *Ars.* Bar-c. *Bell.* Berb. *Canth.* Carb-veg. Caust. *Cham. Chin.* Cina. Colch. Dulc. Hep. *Igt.* Ind. *Kali-c.* Lach. *Lyc.* Mgn-s. *Merc. Nitr.* Nux-m. Nux. Par. Phosp. Phosp-ac. *Puls.* Rhod. *Rhus.* Sass. Sep. *Sil.* Stann. Stront. *Sulph.* Teucr. Thuj. *Verat.* Zinc.
— joints, Kali-c. Merc. Stront. *Teucr.*
— bones, *Agar.* Amm-m. Arg. *Aur.* Bar-c. Chin. *Lyc.* Mgn-s. *Merc. Nitr.* Rhod. *Teucr.*
— os ischium, on rising from seat, Dros.

— hips, Alum. Amm-m. Ars. Calc. Carb-veg. Colch. Euph. *Ferr.* Graph. Kali-c. Mgn-m. Merc. Ntr-c. Par. Phosp-ac. *Rhus.* Sabin. Sep. Stann. Tabac. Zinc.
— — to leg to feet, Kalm.
— hip joint, right, Agn. Cocc-c. Lachn.
— thighs, Alum. Aur. Camph. Caust. Cham. *Chin.* Cinnab. Cist. Clem. Dulc. Euph. Ferr. Hyper. *Kali-c.* Kali-jod. Mgn-s. Merc. Mez. Mur-ac. Ol-an. Plb. Rat. *Rhus.* Sabin. Sass. Sep. Sil. Tereb. Zinc.
— — left, Kali-jod.
— knees, Acon. Amm-caust. Amm-m. Arg. *Arn.* Bell. Bry. Calc. *Caust.* Chenop. *Chin.* Cist. Cocc. Coloc. Con. Croton. Guaj. Igt. Iod. Kali-c. Kali-jod. Lachn. Lact. Laur. *Led. Lyc.* Mang. Merc. Millef. Nitr. *Phosp.* Plb. Rat. Rhod. Sass. Sep. *Sil.* Stann. Sulph. Teucr. Zinc.
— — left, Kali-jod. Lachn.
— above knees, Chenop.
— legs, Alum. *Amm-m.* Ars. Bry. Calc. Camph. Caps. Carb-veg. Caust. Chenop. *Chin.* Chin-sulph. Colch. Croc. Croton. Dulc. Igt. Ip. *Kali-c. Lyc.* Mgn-c. Mez. Millef. Ntr-c. Ntr-m. Ntr-s. Nitr-ac. Ol-an. Phosp. Puls. *Rhod.* Rhus. Sabad. Sass. Sep. Spong. Staph. Sulph. Verb. Zinc.
— — and stinging, as if in periosteum, down to toes, Ars.
— tibia, Amm-c. Ars. Berb. Kali-c. Phosp-ac. Sep. Staph. Zinc.
— — relieved by walking, Grat.
— calf, Bry. Lob. Ntr-s. Sabad. Valer.
— tendo achillis, Berb. Ntrs.
— ankle joints, Alum. Agar. Amm-c. Arg. *Arn.* Berb. Dros. Kali-c. Lac-can. Ntr-c. Samb. Stann. Stront. *Teucr.* Zinc.
— tarsal bones, *Arg. Bism.* Chin. Guaj. Kali-c. Sabin. Staph. *Teucr.*
— feet, Agn. Camph. Caust. Cham. *Chin.* Cocc. *Colch.* Graph. Kali-c. Lyc. Mez. Ntr-c. Ol-an. Phosp. Rat. *Rhod.* Sil. Spong. Stront. Sulph. Verat. Zinc.
— — in pregnant women, Phosp.
— heels, *Amm-m.* Arn. Ntr-s. Sep. Sil.
— soles, Chenop. Coloc. Croton. Nitr. Valer.
— toes, Agn. *Amm-m. Arg.* Aur. Berb. Camph. *Chin.* Cocc. *Colch.* Croc. Graph. Ind. Kali-c. Mgn-s Mez. Ntr-c. Ntr-m. *Ol-an.* Par. Plat. Rat. Sil. Stront. *Teucr.* Valer.
— under nails, Camph,
Rheumatic pains, Actea-r. Ant. Colch. Kali-c. Kalm. Lith. Meph. Nitr. Nitr-ac. Rhus-rad. (compare, Sect. 34.)
— — hips, Kali-b. Led. Mgn-s.

30. LOWER EXTREMITIES.

Rheumatic pains, hips right, Pallad.
— — — left, Lyc. Sang.
— — left leg, Elaps. Mgn-s.
— — inside right thigh, Sang.
— — knees, Gels. Kali-b. Led.
— — — right, Cinnab. Jac-cor. Kali-b. Led. Lob. Nicc. Phosp.
— — tibia, Chenop.
— — ankles, Zinc.
— — feet, Colch.
— — — soles of, Chenop.
— — metatarsal bones, worse from contact, not from motion, Chin.
— — heel, Meph.
— — of small bones, Cauloph.
— — big toes, Croton. Ol-an.
— — — right, Benz-ac. Bry. Cist. Lac-can.
— — — left, Agn. Led.
— — toe-joints, Arg. *Aur.* Kali-c. Stront. *Teucr.*
Restlessness, legs and feet, Actea-r. *Anac.* Ars. Bar-c. Carb-veg. Caust. Chin. Con. Croc. Ferr. Glon. Graph. Kali-c. Lach. Lyc. Mgn-c. Mgn-m. Meph. Merc. Mosch. Ntr-m. Ntr-s. *Nitr-ac.* Ox-ac. Plat. Prun. Psor. Rhus. Sep. Sil. Sulph. Zinc.
— in evening, Kali-c. Nitr-ac. Sec-c. Sep. Tabac.
— at night, Lyc.
Rhagades, cracks in skin, Alum. Aur. Calc. *Hep.* Lach. Petr. Sulph. Zinc.
— heel, Lyc.
Roughness of skin of hams, like tetter, Creos.
Sciatica, Curare. Graph. Lach. Phyt. Plantago-min. Tellur.
— left side, Kali-b.
Senselessness, insensibility, Alum. Carb-veg. Cocc. Graph. Kali-c. Led. Merc. *Nux.* Op. Rhus. Sec-c. Sil. Spong. Sulph. Sulph-ac.
— — at night, Alum.
— thighs, Euph. Ferr. *Graph.* Merc. Nux. Plat.
— legs, Amm-m. Arg. Puls. Sil.
— feet, Arg. Asa-f. Carb-veg. Con. Nitr. *Nux.* Plat. Plb. Puls. Rhus.
— — obstinate, Carb-veg.
— — painful, Puls.
— — when sitting, Plat.
— toes, *Chelid.* Graph. Phosp. Puls.
Separation and drawing together of legs, spasmodic, Lyc.
Shivering, on the legs, Kali-c. Meny.
Shocks, blows, Op. Phosp. Sulph.
— hips, Bell. Verat.
— thighs, Euphr. Sep.
— knees, Sulph-ac. Verat.
— legs, Plat. Sep.
— feet, Phosp. Spig. Stann.
— electric, upward through the thigh, followed by numbness, Euphr.

Shooting in one knee, Nitr-ac.
Shortening of tendons, sensation of, Ambr. Amm-m. Bar-c. Caust. Ntr-c. Phosp. Puls. Sil. Zinc.
— groin, Carb-an.
— hips, Amm-m. Carb-veg. Coloc. Euph.
— thighs, Berb. Carb-veg. Mgn-c. Ol-an. Plat. Puls. Sabin.
— — when sitting down, Sabin.
— knees, Amm-m. Bell. Berb. Carb-an. Carb-veg. Caust. Con. Creos. Euphr. Graph. Lach. Led. Merc. Mez. *Ntr-m.* Nux. *Ol-an.* Petr. Phosp. Rhus. Rhus-rad. Ruta. Samb. *Sulph.* Verat.
— legs, Puls.
— calf, Ars. *Bov.* Caps. Led. Ntr-c. Ntr-m. Puls. Sil.
— tendo achillis, Euphr. Graph.
— heel, Led. Sep.
— feet, Carb-an. *Caust.* Ntr-c. Plat. Sep.
— — left, Cycl.
— toes, Plat.
Shrivelled skin, *Rhod.*
Smarting, (compare Rasping.)
Softening of femur, Sil.
Sore pain, hips, Puls.
— bones, *Led.*
— thighs, Hep. Led. Puls. Sulph.
— knees, Carb-an. Led.
— ankles, Plat.
— heels, Amm-m. Borax. Cycl. Kali-b. Ran-b.
— — right, Euph.
— soles, Arum-trif. Lac-can. Puls.
— toes, Ars. Berb. Cycl. Ntr-c. Nitr-ac. Ran-b.
— big toe, ball of, Led.
Spasm and distortion, Ars. Cina. *Hyosc.* Plb. Sec-c. Spong.
— buttocks, Bar-c. Calc. Nux. Sep.
— hips, Phosp.
— knee, extending up and down, Berb.
— legs, *Jatr.*
— feet, Iod. Sec-c.
— — at night, Iod.
Sprained, as if, hip-joint, Hep.
— knees, Hipp.
— feet, Kalm.
— — left, Hyper. (compare, Wrenching.)
Stability, want of, Acon. Ambr. Bry. Cannab. Hell. Nux.
— hips, Acon. Chin.
— knees, *Acon.* Carb-veg. *Chin.* Lact. Mang.
— feet, Chin.
Stiffness, Acon. Alum. *Anac.* Ang. Bell. Calc. Caps. Cic. Cina. Cocc. Cupr. Dig. Lact. Lyc. Mang. Ntr-m. Nux. Ol-an. Ox-ac. Plat. Rhus. Rhus-rad. *Sep.* Spong. Tereb. Thuj.
— at night, Alum.
— after sitting. Bell. Dig. Nux. Puls. Rhus. *Sep.* Zinc.
— when walking, Ol-an. Thuj.

30. LOWER EXTREMITIES.

Stiffness, by walking relieved, Dig.
— painless, Oleand.
— hips, Acon. Bar-c. Bell. Euphr. Hell. Rheum. Rhus. Staph.
— in morning, Staph.
— — rising up, preventing, Bell.
— thighs, Ars. Amm-m. Aur-s. *Graph.* Merc. Ntr-m. Rhus. Thuj.
— knees, *Amm-m.* Ant. Ars.*Bry.*Carb-veg. Coloc. Elaps. Euph. Ferr-m. *Graph.* Hell. Hyosc. Igt. Lach. *Led.* Lyc. Mez. Ntr-m. Nitr-ac. Nux. Ol-an. Petr. Phosp. Plb. Rheum. Rhus. Sang. Sass. Sep. Spig. Stann. *Sulph.*
— — stretching out, preventing, Ant.
— — squatting, down preventing, *Coloc.* Graph.
— legs, Acon. Aur-m. Bry. Ferr. Rhus. Sass. Zinc.
— ankle joint, Carb-an. Caust. Chelid. Dros. Lyc. Ruta. Sep. Sil. Sulph.
— feet, Ambr. Caps. Chelid. Dros. Graph. Igt. Kali-b. Laur. Led. Petr. Ran-b. Rhus. *Sep.* Sulph. Sulph-ac. Zinc.
— toes, *Graph.* Sil. Sulph.
— sense of, Alum. Arg. Berb. Plat. Pod. Rhod.
— — feet, Asa-f.
Stinging pain, stitches, Ars. Bry. Coloc. Creos. Dros. Euphr. *Grat. Kali-c.* Led. *Merc. Nux.* Phyt. Rhus-rad. *Sass. Sulph. Thuj.*
— joints, Acon. Merc. Nux. Sil. Thuj.
— bones, Merc.
— hip, Acon. Alum. Amm-m. Arg. Ars. *Bell.* Bry. Calc. Carb-an. Colch. Coloc. Euph. Evon. *Ferr.* Hell. Kali-jod. Merc. Merc-cor. Ntr-c. Ntr-m. Nux. Phyt. *Rhus. Sabin.* Sil. Sol-m. Zinc.
— — right, Fluor-ac. Merc-cor. Sep. Sulph.
— — left, Carb-an. Sep.
— thighs, Acon. Arg. *Bry.* Calc. Creos. Ferr. Ferr-m. Mang. Merc. Nux. Oleand. Phyt. Plb. Rhus. Rhus-rad. Sabad. Samb. Sass. *Sep.* Sil. *Spig.* Tar.
— — from, liver, Kobalt.
— knees, Acon. Ant. Aur-m. Bar-c. Berb. Bov. Bry. Calc. Ferr-m. *Hell.* Kali-chl. Kalm. Lach. Laur. Led. Merc. Nitr-ac. Nux. Ol-an. *Petr.* Phyt. Plb. *Puls.* Rheum. Rhus. Rhus-rad. Sabad. Sass. *Sep.* Sil. Spig. *Staph. Sulph.* Sulph-ac. Tabac. Tar. Verb. Viol-tr.
— — left, Gymnoc.
— patella, Lachn.
— — right, Nicc.
— legs, Alum. Ant. Ars. *Bry.* Calc. Caps. Carb-an. Carb-veg. Caust. Chin. Coloc. Dulc. *Kali-c.* Kobalt. Led. *Lyc.* Mgn-c. Ntr-c. Nitr-ac. Rheum. Rhus. Sass. Sep. Sulph. Zinc.
— tibia, Ant. Berb. Samb. Sep. Viol-tr.

— calf, Bry. Tar.
— tendo achillis, Berb. Mur-ac.
— ankle joint, Ambr. Arn. Asar. Bov. Caust. Croton. Dros. Graph. *Hell.* Hep. Igt. Kali-c. Mang. Petr. Puls. Rhus. *Ruta.* Sep. Sil. Spig. Sulph.
— tarsal bones, Aur. Puls.
— heels, Berb. Bry. Calc. Ferr-m. *Graph.* Hep. Hipp-m. Igt. Kali-c. Nitr-ac. Puls. Ran-b. *Sep.* Sil. Sulph. Valer. Zinc.
— — left, Nicc.
— feet, Agar. Bry. *Grat.* Kali-c. Kalm. Meph. Ntr-s. Oleand. Ol-an. Phosp. Rhus. Rhus-rad. Sep. Sil. *Sulph.*Viol-tr.
— instep, *Puls.*
— soles, Borax. Bry. Graph. Igt. Ntr-c. *Puls.* Raph. Tar.
— under soles, in morning, Fluor-ac.
— toes, Agar. *Amm-m.* Aur. Berb. Bry. Carb-veg. Cist. Croton. Ferr-m. Hep. Kali-c. Kalm. Mgn-s. Mez. Ntr-m. Oleand. Par. Phosp. *Puls.* Ran-b. *Ran-sc.* Rhus. Rhus-rad. Sabin. Sil. Tart. *Verat.* Verb. Zinc.
— big toe, Asa-f.
— — right, Benz-ac. Lyc.
— — left, Kalm. Led.
Stinking feet, *Sil.*
Stretching, spasmodic, *Cina.*
To stretch the legs, inclination, Cina. Sulph-ac.
Suppleness, want of, knees, which prevents squatting, *Coloc. Graph.*
Swelling, Ars. Bry. Calc. Carb-veg. Con. Dulc. Iod. Kali-b. Kali-c. Lach. *Led. Lyc.* Merc. Nux. Puls. Rhus. *Sep. Sil. Sulph.*
— buttocks, Croton. Phosp-ac. Sulph.
— thighs, Chin. Led. Merc.
— knees, Acon. Ant. *Bry. Calc.* Chin. *Cocc.* Cocc-c. Cop. Ferr. *Hep. Iod.* Lach. *Led. Lyc.* Merc. Mur-ac. Nux. *Puls.* Sass. Sep. *Sil.* Sulph.
— — right, Chin.
— — fatty, Dig.
— bend of knee, Mgn-c.
— legs, *Acon.* Arn. Borax. *Bry. Calc. Colch.* Dulc. Graph. Kali-c. Lach. *Led. Lyc. Merc.* Ntr-c. Nux. *Puls.* Rhod. Ruta. Sil. Sulph.
— tibia, Phosp.
— calf, Bry. Chin. Mez. Puls.
— tendo achillis, Zinc.
— — lymphatic, Berb.
— ankles, Arn. *Asa-f.* Calc. Eupat. Hep. Lyc. Mang. Phosp. *Stann.* Sulph.
— around ankles, Sacch.
— — with difficult breathing, Hep.
— ankle-joints, Arn. Asa-f. Benz-ac. Calc. Cop. Ferr. Lyc. Sulph.
— tarsal bones, *Merc.* Staph.
— heels, Ant. Merc. Petr.

30. LOWER EXTREMITIES.

Swelling, feet, Acon Ambr. Amm-c. Apis. Arn. Ars. Bar-m. Bell. Berb. Bov. Bry. Calc. Cannab. Carb-an. Caust. Cham. Chin. Chin-sulph. Cocc. Colch. Coloc. Con. Creos. Dig. Eupat. Ferr. Graph. Hyosc. Hyper. Kali-c. Lac-can. Lach. Led. Lyc. Merc. Ntr-c. Ntr-m. Nux. Op. Petr. Phosp. Phosp-ac. Plb. Puls. Rhod. Ruta. Sabad. Sass. Sec-c. Sep. Sil. Stann. Stront. Sulph. Sulph-ac. Verat. Zinc.
— — blue, with red spots, Elaps.
— — up to ankles, Kali-c.
— — by day, diminishing at night, Dig.
— — in morning, Sil.
— — — evening, Stann.
— instep, Bry. Calc. Merc. Puls. Rhus. Staph. Thuj.
— soles, Calc. Cham. Chin. Kali-c. Lyc. Petr. Puls.
— toes, Amm-c. Arn. Bar-c. Carb-an. Carb-veg. Daph. Graph. Led. Merc. Ntr-c. Pæon. Phosp-ac. Plat. Sabin. Sulph. Thuj. Zinc.
— left big toe, Eupat.
— toes, tips, Chin. Mur-ac. Thuj.
— bluish, Lach.
— cold, Asa-f.
— dropsical, Apis. Ars Cact. Chin-sulph. Colch. Creos. Eupat. Iod. Led. Merc. Puls. Rhod. Ruta. Samb. Sulph. (compare Dropsy, Sect. 34.)
— — after scarlet fever, Bar-m.
— erysipelatous, Rhus.
— hard, Ars. Chin. Graph. Led. Mez. Sacch.
— hot, Acon. Amm-c. Arn. Ars. Bry. Calc. Carb-an. Chin. Cocc. Cocc-c. Colch. Graph. Iod. Kali-c. Led. Lyc. Petr. Puls. Sass. Sec-c. Sep. Stann.
— inflammatory, Acon. Calc. Iod. Puls. Rhus. Sil.
— itching, Cocc.
— large, Sulph.
— lymphatic, Bar-c. Berb.
— painful, Acon. Ant. Arn. Ars. Carb-an. Chin. Con. Daph. Lach. Mgn-c. Merc. Nux. Puls. Sep. Sil.
— — burning, Ant. Ars. Mur-ac. Petr. Phosp-ac. Puls.
— — cutting, Phosp-ac.
— — drawing, Arn. Led. Puls.
— — pressing, Led.
— — stinging, stitches, Acon. Ant. Arn. Bry. Carb-veg. Cocc. Graph. Iod. Led. Lyc. Merc. Petr. Puls. Sass.
— — tearing, Colch. Led. Merc. Plat. Puls.
— — tense, Bry. Chin. Led. Sass. Thuj.
— — throbbing, Phosp-ac. Plat.
— red, Acon. Amm-c. Ant. Arn. Bry. Carb-veg. Chin. Hep. Lach. Ntr-c. Nux. Petr. Puls. Sabin. Sass. Sil. Stann. Thuj.
— — spots, Acon. Chin.

— — or blue-black blisters, Ars.
— bright-red, Iod.
— rheumatic, Hep.
— shining, Acon. Arn. Ars. Bry. Merc. Sabin. Sulph.
— soft, Chin. Led.
— transparent, Sulph.
— white, Apis. Ars. Bell. Calc. Creos. Graph. Iod. Lyc. Merc. Nux. Rhus. Sulph.
— in day-time, less at night, Dig.
— — morning, Sil.
— — evening, Amm-c Cocc. Hyper. Phosp. Puls. Rhus. Stann.
— after abuse of china, Puls. Sulph.
— after gout, Eupat.
— — walking in open air, Phosp.
— when walking, increased, Rhus. Sep.
Tenderness, knees, Acon.
— feet, Rumex.
— heels, Zinc.
— when walking on them, Jatr.
— to soles, Sabad. Sass. Sulph.
— toes, Calc.
Tendons, twitching, feet, Iod.
Tension, Ang. Bar-c. Berb. Coloc. Hep. Mang. Nux. Plat. Puls. Rhus. Sulph.
— hams, Lact.
— hips, Coloc. Con. Croton. Ferr-m. Rhus.
— — right, Ntr-ac.
— — left, Lyc.
— thighs, Arn. Berb. Cham. Croton. Guaj. Hell. Mang. Mez. Ol-an. Puls. Rat. Rhus. Sabin. Spig. Sulph.
— knees, Arn. Berb. Bry. Calc. Caps. Caust. Con. Croton. Dig. Euphr. Hell. Led. Merc. Nux. Ol-an. Petr. Puls. Rhus. Stann. Sulph. Tart. Zinc.
— legs, Amm-m. Bar-c. Borax. Bry. Caust. Cham. Igt. Mez. Puls. Rhus. Tabac.
— calves, Alum. Anac. Bar-c. Berb. Bry. Caust. Creos. Cupr. Igt. Mur-ac. Ntr-c. Nux. Puls. Sabad. Valer. Zinc.
— tendo achillis, Caust. Graph. Mgn-c. Mur-ac. Ran-b. Sep. Teucr.
— heels, Caust. Led.
— feet, Cannab. Caust. Mez. Rhus. Sass.
— instep, Bry. Caust. Tart. Thuj.
— toes, Mez.
Throbbing, Sep.
— hips, Hep. Merc.
— thighs, Berb. Murex.
— feet, Arg. Cannab.
— toes, Amm-m. Asa-f. Phosp-ac. Plat. Zinc.
Tickling, soles, Ferr-m. Hep.
— — after scratching, Sil.
Torpor, rigidity, Alum. Cic. Dros. Petr. Sep.
— — at night, Alum.
— ankle-joint, Dros. Sep.
— sensation of, Alum. Arg. Plat. Rhod.
— feet, Asa-f.

30. LOWER EXTREMITIES.

Tottering, legs and knees, Agar. Asar.
Aur Bell. Bry. Cannab. Hell. Mur-ac.
Nux. Plat. Puls.
Treading, prevented, by pain in knees,
Nitr-ac.
— legs, Lyc.
— tarsal bones, Ruta.
Tremor, Agar. Anac. Arg-n. Ars. Bell.
Canth. Caps. Carb-veg. Caust. Chin.
Cic. Cocc. Con. Cupr. Hipp-m. Hyosc.
Iod. Ip. Kobalt. Lach. Lact. Lyc. Ntr-c.
Ntr-m. Nitr-ac. Nux. Oleand. Op. Petr.
Phosp. Puls. Raph. Rhus. Sass. Sec-c.
Seneg. Stram. Sulph. Tibia.
— — in evening and at night, Lyc.
— — after standing for some time, Oleand.
— thighs, Anac. Laur.
— knees, Acon. *Anac.* Bell. Lach. Laur.
Led. Mang. Nux. Oleand. Puls. *Ruta.*
Verb.
— — when sitting and walking, Led.
— legs, Bar c. Coloc. Plat. *Puls. Ruta.*
— — left, Cic.
— feet, Bar-c. Bov. Coff. Ip. Lyc. Nicc.
Ol-an. *Plat.* Sass. *Stram.* Tabac. Verat.
Zinc.
Ulceration, subcutaneous, in buttocks,
Borax.
Ulcers buttocks, Sabin. Sulph.
— thigh, Sil. Thuj.
— legs. Amm-c. *Ars. Calc.* Carb-veg.
Graph. Ip. Jac-cor. Lach. *Lyc.* Mur-ac.
Ntr-ac. Phosp-ac. Psor. Ruta. Selen
Sil. Sulph.
— tibia, Asa-f. *Sabin.*
— ankle, Merc-jod. Sil. Sulph.
— instep, *Sep. Sulph.*
— heel, Ars. Caust. Ntr-c. *Sep.*
— — on a spot of, from rubbing of shoe,
All-cep. Borax.
— — from a spreading blister, Caust.
Laur. Ntr-c. Sep.
— — left, Diad.
— foot, Bar-c. Ip. Sulph.
— on previously inflamed feet, Kali-c.
— — one foot, with stitching pains upward; the other foot burning, Puls.
— sole, Ars. Caust. Lach. Ruta. Sec-c.
— toes, Ars. Carb-veg. Caust. *Graph.* Petr.
Plat. Sep. Sil. Sulph. Thuj.
— — originating in blisters, Petr.
— joint of toe, Sep.
— on border of big toe, Graph.
— on the nail, Caust. Sep. Sil.
— black base, Ip.
— bleeding easily, Carb-veg. Phosp-ac.
— burning, Ars. Lyc. Mgn-c. Sulph. Zinc.
— dirty bottom, Lach.
— elevated margins, Petr.
— fetid, Carb-veg.
— fistulous, Ruta.
— flat, Lach. Selen.
— foul, putrid, Bry. Mur-ac.

— gangrenous, Lach.
— which follow gnawing vesicles, Ntr-c.
Sep.
— irritable, Phyt.
— itching, Lyc. Phosp ac. Psor. Sil.
— obstinate, Petr. Sulph.
— painless, Ars. Carb-veg. Graph. Plat.
Sep. Sil. Sulph.
— painful, at night, Lyc.
— in phagedenic blisters, originating,
Ntr-c. Sep.
— puffy (suety), *Sabin.*
— red base, Petr.
— running, oozing, Petr.
— sanious, Sulph.
— smooth, Selen.
— stinging, Ars. Sabin. Sil.
— superficial, Lach. Petr.
— tearing, Lyc.
Ulcerative pain, buttocks, Phosp. *Puls.*
— hip joints, Puls.
— legs, Puls.
— heels, Amm-c. *Amm-m.* Graph.
Kali-jod. Laur. Ntr-s.
— feet, Bry. Ntr-m. Ntr-s.
— soles, Ambr. Canth. Creos. Graph. Igt.
Phosp. *Puls.*
— toes, Berb. Kali-jod.
— under toe-nails, Lact.
Varices, Ambr. Am. Ars. Calc. Carb-veg.
Ferr. Graph. Lyc. *Puls.* Sulph. Zinc.
— thighs, Lac-can. Puls.
— left leg, Fluor-ac.
— itching, Graph.
— painless, of pregnant women, Millef.
— tensive, Graph.
— tearing, Sulph-ac.
Veins distended, legs, Carb-veg. Puls.
Sulph.
— on soles, net work as if, marbled, Caust.
Lyc. Thuj.
Vesicles, corroding, gnawing, Caust.
Graph. Sep. Sil. Sulph.
— — — buttocks, Borax.
— — — soles, Ars. Sulph.
Vibration, sensation of, Oleand. Mosch.
— leg, Ambr. Berb.
— calves, Phell.
— soles, Oleand.
— swollen, bend of knee, Berb.
Voluptuous tickling on the sole, after
scratching, Sil.
Walking, late and with difficulty, in children, Bell. *Calc.* Calc-ph Sil. Sulph,
— awakened, Sabad. Sil. Verat.
— difficulty, Aur. Chin. Oleand. Tereb.
— drags the feet, in, Nux.
— infirm, Caust. Kali-c. Mgn-c. Ntr-c.
Ol-an. Phosp. Sulph.
— limping, Bell. Carb-an. Dros. Kali-jod
Nitr-ac.
— tottering, Acon. Agar. Aur-s. Bell.
Cannab. Caust. Gels. Glon. Iod. Lact.

234   30. LOWER EXTREMITIES.

Mur-ac. *Ntr-m.* Nux Phosp-ac. Rhus. Ruta. Sacch. Sec-c. Stram. *Sulph.* Teucr. Verat. Verb. (compare Tottering)
Walking almost on the ankle, from inclination of the joint, Bruc.
— feet turn easily when walking, Carb-an.
— — — — on a stone pavement, Agn.
Warts, toes, Spig.
Weakness, *Amm-m. Anac.* Arg-n. Ars. Berb. Borax. *Chin.* Con. Dig. Glon. Guaj. Merc. Murex. Ntr-m. *Nux.* Oleand. *Ol-an.* Op. Ox-ac. Phosp. Phosp-ac. Puls. Rhod. *Sec-c. Sulph.* Thuj. Tilia.
— hips, Chin.
— thighs, Acon. Ars. Carb-an. *Chin.* Croc. Guaj. *Merc.* Mur-ac. Nux. Oleand. *Plat.* Puls. *Ruta.* Staph.
— — left, Chelid. Glon.
— knees, Anac. Arn. Aur. *Chin.* Ferr. Lach. Led. Lith. Mosch. Ntr-m. *Nitr-ac.* Nux-m. Nux. Oleand. Petr. Phosp. Plat. Pod. Puls. *Ruta.* Sabad. *Staph.* Sulph. Sulph-ac. Tart.
— — left, Chelid.
— legs, Agar. All-cep. Aloe Arg-n. Bufo. Camph. *Euph. Merc.* Murex. Ntr-m. *Nitr.* Nux. *Oleand.* Phosp-ac. Puls. Ruta. Sacch. *Staph.* Valer.
— — bones of, Puls.
— calves, Kalm.
— ankle joint, Ntr-c.
— feet, *Chin.* Hipp. Nicc. *Oleand. Ol-an.* Puls. *Tabac.* Zinc.
— in morning, in bed, Tart.
— when ascending steps, Thuj.
— — rising from sitting, Ruta.
— while standing, Agar.
— in making a false step, Phosp-ac.
— when walking and sitting, Led.
— after a walk, Mosch. Nitr.
Weariness, after a walk, of legs, Murex. Ruta.
— — of feet, Alum. Cannab.
Wood, limbs feel as if made of, when walking, Nitr. Plb. Rhus. Thuj.
Wrenching, spraining pain, Arn. Berb. Carb-veg. Caust. Ntr-m. Oleand. Puls. Rhus.
— on sitting down, Ip.
— hips, Amm-m. Arg. Bar-c. *Calc. Caust.* Chin. *Euph.* Hep. Ip. *Ntr-m.* Nitr-ac. Nux. *Phosp.* Psor. Puls. Rhod. Rhus. Rhus-v. Seneg. Stann. Sulph.
— knee, Amm-c. Calc. Caust. Creos. Graph. Hipp. Lach. *Lyc.* Ntr-m. Phosp. Prun. Rhod. Rhus. Spig.
— — right, Nux-m.
— ankle joints, Ang. Ars. Bar-c. Camph. Caust. Cocc. Cycl. Dros. Graph. Hell. Hep. Igt. Lyc. Merc. Mosch. Ntr-m. Nitr-ac. Nux. Phosp. Phosp-ac. Plat. Plb. Puls. Rhus. Ruta. Sil. Sulph. Zinc.

— feet, Ang. Bar-c. *Bry.* Calc. Carb-veg. Caust. Creos. *Cycl. Dros.* Ferr-m. Kalm. Merc. Ntr-m. Nux. Phosp. Prun. Puls. *Rhus.* Sulph. Tilia. Valer. Zinc.
— — left, Hyper.
— toes, *Amm-c.* Berb. Zinc.
— big-toe, pain in first joint of, as if pulled out, Prun.
In morning, pain, Anac. Caust. Sil.
— in bed, Bov. Bry. Nitr-ac. Tart.
— hips, Amm-c. Ferr-m. Staph.
— in hip, worse in forenoon, free after midnight, Prun.
— thighs, Amm-c. Aur. Caust. Viol-tr.
— knees, Tart.
— evening, pain, Ambr. Calc. Ferr-m. Kali-c. Led. *Lyc.* Ntr-s. Nitr-ac. Selen. Sep.
— in bed, Carb-an. Ferr-m. Ind. Phosp. Sulph.
— hips, Ferr. Valer.
— thighs, Aur. Ferr.
— knees, Lyc.
— legs, Cinnab. Lyc.
— calves, Nux.
— ankle joint, Ntr-c.
— feet, Ferr-m. Lyc. Phosp. Puls. Sil. Sulph.
— soles, Berb. Mgn-m. Sil.
— toes, Cist.
At night, pain, Alum. Ambr. Bry. Carb-an. Carb-veg. Cham. Coloc. Eugen. Graph. Hep. Iod. Kali-c. *Lyc.* Mgn-c. Mgn-s. Mang. *Merc.* Nitr-ac. Nux. Phosp. Rhus. Sep. Staph. *Sulph.* Tereb.
— in bed, Sulph.
— bones, Kali-c. Merc.
— hips, Bell. Cham. Ferr. Ferr-m. Lach. Merc. Ntr-s. Prun.
— thigh, Cham. Euph. Ferr. Lach. Merc. Nux.
— knees, Lach. *Lyc.* Merc. Zinc.
— legs, Amm-m. Croc. Lyc. Spong.
— tibia, Phosp-ac.
— calves, Anac. Cham. Lyc. Nux. Sabad. Sulph.
— tendo achillis, Mur-ac.
— feet, Cham. Kali-c. Lyc. Phosp. Sil. Spong.
— soles, Sil. Sulph.
— toes, *Amm-c.* Kali-c. Led. Ntr-c. Plat.
— before midnight, Prun.
After midnight, Nux.
By day, Phosp.
In open air, Graph.
After walking in open air, Phosp.
Alternately with affections of eyes, Creos.
When ascending a hill, Hyosc.
— steps, pain hips, Bry. *Plb.* Rhus. Thuj. Verb.
— — — knees, Alum. Cannab. Nux-m. *Plb.*
— — ankle joint, *Plb.*

30. LOWER EXTREMITIES.

When bending, pain, knees, *Spig*.
— — — foot, Coff. Selen.
When crossing legs, pain, thigh, Dig.
— — — — calf, Dig. Valer.
— descending steps, pain, knees, Arg. Cannab. Verat.
— — — — calf, Arg.
After exertion, pain legs, Igt.
From letting limbs hang down, Puls.
When lying, pain, hips, Coloc. Kali-jod. Murex. Plb.
After lying, pain, hips and thighs, Acon.
— — down, Acon.
During a meal, pain hips and legs, Phosp-ac.
After a meal, Kali-c.
When moving the part, Acon. Berb. Bry. Calc-ph. Cocc. Creos. Mang. Puls. Sulph.
— — pain in bones, *Merc*.
— — hips, Kali-b. Led. Merc. *Ntr-s. Nux.* Sulph.
— — thighs, Cocc. Merc. Spig.
— — knees, Kali-b. Merc. Rheum.
— — legs, Acon. Colch
— — ankle joints, Arn.
— — feet, Acon. Bry. Puls. Thuj.
— — soles, Puls.
— — toes, Amm-c. Thuj.
By motion, pain increased, Bry. Ntr-s. Nux.
— — relieved. Agar. Jac-cor.
Periodically, Lyc.
In rainy weather, pain, Borax.
When raising the foot, pain, preventing flexion, Berb.
During rest, pain, Cupr. Euphr.
— hips, Ferr. Puls. Rhus.
— thighs, Ferr. Puls.
— legs, Coloc.
— calf, Amm-c. Cupr.
— soles, Coloc.
By rest pain increased, Cupr. Euphr. Puls. *Rhod*. Nux. Ruta.
. restlessness pain relieved, Osm.
When rising from sitting, pain, hips, Ntr-s. Phosp-ac. *Rhus*.
— — — — — thighs, Nitr-ac. Phosp-ac.
— — — — — knees, Berb. Nux.
— — — — — heels and soles, Graph.
After scratching, Lach. Sil.
On sitting down, Sabin.
When sitting, pain, Agar. Ant. Calc. Cham. Chin. Croc. Iod. Kobalt. Led. Mgn-m. Oleand. Pæon. Phosp-ac. Plat. Sulph.
— buttocks, Hep. Phosp. Sep. Sulph.
— hips, Phosp-ac. Sulph.
— thighs, Cist. Guaj. Sep.
— knees, Calc. Cist.
— legs, Amm-c.
— heels, *Valer*.
— feet, Alum. Ntr-c. Valer.

After sitting, pain, knees, Bell. Berb. Con· Dig. Nitr-ac. Nux. Sep. Zinc.
In sleep, pain, toes, Led.
After sleep, pain, hips and thighs, Acon.
When squatting, pain, knee, Calc.
— standing, pain, knees, Calc. Nux.
— calf, Euphr.
— toes, Ntr-m.
— soles, Croc.
— — relieved, Euph.
— standing upright, Agar. Bry. Graph. Puls.
— when stepping, pains in hips, Asar. Kali-c. Rhus. Sabin.
— — thighs, Asar.
— — knees, Con.
— — ankle joints, Bry. Ntr-m. Rhus. Sil.
— — heels, Nitr-ac.
— — feet, Bry. Caust. Thuj.
— — soles, Bry. Ntr-c. Sulph.
— — toes, Bry. Led. Thuj.
— — stepping out, stinging pain, Berb.
— — stooping, pain hips, *Ntr-s*.
— stretching, out, pain, hips and legs, Ruta.
— — instep, Bry.
— when touched, pain, Bell. Bry. Chin. Nux. Plat. Puls. Sulph.
— — bones and sinews Berb.
— — hips, Bell. Ruta. Sulph.
— — thighs, Nux.
— — knees, Acon.
— — legs, Acon. Borax. Puls.
— — feet, Acon. Borax. Bry. Chin. Ferr-m.
—.— ankles, Ntr-m.
— — instep and soles, Puls.
— — toes, *Chin*. Phosp-ac.
By touch increased, pain, *Bell. Bry*. Chin. Guaj. Nux. Plat. Puls. Ruta. Sulph.
When undressing, pain, Ntr-s.
After vexation, pain leg, Sep.
When walking, pain hips, Agar. Arg. Asar. Dros. Euph. Mez. Phosp-ac. Sol-m.
— — thighs, Asar. Calc-ph. Cist. Dros. Guaj. Phosp-ac. *Spig*. Staph.
— — knees, Berb. Bry. Calc-ph. Caps. Cist. Euph. Tart.
— — right patella, Cocc-c.
— — legs, Igt. Puls. Tabac.
— — calves, Alum. Anac. Caps. Igt. Lyc. Mur-ac. Nux. Sulph. Zinc.
— — tendo, achillis, Euphr. Mur-ac.
— — ankle. Drcs.
— — bends, Nitr-ac.
— — heel, Berb. Jatr. Kali-b.
— — feet, Agn. Caust. Ferr. Ntr-c. Puls. Sulph. Tart.
— — soles, Ambr. Bar-c. Caust. Igt. Led. Lyc. Phosp. Puls. Sulph.
— — toes, Agn. Ant. Ars. Camph. Caust. Lyc. Ntr-m.
— — under the nails, Camph.
— walking on stone pavement, feet turn easily, Agn. Ant.

After walking, pain, knees, Berb. Cycl.
   Mosch. Nitr. Rhus. Valer.
— — — as if palsied, Berb.
— calf, Amm-m. Cinnab.
By walking increased, pain, Ambr. Anac.
   Ant. Arn. Berb. Bry. Calc-ph. Ferr.
   Ferr-m. Hep. Hyosc. Led. Lyc. Nitr-ac.
   Ol-an. Petr. Phosp. Sep. Stann. Stram.
   Tabac. Thuj. Viol-tr.
— relieved, Amm-c. Dig. Rhus. Sep.

Warmth, sensation of, soles, Berb.
In warmth of bed, pain in legs, Sulph.
— — relieved, Amm-c.
Weather changing, Lach.
— windy, Lach.
With epistaxis, inflammation of leg, Borax.
— colic, Amm-c. Coloc.
— constipation, paralysis, Lyc.
— pain in hip leg shortened, Mez.
— — — — elongated, Coloc. Rhus. Thuj.

31. Sleep and Dreams.

Yawning, *Acon*. Amm-c. Arn. Ars. Brom. Bry. Cannab. Canth. *Caust.* Chelid. *Cina*. Cocc. Cor-r. *Creos. Croc.* Cupr. Elat. Gels. *Igt.* Kali-b. Kali-c. Kali-jod. Laur. Lyc. Mgn-c. Mgn-m. Mang. Meny. Merc. Mosch. Mur-ac. Ntr-m. *Nux.* Oleand. Ol-an. Op. Par. Phosp. Phosp-ac. Plat Puls. Rheum. *Rhus.* Ruta. Sabad. Sass. Sep. Sil. Spong. Stann. *Staph.* Sulph. Tabac. Tart. Tart-ac. *Viol-od.* Zinc.
— frequent, *Acon*. Cor-r. Euph. Grat. Kali-jod. Laur. Lyc. Mgn-c. Meph. Mosch. *Oleand.* Phell. Rhus. Scill. Stann. Sulph. Tabac. Tar. Tabac.
— interrupted, Lyc.
— spasmodic. Ang Bry. Cocc. *Cor-r.* Hep. Igt. Mosch. Nux. *Plat. Rhus.* Sep.
— vehement, Agar. *Cor-r. Hep. Igt.* Mgn-c. *Plat. Rhus.*
— in the morning, Igt. Nux. Viol-od.
— afternoon, Canth. Igt. Plat.
— when walking in open air, *Euph.*
— with chilliness, Oleand. Par. Sep.
— — coldness, Ntr-c.
— — giddiness, Agar.
— — goose skin, Laur. Par.
— — headache and congestion of blood to the head, Glon.
— — lachrymation, Creos. Igt. Meph. Staph. Viol-od.
— — oppression of chest, Stann.
— — pain in articulation of jaw, Cor-r. Igt.
— — shaking, chills, *Mur-ac.*
— — shuddering, Calad. *Cina.* Laur. Oleand.
— — stretching, Alum. Amm-c. Ars. Bell. Calc. Canth. Carb-veg. Caust. Cham. Chin. Graph. Guaj. Ip. Ntr-s. Nux. Ol-an. Puls. Rhus. Ruta. Sabad. Sep. Spong. Staph. Sulph. Tart. Tart-ac.
— — tremor, Cina. Oleand.
— without inclination to sleep, Igt. Plat. *Rhus.* Sep.
Sleepiness, drowsiness, in day time, Acon. Agar. Aeth. Ambr. *Amm-c.* Amm-m. Anac. Ang. *Ant.* Arg-n. Arn. Ars. Asar. Asa-f. *Bar-c. Bell.* Berb. Bry. Calad. *Calc. Camph.* Cannab. Carb-veg. Caust. Chin. Cimex. Cinnab. Clem. Cocc. Colch. Cor-r. Creos. *Croc.* Cycl.

Dig. Dulc. *Euph.* Euphr. *Ferr.* Gels. Graph. Grat. Gum-gut. Hæmatox. Hell. Hep Hipp-m. Hyosc. Hyper. Kali-c. Lac can. Lach. Lachn. Lact. *Laur. Led.* Lyc. *Mgn-c. Mgn-m.* Meph. Merc. Merc-cor. Merc-jod. Mez. Morph. *Mosch.* Mur-ac. Ntr-c. *Ntr-m.* Nitr-ac. *Nitr. Nux-m. Nux.* Ol-an. *Op.* Ox-ac. Par. Petr. Phell. *Phosp. Phosp-ac. Plb.* Pod. Psor. *Puls.* Ran-b. Rat. Rheum. *Rhod.* Rhus. Sabad. *Sec-c. Sep.* Sil. Sol-m. Spig. Stann. *Staph. Stram. Sulph.* Tabac. Tar. *Tart.* Therid. *Verat.* Zinc.
— in morning, Agar. Bism. *Calc.* Caust. Clem. Cocc. Con. Euph. *Graph.* Led. Mgn-m. Merc. Ntr-c. Ntr-m. Ntr-s. *Nux.* Phosp. Phosp-ac. Rhus. *Sep.* Sil. *Spig.* Sulph. Zinc.
— — forenoon, *Ant.* Bism. Cannab. Carb-veg. Mosch. Ntr-c. Ntr-s. Nux. *Sabad.* Sep.
— — — if he smokes tobacco, Bufo.
— — — with rumbling in bowels, Pod.
— at noon, Agar. Aur. Bry. *Chin.* Dros. Ol-an. Tabac.
— afternoon, Acon. Agar. Anac. Bov. Canth. *Chin. Grat.* Guaj. Lach. Nux. Pallad. Phosp. Puls. *Rhus.* Ruta. Staph. *Sulph.* Viol-tr.
— evening, Alum. Anac. *Ang.* Amm-m, Arn. Ars. Bell. Berb. Borax. *Bov. Calc.* Chin. Con. *Croc.* Cycl. Graph. Hep. Ind. *Kali-c.* Lac-can. *Lach.* Laur. Lith. Lyc. Mgn-s. Mang. *Nux.* Par. Petr. *Phosp-ac.* Plat. Ruta. Sass. Sep. *Sil.* Spig. *Sulph.* Tabac. Tart. Thuj.
— — at sunset, Dros.
— — every other, Lach.
— excessive, *Acon. Aeth.* Agn. Ang. *Ant.* Ars. *Asa-f.* Bar-c. Berb. Bism. *Bov. Bry.* Camph. Canth. *Carb-veg. Caust.* Cham. Clem. Con. *Cor-r. Croc.* Dig. Dulc. *Euph.* Ferr. *Graph.* Grat. Guaj. Hep. *Kali-c.* Laur. Led. Mgn-c. Mgn-m. Mang. Merc. Mez. *Mosch.* Mur-ac. Ntr-s. *Nux-m.* Nux. *Ol-an.* Op. Par. Phosp. Phosp-ac. Plat. *Plb.* Puls. Rhod. *Ruta.* Sabad. *Sec-c.* Seneg. *Sep.* Sil. Spig. Stram. Tabac. *Tar. Tart.* Tereb. Thuj. Verat. *Verb.* Zinc.

31. SLEEP AND DREAMS.

Sleepiness, alternately with sleeplessness, Lach.
— with delirium, Arn.
— proceeding from eyes, Euph.
— with burning in eyes, *Rhod.*
— — contraction of eyelids, Con. Croc. Kali-c. Tart.
— when exercising, relieved, Carb-veg. Mur-ac.
— with palpitation of heart, Chin.
— invincible, *Arum.* Cannab. *Cor-r. Lach.* Laur. Ntr-c. *Sulph.* (compare Coma.)
— in open air, Acon. Tart.
— when reading or writing, Brom. Ntr-s.
— in sitting, Petr. Par.
— without sleep, Arn. *Bell.* Borax. *Calad.* Cham. *Chelid.* Coff. *Ntr-m.* Op. *Samb.* Sil. Sol-m.
— with stupidity, Ntr-m.
— tertian type, Lach. Sep.
— during a thunder storm, Sil.
— from weakness, Mez. Merc-sulph. Nitr-ac.
— while working, Sulph.
Sleeplessness at night, Acon. Aeth. Ambr. Amm-c. *Ars.* Bapt. *Bar-c. Bell.* Borax. Bry. Calc. *Camph.* Cannab. Caps. Carb-an. *Carb-veg.* Caust. *Cham. Chin.* Cic. *Cina.* Cinnab. Clem. *Coff.* Coloc. Con. Creos. Daph. Dig. Graph. Hell. *Hep.* Hyosc. Igt. Ip. *Iod.* Iris *Jalap.* *Kali-c.* Kali-jod. Lach. Laur. *Led.* Lyc. *Mgn-c. Mgn-m. Mgn-s.* Merc. Mez. Mosch Ntr-c. Ntr-m. Nux. Op. *Phosp.* Phosp-ac. Plat. Plb. *Puls.* Ran-b. *Ran-sc.* Rhus. Sabad. Sang. Sass. Selen. *Sep. Sil.* Spong. Staph. Sulph. Thea. Thuj. Tilia *Valer.* Verat.
— before midnight, *Alum.* Amm-m. *Ang.* Arn. Ars. Bell. Borax. *Bry.* Calad. *Calc.* Carb-an. *Carb-veg.* Chin Cor-r. Creos. Graph. Hep. Igt. Kali-c. Lach. Led. Lyc. Mgn-m. *Merc.* Mur-ac. *Nux.* *Phosp. Puls.* Ran-b. *Rhus.* Selen. *Sep.* Sil. Spig. Sulph. Teucr. Thuj. Valer.
— after midnight, Ars. Asa-f. Cannab. *Caps. Coff.* Dulc. Hep. *Kali-c.* Mgn-c. Ntr-c. *Nux.* Oleand. Psor. *Ran-sc.* *Rhod.* Rhus. Sep *Sil.* Sulph-ac.
— — 1 A. M. Merc-jod.
— — 2 A. M. Benz-ac. Caust. Coff. Graph. Kali-b. Kali-c. Mgn-c. Mez. Ntr-m. Pallad.
— — 3 A. M., Amm-c. Calc. Coff. Creos Euphr. Graph. Mgn-c. Mgn-m. Mez Nicc. Nux. Ran-sc. Rhus. Selen. Sep. Sulph.
— — 4 A. M., Verb.
— until 4 A. M., Amm-c.
— with sleepiness, Acon. Apis. Arn. Ars. Bell. Bry. Calad. Calc. Caust. Cham. Chelid. Chin. Coff. Con. Daph. Ferr. Hep. Kali-c. Merc. Ntr-c. Ntr-m. Nux.

Op. Phosp. Phosp-ac. Puls. Rhus. Samb. Sep. Sil. Sol-m. Sulph.
— with sensation of refreshment in morning, Cinnab.
— hysterical, Mosch.
— because not able to lie on left side, Colch.
— with inability to open the eyes, Carb-veg.
— — convulsions and concussions as from fright, Hyosc.
— if not retiring early, not sleepy next day, Sep.
— with talkativeness, Lach.
— without restlessness. Merc-jod.
Difficulty of going to sleep late at night and of waking up in the morning, Ntr-c.
Sleep prevented by congestion of blood. Amm-c. Asar. *Puls.*
— — aggregation of ideas, *Chin.* Cinnab. Cocc. Coff. Fluor-ac. Lyc. *Nux. Puls.* Sabad. Sil. *Staph.* Sulph. Tart. Viol-tr.
— — same ideas always repeated, Calc.
— — one fixed idea, Graph.
— — anxiety, Ars. Carb-veg. Cham. Laur. Merc. Merc-cor. Phosp. Sep. Verat.
— — backache, Amm-m.
— — chills, Lyc.
— — coldness of body, Ambr.
— — colic, Plb.
— — cyphers before the eyes, Phosp-ac.
— — delirium, Bry. Sil. *Spong.*
— — dyspnœa, Psor. Ran b.
— — erections, Thuj.
— — excitability, Mosch.
— — fear to go to sleep, that he would die, Nux.
— — flatulent distention of, abdomen, Nux-m.
— — headache, Sil.
— — lancinating, Elaps.
— — heat, dry, Bry. Cannab. Ran-sc. Thuj.
— — hunger, feeling of, Igt.
— — imaginations of fancy, Bell. Carb-veg. Chin. Coff. Led. Merc. Phosp.
— — itching of skin, Arum-trif.
— — — — head, face, neck and shoulders, Gels.
— — jerks in limbs, Ip. Lyc. Merc-cor.
— — — — feet, Phosp.
— — — — whole body, Bell.
— — longing for the company of friends, Plb.
— — mouth, soreness of, Arum-trif.
— — nervousness, Apis. Camph. Lac-can. Phosp.
— — nervous irritation, Hyosc.
— — on account of pains Merc.
— — nightmare, Amm-c.
— — pain in ulcers and tetters, Staph.
— — pains, commence just before loosing himself in sleep, Lil-tigr.

31. SLEEP AND DREAMS.

Sleep prevented by perspiration, *Ars.* Sulph. Tar. Verat.
— — pulsation in head, Cycl.
— — restlessness, Acon. *Ars.* Carb-veg. Cina. Cor-r. Creos. Ferr. *Laur.* Led. *Mgn-m.* Merc. Phosp. Sil. Sulph. Thuj. Valer.
— — — and heat, Bry. Phosp. Rhus. Thuj.
— — — eyes closed, Acon.
— — — restless after a short nap, Phosp.
— — sneezing, Amm-m.
— — stomach, pressure in, Cina.
— — — emptiness in, Dig.
— — starting, Alum. Ambr. Ars. Bell. Bry. Calc. Caust. Chelid. Cor-r. Dulc. Euph. Guaj. Hep. Igt. Kali-c. Lyc. Merc. Merc-cor. Ntr-c. Nitr-ac. Nux. Phosp. Plb. Puls. Ran-sc. Rhus. Selen. Sep. Sil. Stront. Sulph. Thuj.
— — tremor, Euph.
— — twitching of limbs, Ambr. Ars. Bell. Igt. Merc-cor. Puls. Rhus. Selen. Stront.
— — urination, desire for, Thuj.
— — vertigo, Calad. Merc-cor.
— — visions, dreadful, Carb-veg.
— — — as soon as he closes the eyes, Calc.
— — — — — — — — disappear on opening them, Apis. Lach. Thuj.
Falling asleep late, Amm-c. Anac. Apis. *Ars.* Bell. Borax. *Bry.* Calad. *Calc.* Carb-an. Carb-veg. Chelid. *Chin.* Clem. Con. Cycl. Euph. *Ferr.* Ferr-m. Gels. Glon. Graph. Guaj. Hep. Hyosc. Igt. *Kali-c.* Lach. Led. Lith. *Lyc.* Mgn-m. *Merc.* Mur-ac. Ntr-m. Nitr-ac. *Nux.* Ol-an. Petros. Phell. *Phosp.* Phosp-ac. Plb. *Puls.* Ran-b. Rat. *Rhus.* Sabad. Selen. *Sep.* Sil. Spig. *Stann. Staph.* Stront. *Sulph.* Sulph-ac. Tabac. Tart. Tereb. *Thuj.* Valer. Viol-tr. Zinc.
— — every other evening, Lach.
— — when going to bed late, Amm-c.
Sleep anxious, Acon. Ars. Bell. Cast. Cocc. Ferr. Kali-c. Op.
— dizzy, Calad. Graph.
— interrupted, Ars. Cocc. Dig. Par. Zinc.
— too long, Berb. *Borax.* Lact. Merc. Ntr-c. Nux. Ol-an. Phell. Plat. *Sulph.*
— profound, sound, Ars. *Bell.* Berb. Croc. Cupr. Eugen. Hyosc. *Igt.* Laur. Led. *Nux-m. Op. Phosp-ac.* Psor. Puls. *Rhod.* Sec-c. *Seneg.* Sol-m. Spig. Stann. *Stram.* Sulph. *Tart.* Therid. Verat.
— — before midnight, Rhod.
— — in the morning, Bry. Hep. Graph. Nux. Op. Sulph.
— light, Acon. Alum. Ars. Calad. Igt. *Merc.* Igt. Ol-an. *Selen.* Sil. Sulph. Tart.

— restless, Alum. Ambr. Anac. Ang. Arg-n. *Ars.* Aur. *Bar-c.* Bell. Berb. Bov. Bry. Calc. Cast. *Cham. Chin.* Cic. Coloc. Creos. Diad. Dig. Dulc. *Ferr.* Ferr-m. Graph. Hep. Igt. Ind. Ip. Kali-c. Kali-jod. Kali-m. Lact. *Lyc.* Meny. Merc. Mez. Mur-ac. Ntr-c. Ntr-s. Nicc. Nitr-ac. Nitr. Petr. Phosp. Puls. *Rheum. Rhus.* Sabad. *Sabin.* Scill. Seneg. *Sep. Sil. Spig.* Stann. Staph. Stram. Stront. *Sulph.* Tabac. *Tereb.* Teucr. Thuj. Valer. Verb. Viol-tr. Zinc.
— slumber, like, half sleep, Arn. Ars. Bell. Bry. Canth. *Cham.* Cic. Cocc. Dig. Euph. Graph. *Hep.* Kali-c. *Lach.* Merc. Nitr-ac. Op. *Par. Petr.* Ran-sc. Rhus. Sabad. Samb. Selen. Sil.
— somnolency, Bry. Con. Croc. *Nux-m.* Op. Tart.
— soporous, Anac. *Bell.* Bry. Calad. Calc. *Camph.* Cicc. Cocc. Con. Croc. Euph. Graph. Hell. *Hep.* Hyosc. Igt. *Led.* Nitr. *Nux-m.* 'Nux. *Op.* Phosp. Plb. Puls. Sulph. *Tart.* Valer. *Verat. Seneg.* Spig. *Stram.*
— — in the early morning, Bell. Calc. Con. *Graph.* Led. *Nux.* Phosp.
— unrefreshing, Acon. Agar. *Alum.* Ambr. Berb. Bism. *Bry.* Calc. Cannab. Caust. Chelid. Chin. Cic. Clem. Con. Daph. Graph *Hep.* Igt. Kali-b. Kobalt. Lach. Lact. Lyc. Mgn-c. Mgn-m. Mez. Ntr-c. Ntr-m. Nitr-ac. *Op.* Petr. *Phosp.* Pod. Sabad. Selen. Sep. Sil. Spig. Stann. Staph. *Sulph.* Tart. Teucr. *Thuj.* Zinc.
Coma, *Agn. Ant.* Ars. *Asa-f.* Bar-c Bell. Bry. Camph. *Caust.* Coloc. Con. *Croc,* Cupr. *Dig. Laur.* Led. *Nux-m.* Nux. *Op.* Phosp. *Phosp-ac.* Plb. Puls. *Sec-c.* Sep. *Stram.* Tart. Tereb. *Verat.* Zinc. Zing.
— day and night, Bar-c.
— in evening, Ars. Tart.
— — forenoon, Ant.
— with lustreless, glassy eyes, Croc.
— in open air, Tart.
— with snoring, Bell. Camph. Carb-veg. Hyosc. Op. Rhus. Sil. Stram.
— tertian type, Sep.
— with vomiting, Dig.
Coma vigil, *Acon.* Aeth. Agar. Anac. Ars. *Bry. Cham.* Cocc. Con. *Cycl.* Euph. *Hell.* Hep. Hydroc-ac. *Hyosc. Laur. Merc. Mosch.* Nux. Oleand. *Op.* Phosp. Phosp-ac. *Plb. Puls.* Rhus. Spong. Sulph. *Verat.*
— — feverish, Acon. *Cham. Puls.*
During sleep, abdomen, rumbling in, Cupr.
— — anxiety, *Ars. Bell.* Cocc. *Ferr. Hep.* Petr.
— — biting the tongue, Ind. Mez. Phosp-ac. Therid. Zinc.

31. SLEEP AND DREAMS.

During sleep, burning in veins, Ars.
— — called, thinks he is, Sep.
— — chilliness, Borax.
— — clinching of thumbs, Viol-tr.
— — coldness of body, Ambr.
— — congestion of blood, Ntr-c. Sep.
— — — — — to chest, Puls.
— — — — head, Berb.
— — convulsions, Rheum.
— — cough, Arn. Bell. Calc. Cham. Lach. Merc. Verb.
— — — barking, Nitr-ac.
— — — dry, Mgn-s.
— — — loud, Lyc.
— — delirium, Acon. Arn. Aur. Bell. Cact. Camph. Cocc. Coloc. Dig. Dulc. Gels. Hyosc. Lach. Mur-ac. Nux. Op. Puls. Rheum. Sec-c. Sep. Spong. Stram. Sulph. Verat.
— — dyspnoea when falling asleep as if he would suffocate, Graph.
— — epistaxis, Graph. Merc. (compare Sect. 7).
— — eyes, convulsed, Hell. Op. Phosp-ac.
— — — half open, Bell. Bry. Caps. Coloc. Ferr. Ferr-m. Hell. Ip. Op. Phosp-ac. Pod. Samb. Stram. Sulph. Tart. Verat.
— — — staring, Tart.
— — — lids twitching, Rheum.
— — — pupils turned up, Hell.
— — — face cold and pale, Bell.
— — — puffed up, Op.
— — — red, Arn. Op. Viol-tr.
— — — twitching facial muscles, Rheum.
— — fearful moaning, Stann.
— — fever, Amm-c. Amm-m. Bell. Borax. Calc. Hell. Lyc. Mgn-c. Merc. Ntr-c. Nicc. Nitr-ac. Puls. Sulph.
— — grasping with the hands, Arn. Bell. Borax. Cocc. Hyosc. Op. Phosp-ac. Rhus.
— — grinding of the teeth, Acon. Ant. Ars. Bell. Caust. Cina. Coff. Con. Hyosc. Kali-c. Plb. Pod. Sep. Stram. Verat.
— — hallooing, shouting, Borax. Bry. Cham. Cocc. Lyc. Mgn-c. Ruta. Stram. Sulph. (compare Shrieking.)
— — hands cold, Bell. Carb-veg. Merc.
— — — hot, Lach. Staph.
— — head lifted from pillow or starts up and gazes, Stram.
— — headache, Cham. Mgn-m.
— — heat, Dulc. Petr. Viol-tr.
— — — dry, Samb. Thuj.
— — hiccough, Merc-cor.
— — jaw hanging, Nux Op.
— — jerks, Ambr. Ars. Bell. Bry. Cast. Cham. Con. Cupr. Dulc. Hep. Igt. Kali-c. Kobalt Lyc. Merc-cor. Ntr-c. Ntr-m. Ntr-s. Nitr-ac. Op. Phosp. Puls. Ran-sc. Rheum. Selen. Sep. Sil. Stann. Staph. Stront. Sulph.

Sulph-ac. Tart. Thuj. Viol-tr. Zinc.
— — — through the whole body, Cupr. Ip. Mez. Ntr-c. Op. Sulph. Tart. Zinc.
— — — of feet, Phosp.
— — illusions of fancy, Bell. Calc. Cham. Led. Phosp. Puls. Stram.
— — — — auditory nerve, Carb-veg. Cham.
— — laughing aloud, Caust. Croc. Hyosc. Lyc. Sil. Sulph.
— — — and whining, Aur. Cham.
— — — with spasms, Igt.
— — — when lying on the back, waking with screams, Guaj.
— — masticating motion, Calc. Sep.
— — mental labor, Anac. Bry. Igt. Lach. Sabad. Sabin.
— — moaning, Apis. Ars. Aur. Bell. Caust. Cham. Cupr. Igt. Lach. Lyc. Merc. Mur-ac. Nitr-ac. Nux. Pod. Puls. Stram.
— — motion of limbs, Caust.
— — mouth open, Merc. Op. Rhus. Samb.
— — moving about in bed, Acon. Puls. Rheum.
— — nightmare, Acon. Alum. Ambr. Amm-c. Amm-m. Arum-trif. Bell. Bry. Cina. Cinnab. Con. Cycl. Daph. Guaj. Hep. Kali-c. Lvc. Mgn-m. Mez. Ntr-m. Nitr-ac. Nitr. Nux. Op. Phosp. Puls. Ruta. Sil. Sulph. Tabac. Tereb. Valer.
— — numbness of left leg and right arm, Kali-c.
— — palpitation of heart, Ntr-c.
— — perspiration, Carb-an. Cic. Chin. Dros. Euph. Ferr. Jatr. Merc. Nux. Phosp. Puls. Selen. Thuj.
— — — about head when falling asleep, Graph.
— — picking the bed clothes, Arn. Ars. Bell. Chin. Cocc. Hyosc. Op. Phosp. Phosp-ac. Rhus. Stram.
— — redness of face, Arn. Arum. Op. Viol-tr.
— — reveries, Acon. Arn. Bry. Camph. Coloc. Dulc.
— — respiration short, Acon. Cham. Merc. Rhus.
— — inspirations, shorter than expirations Camph.
— — respiration intermittent, Op.
— — — obstruction of, Hep.
— — — slow, Chin. Op.
— — — wheezing, Nux.
— — shrieking, Anac. Bell. Borax. Calc. Cham. Cina. Cocc. Croc. Diad. Jalap. Lyc. Mgn-c. Mgn-m. Puls. Rheum. Ruta. Senna. Sil. Stram. Sulph. Tart. Thuj.
— — — in children. Bell. Borax. Cham. Cina. Coff. Jalap. Ip. Rheum. Senna.

31. SLEEP AND DREAMS.

During sleep, singing, Bell. Croc. Phosp-ac. Sulph.
— — sliding down in bed, Ars. Mur-ac.
— — smiling, Hyosc. Igt. Lyc. Phosp-ac.
— — sneezing, Nitr-ac.
— — snoring, Bell. Camph. *Chin.* Dros. Hyosc. Igt. Laur. Mur-ac. Nux. *Op.* Rheum. Sil. *Stram.* Sulph.
— — — inspirations, respirations puffing, Chin.
— — — moaning, Calc.
— — — suffocative, Bell.
— — — when expiring. Nux. Op. Tart.
— — — — inspiring, Bell. Bry. Caps. Cham. Chin. Hyosc. Igt. Nux. Puls. Rheum.
— — — — inspiring and expiring, Arn. Camph. Chin.
— — — — lying on the back, Dros. Dulc. Kali-c. Mgn-c. Sulph.
— — snuffling, Nux. Samb.
— — sobbing, anxious, Aur. Calad. Hyosc.
— — somnambulism, Acon. Agar. Alum. Anac. *Bry.* Cycl. Kalm. Ntr-m. *Op.* Petr. *Phosp. Sil.* Spong. Sulph.
— — starting, Agn. Arn. *Ars. Bell.* Bism. Borax. Bry. Calad. Caust. *Cham.* Cina. Cor-r. Croc. Daph. Dig. Dros. Euph. Graph. Hep. Hyosc. Ip. Iris. Kali-c. Lach. Led. Lyc. Mgn-c. Merc. Merc-cor. Ntr-c. Ntr-m. Nitr-ac. *Nux.* Op. Petr. Phosp. Plb. *Puls. Rheum.* Rhus. Ruta. Sabad. Sacch. Samb. Sec-c. Selen. Sil. Staph. Stram. Stront. Sulph. Tabac. *Tart.* Thuj. Verat.
— — — as if falling from a height into the water, Dig.
— — — when touched, Stram.
— — — with wild gestures, Stram.
— — suffocative attacks, Op.
— — talking, Acon. Alum. Arn. Ars. Bar-c. Bell. Bry. Calc. Camph. Carb-an. Carb-veg. Cham. Cinnab. Graph. Igt. Kalm. Kali-c. Mgn-c. Mgn-m. Merc. Mur-ac. Ntr-m. Nitr-ac. Nux. Phosp. Phosp-ac. Plb. *Puls.* Raph. Rhus. Sabin. Sep. Sil. Stann. *Sulph.* Tart. Zinc.
— — thirst, Bry. Carb-veg. Caust. Cham. Cycl. Nitr-ac. Sil. Sulph. Sulph-ac.
— — tossing about, Alum. *Ars.* Bell. Bry. Calc. *Cast Cham.* Cic. *Cina.* Cist. Clem. Cocc. Cor-r. Creos. Ferr. Ferr-m. Guaj. Hell. Igt. Lach. Led. Lyc. Mur-ac. Ntr-c. Ntr-m. Op. Par. Phosp. Puls. *Ran-sc.* Rheum. Rhus. Scill. Senna. Sep. Staph. Sulph. Valer. Verat.
— — tremor of, limbs, Tart.
— — twitching of fingers, Rheum. Sulph-ac.
— — — hands, Viol-tr.
— — — convulsive of muscles, Cupr. Hell. Sil.
— — uncovering, Cor-r. Plat.
— — weeping, Alum. Aur. Carb-an. Cham. Cina. Con. Hyosc. Kali-c. Lyc. Mgn-c. Merc. Ntr-m. Nitr-ac. Nux. Phosp. Puls. Rheum. Rhus. Sil. Stann. Stram.
— — — appearance, Phosp-ac.
— — whining, Alum. Arn. Ars. Bar-c. Bell. Borax. Bry. Calad. Carb-an. Cham. Chin. Ip. Lach. Lyc. Mgn-c. Merc. Mur-ac. Nitr-ac. Nux. Op. Phosp-ac. Puls. Rheum. Stram. Sulph. Verat.
Sleep disturbed by abdominal pains, Acon. Ambr. Amm-c. Amm-m. Borax. Gels. Kali-c. Lyc. Mgn-c. Mgn-s. Ntr-c. Nicc. Nitr-ac. Phosp. *Plb. Rhus.* Sep. Sulph. Verat.
— — aggregation of thoughts, Borax. *Calc.* Chin. Coff. Grap. Hep. Kali-c. *Lyc. Nux.* Puls. Sabad. Sil. *Staph. Sulph.* Viol-tr.
— — — peevish, Alum. Graph. Nux.
— — — sorrowful, Graph.
— — anxiety, timorous, Acon. Alum. Amm-c. *Ars.* Bar-c. *Bell.* Bry. Calc. Cannab. Carb-an. Carb-veg. *Caust. Cham.* Cina. *Cocc.* Dis. *Graph.* Hyosc. Kali-c. Lyc. Mgn-c. *Merc.* Nitr-ac. Nux. Petr. *Phosp.* Plb. Ran-sc. Rhus. Sabad. Sep. Sulph. Verat.
— — arms, heaviness in, Diad.
— — — as if enlarged, Diad.
— — — burning in veins, *Ars.*
— — chills, Lyc. *Mur-ac.*
— — coldness, Alum. Ambr. Amm-c. Arg. Ars. Bov. Calc. Carb-veg. Caust. Creos. Daph. Ferr. Mgn-s. Merc. Mur-ac. Ntr-s. Nux. Staph. Tart-ac. Thuj.
— — — of feet, Amm-m. Carb-veg. Zinc.
— — congestion of blood, Amm-c. Asar. Bar-c. Benz-ac. Borax. Bry. Cact. Calc. Croton. Merc. Ntr-c. Nux. Phosp. Psor. *Puls.* Ran-b. Rhus. Sabin. Senna. Sep. Sil.
— — — to chest, Puls.
— — — — head, Amm-c. Cycl. *Psor.* Puls. Sil.
— — — lower legs, Meph.
— — — cough, dry, Sang.
— — — tickling, Lach.
— — cyphers before the eyes, Phosp-ac.
— — dreams, anxious, Bry. Coloc. Mez.
— — — many, Apis.
— — — as soon as he falls asleep, Bell.
— — excitement, nervous, Ambr. Camph. Canth. Caps. Chin. Coff. *Colch.* Hyosc. Lach. Laur. Merc. Mosch. Nitr-ac. Nux. Puls. Ran-b. Sep. Sulph. Sulph-ac. *Teucr.*
— — fear of ghosts, Carb-veg. Cocc.
— — — suffocation, Arum-trif. Carb-veg.
— — formication, Carb-veg. Lyc.

Sleep disturbed by giddiness, vertigo, Amm-c. Calc. Caust. Ntr-c. Phosp. Spong. Sulph. Therid.
— — hawking of mucus, Amm-c.
— — headache, Arg-n. Canth. *Chin.* Gels. Kali-b. Mgn-s. Ntr-m. Nitr-ac. Sil.
— — heat, Ars. Benz-ac. Bry. *Calc.* Carb-an. Carb-veg. *Caust.* Cham. Dulc. *Hep.* Laur. Mgn-c. Merc. Ntr-m. Nicc. Nitr-ac. Nitr. *Petr. Phosp.* Phosp-ac. Puls. Ran-b. Ran-sc. Rhod. Sabin. Samb. Sil. Stront. Tar. Thuj.
— — at 2 A.M., Benz-ac.
— — — 3 A.M., Ang. Euphr.
— — anxious, Kali-b. Ntr-m. Puls.
— — dry, Caust. Phosp. Thuj.
— — in head, Camph. *Sil.*
— — — hands, Staph.
— — with aversion to being uncovered, Mgn-c
— — heaviness of legs, Caust.
— — hunger, Chin. Lyc. Teucr.
— — imaginary forms, Bell. Calc. Carb-veg. Chin. Coff. Led. Merc. Phosp. Sil.
— — — dreadful, Calc. Carb-an.
— — — frightful, Bell. Calc. Carb-veg. Merc. Sil.
— — — voluptuous, Calc-c.
— — itching, Amm-c. Amm-m. Bar-c. Berb. Cocc. Creos. Merc. Mez. Nux. Psor. Puls. Sulph. Thuj.
— — — caused by ascarides, Ferr.
— — jerks, Ambr. Ars. Bell. Carb-veg. Cham. Con. Cor-r. Cupr. Daph. Dulc. Hep. Igt. Ip. Kali-c. Kobalt. Lyc. Ntr-c. Ntr-s. Op. Phosp. Puls. Rheum. Rhus. Selen. Sep. Sil. Staph. Stront. Sulph. Sulph-ac. Tart. Thuj. Viol-tr.
— — — eyes, Cocc. Puls.
— — — face, Op. Rheum.
— — — feet, Phosp.
— — — fingers, Anac. Ars. Cocc. Rheum. Sulph-ac.
— — — head, Cocc.
— — — mouth, Anac. Op. Puls.
— — — upwards from larynx, with saltish mucus, Spong.
— — moaning, Cina.
— — nausea, Alum. Amm-c. Con. Kali-b. Nitr-ac. Phosp. Rhus. Sil.
— — oppression of chest, Acon. Alum. Ars. Calc. Carb-veg. Cham. Graph. Kali-c. Lact. Lyc. Mgn-c. Op. Phosp. Psor. Ran-b. Seneg. Spong. Sulph.
— — pains, Lil-tigr.
— — — in back, Diad.
— — — chest, Alum. Amm-c. Amm-m. Graph. Sabad. Seneg.
— — — face, Mez. Nicc.
— — — gums, Dolich.
— — — as if the menses were coming on, Murex.
— — — sacral region, Mgn-s.
— — — stomach, Graph. Rhus. Seneg.
— — — calves of legs, Staph.
— — — toes, Amm-c.
— — — in tetters and ulcers, Staph.
— — — on part on which he lies, Hep. Thuj.
— — perspiration, Cic. Kali-b. Sabin.
— — restlessness, Agar. *Ars.* Bell. Bry. *Calc. Carb-an. Carb-veg.* Caust. *Cham.* Chin. Clem. *Cocc.* Con. Dig. Guaj. Hell. *Jalap.* Laur. Led. Mgn-c. *Mgn-m.* Merc. Ntr-c. Ntr-s. Nicc. Nux. Oleand. Op. *Phosp.* Phosp-ac. Plat. *Ran-b. Rhod. Rhus.* Ruta. *Senna. Sil.* Spig. Stann. Sulph. Thuj. Tilia.
— — — in children, Bell. *Cham. Cina.* Coff. Ip. *Jalap. Rheum.* Senna.
— — — after midnight, Ferr.
— — — towards morning, Rhod.
— — — the side on which he lies becomes sore, must move, Hep.
— — sadness, Murex.
— — shrill shrieks, (in hydrocephalus), Apis.
— — sighing, Lach. Merc.
— — sore, pain as from a, in urethra, Cinnab.
— — throat, Amm-c.
— — sorrowful thoughts, Graph.
— — sprained pain on the parts lain on, Mosch.
— — stitches here and there, Berb. Cannab. Euph.
— — suffocative fit, Graph. Kali-c. Samb.
— — thirst, Berb. *Bry.* Calc. Cham. Coff. Colch. Mgn-m. Nitr-ac. Sulph.
— — tightness of chest, Calc.
— — tingling in skin, Bar-c. Carb-veg. Lyc.
— — throat, dry, Cist.
— — toothache, Bar-c. Mgn-c. Mgn-m.
— — tossing about, Acon. Alum. Ars. Asa-f. Bell. Calc. Cham. Croton. Creos. Guaj. Hell. Lach. Sulph.
— — tremor, Euph.
— — internal, Ntr-m.
— — twitches, Alum. Ars. Bell. Calc. Cast. Igt. Kali-c. Puls. Rhus. Selen. Sep.
— — urinate, desire to, Amm-c. Dig. Kali-b. Lach. Lith. Rhus.
— — visions, Alum. Chin. Igt. Led. Op. Phosp. Phosp-ac. Rhus. Spong.
— — — dreadful, Bell. Calc. Carb-an. Merc. Sil. Sulph.
— — vomiting, Nitr-ac. Sil.
Positions in sleep.
— on the abdomen, Bell. Cina. Cocc. Coloc. Puls. Stram.
— arms over the head, Euph. Nux. Puls. Rheum. Verat.
— — crossed on abdomen, Puls.

31. SLEEP AND DREAMS.

Positions in sleep, hands under head, Colco. Nux. Tait. Viol-od.
— head bent backwards, Bell. Calc. Cina. Spong.
— — low, Spong.
— knees apart, Cham.
— — bent, Viol-od.
— kneeling, Stram,
— legs crossed, Rhod.
— — stretched apart, Cham.
— — drawn up, Plat. Puls.
— — one drawn up, the other stretched out, Stann.
— inclined to have, uncovered, Plat.
— on left side, Bar-c. Sabin.
— — — impossible, Lyc.
— — right side, impossible, Bry. Psor.
— — either side, impossible, Acon. Ferr. Ferr-m. Mosch. Phosp. Ran-b. Rhus. Sabad. Sulph.
— lying intolerable, Lyc. Sulph.
— — on one side, Bar-c. Colch. Phosp.
— sitting, Ars. Cina. Lyc. Rhus. Sulph.
— supine, on the back, *Bry.* Calc. Cic. Colch. Dros. Ferr. Igt. Lyc. Nux. Plat. *Puls. Rhus.* Stram. Sulph. Viol-od.
Dreams, Acon. *Alum.* Arn. *Bry.* Calc. *Chin.* Cic. Con. Graph. Igt. Lach. *Mgn-c.* Merc. Ntr-c. Ntr-m. *Nux. Phosp.* Phosp-ac. *Puls. Rhus.* Sabad. Sep. *Sil.* Stann. Staph. *Sulph.* Tar. Tart. Tereb. Therid. Thuj.
— fatal accidents of, Amm-m. Arn. Bell. Cham. Chin. *Graph.* Kali-c. Lyc. *Nux. Puls.* Sass. Sulph. *Sulph-ac.* Thuj.
— of the adventures of the day, Bry. Cic. Rhus.
— alarming, even after waking, Calc. Chin. *Phosp-ac.* Psor.
— animals of, Amm-m. *Arn.* Nux.
— — — which bite, Merc. Phosp. Puls.
— amorous, Ant. Canth. Con. Graph. Igt. Lach. *Ntr-c. Nux.* Oleand. Phosp. Plat. Puls. Sabad. Sep. Sil. *Staph. Viol-tr.* (compare Voluptuous.)
— anxious, Acon. *Alum.* Ambr. *Amm-m.* Anac. Arg. *Arn.* Ars. Aur. Bar-c. Bell. Berb. Bov. Bry. Calc. Carb-veg. Cast. *Caust. Chin. Cocc.* Con. Cor-r. Creos. Dig. *Graph.* Hell. Hep. Igt. Iod. *Kali-c. Laur.* Led. Lyc. *Mgn-c.* Mgn-m. Mgn-s. *Mang.* Merc. Ntr-c. Ntr-m. Nicc. Nitr-ac. Nitr. *Nux.* Op. Petr. Petros. *Phosp. Phosp-ac.* Plat. Plb. *Puls. Ran-b. Ran-sc.* Rheum. Rhus. Sass. *Sep. Sil.* Spong. Stann. Staph. Stram. *Sulph.* Sulph-ac. *Thuj.* Valer. *Verat.* Verb.
— — — if he lies on the left side, Lyc. Phosp. Puls. Sep. Thuj.
— apprehensive, Phosp.
— arrested, as if he would be, Clem.
— black forms, Arn. Ars. Puls.
— business, Anac. Bell. *Bry.* Chelid. Cic.

Croc. Elaps. Kali-c. *Lach.* Lyc. Merc. Nux. Phosp. Rhus. Sass. *Sil.* Staph.
— — of the day, Bry. Mgn-c. Nux. Puls. Rhus.
— calling out, Kali-c. Thuj.
— cats of, Arn. Ars. Daph. Hyosc. Lac-can. Puls.
— cellar, of being confined in a, Bov.
— choked, of being, Phosp. Zinc.
— clairvoyant, Acon. Phosp.
— confused, Bar-c. Bry. Cannab. *Chin.* Cic. Eugen. Hell. Ntr-c. Puls. Stann. Valer.
— — after midnight, *Chin.*
— full of confusion and agitation, Nux.
— continued after waking, Calc. *Chin.* Igt. Ntr-c. Ntr-m.
— corpses of, and dead people, Amm-c. Anac. Arn. *Ars.* Elaps. Graph. Kali-c. *Mgn-c.* Phosp. Plat. *Thuj.* Verb.
— cruel, Nux. Selen. Sil.
— danger of, Anac. Calc-ph. Con. Hep. Kali-c. Nitr. Ran-b. Thuj.
— — deadly, Thuj. (compare Accidents.)
— defamatory, Mosch.
— devils of, Kali-c. Lac-can. Ntr-c. Nicc.
— diseases, of, Calc. Creos. Kali c. *Nux.* Sulph. Verat. Zinc.
— dogs, of, Arn. Calc. Lyc. Merc. Sil. Sulph. Verat. Zinc.
— dreadful, Cast. *Nux.* Psor. Ran-sc. Verb. Zinc.
— drowning, of, Alum. Igt. Merc. Ran-b. Samb.
— emaciated, of being, Creos.
— embarrassment, with, *Amm-m. Ars.* Graph. Mgn-c. Phosp.
— enemies, pursued by, Con.
— escaping recollection, Aur. Bell. Cic. Hell. Lyc. Merc. Meny. Selen. Spig. Tar. Verat.
— falling, of, Amm-m. Dig. Kali-c. *Thuj.* Zinc-ox.
— fanciful, Calc. Kali-c. Lach. Spong.
— fearful, Con.
— fire, of, Anac. Hep. Mgn-c. Mgn-m. Phosp.
— firing, shooting, of, Amm-m.
— fixed upon one subject, Igt.
— flying, of, Lyc. Ntr-s.
— forest, of a, Canth. Mgn-m. Sep.
— frightful, *Amm-m.* Aur. *Bell.* Bov. Diad. Dig. Euphr. Graph. Jac-cor. Mgn-m. Merc. Merc-jod. Ntr-c. Ntr-m. Ntr-s. Nicc. Ox-ac. *Phosp.* Plat. Ran-sc. Sass. Sep. Sulph. Zinc.
— furunculi, of, Prun.
— ghosts of, *Carb-veg.* Igt,
— graves, pits, of, Anac. Arn.
— hæmoptisis, of, Meph.
— hammorhages, of, Phosp.
— heavy, *Chin.* Dulc. *Laur.* Ntr-m. Ntr-s. Nux. Sass. Thuj.
— — towards morning, *Nux.*

31. SLEEP AND DREAMS.

Dreams, help, calling for, Kali-c.
— historical, Amm-c. Mgn-c. Merc. Phosp.
— horrible, Cast. *Nux. Psor.* Ran-sc. Verb. Zinc.
— horses, of, Alum.
— indifferent, Bry. Chin. Mgn-c. Nux. Phosp-ac. Puls. Rhus. Sep. Sulph.
— interrupted, Rhus.
— invention, full of, Lach. Sabin.
— jocose and joyful, Croc.
— lasting long, Acon. Bry. Calc. Chin. *Igt.* Ntr-c. Puls.
— lice, of, Amm-c. Mur-ac. Nux. Phosp.
— loathsome, Anac. Nux. Puls. Zinc.
— lying in bed, as if some body were, Petr.
— many, Acon. *Alum.* Ang. Arn. Asa-f. Bar-c. Bell. Bov. *Bry.* Calc. Caps. *Chin.* Cic. Clem. Coloc. Ferr. Ferr-m. Graph. Igt. *Kali-c.* Lach. Lyc. Mgn-c. Mgn-s. *Mang.* Merc. Ntr-c. Ntr-m. Nitr-ac. *Nux. Par.* Petr. *Phosp.* Phosp-ac. Plb. *Puls. Rhus.* Sabad. *Sep. Sil. Stann.* Staph. Stram. Stront. *Sulph.* Tar. Tart. *Tereb.* Therid. Thuj.
— marriage of, Alum.
— mental exertion, with, Acon. Anac. •Bry. *Igt.* Lach. Rhus. Sabad. Sabin. Thuj.
— merry, Asa-f. Croc. Lach. *Op.*
— mice, of, Colch.
— mind, affecting the, Bry. Chin. *Igt.* Lach. Ntr-m. Nux. Oleand. Phosp. Phosp-ac. Sabad. Sabin. Sulph. Thuj. Viol-tr.
— miscarrying undertakings, of, Dig. Mosch.
— money, Alum. Cycl. Mgn-c. Puls.
— — counterfeit, Zinc-ox.
— murder, of, Amm-c. Calc. Carb-an. Guaj. Igt. Kali-jod. Lach. Lact. Led. Lyc. Merc. Ntr-c. *Ntr-m.* Ol-an. *Petr.* Rhus. Sil. Spong. *Staph.* Zinc.
— murdered, of being, Amm-m. Guaj. Igt. Kali-jod. Lact. Lyc. Merc. Zinc.
— peevish, Ant. Asar. Bry. Caust. Mgn-s.
— people, of, Bell. Merc.
— phantastical, *Calc.* Carb-an. Con. Graph. Kali-c. Ntr-c. *Ntr-m. Op.* Sep. Sulph.
— pleasant, Ant. Aur. *Calc.* Carb-an. Coff. Croc. Graph. Kali-c. Lach. Mgn-c. *Ntr-c.* Ntr-m. Nux. *Op.* Phosp. Phosp-ac. Plat. *Puls.* Sabad. *Sep.* Sil. Staph. Sulph. *Viol-tr.*
— poisoned, of being, Creos. Ntr-m.
— quarrelling, about, Ant. Aur. Bry. Caust. Mgn-c. Nicc. Nux. Phosp. Selen. Stann.
— recalling things forgotten, Calad.
— recollected, *Mang.* Meph.
— restless, Led. Nitr. *Oleand.* Sulph. Zinc.
— revelling, rioting, of, Graph. Kali-c.

Lyc. Ntr-c. Ntr-m. Nux. Petr. Sil. Sulph. Zinc.
— reverie, full of, *Ambr.* Ars. Bar-c. Calc. Carb-an. Carb-veg. Con. *Graph.* Kali-c. Led. Lyc. Ntr-c. Ntr-m. Nitr. Petr. Psor. Sep. *Sil.* Spong. Stront. *Sulph. Tart.* Zinc.
— — when falling asleep, Spong.
— riots, of, Bry. Con. Guaj. Ind. Kali-c. Lyc. Ntr-c. Ntr-m. Phosp. Puls. Stann.
— sad, Lyc. *Rheum.* Spong.
— serpents, of, Alum. Bov. Grat. Kali-c. Ran-sc. Rat. Sil.
— sick people, Calc. Rat.
— snow, Creos.
— sorrowful, Ars. Graph.
— spinning, Sass.
— stab, dread of being, while dreaming, Lach.
— swimming of, Iod. Lyc. Ran-b.
— teeth falling out, Nux.
— theives, of, Alum. *Mgn-c.* Merc. Ntr-c. Ntr-m. Sil.
— thirsty, of being, Ntr-m.
— thoughts of the day, continuation of, Igt.
— thunder storms, of, Arn. Ars.
— troublesome, Rhus.
— true, seeming, on waking, Ntr-c. Ntr-m.
— unmeaning, Chin.
— urinating, of, Creos. Lac-can. Merc-jod.
— vermin, of, Amm-c. Lac-can. Mur-ac. Nux. Phosp.
— vexatious, Alum. Ars. Asar. Bry. Caust. Con. Igt. Mgn-s. Mosch. Nux. Rhus. Staph. Sulph.
— vivid, Acon. Anac. Arn. Bell. Bry. Carb-veg. Cic. Clem. Cocc. Coloc. Ferr. Igt. Iod. Lyc. Mgn-c. *Mang.* Meny. Merc. Meph. Mez. Mosch. Mur-ac. Ntr-c. Ntr-m. Nux. Petr. *Phosp.* Phosp-ac. Ran-sc. Rheum. Rhus. Sabad. Sep. *Sil.* Stann. Stram. *Sulph.* Teucr. Viol-tr.
— voluptuous, Ant. Bism. Canth. Coloc. Con. Graph. Igt. Lach. Led. Lith. Lyc. Merc. Ntr-c. Ntr-m. Nitr-ac. *Nux.* Oleand. Op. Par. Phosp. Phosp-ac. Plat. Plb. Puls. Ran-b. Sabad. Samb. Sep. Sil. Staph. Thuj. Viol-tr.
— waking, during, Arn. Bell. Cham. Hep. Merc. Nux. Phosp-ac.
— war and bloodshed, of Plat. Thuj. Verb.
— water, of, *Amm-m.* Ars. Dig. Graph. Mgn-c. Ran-b.
— wedding of a, Alum. Mgn-m. Ntr-c.
— world, sees the end of the, Rhus.
— worms, creeping, Amm-c. Mur-ac. Nux. Phosp.

Wakefulness at night, Aur. Dulc. *Ntr-m.* Puls. *Ran-b.* Rat. Sep. Sil. Sulph. (compare Sleeplessness.)

31. SLEEP AND DREAMS.

After waking once, inability to sleep again, Amm-c. Ars. Aur. Borax. Dulc. Ferr. Ferr-m. Mgn-c. Merc. *Ntr-m.* Ol-an. Phosp. Puls. *Ran-b.* Ran-sc. Rat. Sass. Sep. *Sil* Sulph.

Awaking often at night, Ambr. Ars. *Calc.* Carb-an. Caust. Chin. *Hep.* Igt. Kali-c. Lyc. Merc. Nitr-ac. Nux. *Phosp. Puls.* Ran-b. Rhus. *Sep.* Sil. Staph. *Sulph.* (compare Sleep disturbed).
— from air wanting, Hep. Ip. Samb. Seneg.
— anxiety, with, Calc. Con. Plat. *Puls.* Rat. Samb.
— chills, from, Mur-ac. Ntr-s.
— colic, from, Ox-ac.
— contraction of chest after midnight, wheezing breathing, Lach.
— cough, Caust. Hep. Kali-c. Mgn-m. Nitr. Stront.
— — tickling, Lach.
— difficult, Berb. Calad. Ntr-c. Nux. Phell. Phosp-ac. Tabac. Teucr. Viol-tr.
— too early, Amm-m. Ars. Aur. Borax. Caps. Coff. *Dulc.* Graph. Guaj. *Kali-c.* Mgn c. *Merc.* Mez. *Mur-ac.* *Ntr-c.* Nitr-ac. *Nux.* Ol-an. Phell. Phosp-ac. *Ran-b.* Ran-sc. *Selen.* Sep. Sil. Staph. Sulph-ac. Verb.
— as from an electric shock above larynx, Hipp-m.
— with erection and desire to urinate, Hep. S.l.
— frequent, Ambr. Ars. Bar-c. Berb. Bism. Borax. *Calc.* Canth. Carb-an. Cast Caust. Chelid. Chin. Cic. Colch. Diad. Dig. Euph. Euphr. Graph. Guaj. *Hep.* Igt. Kali-c. *Lyc.* Merc. Mur-ac. Nicc. *Nitr-ac.* Nitr. Nux. Ol-an. Petr. Phell. *Phosp. Puls.* *Ran-b.* Rhus. Ruta. Sabin. Samb. Sass. Scill. Selen. *Sep.* Sil. Staph. *Stront. Sulph.* Tart. Tert b. Viol-tr. Zinc.
— — without any cause, Mgn-c. Sep.
— frightened, starting, Agn. Alum. Amm-c. Ant. Arn. Ars. Bell. Bism. Bry. Calc. Carb-veg. Cast. Caust. Cham. Cocc. Colch. Croc. Dig. Dros. Euph. Graph. Guaj. Hep.

Hyosc. Ind. Ip. Kali-b. Kali-jod. Lyc. Ntr-m. Nitr-ac. Petr. Phosp. Puls. Rat. Rheum. Ruta. Samb. Sass. Sep. Sil. Staph. Sulph. Tabac. Thuj. Zinc.
— at a certain hour, Selen.
— hunger, from, Lyc.
— itching of lobe of right ear, Kali-b.
— lewed dreams and emissions, with, Kobalt.
— least noise from, Selen.
— oppression of breathing, from, Graph. Kali-c.
— partial, Con.
— pressure in chest, Kali-b.
— touched, when, Ruta.
— unconsciousness, with, Chin. Plat. Puls. Rheum. Sol-nig.
— vomiting from, Dig.

On awaking, air wanting, Hep. Samb.
— anxiety, Calc. Con. Plat. Puls. Rat. Samb.
— chill in morning early, Mur-ac.
— cough, Acon. Ambr. Bell. Caust. Chin. Cina. Creos. Dig. Euphr. Lach. Nux. Phosp-ac. Rhus. Scill. Stram. Sulph-ac,
— cries, sudden, shrill, Apis.
— delirium, Bry. Cact. Sep.
— expression, serious, Stram.
— headache, Anac. Ntr-m. Rheum.
— does not know where he is, Chin. Plat. Puls. Sol-m.
— mouth offensive, Rheum.
— — dry, Rhus.
— perspiration, Anac. Berb. Chelid. Cic. Clem. Dros. Ntr-m. Nitr-ac. Samb.
— soreness in limbs, Lach. Viol-od.
— stiffness of limbs, Lach.
— taste bitter, Bry. Rhus.
— — putrid, Rheum.
— thirst, Berb. Phosp-ac. Rat. Sulph.
— tremor, Rat. Samb.
— to be uncovered, aversion, Clem.
— urinate, urgency to, Caust. Dig. Hep. Sil. Tart.
— weariness, Dros. Pod,
— aggravation of sufferings, Bell. Lach. Nux.

32. Fever.

CHILLS, COLDNESS, SHUDDERING, SHIVERING, HEAT, PULSE, AND THIRST DURING FEVERS.

Autumn, Bry. Chin. Nux. Rhus. Verat.
Bilious, Ars Bry. Calc. Cham. Chin. Igt. Ip. Nux. Puls. Tar. (compare, Sect. 34.)
— after anger, Cham. Coloc.
Catarrhal, Amm-c. Anac. *Bell.* Calad. *Cham.* Chin. Con. *Dulc.* Eugen. Hep. Igt. Mgn-c. Mang. Merc. Nux. Puls. Ruta. Spig. Sulph.
Coldness prevailing, Alum. *Bry.* Canth. *Caps.* Diad. *Ip.* Puls. Ran-b. *Sabad. Staph. Verat.*
Consumptive, (compare, Hectic.)
Exanthamatous, Acon. Apis. Arn. Ars. Bell. Bry. Calc. Canth. Carb-veg. Hyosc Ip. Lach. Merc. Mur-ac. Nux-m. Phosp. Phosp-ac. Rhus. Sec-c. Stram.
Gastric, Ars. Asar. Bell. Bry. Cham. Chin. Daph. Dig. Igt. Ip. Nux. Puls. Stram. Sulph. Tar. (compare, Sect. 34.)
Heat prevailing, *Acon. Bell. Bry.* Ip. *Nux* Sabad. *Sil. Valer.* Verat. (compare inflammatory.)
Hectic, Ars. Bar-c. Chin. Con. Cupr. Iod. Merc. Nux. Phosp. Puls. Stann. Sulph.
— in children, Merc.
Inflammatory, Acon. Bell. Bry. Cham. Merc. Puls.
Intermittent, *Ant. Arn. Ars.* Bell. Bov. Bry. Calc. *Caps. Carb-veg. Chin. Cina.* Cocc. *Diad.* Dros. Ferr. Igt. *Ip.* Lyc. Meny. *Ntr-m.* Nux-m. Nux. Petr. Puls. Ran-b. Ran-sc. Rhus. *Sabad.* Samb. Sang. *Sep. Sil.* Spig. *Staph.* Sulph. Thuj. Valer. *Verat.*
— malignant, Ars. Chin. Nux-m.
— marsh, Arn. *Ars.* Carb-veg. *Chin.* Cina. Ferr. *Ip.* Ntr-m. Rhus.
— in damp and cold seasons, Calc. Carb-Chin. Lach. Nux-m. Puls. Rhus. Sulph. Verat.
— in spring and summer and warm seasons, generally, Ant. *Ars. Bell.* Bry. *Calc. Caps.* Carb-veg. *Cina. Ip. Lach.* Ntr-m. Puls. *Sulph.* Thuj. *Verat.*
— after abuse of quinine, *Arn. Ars. Bell.* Calc. Caps. Carb-veg. Cina. *Ferr. Ip.* Lach. Meny. Merc. *Ntr-m.* Nux-m. Nux. *Puls.* Sacch. Sulph. *Verat*
— masked, *Ars.* Spig.

Malignant plague, Sacch.
Mercurial. Chin. Hep. Lach. Sulph.
Milk-fever, Acon. *Arn. Bell. Bry.* Cham. Coff. Igt. Merc. Op. Rhus.
Mucus, Ars. Bell. Bry. Cham. Chin. Cina. Dig. *Dulc.* Ip. *Merc.* Nux. *Puls.* Rheum. *Rhus.* Spig. Sulph-ac.
Nervous, Acon. Arn. *Ars.* Bapt. *Bell. Bry.* Camph. *Canth.* Carb-veg. Cham. *Chin. Cocc.* Croton. Cupr. Daph. Gels. *Hell. Hyosc.* Lach. Lact. *Lyc.* Merc. *Mur-ac. Ntr-m. Nux.* Op. *Phosp-ac.* Puls. *Rhus.* Sang. *Stram.* Sulph. Verat.
— slow, Ars. Asar. Bell. Camph. Canth. Chin. *Cocc.* Con. Cupr. Dig. *Hell.* Igt. Merc. Phosp-ac. Plb. Stann. Verat.
Postponing, Chin. Cina.
Anticipating, Ars. Chin. Igt. Ntr-m. Nux.
Pectoral forms, Pneumethorax, Bry. Carb-veg. Hyosc. Phosp. Rhus. Tart.
Puerperal, *Acon.* Actea-r. Arn. Ars. *Bell. Bry. Cham.* Coff. Coloc. Cupr. Gels. Hyosc. Igt. Ip. Kali-c. Lach. Nux. Op. Phosp. Plat. *Puls. Rhus.* Sec-c. Spig. Stram. Tilia. Verat. Verat-virid. Zinc.
— with fulness of breasts, Bry.
Putrid, *Ars.* Bell. Chin. Hyosc. Ip. Merc. Mur-ac. Nux-m. *Nux.* Op. Phosp-ac. *Rhus.* Sulph.
Quartan, Acon. Anac. Arn. *Ars.* Bell. Bry. Carb-veg. Cina. Clem. Clem. *Hyosc.* Igt. Iod. Ip. Lach. Lyc. Ntr-m. Nux-m. Nux. *Puls.* Rhus. *Sabad. Verat.*
— double, Bell. Chin. Graph. Puls. Stram, Spig Scill. Sulph.
— at same hour, Sabad.
Quotidian, Acon. Ars. Bell. Bry. Cact. Calc. Caps. Carb-veg. Chin. Cic. Cina. Diad. Dros. Gels. Graph. Igt. Ip. Kali-c. Lach. Lyc. Ntr-m. Nitr-ac. Nux. Puls. Rhus. Sabad. Spig. Stann. Staph. Stram. Sulph.
— double, Bell. Chin. Graph. Stram. Sulph.
— at same hour, Cact. Diad. Gels. Stann.
— — 11 A.M. to 4 P.M., Gels.
— — 3 P.M. Ang.
Spring, Lach.
Sweating, Merc. Op. Samb.

32. FEVER.

-Tertian, Alum. Anac. Ant. *Ars*. Bar-m. *Bell*. Borax. *Bry*. Calc. *Canth*. Caps. Carb-an. Carb-veg. Cham. *Chin*. Cic. Cina. Croton. Daph. Dros. Dulc Eupat. Ferr. Gels. Hyosc. Igt. *Ip*. Lach. *Lyc*. Mez. Ntr-m. Nux-m. *Nux*. *Puls*. *Rhus*. Sabad. Sulph. Verat.
— double, Ars. Chin. Dulc. Nux-m. *Rhus*.
Typhus, Bry. *Hyosc*. Hipp-m. Nux-m. Nux. *Rhus*. (compare, Putrid and nervous fevers.)
— abdominalis, Apis. Ars. Bell. Bry. Calc. Carb-veg. Chin. Colch. Gins. Ip. Lyc. Mur-ac. Nitr-ac. Nux. Phosp. Phosp-ac. Rhus. Sec-c. Sulph. Verat.
— apoplectic, Gels. Glon. Lach. Sang. Verat-virid.
— bilious, Bell. Cham. Merc.
— cerebral, Arn. Bapt. Bell. Bry. Hyosc. Lach. Nux-m. Op. Phosp. Rhus. Stram. Verat.
— mucus, Merc. Puls. Rhus.
— stupid, Arn. Ars. Bell. Bry. Carb-veg. Chin Cocc. Hell Hyosc. Lach. Mur-ac. Nitr. Nux. Op. Phosp. Phosp-ac. Rhus. Sec-c. Stram. Verat.
— versatile, Bell. Bry. Cham. Cina. Dig. Hyosc. Igt. Lyc. Mur-ac. Nux. Op. Phosp-ac. Puls. Rhus. Stram.
Worm fever, Acon. Cic. Cina. Dig. Filix. Hyosc. Merc. Nux. Sabad. *Sil*. *Spig*. Stann. Stram. Valer. Sulph.
In morning, Ambr. Ang. Arn. Bell Bry. Calc. Carb-veg. Chin. Con. Eupat. Euphr. Gels. Graph. Hep. Kali-b. Lach. Lam. Lyc. Mgn-c. Merc. Ntr-m. Nicc. Nitr-ac. Nux. Sabad. Sep. Spig. Spong. Staph. Sulph.
— forenoon, Calc. Chin. Cop. Ntr-m. Sabad.
— noon, Ant. Asar. Borax. Calc. Kali-c. Lob. Mgn-c. Spig. Stram.
— afternoon, Alum. Ant. *Ars*. Calc. Caust. Chin. Coff. Dig. Hyosc. Lach. Ntr-m. Nitr-ac. Nux. Phosp. Puls. *Ran-b*. Spong. Staph. Sulph.
— evening, Acon. *Alum*. Ant. *Arn*. Ars. *Bell*. Bov. Bry. *Calad*. Calc. Carb-veg. Cham. Chin. Cycl. Hell. Igt. Ip. Lach. Led. Lyc. Nitr-ac. Nux. Petr. *Phosp*. Phosp-ac. Puls. *Ran-b*. Rhod. *Rhus*. Sabad. Sabin. Sep. Spig. *Staph*. Sulph. Thuj.
— — 5 P.M., Con. Ntr-o. Rhus. Sabad. Sulph.
— — 6 P.M., Cocc. Kali-c. Rhod. Tart.
— — 7 P.M., Bov. Lyc. Mgn-c. Mgn-s. Petr. Rhus.
— — 8 P.M., Coff. Hep. Mur-ac. Sulph. Tart.
— — 9 P.M. Mgn-s. Nitr-ac.
— — 10 P.M., Lach. Petr. Sabad.
— — 12 M. to 4 A.M., Actea-r.

— — paroxysm lasts all night, Lyc. Puls. Rhus.
— night, Amm-c. Ang. Ars. Bar-c. Bell. Borax. Caps. Carb-an. Carb-veg. Caust. *Cham*. Hep. Lach. Mgn-s. Merc. Nux. Phosp. Puls. Ran-sc. Rhus. Sabad. Scill. Sep. Sil. Staph. Stram. Sulph.
— midnight, Rhus.
— — before, Verat.
— — after, Amm-m. Borax. *Ran-sc*. Thuj.
— — — 2 A.M Borax. Taxus.
— — — 3 A.M., Thuj.
— from a cold, Dulc. Kali-c. Nitr-ac. (compare, Sect. 34.)
Preceded by, anguish, Chin.
— back, pain in, Ars. Ip.
— bleeding of gum, Merc.
— bones, pain in, Arn. Carb-veg. Ntr-m. Nitr. Therid.
— burning in eyes, Rhus.
— chest, pain in, Ars.
— chilliness, Puls.
— coldness (before chills.) Puls. Sulph.
— complaints in general, Ars. Chin. Rhus.
— cries, Bell. Lach. Lyc.
— diarrhœa, Rhus.
— — slimy, Puls.
— drowsiness, Puls.
— fainting fit, Ars.
— faintishness, Ars. Calc.
— feet cold, Carb-veg.
— headache, Ars. Bell. Bry. Carb-veg. Chin Lach. Ntr-m. Nitr. Puls. Rhus.
— — head, heaviness in, Calc.
— lie down, inclination to, Ars.
— limbs, pain in, Bry. Cina. Carb-veg. Chin. Sulph.
— — heaviness in, Calc.
— mucus increased in mouth, Rhus.
— nails blue, Cocc.
— nails (of great toes) pain in, Eupat.
— nausea, Chin. Cina. Lyc. Puls.
— palpitation of heart, China.
— ravenous hunger, Cina. Phosp. Staph.
— shuddering, Bry. Cocc.
— sleeplessness, Chin. Puls. Rhod. Rhus.
— sneezing, Chin.
— stretching, Acon. Alum. Ang. Ars. Bell. Bry. Calc. Carb-veg. Cham. Chin. Cina. Igt. Ip. Rhus. Stran.
— stupefaction, Ars.
— sweat, Samb.
— taste bitter, Hep.
— tearing pain, in joints, Calc.
— — — limbs, Ars. Cina.
— thirst, Arn. Ars. Bell. Caps. Chin. Cina. Eupat. Lach. Nux. Puls. Sep. Sulph.
— toothache, Carb-veg.
— uncomfortableness, Ip.
— vertigo, Ars. *Bry*. Puls.
— vomiting, Chin. Cina. Lyc. Puls.
— want of appetite, Puls.

32. FEVER.

Ppeceded by weakness, Ntr-m. Nux.
— weariness and drowsiness, Rhus.
— yawning, Ars. Rhus.
During the fever, abdomen, coldness in, Meny.
— — distention of, Ferr.
— anxiety, Ars. Calc. Chin. Coff. Lach. Nux. Rheum. Verat.
— apopletic fit, Nux.
— appetite, want of, Ant. Chin. Con. Daph. Kali-c. Lach. Ntr-m. Puls. Sabad. Staph.
— asthma, Mez.
— aversion to all food, Amm-c. Ant. Ars. Kali-c. Ip. Rheum.
— back, pain in, Ars. Bell. Calc. Caust. Chin. Cocc. Lach. Lyc. Ntr-m. Ntr-s. Rhus.
— bilious complaints, Ant. Ars. Bry. Cham. Chin. Cocc. Dig. Igt. Nux. Puls.
— bitterness of mouth, Alum. Ant. Ars. Phosp. Sep.
— blood, congestion of, Ars. Bov. Ferr. Mosch. Phosp. Phosp-ac. Sass. Sep. Staph. Sulph.
— — towards head, Ars. Ferr. Phosp. Sep. Sulph.
— blood vessels, distention of, Aloe. Chin. Ferr. Hyosc. Puls.
— — throbbing in, Bell.
— bones, pain in, Arn. Ars. Chin. Mgn-c. Mur-ac. Ntr-m. Puls.
— brain, paralytic affection of, Ars. Lyc.
— breast, swelling of, Puls.
— breath, difficult, Ars.
— — hot, Zinc.
— — offensive, Arn.
— — panting, Calad.
— — short, Ferr. Zinc.
— carphalogia, Ars. Iod. Op. Phosp. Phosp-ac. Rhus. Sulph. (compare Sect. 34.)
— chest, oppression of, Bry. Ip. Lach.
— — pain in, Acon. Ars. Bry. Calad. Daph. Ip. Kali-c. Sabad.
— colic, Ant. Ars. Bov. Bry. Calc. Cham. Cocc. Ferr. Phosp. Ran-b. Rhus. Sep. Sulph.
— coma, Op. Tart.
— constipation, Bell. Cimex. Cocc. Lyc. Nux. Op. Puls. Staph. Verat.
— coryza, Calad. Rhus.
— cough, Ars. Bry. Calc. Chin. Con. Ip. Kali-c. Lact. Phosp. Puls. Sabad. Sulph.
— — with remitting fever, Pod.
— — dry, Bry.
— — hooping, Kali-c.
— — nightly, Hyosc.
— — with vomiting, Bry.
— deafness, Lachn. Rhus.
— delirium, *Acon.* Ars. *Bell.* Bry. Calc. *Cham.* Chin. Cina. Dulc. Hyosc. Igt.

Lachn. Nux. Op. Phosp-ac. Plat. Pod. Samb. Sang. *Stram.* Sulph. Verat.
— diarrhœa, Alum. Amm-c. Ant. Apis. Arg. Arn. *Ars.* Bapt. Bell. Bry. Caps. Cham. Cina. Con. Gels. Hydroph. Hyosc. Lach. Mur-ac. *Ntr-m.* Nitr-ac. Nux-m. *Nux.* Op. Phosp. Phosp-ac. Puls. Rhus. Ruta. Sec-c. Stram. Sulph. Tereb. Thuj. *Valer. Verat.*
— ears, buzzing in, Ars.
— — pain in, *Calad.*
— epistaxis, Puls.
— epilepsy, Hyosc.
— eructations, Alum. Ant. Carb-veg. Nux.
— eyes, burning in, Lact.
— — painful, Creos. Led. Rhod.
— face bloated, Lyc.
— — about eyes, Ferr.
— — pain in, Lact. Spig.
— — pale, Igt. Mez. Puls. Rhus.
— — red, Acon. Bar-m. Cham. Chin. Cocc. Creos. Lach. Merc. Op. Puls. Rhus. Verat.
— — yellow, Chin. Lach. Ntr-m. Rhus.
— feet cold, Acon. Cist. Kali-chl. Lach. Merc. Puls. Rhod.
— gastric complaints, *Ant.* Cham. Cocc. Diad. *Igt.* Ip. *Nux.* Puls. Rhus. Sabad.
— gums, bleeding of, Staph.
— hands cold, Acon. Agar. Agn. Dros. Merc. Puls. Sulph.
— — hot, Berb. Carb-veg. Ip. Lach. Merc. Ntr-c. Nux. Puls. Sabad. Stann. Sulph.
— headache, Ang. Ars. *Bell.* Bry. Calc. Chin. Daph. Dros. Graph. Hell. Hep. Ip. Kali-c. Lach. Led. Lyc. Mang. Mez. *Ntr-m.* Petr. Phosp. Ruta. *Sep.* Spig. Tar.
— head, heat in, Rhod.
— — obtusion of, Kali-c. Phosp. Sep. Valer.
— hiccough, Lach.
— inability to recollect, Ars. Ntr-m. Phosp-ac. Sep.
— jaundice, Chin. Rhus.
— jerks, Rhus.
— joints, pain in, Ars. Calc. Carb-veg. Chin. Hell. Lact. Lyc. Phosp. Sep. Sulph.
— — knee, Hell.
— legs, lassitude of, Ars. Chin.
— — sorenesss in, Nitr.
— lie down, desire to, Bry. Calc. Dros.
— limbs, painfulness of, Ars. Bry. Chin. Hell. Lach. Nitr. Nux. Phosp. Rhus. Sep. Sulph.
— — as if beaten, Caps. Carb-veg. Rhus.
— — drawing pain in, Ntr-m.
— — soreness in, Rhod.
— lips dry, black, Ars. Chin. Merc. Tart. Verat.

32. FEVER.

During fever, lips dry, black, open mouth, Phosp.
— — dry, Ars. Cham. Chin. Igt. Lach. Lyc. Phosp Rhus.
— — eruption on, Ars. Ntr-m. Nux.
— — thin brown streak along upper lip, at junction of lower, Ars.
— liver, pain in, Ars. *Chin.* Kali-c.
— loathing of food, Amm-c. Ant. Ars. Ip. Kali-c. Rheum.
— micturition, painful, Cham.
— mouth, dryness of, Nux-m. Thuj.
— — open, Lyc. Op. Phosp.
— nausea, Ant. Ars. Bry. Cham. Chin. Dros. Ip. Lyc. Nux. Phosp. Sep. Verat.
— nettle rash, Igt. Rhus.
— nose, pain in, Rhod.
— — obstruction, Sulph.
— — scabs in, Sulph.
— olailga, Calad.
— pains intolerable, *Ars. Cham. Coff.*
— palpitation of heart, Aloe. Lach. Mez. Rhus. Siss. Sep. Spig. Sulph.
— paralytic, condition, Ars.
— — feeling in limbs, Nux.
— — weakness, Ars. Led. Lyc.
— perspiration on hot body, Op.
— pit of stomach, pain in, Rhus.
— ptyalism, Nitr-ac.
— pressure at stomach, Ferr. Rhus. Sep.
— pupils contracted, Arn.
— rattling in throat, Ars. Carb-veg. Nux-m.
— restlessness, Acon. Arn. Ars. Bell. Cham. Cina.
— rheumatic pains, Ars. Led. Lyc.
— scorbutic complaints, Staph.
— shrieking, Bell.
— sighing, Bry. Ip.
— skin, burning in, Acon. Petr.
— sleepiness, Ant. Ars. *Calad.* Daph. Lachn. Ntr-m. *Nux-m.* Op. Phosp. Sep. Stram. *Tart.* Verat.
— sleeplessness, Chin. Puls. Rhod. Rhus.
— snoring, Igt. Op. Rhus.
— somnolence, Bell. Carb-veg. Igt. Lyc. Merc. Op. Phosp. Puls. Tart.
— spasms, Cocc.
— spleen, pain in, Ars. Berb. Mez.
— stitches in side, Bry. Nux.
— stomach, pain in, Ars. Cocc. Lyc. Ntr-m. Nux. Sabad. Sep. Sil. Sulph.
— — spasms of, Cocc.
— — pit of, pain in, Ant. Ars. Cham. Igt. Ntr-m. Rhus.
— submaxillary, glands, swollen, Calad.
— sweat predominant, *Samb.*
— swelling of pit of stomach, Rhus.
— — — spleen, Caps. Chin. Ferr. Mez.
— taste, bitter, Alum. Ant. Ars. Calc. Chin. Ntr-m. Phosp. Puls. Sep.
— — putrid, Puls. Staph. Zinc.
— thirst, Acon. Aloe. Arn. *Ars.* Bell. Bry. Calad. Calc. *Caps.* Cham. Diad. Merc.

Ntr-m. Nux. Puls. Rhus. Ruta. Tereb. Thuj. *Valer. Verat.*
— thirstlessness, Amm-m. Ant. *Ars.* Bell. Calc. Camph. Caps. Carb-veg. Caust. Chin. Hell. Hep. Ntr-m. Nux-m. Nux. *Puls.* Rhod. *Sabad.* Sep. Spig. *Tart.*
— throat, inflammation of, Con. Dios.
— throbbing sense through body, Zinc.
— tongue coated, Ant. Nux. Phosp.
— — dry, Ars. Cham. Lach. Lyc. Ntr-m. Phosp. Rhus.
— — white, Igt. Nux-m.
— toothache, Graph. Kali-c.
— tossing about, Bell.
— tremor, Ars. Calc. Cist. Con. Ntr-m. Sep. Zinc.
— — of lower jaw, Alum.
— unconsciousness, Arn. *Bell.* Cocc. *Hell.* Hyosc. *Mur-ac. Ntr-m. Op. Phosp-ac.* Puls. *Stram.*
— urine dark, Sep. Verat.
— — frequent, Lyc.
— — offensive and brown, Sep.
— — turbid, Phosp.
— vertigo, Ars. Bry Chin. Nux. Verat.
— vomiting, *Ant.* Ars. Chin. Cina. Con. Ferr. Hep. Igt. Ip. Lach. Lyc. Nux. Puls. Stram. Sulph. Verat.
— — bilious, *Ant.* Ars. Cham. *Chin.* Igt. *Nux.*
— — mucus, Igt. Puls.
— — sour, Lyc.
— — of what had been eaten, *Cina.* Ferr. Igt.
— — with clean tongue, Cina.
— — inclination for, Cham. Dros. Sep. Verat.
— weakness, *Ars.* Chin. Ferr. Ip. Merc. *Ntr-m.* Puls. Sabad. Sulph. Verat.
After the fever coldness, Verat.
— debility, Dig.
— dreams, frightful, Ars.
— headache, Ars. Carb-veg. Cina. Hep.
— hungry, ravenous, Staph.
— pains in limbs, Crotal. Sabad.
— perspiration, Ars.
— sleep, Apis. Ars.
— thirst, Ant. Ars. Chin. Ntr-m. Nux.
— thirstlessness, Igt.
— vomiting, Chin. Cina. Hep.
Chills, Aeth. *Alum. Ambr.* Amm-c. *Anac. Arg. Arn. Ars.* Asar. Bell. Berb. Bov. *Bry.* Calad. Calc. *Cannab.* Canth. *Caps.* Carb-an. Carb-veg. Caust. Cham. Chin. Cina. Cocc. Coff. Colch. Coloc. Con. Creos. Cupr. Cycl. Daph. Diad. Dig. Dros. Euph. Evon. Graph. Guaj. Hell. *Hep.* Hyosc. Kali-c. Kali-jod. Igt. Ip. Led. *Lyc.* Mgn-m. Mgn-s. Mang. Meny. *Merc. Merc-cor.* Mez. *Mur-ac.* Ntr-c. Nitr. *Nux-m. Nux.* Ol-an. Op. Petr. Phell. *Phosp. Phosp-ac. Puls.* Ran-b. Rhus. *Ruta. Sabad.* Sabin. Samb. Sass.

32. FEVER.

Sep. Sil. Spig. Spong. Stann. *Staph.*
Stram. *Sulph.* Tar. *Tart* Therid. Thuj.
Valer. *Verat.*
Chills, of the different parts is found under the appropriate sections.
— as if dashed with cold water, Ars. Bry. Lyc. Merc. Mez. Phosp. Puls. Rhus. Spig. Thuj. Verat. Verb.
— external, Acon. Ars. Bell. Calc. Camph. Carb-veg. Chin. Dig. Euph. Ferr. Igt. Merc. Mosch. Nux. Oleand. Rhus. Sil. Zinc.
— flying, Bar-c. Cham. Ferr.
— internal, Agar. *Agn. Anac.* Arn. Ars. Bell. Bry. *Calc.* Caust. Cham. Chin. Coff. Daph. Hell. Igt. Iod. Ip. Guaj. Kali-c. Lac-can. Lach. Laur. Lvc. Merc. Ntr-m. Ntr-s. Nux. Phosp. Plb. Puls. Scill. Sep. Sil. Spig. Thuj. Verat.
— in single parts, Ars. Bell. Bry. Chin. Creos. Hep. *Igt.* Lyc. *Nux.* Par. *Puls.* Rhus. *Sep.* Sil. *Spig.* Verat.
— one-sided, Bar-c. Bry. Caust Chelid. Dig. Lyc. Ntr-c. Nux. Puls. Rhus. Thuj. Verb.
— — right, Bry. Caust. Nux. Rhus. Thuj.
— partial, Bry. Caps. Caust. Chin. Graph. Hell. Hep. Igt. Rhus. Sabin. Samb. Spig. Spong. Thuj.
— shaking, Acon. Agar. Amm-c. Anac. Bell. Berb. *Bry.* Camph. Canth. Caps. Cast. *Chin.* Cocc. Creos. Igt. Iod. Ip. Laur. Lyc. Mang. *Mur-ac.* Ntr-s Nux. Petr. Phell. *Phosp-ac.* Puls. *Rhus.* Samb. Stram. Sulph. Verat.
— with goose-flesh, Bell. Bry. Camph. Cannab. Croc. Nux. Sabad. Thuj.
— in the morning, Ang. Arn. Calc. Con. Cycl. Dros. Eupat. Gels. Graph. Kali-c. Led. Ntr-s. Phosp. Phyt. Spig. Therid. Thuj.
— — forenoon, Ambr. Ang. Arn. Con. Cop. Euph. Guaj. Led. Stann. Stront.
— — afternoon, Arg. Ars. Bry. Chin. Cocc. Croc. Dig. Lach. Nitr-ac. Phosp. Puls. Sulph.
— evening, Acon. Agar. Alum. Amm-c. *Amm-m.* Arn. Ars. Bov. Bry. Carb an. Carb-veg. Cham. Chin. Cina. Cocc. Cycl. Dulc. Ferr. Graph. Guaj. *Hep. Kali-c.* Lach. *Lvc.* Mgn-c. *Mgn-m.* Mang. Merc. Ntr-s. Nitr-ac. Nitr. *Nux.* Petr. *Phosp.* Phosp-ac. Plat. *Puls. Rhus.* Samb. Sep. Sil. Stann. Stront. Sulph. Tabac. Teucr. Tilia.
— — in bed, Alum. Amm-c. Bov. Carb-an. Chin. Ferr. Mur-ac. Nux. *Phosp.* Sil. Sulph.
— every other day, Lyc.

— — with the pains, Igt. *Puls.*
— — lasting all night, Lyc. Puls. Rhus.
— at night, Alum. Arg. Bov. Carb veg. Caust. Ferr. Hep. Iris. Mgn-s. *Merc.* Mur ac. Ntr-s. *Nux.* Staph. Thuj.
— after midnight, Thuj.
— during day, fever at night, Alum.
— day and night. Sass.
— at 3 A. M., Thuj.
— — 6 A. M., Nux.
— — 7 A. M., Pod.
— — 7 A. M. to 9 A. M., Pod.
— — 9 A. M., Kali-c. Ntr-m.
— — 10 A. M., Ars. Cact. Ntr-m. Petr. Rhus. Sacch. Stann. Sulph.
— — 10 A. M., fever, but no chill, tertian, Gels
— — 10:30 A. M., Lob.
— — 10 A. M. to 11 A. M., Ars Ntr-m.
— — 10 A. M. to 2 P. M., Merc-sulph.
— — 10 A. M., to 3 P. M., Sil. Sulph.
— — 11 A. M., Hyosc. Ip. Op.
— — 11 A. M. to 12 A. M., Kali-c. Kobalt.
— — 11 A. M. to 4 P. M., Gels.
— — 11 A. M to 11 P. M., Cact.
— — morning to noon, Ntr-m.
— — noon, Elaps. Lob.
— — to 2 P. M , Lach.
— — 1 P. M., Cact.
— — 1 P. M. to 2 P. M., Ars. Eupat.
— — 2 P. M., Calc.
— — 3 P. M., Ang. Apis. Con. Staph. Thuj.
— — 3 P. M. to 4 P. M., Apis. Lach.
— — 3 P. M. to 6 P. M., Ars.
— — 4 P. M., Puls.
— — 4 P. M. to 5 P. M., Kobalt.
— — 4 P. M. to 7 P. M., Kali-jod.
— — 4 P. M. to 8 P. M., Bov.Graph.Hell. Hep. Lyc. Mgn-m Ntr-s.
— — after 4 P. M., Graph.
— — 5 P. M., Con. Kali-c.
— — 5 P. M. to 6 P. M., Phosp. Sulph.
— — 5 P. M. to 7 P. M. 8 P. M., Hep.
— — 6 P. M., Arg n. Nux.
— — 6 P. M. to 8 P., Kali-jod. Sulph.
— — 6 P. M., to midnight, Lachn.
— — 7 P. M., Lyc. Petr. Rhus.
— — 7 P. M. to 8 P. M., Sulph.
— — 9 P. M. to 10 A. M., Mgn-s.
— — at same hour, Ant. Apis. Bov. Cact. China. Cina. Con. Diad. Gels.Graph. Hell. Hep. Kali-c. Lyc. Mgn-m. Phosp. Sabad. Spig. Stann. Staph. Thuj
— every 14 days, Ars. Calc. Chin. Puls.
— — year, Ars. Carb-veg. Lach. Sulph. Thuj.
— anticipating, Ars. Chin. Igt. Ntr-m. Nux.
— postponing, Chin. Cina.
— anger, from, *Bry.* Nux.

32. FEVER.

Chills, bed, in, Alum. Amm-c. Bov. Calc. Carb-an. Chin. Dros. Ferr. Hep. Laur. Nux. *Phosp.* Rhod.
— — relieved, Caust. Hell. Mgn-m. Mgn-s. Merc. Ntr-c.
— — getting out of, ameliorated, Lyc.
— cold, after, a, Lyc. Sep.
— — air, as of, blowing on uncovered parts, Mosch.
— — — — around waist, Sil.
— dinner, before, Berb.
— drinking after, Ars. Asar. Cannab. Caps. Chin. Eupat. Lob. Mez. Nux. Sil. Tar. Verat.
— — — less, Caust.
— eat, when beginning to, Euph.
— epileptic paroxysms, after, Cupr.
— exercising, when, Apis. Bry. Coff. Lachn. *Merc-cor.* Nitr. *Nux.* Plb. Rhus. Sil. *Spig.*
— — ameliorated, Puls. Staph. Sulph-ac.
— meals, after, dinner, ameliorated, Ambr. Ntr-c. Phosp.
— — during, Euph. Ran-sc. (compare Sect. 13.)
— moving, on, Apis. Arn. Asar. Bell. Cycl. Merc. Mez. Nitr-ac. Nux. Pod. Rhus. Sil. Spig.
— nervous, skin warm, wants to be held to prevent shaking, Gels.
— open air, in, Agar. Anac. Hep. Kali-chl. Merc-cor. Mosch. *Nux-m.* *Nux.* Petr. Plat. Plb. Ran-b. Rhus. Seneg. Sep. Zinc. Zing.
— — — — ameliorated, Phosp. Puls. Sulph-ac.
— pains, with the. Ars. Bry. Dulc. Graph. Led. Lyc. *Mez.* Ntr-m. *Puls.* Rhus.
— — after the, Kali-c.
— periodically, Oleand.
— rising from stooping, when, Merc-cor.
— room, in a, Ars. Bry. (compare Warmth.)
— sitting, when, ameliorated, Nux.
— sleep after, Bry. Calc.
— streaks, in, Acon.
— sunshine, in, amelioration, Anac. Con.
— touched, when, Acon.
— uncovering, when, Acon. Agar. Bell. Clem. Cor-r. Mercurial. Nux-m. Stram.
— walking in open air, Alum. Amm-c. Ars. Caust. Chelid. Chin. Kali-chl. Merc. Merc-cor. Nitr-ac. Nux. Petr. Rhus. Tabac.
— walk, after a, Ntr-s.
— — in open air, *Nux.* Ol-an.
— warmth, in, Alum. Anac. Ant. Bell. Bov. Canth. Caust. Cic. Cina. Cinnab. Cocc. Creos. Dulc. Grat. Guaj. Iod. Ip. Lact. Lam. Laur. Mgn-m. Meny. Merc. Mez. Nux. Phosp. Puls. Rheum. Ruta. Sil. Staph. Spong.
— — ameliorated, Bar-c. Camph. Carb-an. Cic. Con. Cor-r. Hipp. Igt. Kali-c.

Meny. Nux-m.
— — by wrapping up, followed by severe fever and sweat, Sil.
— weakness in legs, from, Seneg.
— weather, stormy, in, Diad. Zinc.
— wet when becoming, *Sep.*
Chills with abdominal pains, Ars. Bov. Calad. Calc. Chin. Coff. Diad. Igt. Lach. Meph. Merc-cor. Nitr-ac. Nux. Pallad. Phosp. Pod. Puls. Rumex. Sep.
— — — in pit of, Eupat.
— coldness, Ars. Phosp-ac.
— anxiety, Acon. Ars. Caps. Chin. Nux. Puls. Verat.
— asthma, Mez.
— back, pains in, Ars. Bell. Calc. Caps. Caust. Eupat. Hyosc. Igt. Lach. Mosch. Ntr-m. Nux. Pallad. Puls. Zinc.
— blood, congestion of, to head, Chin. Nux.
— bones, pains in, Ars. Eupat. Ntr-m. Sabad.
— breath, hot, Anac.
— breathing, difficult, Ars. Gels. Kali-c. Mez. Ntr-m. Puls. Seneg. *Zinc.*
— — wheezing, Calad.
— chattering of teeth, Cact. Camph. Caps. Hep. Lach. Ntr-m. Ntr-s. Nux. Plat. Phosp. Ran-b. Sabad Tabac.
— cheeks, heat of, Calc. Cham.
— chest, oppression of, Ars. Bry. Cimex. Daph. Ip. Puls.
— — pain in, Ars. Bell. Lach. Sabad. Seneg.
— — stitches in, Bry. Kali-c. Rumex.
— coryza, Calad.
— cough, Bry. Calc. Creos. Phosp. Sulph.
— — spasmodic, Sabad.
— convulsions, Lach. Merc.
— delirium, Sulph.
— diarrhœa, Ars. Phosp.
— dulness of mind, Caps.
— ear-ache, Graph. Gum-gut.
— ears, heat in, Acon. Ran-b.
— epistaxis, Creos.
— eructations, Alum. Gum-gut. Ran-sc. Rhus.
— eyes, fixed, Acon.
— — pain in, Seneg.
— face, coldness of, Cina. Dros. Ip. Ntr-c. Petr.
— — heat in, Acon. Agar. Alum. Anac. Apis. Bell. Berb. Bry. Calc. Cannab. Cham. Chin. Coloc. Creos. Dig. Euph. Ferr. Hell. Hyosc. Jatr. Lach. Lact. Led. Lyc. Merc. Mercurial. Mur-ac. Ntr-c. Nux. Oleand. Puls. Ran-b. Rhus. Sabad. Seneg. Staph. Sulph.
— — pale, Bell. Camph. Canth. Chin. Cina. Dros. *Nux-m.* Nux. *Puls.* Sulph. Tart.

32. FEVER.

Chill with, face puffed, Bell.
— — red, Acon. Arn. Ars. Bry. Cham. Chin. Creos. Igt. Ferr. Lyc. Merc. Nux. Ox ac. Plb. Puls. Rhus. Stram. Sulph.
— — — and pale alternately, with redness and heat, Rhus.
— — — followed by paleness without coldness, Scill.
— — tension, Bar-c.
— feet, coldness of, Berb. Brom. Chin. Cop. Creos. Dros. Gels. Hep. Lach. Mang. Merc. Mez. Ntr-m. Pallad. Samb. Sep.
— — cramps in, Nux.
— — heat in, Ca'ad. Kali-chl.
— — numbness in, Lyc.
— — pain in, Cop.
— fingers, torpor deadness of, Croton. Sep. Stann.
— fluids disgusting, Hell.
— forehead, heat in, Acon. Calc. Chin. Ntr-s.
— — perspiration on, Bry. Dig.
— goose-skin, Bar-c. Canth. Croton. Hell. Laur.
— hair, bristling, Bar-c. Grat. Meny.
— hands, blue, Gels. Jatr. Nux.
— — cold, Agar. Agn. Chin. Dros. Euph. Gels. Ind. Jatr. Mang. Mez. Ntr-c. Ntr-m. Oleand. Pallad. Petr. Phosp ac. Sep.
— — heat in, Apis Cina. Kali-c. Ip. Nux. Ntr-c. Ntr-s. Sabad.
— — stiffness of, Kali-c.
— — torpor, deadness, Lyc. Sep.
— — palms, moist, Nicc.
— head, bewilderment of, Caps. Hydroc-ac.
— headache, Acon. Anac. Ars. Berb. Borax. Bry. Caps. Chin. Cimex. Cina. Cor-r. Creos. Daph. Dros. Elat. Eupat. Ferr. Gels. Graph. Ind. Mang. Mez. Ntr-m. Nux. Petr. Puls. Sang. Sep. Sulph. Tart.
— head, externally painful, Hell.
— — heat of, Acon. Arn. Asar. Bell. Berb. Bry. Cina. Mang. Meph. Ntr-s. Nux. Rhod. Verat.
— — — burning, Arn. Verat.
— — pressure, Puls.
— — throbbing in, Seneg.
— hip, pain in, Rhus.
— hoarseness, Hep.
— hunger, Nux. Phosp.
— ill-humor, Anac. Caps. Creos.
— joints, pain in, Cimex. Hell. Raph.
— kidneys, pain in, Millef.
— knees, elbows and wrists, aching in, Pod.
— legs, cold, Bell. Berb. Nux. Puls.
— — disabled, Igt.
— limbs, benumbed, Nux.
— — contraction of, Caps. Cimex.

— — heavy, Therid.
— — pain in, Acon. Ars. Bell. Bry. Caps. Cinnab. Hell. Lach. Lyc. Nitr. Nux. Puls. Rhus. Sabad. Sep. Sulph.
— — shaking of, Bell. Sabad.
— — soreness of, Bell.
— — tearing in, Bry. Caps. Lyc. Phosp. Rhus. Sabad.
— — twitching of, Stram.
— — weariness, painful of, Rhus.
— lie down, obliging one to, Bry. Dros. Merc. Nux. Puls. Therid.
— loathing of food and drink, Bry. Kali-c.
— liver, pains in, Ars. Chin. Nux. Verat.
— loins, pain in, Ars. Creos. Lach. Nux. Verat.
— low spirits, Sacch.
— — ceasing during the heat, Plat.
— moaning, Eupat.
— mouth dry, Berb. Thuj.
— — foam, at, Therid.
— muscles, tremor in, Merc. Oleand.
— nails, blue, Aur. Cocc. Dros. Ntr-m. Nux. Petr.
— nausea, Arg-n. Ars. Bell. Bry. Chin. Cina. Con. Eupat Igt. Kali-b. Kali-c. Kobalt. Merc-sulph. Rumex. Sang. Sep. Verat.
— — with inclination to vomit, Ars. Aur. Rhus. Sabad.
— noise is intolererable, Caps.
— obtusion of head, Calc. Kali-c.
— pain, paroxysms of, Ars. Chin. Nitr. Puls. Rhus.
— — aching, Eupat.
— palpitation of heart, Gels. Phosp-ac.
— paralysis, sense of, in legs, Ars. Igt.
— perspiration, Ars. Euph. Sulph.
— photophobia, Hep.
— pulse weak, Gels.
— — slow, Meny.
— pupils contracted, Acon.
— — dilated, Acon. Op.
— rage, Cimex.
— recollect, inability to, Ars. Caps. Stram.
— ribs pain in, Sabad.
— sacral region, pain in, Ars. Gum-gut. Hyosc. Nux. Verat.
— sensation, loss of, Lach.
— sensitiveness to cold, Cycl. Merc.
— sight, obscuration of, Bell. Cic. Hydroc-ac. Sabad.
— skin blue, Merc. Nux.
— — contracted, sensation as if, Par.
— — cold, damp, clammy, Lachn.
— — dry, parchment like, Ars. Asa-f. Iod.
— — painful, Nux.
— — stinging, Samb.
— — tingling, Samb.
— sleepiness, Aeth. Ambr. Borax. Cimex. Daph. Hell. Kali-b. Mez. Ntr-m. Nux-m. Nux. Op. Phosp. Tart.
— sneezing, Ox-ac.

32. FEVER.

Chills, with, spasms, chronic, Calc.
— — of chest, Ars.
— spitting saliva Alum. Caps. Rhus.
— staggering, Caps.
— staring, Cic.
— stiffness and rigidity of the body, Op.
— stomach, pain in, Ars. Lyc. Sil. Sulph.
— — pit of, pain in, Ars.
— stretching, Ars. Bry. Caps. Coff. Creos. Ip. Laur. Mur-ac. Ntr-c. Nux. Prun.
— stupefaction, Ntr-m. Op. Puls.
— swelling of spleen, Caps.
— taste, bitter, Alum. Ars. Hep.
— — insipid, Aur.
— tastelessness of food, Ars.
— tenesmus, Merc-cor.
— thirst, *Acon.* Ant. *Arn.* Ars Bell. Borax. *Bov.* Bruc. *Bry.* Calad. Calc. *Cannab.* Caps. Carb-veg. *Cham* Chin. Cina. Cor-r. Croc Daph. Diad. Dulc. *Eugen.* Ferr. Gum-gut. *Igt. Ip.* Kali-c. Kali jod. Led. Lob. Lyc. Mgn-s Merc. *Mez.* Mur-ac. Ntr-c. Ntr-m. Ntr-s. Nitr. *Nux.* Plb. Pol. Psor. Puls. Ran-b. Rhus. Ruta. Sabad. Sec-c. Spong. Stann. Sulph. Thuj. *Verat.*
— — before the chill, Amm-m. Arn. Caps. Chin. Cimex. Eupat. Lob. Nux. Puls.
— — between the chill and fever, Chin. Sabad.
— — drinking a good deal, Arn.
— thirstlessness, Agar. Agn. An-c. Ant Ars. Asar Aur. Bell. Bov. Bry. Calad. Calc. Camph Caps. Carb-veg. Caust. *Chin.* Cina. Cocc. Coloc. Con. Cycl. Dros. Elaps. Euph. Guaj. *Hell.* Hep. Hyosc. Ip. Lach. Lam. Lyc. Mang. Merc. *Mur-ac* Ntr-c. Ntr-m. Ntr s. Nitr-ac. Nitr. Nux m. *Nux.* Oleand Op. Petr. Phosp. Phosp-ac. *Puls.* Rhus. *Sabad.* Samb. Sep. Spig. Staph. S.ram. Sulph. Tart. Therid. Thuj.
— throbbing through the body, Zinc.
— — in head, Seneg.
— tongue, coated thick, Gels.
— toothache, Kali-c. Gra h. Rhus.
— torpor of affected side, Puls.
— tremor. *Agn.* Anac. Ars. Bell. Borax. Cina. Cocc. Croc. Con. Eupat. Gels. Merc-jod. *Par.* Plat. Sabad. Tart. Teucr. Zinc.
— trismus, Lach.
— uneasiness, Calc. Cannab. Caps. Hyosc. Sil.
— urine, dark, Verat.
— urinate, constant desire to, Ind. Meph. Merc.
— veins on hands, swollen, Phosp.
— vertigo, Alum. Calc. Caps. Chin. Kali-b. Ntr-m. Phosp. Puls. Rhus. Sulph. Verat.
— vomit. inclination to, Ars. Aur. Cina. Igt. Kali-c. Puls. Rhus. *Sabad.*

— vomiting, Borax. Caps. Puls.
— — bilious, Ars. Chin. Cina. Igt.
— — of what has been eaten, Igt.
— — mucus, Caps, Igt. Puls.
— weakness, Ambr. Ars. Borax. Calc. Carb-veg. Caust. Dros. Lach. Lam. Op. Phosp.
— yawning, Ars. Bry. Calad. Caps. Caust. *Cina.* Elat. Gum-gut. Kobalt. Laur. Merc-sulph. *Mur-ac.* Murex. Ntr-m. Ntr-s. *Oleand.* Par. Phosp. Sil. Thuj.
— preceded by, head, congestion to, Chin.
— — headache, Rhus.
— — nausea and vomiting, then perspiration, no heat. Lyc.
— — pain in back, Pod.
— — in bones, as if broken, Eupat. Therid.
— — sleepiness, Therid.
— — thirst, Ang. Arn. Borax. Chin. Cimex. Eupat Nux Puls. Sulph.
— — yawning, Elat. Nicc.
— — succeeded by, feet, coldness of, Petr.
— — hands and face, bloatedness of, Lyc.
— — itching of body, Petr.
— — nausea, Acon.
— — sleep, Ars. Mez. Nux. Sabin.
— — tired feeling and cough, worse from drinking, Cimex.
— — thirst, Ars. Chin. Cimex. Creos. Dios. Hep. Mgn-s. Ntr-c. Puls. Sabad. Thuj.
— — vomiting, bitter, Eupat.
— — sour, Lyc.
— — weakness, Ars.
Chilliness, *Agar.* Agn. *Alum.* Anac. Ars. Asar. *Bar-c.* Bov. Bruc. *Bry. Calc.* Carb-an. *Carb-veg.* Cast. *Caust.* Cham. *Chelid.* Chin. *Cic.* Coff. Creos. Euphr. Ferr-m. Grat. Hep. Ip. Laur. Lyc. Meny. Merc-cor. *Mez.* Mosch. *Ntr-m. Nitr-ac.* Nux-m. Nux. Ol-an. Petr. *Phosp. Plb. Puis.* Ran-b. Rat. Rhus. Scill. *Sil. Spig. Sulph. Tabac. Tart.* Teucr. Viol-tr.
— on left side of breast, Ferr-m.
— in damp weather, Ferr-m.
Chilly shivering, Agn. Canth. Cocc. Coff. Dulc. Ferr-m. Guaj. Hell. Ntr-s. Nux-m. Par. Phosp. Plat. Ran-sc. Sabad. Seneg. Sep. Spig. Stann. Teucr. Thuj. Zinc.
Coldness in general, Acon. Aeth. *Ars.* Asar. *Aur.* Borax. *Bry. Camph. Cannab. Canth. Caps. Carb-veg.* Caust. Cham. Chelid. *Chin.* Cic. Coloc. Con. Cycl. Diad. *Dig.* Dulc. Eugen. Euph. Hell. Igt. Iod. *Ip.* Jatr. Kali-jod. Lach. *Laur. Led.* Lyc. Merc. Mez. *Ntr-m. Ntr-s* Nicc. Nitr-ac. *Nitr. Nux.* Ol-an. Op. *Par.* Phosp. *Plb.* Puls. Ran-b. *Rhus. Ruta. Sabad. Sass.* Sec-c. Sep. *Stram.* Sulph. Tabac. *Tart.* Teucr. Thuj. *Verat. Verb.*
— of limbs, Acon. Aeth. Ambr. Arn. *Ars.*

32. FEVER

Aur. Bell. *Calad.* Calc. *Camph.* Carb-an. *Carb-veg. Caust.* Chelid. Chin. Cic. Coloc. Con. Dig. Graph. *Hell.* Hydroc-ac. Hyosc. *Ip.* Jatr. Kali-c. Laur. *Led.* Lyc. Merc. Mez. Ntr-m. Nitr-ac. Nitr. Nux. Op. Pæon. Phosp. *Plb.* Puls. *Rhus.* Scill. Sec-c. *Sep. Stram. Sulph.* Tart. Thuj. *Verat.* Verb.
Coldness, sensation of, Cocc. Mosch. Phosp-ac. Sulph. Tart-ac.
— in single parts, compare different sections.
— inward, Ntr-s. *Par.* Thuj.
— external, Arn. Calc. Chin. Dig. Sabad. Sil.
— one sided, Caust. Dig. Nux. *Puls. Rhus.*
— in morning, Ntr-s.
— — forenoon, Cop.
— at noon, *Ran-b.*
— in afternoon, *Borax. Nitr. Ran-b.*
— — evening, *Amm-m.* Bry. Dulc. Ntr-s. Petr. Rhus. Tart-ac.
— — — in bed, Bry. Tart-ac.
— at night, Ambr. Ntr-s. Tart-ac. Thuj.
— from affections of internal organs, Euph.
— after meals, *Ran-b.* (compare Sect. 13.)
— in open air, Laur.
— after walking, Ntr-s.
— in warmth of room, Dulc. Ruta.
Shuddering, shivering, Acon. Anac. Ang. *Arg. Ars.* Bar-c. Bell. Calad Cannab. Cast. Caust. *Cham.* Chelid. Chin. Cina. Cocc. Con. Evon. Ferr. Guaj. Hep. Hyosc. *Igt. Ip. Kali-c.* Laur. *Led.* Mgn-s. Meny. *Merc.* Merc-cor. Mosch. Ntr-c. Nux. *Oleand.* Ol-an. Phell. Phosp. *Phosp-ac.* Plat. Puls. Rat. Rheum. *Rhus. Ruta.* Sabad. *Sabin.* Samb. Seneg. Sep. Sil. Stann. Staph. Sulph. Tabac. Verat. *Verb.* Viol-od. Zinc.
— one sided, Bell. Caust. Cocc. Lyc. Nux. *Puls. Rhus.* Thuj. *Verb.*
— partial, Ars. *Bell.* Caust. *Cham.* Chin. Cocc. Graph. *Puls.* Staph. *Verat.*
— wandering, Nux.
— forenoon, in, Ars. Stann.
— afternoon, in, Arg. Dig. Nux.
— evening, in, Acon. Ars. Aur. Bov. Cham. Diad. Mgn-s. Merc. Phell. Phosp. Phosp-ac. Rat.
— day and night, Sass.
— night, at, Arg. Merc. Staph.
— midnight, after, Thuj.
— day time, in, Kali-c.
— alternate day, every, Lyc.
— with affections of internal organs, Euph.
— anger, after, Nux.
— bed, in, Ars. Alum. Aur. Borax. Carb-an. Ferr. Laur. Merc. Nux. Phosp.
— — relieved, Mgn-s. Mgn-m.
— chill, after a, Lyc. Sep.
— cold temperature, in, Cham.

— drinking, after, Ars. Caps. Chin. Eupat. Nux. Verat.
— epileptic fit, after, Cupr.
— exercising, when, Ars. Merc. Nux. Sil. Sulph.
— meals, after, Ars. Rhus.
— — — relieved, Ambr.
— open air, in, Agar. Hep. Laur. Merc-cor. Mosch. Nux-m. Petr. Plat. Rhus. Seneg.
— pains, with the, Ars. Bar-c. Mez. Puls. Ran-b. Sep.
— parts affected, on the, Ars.
— rest, when at, Bruc.
— room, in the, Ars.
— touched, when, Spig.
— urinate, with desire to, Hyper.
— warmth, in, Alum. Anac. Bov. Dulc. Guaj. Iod. Lact. Lam. Laur. Merc. Ruta.
— — relieved, Nux.
Heat in general, *Acon.* Anac. Arn. *Ars. Bell.* Borax. *Bov. Bry.* Calc. Camph. Caps Carb-veg. *Casc.* Caust. *Cham. Chin.* Cina. *Coff.* Con. Cycl. Dig. Dros. Ferr. Graph. Hell. *Hep. Hyosc. Igt. Iod.* Ip. Kali-c. Led. Lyc. Mgn-c. Mgn-s. Mang. Meny. *Merc.* Mosch. *Mur-ac.* Ntr-m. Nicc. Nitr-ac. Nux. Op. Petr. *Phosp.* Phosp-ac. Plb. *Puls.* Rhod. Rhus. Sabad. Sabin. *Samb. Sep.* Sil. Spig. Spong. *Stann.* Staph. Stram. Stront. *Sulph.* Sulph-ac. Tar. *Tart.* Tereb Zinc.
— sensation of, Cham. Igt. Mgn-c. Oleand. Sil. Stann.
— of different parts, compare the Sections.
— anxious, *Acon.* Arn. *Ars.* Bell. Bry. Calc. Carb-veg. Igt. *Merc.* Ntr-m. Nitr-ac. *Nux.* Petr. *Phosp.* Phosp-ac. Puls. Rhus. Sep. Spong. Stann. Stram. Sulph.
— burning, *Acon. Ars. Bell.* Bry. *Cham. Dulc.* Hell. Laur. *Lyc.* Merc. Mosch. Op. Puls. Sabin. *Scill.* Stann. Staph.
— dry, *Acon.* Arn. *Ars.* Arum-trif. Bar-m. *Bell.* Bry. Calc. Caust. Clem. Cocc. Coff. Coloc. Con. *Dulc.* Hell. *Hep.* Ip. Kali-c. *Lach.* Led. *Lyc.* Merc. Ntr-s. Nitr-ac Nitr. *Nux.* Op. *Phosp.* Phosp-ac. *Puls.* Rhus. Samb. Scill. Sec-c. Sep. Sil. Stann. Staph. Stront. *Sulph.*
— — of covered parts, Thuj.
— external, *Acon. Anac.* Arn. *Ars.* Bell. Bry. Calc. Caps. Carb-veg. Cham. Cocc. Coloc. Cor-r. Dig. Euph. Hell. Hyosc. *Igt.* Kali-c. Lach Lyc. Merc. Nux. Op. Phosp. Puls. *Rhus.* Scill. Sep. *Sil.* Spig. Sulph.
— flushes of, Agn. Ambr. Amm-m. Arn. Bar-c. Bism. Borax. Calc. *Carb-veg.* Cocc. Coloc. Creos. Croc. Cupr. Dig. *Graph.* Hep. Igt. Iod. Kali-c. Kali-jod. Lach. *Lyc.* Mgn-c. Ntr-c. Ntr-m. Nitr-ac. Nux-jug. Nux. Oleand. Ol-an. Petr.

32. FEVER.

Phosp. Rumex. Ruta. Seneg. *Sep.* Sil. Spig. Spong Stann. Sulph. Sulph-ac. Teucr. *Thuj* Valer.
Heat, internal, *Acon.* Arn. Ars. *Bell.* Bry. Calc. Cham. Chelid Ferr-m Hell.Nux. Phosp. *Phosp-ac.* Puls. *Rhus.* Sabad. Sep. Spig. Stann. Verat. Zinc.
— of single parts, Acon. Arn. *Ars.* Bar-c. *Bell. Bry.* Calc. Canth. Carb-veg.Cham. Graph. Laur. Lyc. *Merc.* Mez. Nux. *Phosp. Phosp-ac.* Puls. Sabad. Sep. Stann. *Sulph.*
— — — outer parts, Acon. Arn. *Ars.* Bar-c. *Bell.* Bry. Calc. Carb-veg. Caust. Graph. Kali-c. Lyc. *Merc.* Nux. *Phosp. Phosp-ac.* Sep. Spig. Stann. Staph. *Sulph.*
— — — inner parts, *Acon.* Arn. Ars. *Bell. Bry.* Calc. Camph. *Canth.* Carb-veg. Cham. Euph. *Laur.*Lyc. *Merc.* Mez. Nux. *Phosp.*Phosp-ac. Puls. Sabad. Sec-c. Sep. *Sulph.*
— one side only, Bell. *Bry.* Lyc. Nux. Phosp Phosp-ac. *Puls.* Sulph.
— periodical, from bodily or mental exertion, Oleand.
— ascending, Alum.
— descending, Sep.
— from mouth and nose, coming, Stront.
— — face, Alum.
— day and night, Bar-m.
— — only, Sep. Tart.
— morning, in, Borax. Euph. Kali-c. Mgn-c. *Sulph.*
— — 3 A. M., Ang.
— forenoon, in, Berb. Sass.
— — 9 A. M., Kali-c.
— — 10 A. M., Rhus.
— — fever, no chill, tertian, Gels.
— afternoon, in, Anac. Ars. Berb. Bry. Canth. Chin. Cop. Graph. Lach. Lyc. Ntr-s. Puls. Spig. Stann.
— — 3 P. M., Nicc.
— — 4 P. M., Anac. Stann.
— — 5 P. M., Kali-c.
— — 6 P. M., Caust.
— evening, in, Agn. Alum. Ambr. Ang. Berb. *Chin.* Ferr. Hell. *Hep.* Hipp. Hyosc. Lach. Mgn-c. Merc. Mosch. Mur-ac. Nicc. Ol-an. Phosp. Phosp-ac. Psor. Ran-sc. Sacch. Sass. Sulph. *Thuj.*
— night, at, Alum Ant. Ars. Berb. Bry. *Calc.* Carb-an. Carb-veg. Cham. Cic. Cina. Coff. Dros. Dulc. *Hep.* Laur. Mgn-c. Mgn-m. Mgn-s. Merc. Ntr-m. Nicc. Nitr-ac. Nitr. *Petr.* Phosp. Phosp-ac. Psor. Puls. Ran-b. Ran-sc. Rhod. Rhus. Sabin. Sil. Stront. Sulph. Thuj. Viol-tr.
— — burning, dry, *Acon.* Anac. Arn. Ars. Bar-c. *Bry.* Calc. Coff. Dulc. Graph. Lach. Lyc. Nitr. *Nux. Phosp.* Puls.

Ran-sc. Rhod. Spig.
— — without thirst or perspiration, Ars.
— midnight, before, Ant. Eugen.
— — at, quotidian, Rhus.
— artificial heat, relieved by, Cor-r.
— bed, in., Agn. Hell. Kali-c. Mgn-m. Mgn-s. Sulph-ac. (compare At Night).
— conversation, serious, during a, Sep.
— drinking, worse from, Calc.
— exercising, when, Ant. Camph. Nux. Ox-ac. Sep. Stann. Tart.
— — after, Amm-c. Brom. Fluor-ac. Sep.
— meals, after, less, Chin.
— occupied, when busily, Oleand.
— pains, during the, Carb-veg.
— parts affected, of, Acon. Bry. Sulph.
— riding in a carriage, when, Graph. Psor.
— sitting, in, Phosp. Sep.
— — relieved, Nux.
— sleep, in, Dulc. Petr. Viol-tr.
— — after, Cina.
— stooping, when, Merc-cor.
— vexation, after, Petr. Sep.
— warmth of room, in, Amm-m. Ip.
Heat, with abdomen, burning, in, Selen. Spig.
— — coldness, in, Zinc.
— — inflated, Ars.
— — pain in, Ars. Caps. Carb-veg. Cina.
— — pulsations in, Kali-c.
— anxiety, Acon. Ambr. Ars. Asa-f. Berb. Bov. Calc. Canth. Cham. Cycl. Ferr. Igt. Ip. Mgn-c. Merc Ntr-m. Nux. Op. Phosp. Phosp-ac. Puls. Ruta. Sep. Spong. Stann. Stram. Sulph.
— back, pain in, Arn. Ars. Caps. Chin. Hyosc. Igt. Lach. Ntr-m.
— — burning in, and loins, Kalm.
— — tearing in, Ars. Lach. Laur.
— bewilderment of head, Ang. Ars. Bry. Valer. Verat.
— blood. congestion of, Ferr. Phosp-ac. Sass. Staph.
— — to head, *Bell.* Hyosc.
— blood vessels, burning in, Ars.
— — distention of, Bell. Camph. Chin. Puls.
— — pulsation in, Zinc.
— bones, pain in, Ars. Igt. Mgn-c. Ntr-m. Puls.
— breath anxious and rapid, Acon. Puls.
— chest, burning in, Cham. Puls. Seneg. Sulph.
— — oppression of, Acon. Ars. Berb. Bov. Carb-veg. Ip. Kali-c. Merc.
— — pain in, Ars. Caps. Carb-veg. Cina. Kali-c. Nux.
— — sensation of heat in, Amm-m.
— colic, Caps. Carb-veg. Elat. Rhus.
— coryza, fluent, Kali-c.
— cough, Dros. Sulph.
— cries, Lach.
— deafness, Lachn.

32. FEVER.

Heat, with delirium, Ars. Bell. Bufo. Carb-veg. Chin. Cina. Hyper. Igt. Lach. Nitr-ac. Op. Pod. Sabad. Sang. Spong. Verat.
— diarrhœa, Con. Puls. Rhus
— dizziness, Ang. Ars. Bry. Valer. Verat.
— drink, repugnance to, Nux.
— dryness of lips, Kali-b. Rhus.
— — mouth, Kali-b. Nux-m. Psor.
— dullness of mind, Ntr-m.
— dyspnœa, Acon. Anac. Ars. Bov. Cact. Camph. Carb-veg. Crotal. Elaps. Igt. Ip. Kali-c. Lob. Lyc. Phosp. Puls. Ruta. Sep.
— ears burning, Caps. Chin. Dig,
— — coldness, Ip.
— — humming, Nux.
— — pain, Calad.
— — redness of, Camph. Cist. Elaps.
— eructations, Lach.
— eyes, weakness of, Carb-veg. Ntr-m. Sep.
— face, bloated, Amm-m. Ars. Bell. Puls.
— — burning, Cham. Cocc. Laur. Sabin. Verat.
— — — at night, Cham.
— — — without being red, Plat.
— — cold, Ip. Rheum.
— — livid, Rhus.
— — pale, Ars. Cina. Croc. Ip. Lyc. Rhus. Sep.
— — red, Acon. Alum. Amm-m. Bar-m. Bell. Bry. Calc. Camph. Carb-veg. Cham. Chin. Cocc. Coff. Con. Creos. Cycl. Dulc. Elaps. Euphr. Ferr. Grat. Hep. Hyper. Igt. Lyc. Mgn-s. Ntr-m. Nux. Op. Plb. Puls. Rhus. Sep. Sil Spig. Spong. Stram. Sulph. Tar. Verat.
— — — followed by paleness without coldness, Scill.
— — — and pale alternately, Acon. Bell Bov. Caps. Nux. Op. Phosp. Puls.
— — sweat of, Puls. Sulph.
— — swelling, Ars.
— — yellow, Ars. Cina. Ntr-m.
— faintishness, Anac. Bell. Calc. Merc. Ntr-m. Nux. Phosp.
— feet, cold, Ant. Anac. Calad. Cocc. Graph. Hydroc-ac. Igt. Ip. Lach. Lact. Meny. Nux. Petr. Phosp-ac. Puls.
— fingers, deadness of, Thuj.
— forehead, coldness of, Chin. Cina. Puls.
— — sweat on, Ip. Mgn-s. Sass.
— hands burning, Agar. B.ll. Lach. Led. Nux. Petr. Phosp. Puls. Ran-b. Rheum. Stann. Sulph. Taxus.
— — cold, Euphr. Ip.
— — perspiration on, Nitr-ac.
— head, heaviness in, Ars. Cham. Phosp. Sep. Valer.
— headache, Acon. Agar. *Ang.* Ars. *Bell.* Berb. Borax. Bry. Cact. Calc. Caps.
Carb-veg. Chin. Cina. Coloc. Croton. Dros. Dulc. Elat. Eupat. Graph. Hipp. *Igt.* Kali-b. Lach. Lob. *Ntr-m.* Nux. Puls. Ruta. Sabad. Sep. Sil. Sulph. Tart. Valer.
— heart, palpitation of, Calc. Merc. Sass. Sep. Sulph.
— heat on palate, Dulc.
— itching of body, Igt.
— knee cold, Agn.
— labor like pains, Puls.
— legs cold, Meph.
— — pain in, Caps. Carb-veg. Lact.
— lie down, necessity to, Calc. Ferr-m.
— limbs, heaviness in, Calc.
— — pain, Ars. Calc. Caps. Carb-veg. Puls. Sep. Sulph.
— lips, burning in, Chin.
— liver, pain in, Ars. Elat.
— loins, pain in, Crotal. Kali-c.
— milk, desire for, Merc.
— moaning, Acon. Cham. Lach. Puls.
— mouth, burning in, Petr.
— nausea, Anac. Ant. Ars. Borax. Bry. Carb veg. Chin. Dros. Fluor-ac. Ip. Lyc. Nitr-ac. Nux. Op. Phosp. Sabad. Sep. Verat.
— nettle rash, Igt.
— pains shooting to tips of fingers and back again, Elat.
— — on corona glans, and prepuce red, and burning, relieved by perspiration, Prun.
— — worse, Merc.
— painfulness of body, when touched, Mang. Puls. Stram.
— — when uncovered, Merc.
— pulse slow, Ferr-m.
— recollect, inability to, Ars. Ntr-m. Phosp-ac. Sep.
— restlessness, Acon. Amm-c. Ars. Bar-c. Bell. Cham. Chin. Hipp. Ip. Mgn-m. Rhus.
— sacral region, pain in, Kali-c.
— shiverings, internal, Igt.
— sick feeling, internal, Sulph.
— skin, damp, Op.
— — dry, Acon. Ip.
— — red, Ars.
— — tingling in, Croc. Hipp-m.
— — yellow, Merc-cor.
— sighing, Puls.
— sight clouded, Ntr-m. Puls.
— weak, Carb-veg. Ntr-m.
— sleepiness, Apis. Asa f. Hep. Igt. Ntr-c. Op. Phosp. Plb. Puls. Stram. Verat.
— sleeplessness, Ntr-c. Puls. Rhod.
— sopor, Op. Tart.
— sore throat when swallowing, Berb. Phosp-ac.
— spleen, hard and painful, Ars.
— starting in sleep, Cham. Lyc.
— — when falling asleep, Puls.

32. FEVER.

Heat, with, stomach, pain, Carb-veg. Cina. Sep.
— — pit, of, pain, Kali-c.
— stool, to urgency, Caps.
— — frequent, Lach.
— stretching, Calc. Rhus. Sabad.
— swelling and redness of glands below ear and in throat, Cist.
— talking, continuous, Lach. Pod. Teucr.
— taste, bitter, Ars. Bry. Phosp. Sep.
— — nauseous, Caps.
— — putrid, Hyosc.
— thighs, numb and chilly, Spong.
— thirst, *Acon.* Amm-c. Ang. Arn. Ars. *Bell.* Bov. Bry. *Calc. Caps.* Carb-an. Carb-veg. Casc. Cham. *Chin. Cina.* Cist. Coff. Colch. Con. Cop. Dros. Dulc. Eupat. *Hep.* Hyosc. Ip. Lach. Lob. Mgn-m. Merc. *Ntr-m.* Nitr ac. *Nux.* Petr. Phosp. Pod. Psor. Puls. Ran-sc. *Rhus.* Sabad. *Sec-c. Sep.* Sil. Spig. Stann. Stram. Stront. *Sulph.* Tart. Valer. Verat.
— drinks little, Arn. Lyc.
— thirstlessness, Agn. Ars. Asa-f. Bell. Berb. Bry. Calc. Camph. Caps. *Carb-veg.* Chin. Cina. Coff. Cycl. Diad. Dulc. *Hell. Igt. Ip.* Kali-c. Led. Mgn c. Mang. Merc. *Meny. Mur-ac.* Ntr-m. Nitr-ac. Nitr. Nux-m. Phosp-ac. Plb. *Puls. Sabad.* Sabin. Samb. Scill. Sep. *Spig.* Staph. Stram. Stront. Sulph. Tar. Thuj.
— throat, dryness of, Lach. Nitr-ac. Nux-m.
— — pain in, Phosp. Phosp-ac. Sep.
— tongue dry, Ars.
— — coated, Ars. Phosp.
— tremor, Ars. Calc. Cist. Eupat. Mgn-c. Sep.
— unconsciousness, stupor, Ars. Dulc. Hipp-m. Ntr-m. Phosp-ac. Sep.
— uncovered, aversion to be, Ars. Aur. Clem. Colch. Con. Hep. Mgn-c. Nux-m. *Nux.* Rhus. *Samb. Scill.* Sil. *Stront.*
— — inclination to be, Acon. Calc. Ferr. Iod. Lyc. Mur-ac. Op. Plat. Spig. Verat.
— urine, red, Nux.
— urination profuse, Hipp-m. Ind.
— vertigo, Ars. Bell. Berb. Bry. Carb-veg. Igt. Ip. Mgn-s. Merc. Ntr-m. Nux. Phosp. Puls. Sep.
— vomit, inclination to, Borax. Cimex.
— vomiting, Ars. Con. Ip. Lach. Nux. Stram.
— — bilious, Cina.
— — — or mucus or water or what has been eaten, Nux.
— weakness, Anac. Ars. Bry. Calc. Eupat. Igt. Ntr-c. *Ntr-m.* Phosp. Sulph.
— weeping, Spong.
— yawning, Calc. Kali-c. Sabad.
— yellowness, of buccal cavity, Plb.

Heat preceded by cough, Calc.
— — — thirst, Chin. Ntr-m. Puls. Sabad.
— — yawning, Calc.
— succeeded by face, pale, Scill.
— — — headache, Ars.
— — — hunger, Dulc.
— — — sleep, Apis. Eupat. Lob.
— — — — with snoring, Op.
— — — thirst, Amm-m. Cact. Chin. Coff. Cycl. Nux. Op. Puls. Stann. Stram.
— — — thirstlessness, Op.
— — — vomiting of bile, Eupat.
— — — — and headache, Calc.
— — — weakness, Dig.
Perspiration, Acon. Anac. Ars. *Bell.* Bry. *Calc.* Canth. Caps. Carb-veg. Caust. Cham. *Chin.* Cina. Coff. Dig. *Dulc.* Eupion. Ferr. Graph. *Guaj.* Hell. *Hep.* Hyosc. Izi. Ip. Kali-c. Lach. Led. Lyc. *Merc.* Ntr-c. Ntr-m. Nitr-ac. *Nux.* Op. Phosp. Phosp-ac. Plb. Puls. Rheum. *Rhus.* Salad. Sabin. Samb. *Selen. Sep.* Sil. Spong. Stann. **Staph.** Stram. *Sulph.* Tart. Thuj. *Verat.*
— of single parts, *Acon.* Bar-c. Bell. Bry. *Calc.* Caps. Caust. Cham. Chin. Graph. Hell. Hep. Igt. Ip. Led. *Lyc.* Merc. Nux. Phosp. Puls. Rheum. Rhus. Sabin. Samb. *Selen. Sep.* Sil. Spig. Spong. *Sulph.* Thuj.
— — different parts, (compare the Sections).
— easy, Bry. Calc. Ferr. Graph. Kali-c. Lyc. *Ntr-c.* Ntr-m. Selen. *Sep.* Sulph. Sulph-ac. Tart. (compare During the day).
— suppressed, Acon. Amm-c. Arn. Ars. *Bell.* Bism. Bry. *Calc.* Cannab. *Cham.* Chin. Coff. *Colch. Dulc.* Hyosc. Iod. Ip. *Kali-c.* Lach. *Led. Lyc.* Mgn-c. Merc. Ntr-c. Nitr-ac. *Nux-m.* Nux. *Oleand.* Op. *Phosp.* Phosp-ac. Plat. Psor. Puls. Rhus. Sabad. Scill. *Sec-c. Seneg. Sil.* Spong. Staph. *Sulph. Teucr.* Verb. Viol-od.
— — with dry burning heat of skin, *Acon.* Arn. Ars. Bell. *Bry.* Calc. Cocc. Coff. Dulc. Hell. Kali-c. *Lach.* Led. *Lyc.* Merc. *Nux.* **Op.** *Phosp.* Phosp-ac. *Puls. Rhus.* Samb. Scill. Sec-c. Sep. Sil. Stann. Staph. Sulph.
— acrid, Cham. Con. Tar.
— bloody, Calc. Clem. Crotal. Lach. Lyc. Nux-m. Nux.
— clammy, viscous, Acon. Anac. Ars. Calc. Cham. Daph. Dig. Ferr. Fluor-ac. Hell. Hep. Iod. Jatr. *Lyc.* Lupulus. Merc. Mosch. Nux. Op. Ox-ac. *Phosp.* Phosp-ac. Plb. Tart. *Verat.*
— cold, Anac. Ars. Bar-m. Bry. Calad. Cannab. Caps. Chin. *Cina.* Cocc. Cupr. Dig. Dulc. Elaps. Gels. *Hep.* Hyosc. *Ip.* Jatr. Kalm. Lyc. Merc.

32. FEVER.

Merc-cor. Mez. Ntr-c. Nux. Ox-ac. Plb.
Puls. Rheum. Ruta. Sec-c. Sep. Sil.
Spig. Stann. Staph. Stram. Sulph.
Sulph-ac. *Tart.* Thuj. *Verat.*
Perspiration, critical, Bry.
— debilitating, Ambr. Ars. Bry. Calc.
Camph. *Carb-an.* Chin. Cocc. Croc.
Dig. Ferr. Graph. Hyosc. Iod. Lyc.
Merc. Ntr-m. *Nitr.* Phosp. Samb. Sep.
Sil. *Stann.* Sulph
— — at night, Ars. Bry. Carb-an. Chin.
Eupion. Merc. Samb. Stann.
— greasy, Bry. Chin. Mgn-c. Merc.
— insects, attracting, Calad.
— itching, Coloc. Fluor-ac. Mang. Par. Rhod.
— one-sided, Ambr. *Bar-c.* Bry. Cham. Lyc. Nux-m. Nux. *Puls.* Rhus. Sulph.
— — right, side, Nux. Puls.
— — left-sided, Phosp.
— — on forepart of body, Arg. *Calc.* Merc. *Selen.*
— — — back part of body, Chin. *Nux.* Puls. Sep. *Sulph.*
— — — upper part of body, Arg. Asar. *Cham.* Chin. Cina. Dulc. Laur. *Rheum.* Sep. Spig. Sulph-ac. Valer. Verat.
— — — lower part of body, Cinnab. Croc. Cycl. Euph.
— spots, on small, Merc.
— smelling. Bell. Canth. Hep. Led. *Lyc.* Mgn-c. Merc. *Nitr-ac.* Nux. Puls. *Rhus.* Sep. Staph. Sulph. Verat.
— — acrid, Rhus.
— — aromatic, Cop. Rhod.
— — bitter, Verat.
— — blood, like, Lyc.
— — camphor, Camph,
— — cheese, Plb.
— — eggs, rotten, Sulph.
— — empyreumatical, Bell.
— — honey, Thuj.
— — lilac, Sep.
— — mouldy, Puls. Rhus. Stann.
— — musk, Puls. Sulph.
— — offensive, Ars. *Bar-c.* Bell. Canth. Carb-an. Con. *Dulc.* Euphr. *Graph.* Guaj. Hep. Kali-c. Led. *Lyc.* Mgn-c. Merc. Nitr-ac. *Nux.* Phosp. Puls. Rhus. Sep. Spig. Staph. Sulph. Zinc.
— — onions, Bov. Lyc.
— — putrid, Carb-veg. Daph. Led. Rhus. *Staph.* Stram. Verat.
— — rhubarb, Rheum.
— — sour, Acon. Arn. Ars. Asar. Bry. Calc. Carb-veg. Caust. *Cham.* Hep. Iod. Ip. Led. Lyc. Mgn-c. Merc. Nitr-ac. Nux. Rhus. *Sep. Sil. Sulph.* Verat.
— — sweet, sour, Bry.
— — sourish, like in measles, Ferr-m.
— — sulphur, Phosp.

— — urine, Berb. Canth. Coloc. Nitr-ac.
— staining, Graph. Merc. Nux. Selen.
— — red, Arn. Dulc. Nux.
— — spotted, Selen.
— — yellow, Carb-an. *Graph. Merc.*
— stiffening the linen, Merc. Selen.
— warm, Ant. Cham. Op. Phosp. Sep. Stram.
— — causing uneasiness, *Calc.*Cham.Nux. *Puls. Sep. Sulph.*
— colliquative, Nitr.
— — in tuberculosis, Eupion.
— favors soreness of skin and decubitus, Fluor-ac.
— in the morning. Alum. Amm-c. Ang. Ant. Arg-n. Aur. Borax. Bov. Bry. Calc. Carb-an. Carb-veg. Caust. Chelid. Cic. Clem. Cocc. Creos. Dros. Eugen. Euph. Ferr-m. Graph. Hell. Hep. Iod. Lyc. Mgn-c. Mgn-m. Mgn-s. Merc. Mercurial. Mosch. Mur-ac. Ntr-c. Ntr-m. Ntr-s. Nicc. Nitr. Nux. Par. Phosp. Phosp-ac. Ran-b. Rhus. Sep. Spong. Stann. Sulph. Sulph-ac.
— — 6 A.M., Sil.
— — every other morning, Ant.
— — to noon, every other day, Ferr.
— during the day, Agar. Ambr. Anac. Bell. Bry. *Calc. Carb-an. Chin. Dulc. Ferr. Graph.* Guaj. Hep. Kali-c. Lach. Laur. Led. *Lyc. Ntr-c. Ntr-m.* Nitr-ac. Phosp-ac. Puls. *Rheum. Selen. Sep.* Sil. *Staph. Stram. Sulph.* Sulph-ac. *Tart.* Verat. Zinc.
— — while awake, Samb.
— at noon, Cinnab.
— in the afternoon, Berb. Mgn-m. Mgn-s.
— — evening, Mur-ac. Sulph.
— — — 3 to 5 P.M., Sil.
— — every other evening, Bar-c.
— at night, night sweats, Acon. Alum. *Ambr.* Amm-c. *Amm-m. Anac.* Arg.Arn. Ars. Aur. Bar-c. Bell. Bry. *Calc.*Camph. Carb-an. *Carb-veg.* Caust. Chin. Cic. Cina. Cist. Cocc. *Coloc. Con.* Cupr. Cycl. Dig. *Dulc.* Eupat. Euphr. Eupion. Ferr. *Graph.* Guaj. Gum-gut. *Hep.* Hell. Ip. Iod. *Kali-c.* Lach. Laur. Led. Lyc. *Mgn-c.* Mgn-m. Mgn-s. Mang. *Merc.* Merc-cor. *Mur-ac. Ntr-c.* Ntr-m. Ntr-s. *Nitr-ac.* Nitr. Nux. Ox-ac. Petr. Phosp. *Phosp-ac.* Plb. Puls. Rhus. Sabad.*Samb. Sep. Sil.* Spong. *Stann. Staph.* Stram. *Stront. Sulph.* Tabac. Tart. Tilia. Verat. Viol-od. Viol-tr. Zinc.
— — at 11 P.M., Sil.
— — after 3 A.M., Calc.
— — with miliary itching eruption, Rhus.
— — — stupor, Puls.
— — alternating, with dryness of skin, Apis. *Ntr-c.*

32. FEVER.

Perspiration, before midnight, Mur-ac.
— after midnight, Alum. Ambr. Amm-m. Clem. Dros. Mgn-m. Nux. Phosp.
— in the cold open air, Bry. Calc.
— bed, when getting out of, Lach.
— — — relieved, Hell.
— cough, with the, Ars.
— exertion, with, moderate of body, Agar. Graph. Kali-c. Lyc. *Ntr-c. Rheum. Sulph.*
— exercise, slight, with, Ambr. Asar. Bell. Berb. Brom. *Calc.* Carb-veg. *Chin. Cocc.* Eupion. *Ferr.* Ferr-m. *Graph.* Kali-c. Led. Lyc. Merc. *Ntr-c.* Ntr-m. Nitr. Op. *Psor. Sep.* Sil. *Stann.* Sulph. Sulph ac. Verat.
— inflamed surfaces on, standing out in drops, Graph.
— lying down, after, Mgn-s. Meny.
— meals, after, Lyc. Nitr-ac. Sep. (compare, Sect. 13.)
— — — less, Chin. Fluor-ac. Lach. Phosp.
— meals, during, Borax. Calc. Carb-an. Carb-veg. Con. Graph. Ntr-m. Nux. Ol-an. Phosp. Sass. *Sep.* Sulph-ac. (compare, Sect. 13.)
— mental exertion, from, Hep. Kali-c.
— pains, with the, *Merc.Ntr-c.*Rhus.Tabac. Tilia.
— paroxysms of madness, after, Cupr.
— parts affected, on the, Fluor-ac. Merc. Sep. Sil. Tart.
— room, in the, Fluor-ac.
— side affected, on the, Ambr. Nux.
— sitting, when, Anac. Rhus. Sep. Staph.
— sleep, in first, Calc.
— — when commencing to, Amm-c. Ars. Con. Mur-ac. Tabac. Thuj. Verat.
— sleep in, Bell. Carb-an. Chelid. Cic. Chin. Cycl. Euphr. Ferr. Hyosc. Mez. Mur-ac. Nitr-ac. Phosp. Plat.Pod.Psor. Puls. Selen.
— — — less, Nux. Rumex. Samb.
— — in morning, Borax. Lachn.
— stool, before, Merc.
— talking, when, Graph. Iod.
— walking, when, Agar. Ambr. Bruc. Cocc-c Kali-c. Led. *Ntr-m.* Selen. Sil.
— — in open air, Bry. *Carb-an.Caust.*Guaj. Ruta.
— — relieved, Alum. Graph.
— warm food, after, Kali-c. Phosp. Sulph-ac.
— attended by,
— anxiety, Arn. Berb. Bry. Calc. Cocc. Ferr. Mang. *Ntr-c.* Nitr. Nux. Phosp. Puls. Sep. Sulph.
— chest, pain in, Bry.
— chilliness, Eupat. Nux.
— colic, Nux.
— congestion of blood to head, Thuj.
— cough, Bry.

— diarrhoea, Acon.
— dreams, many, Puls.
— dyspnoea, Anac. Merc.
— ears, roaring in, Ars. Igt.
— earache, Igt.
— eruption, itching of, Rhus.
— face, cold, Lach.
— — heat, Nux.
— — pale, Verat.
— — red, Puls.
— faintishness, Anac. Ars. Chin. Sulph.
— feet, cramps in, Puls.
— pain in, Staph.
— fingers become shrivelled, Ant. Merc. Phosp-ac,
— formication, Led. Nux. *Rhod.*
— hands, cramps in, Puls.
— — hot, Nux.
— head, heaviness in, Ars. Caust.
— — pain in, Ferr. Rhus.
— — roaring in, Caust.
— hunger, Cimex.
— langor, Ars.
— legs, paralyzed, Ars.
— limbs, pain in, Nux.
— lips dry, Nux.
— miliaria, Rhus.
— nausea, Glon. Merc. Thuj.
— pain on limbs on which he lies, Nux.
— — when uncovered, Stront.
— palpitation of heart, Merc.
— restlessness, Bry. Lachn.
— shaking, Nux.
— sighing, Bry.
— sleep, Ars. Cina. Kali-c. Nitr-ac. Phosp-ac. Puls. Rhus. Sabad.
— stiches in side, Merc.
— taciturn, Mur-ac. Op.
— tenesmus, Sulph.
— thirst, Acon. Anac. Ars. Cact. Chin. Chin. Coff. Con. Eugen. Gels. Hep. Iod. Merc. Ntr-m. Puls. Rhus. Sec-c. Stram. Verat.
— thirstlessness, *Ars.* Bry. Caps. Carb-veg. Caust. Euph. *Hell. Igt. Ip.* Phosp. Puls. Sabad. *Samb.* Sep. *Spig.* Stram. Tart. Verat.
— toothache, Chin.
— tremor, with, Ars. Nux.
— uncovered, to be, inclination to, *Acon.* Calc. Ferr. Iod. Mur-ac. Op. Spig. Verat.
— — aversion to be, Ars. Aur. Chin. Clem. Colch. Con. Hep. Nux-m. *Nux.* Rhus. *Samb. Scill.*Sil.*Stront.*
— urine copious, Acon. Dulc. Phosp.
— — turbid, Phosp.
— vertigo, Ox-ac.
— vomiting, Sulph.
— waking, up, Anac. Ntr-m. Nitr-ac.
— weakness, Ars. Ox-ac. Phosp. Puls.
Perspiration, commencing with thirst,Coff. Thuj.

32. FEVER.

Perspiration commening with headache, Ferr.
— — hunger, Staph.
— followed by cough, Sil.
— — — loose, Eupat.
— — — diarrhoea, Puls.
— — — hunger, Staph.
— — — sleep, Nux-m.
— — thirst, Bell. Borax. Lyc. Nux. Sabad.
— — vomiting, of food, Cina.
Apyrexia, ailments during the;
— apathy, Igt. Phosp-ac.
— appetite, want of, Ars. Caps. Carb-veg. Chin. Cocc. Cycl. Ip. Kali-c. Ntr-m. Nux. Puls. Sabad.
— breathing, difficulty of, in night, Ars. Igt. Merc. Nux. Op. Rhus. Samb. Sulph.
— chilliness, Anac. Bry. Caps. Cocc. Daph. Dig. Led. Ntr-m. Ran-sc. Sabad. Sil. Verat.
— congestion of blood, Acon. Lyc. Petr. Puls. Sep. Sil.
— — — — to head, Acon. Arn. Chin. Lyc. Nux. Phosp. Sep. Sulph.
— constipation, Alum. Anac. Bry. Calc. Carb-veg. Chin. Cocc. Con. Ferr. Graph. Led. Lyc. Ntr-m. Nux. Op. Plb. Sabad Sil. Staph. Stram. Sulph Verat.
— coryza, dry, Calc. Carb-veg. Graph. Kali-c. Ntr-m. Nitr-ac. Phosp. Puls. Rhus. Sep. Sil. Spong. Sulph.
— convulsions, Alum. Ars. Bell. Calc. Caust. Cham. Cina. Dros. Dig. Hyosc. Igt. Merc. Nux. Op. Phosp-ac. Stann. Stram. Valer. Verat.
— cough, Arn. Ars. Bell. Bry. Chin. Cina. Cocc. Con. Dros. Eupat. Hep. Hyosc. Igt. Ip. Merc. Ntr-m. Nux. Op. Phosp. Plb. Puls. Sep. Sil. Spong. Stann. Sulph. Tart.
— — hooping, Arn. Bell. Calc. Caust. Cham. Cina. Dros. Dig. Hyosc. Igt. Merc. Nux. Op. Phosp-ac. Stann. Stram. Valer. Verat.
— diarrhœa, Ars. Cham. Chin. Dig. Dros. Gels. Igt. Merc. Nitr-ac. Phosp. Phosp-ac. Puls. Rhus. Sabin. Tart. Valer. Verat.
— dim-sightedness, Calc. Cocc. Cycl. Dig. Lyc. Merc. Ntr-m. Phosp. Sep. Sil. Stann. Sulph. Thuj.
— ears, pain in, Bell. Nitr-ac. Phosp-ac. Puls. Ran-b. Samb. Spig. Staph Sulph.
— — painful straining in, Bell. Chin Cina. Phosp. Phosp-ac. Rhus. Spig.
— emaciation, Ars. Carb-veg. Chin. Ferr. Merc. Nux. Op. Phosp-ac. Plb.
— epistaxis, Ntr-m.
— eructations, empty, Acon. Arn. Ars Bry. Calc. Carb-veg. Cocc. Con. Daph Graph. Lyc. Nitr-ac. Phosp. Sep. Stann.
— — bitter, Arn. Bry. Calc. Puls.
— — putrid, Arn. Nux. Puls. Sulph.

— — sour, Lyc. Ntr-m. Nux. Phosp. Sulph.
— — tasting of ingesta, Phosp. Puls Sil.
— eyes, affections of, Bell. Kali-c. Ntr-m. Nitr-ac Rhus. Sep. Staph. Tart. Valer.
— exercise, aversion to. Bell. Bry. Caps. Cham. Chin Cocc. Ferr. Igt. Merc. Nux. Op. Puls. Rhus. Sabad. Spig. Stram. Sulph. Verat.
— face, paleness of, Anac. Carb-veg. Chin. Cina. Daph. Igt. Lyc. Petr. Phosp. Plb. Puls. Spong Stann. Sulph. Verat
— — blueness of, Bell. Hyosc. Op. Samb.
— — bloatedness of, Ars. Bry. Hyosc. Lyc. Nux. Sep.
— — heat of, Arn. Cham. Graph. Lyc. Nux. Petr. Sabad. Spig. Verat.
— — redness of, Acon Bell. Bry. Caps. Graph. Hyosc. Op. Rhus. Samb. Stram. Verat.
— — yellowness of, Ars. Caps. Chin. Ferr. Ntr-m Nux. Petr. Rhus. Sep.
— faintishness, Arn. Ars. Calc. Carb-veg. Caust. Chin. Cina. Cocc. Con. Dig. Igt. Ip. Lyc. Ntr m. Nitr ac. Nux. Op. Puls. Sabad Verat.
— feet, coldness of, Carb-veg. Graph. Hyosc. Lyc. Rhus. Sep. Sil.
— — swelling of, Bry Caps. Caust. Chin. Ferr. Lyc. Nux. Puls. Sep. Sil.
— fits, fainting, Acon. Cham. Chin. Graph. Nux. Puls. Stram.
— — suffocating, Ars Bell. Ip. Samb. Verat.
— gastric symptoms, Acon. Ant. Bell. Bry. Cham. Coff. Dig. Igt. Ip. Nux. Puls. Rhus.
— glandular affections, Bell. Cocc. Con. Spong. Staph Sulph.
— gums, bleeding of, Calc. Carb-veg. Graph. Merc. Ntr-m. Nitr-ac. Phosp. Phosp-ac. Sep. Staph. Sulph.
— hands, coldness of, Carb-veg. Nitr-ac. Rhus. Spig.
— — swelling of, Calc. Dig. Lyc. Stann.
— head, heat in, Arn. Igt. Lyc. Sil. Spig.
— headache, Ars. Bell. Bry. Caps. Carb-veg. Chin. Cocc. Dros. Igt. Ntr-m. Nux. Op Phosp-ac. Puls. Rhus. Sep. Spong. Stann. Valer.
— hearing, sensitiveness of, Anac. Arn. Bell. Coff. Igt. Merc. Phosp-ac. Sep. Spig.
— — hardness of, Calc. Lyc. Nitr-ac. Petr. Rhus.
— heartburn, Calc. Caps. Lyc. Nux. Petr. Sep Sil. Spong. Sulph.
— hoarseness, Bry. Calc. Caps. Carb-veg. Cham. Lyc. Ntr-m. Nitr-ac. Petr. Phosp. Phosp-ac. Puls. Sep Spig. Spong.
— hunger, Carb-veg. Chin. Cina. Graph. Lyc. Stann. Sulph. Verat.
— jaundice, Acon. Ars. Bell. Cham. Chin. Dig. Ferr. Merc. Nux. Puls. Rhus. Sulph.

32. FEVER.

Apyexia, lie down, inclination to, Acon. Bell. Caps. Ferr. Nux.
— limbs, sense of paralysis in, Acon. Arn Carb-veg. Chin. Cocc. Cycl. Dros. Nux. Plb. Sil. Verat.
— — stiffness of, Cocc. Lyc. Sabad.
— — tearing pain in, Calc Caps. Carb-veg. Caust. Ch n. Dros. Graph. Lyc. Nitr-ac Puls. Sabin.
— loathing of food, Arn. Bell. Phosp-ac. Puls.
— mammæ, swelling of, Bry. Calc. Pu's.
— menses too early, Acon. Alum. Ars. Bell. Bry. Calc. Carb-veg. Cham Cocc. Ferr. Hyosc. Igt. Kali-c. Led. Lyc. Merc. Nux. Petr. Phosp. Rhus. Sabin. Sep. Spong. Staph. Sulph. Verat
— — too scanty, Alum. Con. Graph. Lyc Ntr-m. Phosp. Puls. Sabad. Sil Sulph. Verat.
— — too late, Bell. Caust. Chin. Con. Ferr. Graph. Hyosc. Igt Ip. Kali-c. Lyc. Ntr-m. Puls. Sabad. Sil. Sulph.
— — too profuse, A on. Ars. Bell. Calc. Cham. Chin. Cina. Ferr Hyosc. Igt. Ip. Led. Lyc. Merc. Ntr-m. Nux. Op Phosp. Sa in. Sep. Sil. Spong. Stann. Stram. Sulph.
— — suppressed, Ars. Ca'c. Cham. Chin. Con. Ferr. Graph. Kali-c. Lyc. Merc. Nux. Puls. Sep. Sil. Sulph.
— mouth. offensive odor from, Arn. Cham. Merc. Nux. Petr. Sep. Sil. Sulph.
— nausea, Ars. Graph. Hep. Hyosc. Ip. Nux. Rhus. Sibad. Sil.
— oppression of chest, Ars. Caps. Carb-veg. Cocc. Igt. Ntr-m. Plb. Sabad. Samb. Spig. Stann. Stram. Sulph. Verat.
— pain in chest, Bry. Puls. Ran-b. Rhus. Sabad. Spig. Stann.
— — joints, Arn. Ars. Bry. Caust. Cham. Chin. Cocc. Igt. Ip. Phosp-ac. Plb. Puls. Rhus. Sabin. Sulph.
— — stomach, pit of, Bell. Bry. Calc. Chin. Lyc. Merc. Nt -m. Nux. Phosp. Puls. Sabad. Sep. Sil. Spig. Stann. Verat.
— — hip, Ars. Bell. Cham. Merc. Nux. Puls. Rhus.
— — liver, Bell. Bry. Cham. Lyc. Merc. Nux Puls.
— — abdomen, Led. Plb. Ran-b. Sulph. Tart.
— — kidneys, Bell Chin. Hep. Lyc. Staph.
— — back, Arn. Ars. Ca'c. Caps Cham. Cina. Igt. Ntr-ac. Nux. Petr. Samb. Sep. Sil. Spig. Stram. Thuj. Verat.
— — rheumatic, Acon. Arn. Bell. Bry. Carb-veg. Caust. C am. Nux. Puls. Rhus. Tart. Thuj Valer. Verat.
— — labor-like, Bell. Op. Puls.
— — in stomach, Acon Arn. Ars. Calc. Caust. Cocc. Con. Ferr. Igt. Lyc. Ntr-m. Nux. Puls. Sabad. Sep. Sil. Stann.

— painlessness, Con. Hell. Op. Phosp-ac. Stram.
— palpitation of heart, Acon. Igt. Merc. Ntr-m. Sep. Spig. Sulph. Verat.
— ptyalism, Cham. Dig. Dros. Hyosc. Led. Merc. Nitr-ac. Rhus. Spig. Verat.
— redness of cheeks, Caps. Cham. Chin.
— repugnance to beer, Alum. Bell. Cham.
— — bread, Bell. Con. Cycl. Igt. Kali-c. Lyc. Nitr-m. Nitr-ac. Nux. Phosp. Phosp-ac. Puls. Rhus.
— — coffee, Bell. Carb-veg. Cham. Chin. Coff. Merc. Ntr-m. Nux. Rhus. Sabad. Spig.
— — fat food, Hell. Hep. Ntr-m. Petr.
— — meat, Alum. Arn. Ars. Bell. Calc. Carb-veg. Cham. Daph. Ferr. Graph. Igt. Lyc. Merc. Nitr-ac. Op. Petr. Puls. Rhus. Sabad. Sep. Sil Sulph.
— — milk, Arn. Bell. Calc. Igt. Sep. Sil. Stann.
— — sour food, Bell. Igt. Phosp-ac.
— — sweet things, Arn. Ars. Caust. Graph. Igt. Merc. Nitr-ac. Verat.
— — tobacco, Alum. Arn. Bell. Calc. Chin. Daph. Igt. Led. Ntr-m. Nux. Phosp. Rhus. Sep. Spig. Stann.
— — warm food, Anac. Ars. Bell. Cham. Chin. Cocc. Coff. Cycl. Ferr. Graph. Hell. Igt. Lyc. Merc Nux. Puls. Sabad. Sil. Sulph. Tart. Verat.
— senses, irritability of, Acon. Bell. Cham. Chin. Coff. Igt. Merc. Nux. Puls. Valer.
— — weakness of, Anac. Caps. Cham. Cycl. Hell. Plb. Puls. Sil.
— sleepiness, Acon. Arn. Bell. Bry. Calc. Carb-veg. Hyosc. Merc. Op. Sabad. Spig. Stann. Stram. Sulph. Valer.
— sleeplessness, Ars. Bell. Bry. Carb-veg. Chin Cina. Coff. Hyosc. Ip. Led. Merc. Ntr-m Nitr-ac. Op. Puls. Ran-b. Rhus. Sil. Spig.
— smell, loss of, Anac. Cycl. Daph. Hyosc. Nux. Op. Puls. Sep. Sil. Tart.
— sensitiveness of, Acon. Bell. Dros. Nux.
— skin, desquamation of, Acon. Daph. Dig. Hell. Merc. Phosp-ac. Rhus. Sabad Sulph. Verat.
— — distention of, Ars. Bell. Bry. Chin. Con. Dig. Ferr. Hell. Hyosc. Op. Plb. Rhus. Samb. Sep.
— somnolence, Bell. Cham. Cocc. Hyosc. Op. Puls. Rhus. Tart.
— sopor, Cham. Op. Puls. Verat.
— spasms in stomach, Ars. Bell. Bry. Carb-veg. Cham. Cocc. Ferr. Igt. Ntr-m. Nux. Puls. Sil. Stann. Sulph. Valer.
— — uterine, Bry. Cocc. Con. Igt.
— stupefaction, Acon. Bell. Cocc. Daph. Kali-c. Op. Stram.

32. FEVER.

Apyrexia, sweat too copious, Ars. Calc. Chin.Ferr. Graph. Nux. Samb. Valer.
— — dificient, Kali-c. Lyc.
— swelling of cheeks, Cham. Rhus.
— tips of fingers, Thuj.
— — pit of stomach, Bry. Carb-veg.Cham. Cic. Coff. Hell. Lyc. Nux. Op. Puls. Sabad.
— — spleen, Caps. Nitr-ac. Nux.
— tongue, Ars. Bell. Chin. Merc. Nitr-ac.
— taste bitter, Ars. Bry. Calc. Carb-veg. Cham. Lyc. Merc. Ntr-m. Nitr-ac. Petr. Phosp-ac. Puls. Sabin. Sulph.
— — — of food, Cham. Ip. Phosp-ac.
— — flat, Bry. Cycl. Nux.
— lost, Lyc. Puls. Sil. Verat.
— — metallic, Cocc. Merc. Nux. Rhus.
— — nauseating, Ip. Kali-c.
— — putrid, Bell. Merc. Nux. Puls.
— — saltish, Ars. Carb-veg. Chin. Merc.
— — sour, Calc. Igt. Nux. Petr. Phosp. Sep.
— throat, inflammation of, Acon. Alum. Bell. Cham. Merc. Nux. Puls. Rhus. Samb.
— — roughness of, Kali-c. Nitr-ac. Phosp. Ran-b. Stann.
— — sore, Bell. Caps. Hep. Igt. Led. Nitr-ac. Nux. Phosp. Plb. Ran-b. Sabad. Sabin. Spong.
— tremor, Arn. Bry. Chin. Cocc. Con. Graph. Igt. Nux. Op. Puls. Rhus. Sabad.
— uneasiness, Acon. Ars. Bell. Cham. Cina. Dros. Phosp. Sil. Spig.
— urine, difficulty of passing the, Caps. Caust. Dig. Staph.
— — urgent desire to pass, Dros. Hell. Hyosc. Lyc. Phosp. Phosp-ac. Tart. Thuj.
— — dark, Bry. Calc. Carb-veg. Chin. Merc. Sep.
— — light colored, Phosp-ac. Thuj.
— — turbid, Chin. Dulc. Graph. Ip. Merc. Tart.
— vertigo, Acon. Arn. Ars. Bell. Calc. Caust. Cham. Cocc. Con. Daph. Hyosc. Lyc. Nitr-ac. Nux. Op. Petr. Phosp. Puls. Ran-b. Sep. Sil.
— vomiting, Chin. Cina. Ferr. Hyosc. Ip. Merc. Nux. Sep. Sil. Tart.
— — bilious, Ars. Ip. Merc. Nux. Stram. Verat.
— — mucus, Merc. Nux. Puls.
— — of ingesta, Ars. Cham. Ferr. Ip. Nux. Puls.
— weakness, Ars. Chin. Dig. Ferr. Lyc. Nitr-ac. Verat.
— — nervous, Bell. Cham. Chin. Coff. Igt. Nux. Puls. Valer.
Compound fevers, Acon. Ars. Bell. Bry. Calc. Caps. Cham. Chin. Graph. Hell.

Hep. Igt. Merc. *Nux*. Phosp. Puls. *Rhus*. Sabad. Sep. *Sulph*. Verat.
— chills with heat, Acon. Anac. *Ars*. Bell. *Calc*. Cham. Cocc. Coloc. Hell. *Igt*. Merc. Ntr-m. Nitr-ac. Nux. Oleand. Petr. Plb. Puls. Ran-b. Rhus Sabad. Sabin. Sep Sil. Staph. Thuj. Verat.
— — — on single parts, Ol-an. Sabad.
— — — sensation of, Oleand.
— — partial with heat, Bell. Nux. Rhus.
— — with heat, then perspiration, Calc. Caps. Sulph.
— — — and perspiration, Nux.
— — external, heat internal, Arn. Chelid. *Mosch*. Phosp-ac. Rhus. Sec-c. Verat.
— — internal; heat external, Acon. Anac. Ars. Bell. *Calc*. Coff. Igt. Lach. *Laur*. Lyc. Meny. Nitr. *Nux*. Par. Phosp. Scill. *Sep*. Sil. Sulph.
— — alternating with heat, Acon. Agn. Ars. Bell. *Bry*. Calc. Chin. Coloc. Hep. Iod. Kali-b. Kali-c. Lach. Lyc. *Merc*. Ntr-m. Nux. Phosp. Phosp-ac. Rheum. Rhod. Sabad. Sang. Selen. Spig. Sulph. Tart. Verat.
—, — — — followed by perspiration,Kali-c. Meny. Verat.
— — — — then heat, finally perspiration, Bry.
— — — — — followed by perspiration, Kali-c.
— — followed by heat, Acon. Alum. Amm-m. Arn. Bar-c. Bell. Berb. Borax. Bry. *Caps*. Carb-veg. Caust. Cham. Chin. *Cina*. Coff. Cop. Croc. Cycl. Dros. Dulc. Graph. Hep. *Igt*. *Ip*. Kali-c. Lach. Lyc. Meny. Merc. Ntr-m. Nitr-ac. *Nux*. Op. Phosp. Phosp-ac. *Puls*. Rhus. *Sabad*. Sec-c. Sep. Sil. Spig. Stram. *Sulph*. Valer. Verat.
— — — partial heat, Cycl.
— — — partial heat in face, Ambr. Cycl. Petr.
— — — heat in head, Ip.
— — — — then cold, Sulph.
— — followed by heat, with perspiration, Acon. Alum. Anac. Bell. Caps. *Cham*. Chin. Cina. Graph.Hell.Hep. Igt. Kali-c. Ntr-m. Nitr-ac. Nux. *Op*. Phosp. Puls. Rhus. Sabad. Spig. Sulph.
— — — with partial perspiration, Hep.
— followed by heat, then perspiration, Ars. Bry. Caps. Carb-veg. Caust. Chin. Cina. Dig. Dros. Graph. Hep. Igt. Ip. Kali-c. Lyc. Ntr-m. Nitr-ac. Nux. Op. Phosp. Plb. Puls. Rhus. Sabad. Sabin. Samb. Spong. Staph. Sulph. Verat.
— — — without perspiration, Graph.
— — with perspiration, Euph. Lyc. Puls. Sulph.

32. FEVER.

Compound fevers, chills followed by perspiration, Bry. Caps. Carb-an. *Caust.* Cham. Dig. Lyc. Mgn-s. Mez. Ntr-m. Op. Petr. Phosp. Phosp-ac. Rhus. Sabad. Sep. Sulph. Thuj. Verat.
— shuddering, with heat. *Bell. Cham. Hell.* Igt. Nux. Rheum. Rhus. Zinc.
— — with flashes of heat, Zinc.
— — alternating with heat, *Ars.* Bell. *Bry*. Cham. Cocc. Mgn-s. *Merc*. Mosch. Nux. Sep.
— — followed by heat, Bell. Igt. Laur. Sep. Sulph.
— — — perspiration, Clem. Dig. Ntr-m. Rhus.
— heat in hands and face, and cool face, Rheum.
— — partial with coldness of limbs, Pæon.
— — in head or face, with coldness of hands and feet. Amm-c. Arn. Aur. Bell. Brom. Kali-c. Lact. Ran-b. Rhod. Ruta. Sabin. Scill. Stram.
— — followed by chills, Bry. Calc. Caps. Caust. Chin. Igt. Meny. Merc. Ntr-m. Nicc. Nux. Petr. Phosp. Puls. Sep. Stann. Sulph. Thuj.
— — — — then heat, Stram.
— — — — then heat, with perspiration, Rhus.
— — followed by coldness of hands, Calc. Iris.
— — in head, followed by coldness and finally heat, Stram.
— — — face, followed by chills, Calc.
— — with shuddering, Acon. Bell. Cham. Hell. Igt. Lach. Merc. Rhus. Sep.
— — — perspiration, Bell. Berb. Bry. Caps. Cham. Chin. Cina. Con. Eupat. Euph. Ferr-m. Grat. Hell. Hydroc-ac. Igt. Kobalt. Lac-can. Mgn-c. Mgn-m. Merc. Ntr-c. Nux. *Op.* Ox-ac. Par. Phosp. Puls. Rhus. Sabad. Stann. Stram.
— — — — partial, Alum. Chin. Ol-an. Puls. Sep. Tart.
— — — — then chills, Phosp. Stann.
— — — — alternately, Bell. Led.
— — followed by perspiration, Aloe. Amm-c. Ant. Calad. Calc. Carb-veg. Hell. Igt. Ran-sc. Sil. Tart.
— — without thirst then chill with thirst, Igt.
— perspiration followed by chills, Carb-veg. Hep.
— followed by chills then perspiration, Nux.
— — followed by heat, Nux.
— — — by thirst, Lyc.
Pulse changed, in general, *Acon.* Arn. Ars. Bell. Bry. Carb-veg. Chin. Con. *Creos.* Cupr. Dig. Hep. *Hyosc. Iod.* Kali-c. Laur. Merc. *Op. Phosp. Phosp-ac. Rhus.* Samb. Sec-c. Sep. *Sil. Stram.* Sulph.

Tart. *Verat.*
— unchanged, Alum. Anac. Ang. Ant. Asa-f. Borax. Caps. Chin. Clem. Cycl. *Dros.* Euph. *Euphr. Mgn-c. Ntr-c.* Oleand. Par. Ran-sc. Rheum. Ruta. Sec-c. Tar. Teucr. Verb.
— audible, Tart.
— contracted, Acon. Arn. Asa-f. Bism. Kali-b. Laur. Plb. Sec-c.
— double heat, Cycl.
— empty, Camph. Chin.
— fluttering, Apis. Phosp-ac.
— frequent, Acon. Apis. Arg. Arn. Ars. Bar-m. Bell. Bry. Calad. Canth. Carb-veg. Cham. Chin. Cina. Colch. Cupr. Igt. Iod. Mosch. Nitr. Nux. Oleand. Phosp-ac. Plb. Samb. Seneg. Sil. Stann. Stram. Viol-od.
— — and intermittent, Hyosc.
— — and rapid, Tart.
— — and small, Ars. Aur. Bell. Colch. Glon. Iod. Igt. Lach. *Phosp. Sil. Stann.* Stram. Sulph-ac. Zinc.
— strong and small, Iod. Phosp.
— full, *Acon.* All-cep. Alum. Arg. Arn. Asa-f. Bapt. Bar-m. *Bell.* Bry. Camph. Canth. Chelid. Chin. Chin-sulph. Colch. Coloc. Cor-r. Cupr. Daph. *Lig.* Dulc. Ferr. Igt. Iod. *Hyosc.* Lach. Led. Merc. Mosch. Mur-ac. Ntr-m. *Nitr.* Oleand. Op. Petr. Phosp. Phosp-ac. Plb. Ran-b. Ran-sc. Samb. Sil. Spong. *Stram.* Sulph. Tart. Verat.
— — and empty, Mosch.
— — and fast, Coloc.
— — — frequent, Cham. Mosch. Spong. Tart.
— — — hard, Acon. Bell. Canth. Chelid. Ferr. Glon. Graph. Phosp. Stram.
— — — large, Iod.
— — — — and frequent, Mosch.
— — — sluggish, Samb.
— — — strong and slow, Stram.
— hard, *Acon.* Aeth. Amm-c. Ant. Arn. Ars. Bar-c. *Bell.* Bism. *Bry.* Calad. Camph. Canth. Chin. *Chelid.* Colch. Coloc. Cor-r. Cupr. Daph. Dig. Dulc. Ferr. Hep. *Hyosc.* Igt. Iod. Led. Merc. Mez. Mosch. Nitr. Nux. Op. Phosp. Phosp-ac. Plb. Sabin. Scill. Seneg. Sep. Sil. Sol-m. Spig. Spong. *Stram.* Sulph. Tart.
— — frequent, Seneg.
— — and full, Nitr.
— — full and large, Colch.
— — intermitting, Mez.
— — small, Cocc.
— — — frequent, Dig.
— — — metallic, Scill.
— — and uneven, Canth.
— heavy, Phosp.
— imperceptible, *Acon.* Agn. Ars. Cannab. Carb-veg. Cicc. Cocc. *Cupr.* Ferr. Hell.

32. FEVER.

Hyosc. Ip. Kalm. Laur. Merc. Nux. Op. Phosp-ac. Plat. Puls. Rhus. Sec-c. *Sil.* Stann. Stram. Sulph. Tart. *Verat.*
Pulse, intermitting, Acon. Agar. Ang. Apis. Ars. Brom. Bry. Canth. Caps. Carb-veg. Chin. Daph. *Dig.* Glon. Hep. Hyosc. Kali-c. Lach. Laur. Mur-ac. *Ntr-m.* Op. *Phosp-ac.* Plb. Rhus. Sabin. Sec-c Sep. Stram. Sulph. Tabac. Thuj. Verat. Zinc.
— — entirely, Plb.
— — every 1 or 2 beats, Phosp-ac.
— — — other beat, Dig.
— — — 3 beats, Mur-ac.
— — — 4th beat, Nitr-ac.
— — — 3d, 5th or 30th, Crotal.
— — — 4th or 5th, Nux.
— — — 10th to 30th beat, Lach.
— — in apoplexy, Lach.
— — better in morning after drinking, coffee, Ang.
— — fast, Hyosc.
— — hard, Mez. Plb.
— — hard and tense, Mez.
—,— irregular, weak and tremulous, Stram.
— — small, Ars. Bism. Grat. *Hyosc.* Nux. *Plb.* Sec-c. Vipra-torv.
— — — and fast, Ars. Asa-f. Stram.
— — spasmodic and fast Sec-c.
— — and fast, Hyosc. Plb. Sec-c.
— — — weak. Plb.
— — — — uneven and contracted, Vipra-torv.
— — slow, Dig. Sec-c.
— — rapid, Ars. Hyosc. Ophist. Plb. Sec-c. Stram. Vipra-torv.
— — small, Ars. Hyosc. Plb. Sec-c. Vipra-torv.
— — uneven, Agar. Ars. Vipra-torv.
— — especially when lying on the left side. Ntr-m.
— — and then the second double stroke of heart is heard, Gels.
— irregular, Acon. Agar. Ang. Asa-f Bell. Bry. Caps. Carb-veg. Chin. Dig. Gels. Glon. Hydroc-ac. Igt. Kali-b Lach. Ntr-m. Op. *Phosp-ac.* Plb. Rhus. Sacch. Samb. Sec-c. Sep. Stram. Sulph. Verat.
— — beating with slow pulse, Laur.
— — and strong. Laur. Seneg.
— — soft, Seneg.
— irritable, Colch. Meny.
— quick, *Acon.* Aeth. All-cep. Alum. Amm-c. Amm-m. Apis. Arn. Ars. Aur. Bell. *Bry.* Canth. Carb-veg. Chin. Colch. Cupr. Daph. Glon. Guaj. Gymnoc. Hep. Hyosc Igt. *Iod.* Ip. Kali-b. Kali-jod. Lach. Lyc. Meny.

Merc. Mosch. Nitr. Op. Petr. Phell. *Phosp. Phosp-ac.* Puls. Ran-b. Sabin. Samb. Seneg. *Sil.* Spong. *Stann.* Staph. *Stram.* Sulph-ac. Thuj. Valer. Verat. Viol-od.
— — in morning, Agar. Ars. Kali-c. Sulph. Thuj.
— — — afternoon, Lyc.
— — when moving about slow when at rest, Dig. Gels.
— — in evening, Cinnab. Ran-b.
— — at night, slow during the day, Bry.
— — at one time, and weak and another, slow and full, Ntr-m.
— quicker than the beating of the heart, Acon. Arn. Rhus. Spig.
— slower than beating of heart, Dig. Hell. Laur. Verat.
— not synochrous with heart, Kali-chl.
— quivering, *Calad.*
— sensation as if circulation was suspended, Sabad.
— shaking the whole body, Ntr-c.
— slow, Bell. Berb. Camph. Cannab. Con. Cupr. *Dig.* Hell. Ferr-m. Lact. Laur. Op. Sep. *Stram* Verat.
— — when, almost imperceptible, thread-like, Ars.
— — — is weak, Arn.: reverse, Bell.
— — in morning, rapid in afternoon, Nitr.
— — after meals, Chin.
— small, *Acon.* Aeth. Apis. Ars. Aur. Bell. Bry. Calad. Camph. *Carb-veg.* Cham. Chin. Cocc. Creos. *Cupr.* Dig. Dulc. *Guaj.* Hipp-m. Hydroc-ac. Hyosc. Kali-b. Kali-c. *Laur.* Lob. Merc Op. Phosp. Phosp-ac. Plat. Puls. Rhus. Samb. Sec-c. *Sil.* Stann. Staph. *Stram.* Sulph. Sulph-ac. *Verat.*
— — slow, Hyosc.
— — — and rapid, Ars. Aur. Bell. Cupr. Hyosc. Iod. Lach. Phosp. Puls. *Sil. Stann.* Stram. Sulph-ac. Zinc.
— — — frequent, Agn. Cupr. Hyosc. Iod. Tabac. Valer.
— — — vermifious, Iod. *Verat.*
— — week and feeble, Nitr.
— soft, Acon. Bapt. Bell. *Carb-veg.* Cupr. Ferr. Laur. Merc. Phosp. Plat. Ran-sc. *Verat*
— — and small, Nitr.
— — — uneven, Seneg.
— suppressed, Acon. Ars. Carb-veg. Nux. Op. Sil. Stram. Tart. (compare Imperceptible).
— tense, Amm-c. Bell. Bry. Camph. Cham. Daph. Dulc. Sabin. Sec-c. Valer.
— tremulous, Apis. Ars. Bell. *Calc.* Cic. Creos. Rhus. Sabin. Sep. *Spig.* Staph.
— weak, (compare small).

33. Skin.

Abscesses, Ant. Asa-f. Calc. Dulc. Hep. Kali-c. Lach. Merc. Ntr-c. Puls. Sep. Sil. Sulph.
Adhesion of skin, Arn. Par.
Bites, Arn. Bell. Calad. Led. Sulph-ac.
— of venomous, animals, Aur. Ars. Bell. Lach. Seneg.
— stings, Arn. Bry. Bufo.
Biting on skin, Amm-m. Berb. Bry. Calc. Carb-veg. Caust. Colch. *Euph.* Ip. Lach. *Led.* Mez. Nux. Oleand. Ol-an. Phell. *Puls.* Ran-sc. Spong. Sulph.
Bladders, *Amm-m* Ant. *Ars. Bell.* Bry. Canth. Carb-veg. Caust. Chin. Clem. Creos. *Dulc.* Graph. Hell. Hep. Kali-c. Lach. *Merc.* Ntr-c Phosp. Plat. *Ran-b.* Ran-sc. *Rhus.* Sep Sil. Sol-m. *Sulph.* (compare Vesicles).
— forming, scabs, Amm-m.
Blood oozing from skin, Lach.
— blisters, *Ars.* Aur. Fluor-ac. Ntr-c. Ntr-m. *Sec-c.* Sulph.
— — black, Arg-n. Lach.
— — brown, Ant. Carb-veg. Lyc. Mez. Ntr-ac. Phosp. Sep. Thuj.
Boils, Acon. Ant. Apis *Arn. Bell.* Brom. Calc. Caust. *Euph.* Hep. Hyosc. Ind. Lach. Led. Lyc. Mgn-c Mgn-m Merc. Mez. Mur-ac. Ntr-m. *Nitr-ac.* Nitr. Nux-m. *Phosp. Phosp-ac.* Sec-c. Sep. Sil. Staph. Sulph. Sulph-ac. *Thuj.* Zinc.
— blood, Arn Bell. Euph. Hyosc. Iris. Led. Lyc. Mgn-m. Mur ac. Ntr-m. Ntr-ac. Nux-jug. Phosp. Phosp-ac. Sep Sil. Sulph. Thuj.
— blue. Lach.
— large, Hep. Hyosc. Lyc. Nitr-ac. Nux. Sil.
— periodical. Hyosc. Lyc. Nitr-ac. Staph
— small, Arn. Kali-jod. Mgn-c. Sulph. Zinc.
— in the spring, Bell.
— stinging when touched, Mur-ac. Sil.
Bran like, furfuraceous, covering of skin, Ars. Calc. Carb-an. Carb-veg. Lach. Lyc. Merc. Nitr-ac. Sil. Sulph.
Bubbling in skin, Calc.
Burning, *Acon. Agar.* All-cep. *Ambr.* Anac. Arg. Arn. *Ars. Bell.* Berb. Bry. Calad Calc. Caps. *Carb-veg* Caust. Cic. Cop. Dig. Dulc. *Euph. Hep.* Hyosc. Igt.

Kali-c. Lach. Lyc. Mang. Merc. Mez. Nitr. Nux. Ol-an. Op. *Phosp.* Puls. Ran-b. *Rhus.* Sabad. Scill. Selen. *Sep. Sil.* Stann. Sulph.
— in evening, after rising from bed, Mang.
— itching, Anac. Arg. Calc. Cic. Colch. Dig. Euph. Hep. Kali-c. Nux. Ol-an. Phell. Plat. Puls. Rhus. Scill. Stann. (compare, Itching—burning.)
— in skin after itching, Sep.
— after mental affections, Bry.
— at night, *Ars.* Cinnab.
— on parts affected, Acon. Sabin.
— prickling, Bar-c. Lact. Plat.
— when scratched, Anum c. Evon. Grat. Led. *Merc.* Ntr-s. Sep. Sil. Sulph.
— stinging, *Bar-c.* Bry. Cannab. Sabad.
— when touched, Ferr. Sabin.
— with desire to touch the part, Calad.
— in cavities of the body, Canth.
— as from flames, Viol-tr.
— — — sparks, Sec-c. Selen.
— vesicular, Kali-c.
— in small spots, Fluor-ac.
Burnings, *Ars.* Carb-veg. *Caust.* Creos. Stram.
Burnt, pain as if, Ars. Caust. Puls. Sec-c. Sulph-ac. Urt-ur.
Callosites, Ant. *Graph.* Phosp. Ran-b. *Sep.* Sil
— horny, Ant. Graph.
— red, Sabad.
Carbuncle, *Ars. Bell.* Bufo. Sec-c. *Sil.*
— with burning pains, Ars. Coloc.
— — and stinging pains, Apis.
— purple, with many small blisters, around, Lach.
— soreness in, Hep.
Chafing, *Amm-c.* Arn. Ars. *Bar-c.* Calc. *Caust. Cham. Chin. Graph.* Hep. *Igt.* Kali-c. Lach *Lyc.* Mang. Merc. Ol-an. *Petr.* Phosp. Plb. Puls. Ruta. Scill. *Sep.* Sulph. Sulph-ac.
— pain as from, Acon. Ferr. Hep. Nux. Par. Plat
— — — when touched, Ferr. Hep. Par.
— in bends of joints, Bell. Caust. Lyc. *Mang.* Ol-an. Petr. Sep. Sulph.
— — children, Amm-c. Calc. *Carb-veg.* Caust. *Cham.* Chin. Graph. *Igt.* Kali-c. Lyc. Ruta. Scill. Sep. *Sulph.*

33. SKIN.

Chafing, with gangrenous ulceration, becomes easily chafed with walking or riding, Sulph-ac.
— itching, Petr.
— between the limbs, Scill.
— moist, *Bar-c.* Lyc. *Petr.*
— rasping, Phosp.
— stinging, Phosp.
Chicken-pox, *Ant.* Led. *Puls.* Rhus. Sil. *Sol-m. Tart.*
Chilblains, *Agar.* Ant. Ars. Bell. Bry. *Carb-an. Carb-veg.* Cham. Chin. *Croc.* Cycl Hyosc. Igt. Lyc. Nitr-ac. *Nitr.* Nux-m. *Nux.* Op. *Petr. Phosp.* Phosp-ac. *Puls.* Rhus. Sep. Stann. Staph. Sulph-ac. Thuj. Zinc.
— bluish, Arn. Bell. Kali-c. Puls.
— — burning, Nux. Puls. Spig.
— cracked, Nux. Petr.
— inflamed, Ars. Nitr-ac. *Puls.* Sulph.
— itching, Agar. Berb. Colch. Lyc. Nitr-ac. Nux. Sulph.
— — from slight cold, with cracking of skin, Nitr-ac.
— — in warmth, Sulph.
— inflamed, burning, Carb-an.
— — — itching, Agar. Berb. Hep. Puls. Sulph.
— painful, *Nitr-ac.* Petr. Phosp. Puls.
— pustulous, Nitr-ac. *Rhus.*
— red, Agar. Ant. Arn. *Ars. Bell.* Berb. Bry. *Carb-an.* Cham. Colch. Cycl. Hep. Hyosc. Lyc. *Nitr-ac. Nux. Petr.* Phosp. Phosp-ac. *Puls. Rhus.* Staph. *Sulph.* Sulph-ac. *Thuj.*
— tickling, *Rhus.*
— aggravated in warm weather, Fragaria-vesca.
Cicatrices, Lach. Nitr-ac. Phosp. Sil.
— cicatrized skin, Sabin.
— aching in, Nux.
— bleeding, Lach. Phosp.
— breaking open, Carb-veg. Croc. Crotal. Lach. Ntr-m. Phosp. Sil.
— — and suppurating, Croc.
— brown, Lach.
— burning in, Ars. Carb-veg. Graph. Lach.
— itching, Fluor-ac. Iod.
— painful, Lach. Nitr-ac. Nux.
— — on change of weather, Carb-veg. Nitr-ac.
— red, *Merc.*
— — with itching vesicles, Fluor-ac.
— pimples, itching in, Iod.
— sore, Nux.
— — becoming, Caust.
— contractive pain, Phosp.
— stinging, Carb-an.
— fissure in cicatrix of an old issue, Kali-c.
Clammy skin, Acon. Bry. Cham. Iod. Lyc. Merc. Phosp. Phosp-ac. Verat.
Coldness of skin, Arn. *Ars.* Bell. Calc. Camph. Caust. Chelid. Chin. *Ip.* Lyc. Merc. Mez. Nitr-ac. *Nux-m.* Nux. Phosp. *Plat.* Puls. *Rhus.* Ruta. Samb. *Sec-c.* Sep. *Sulph.* Tart. *Verat.* (compare, Fever.)
— sensation of external, Arn. Calc. Caust. Chelid. *Merc. Mosch. Plat.* Puls. *Rhus. Sec-c. Verat.*
Color of skin, blackish, Arg-n. Lach.
— bluish, Amm-c. *Ars.* Bell. Camph. Carb-veg. Chin. Con. Cupr. *Dig.* Hydroc-ac. *Lach.* Laur. Nux. *Op.* Phosp. Plb. Sec-c. Sulph. *Verat.*
— — gray, Arg-n.
— brown, Ant. Carb. Lyc. Mez. Nitr-ac. Phosp. Sep. Thuj.
— dirty, Ferr. Iod. Merc.
— — brown, Ferr. Iod. Thuj. (compare, the colors.)
Condylomata, Calc. Cham. Cinnab. Euph. Euphr. Lyc. Nitr-ac. Phosp-ac. Phyt. Sabin. Staph. *Thuj.*
Corns, *Amm-c. Ant.* Bov. Bry. *Calc.* Caust. Igt. *Lyc.* Nitr-ac. *Petr. Phosp. Phosp-ac.* Ran-sc. Rhus. Sep. *Sil.* Sraph. Sulph.
— aching, Ant. Lyc. Sep. Sil. Sulph.
— boring, Ran-sc. Sep. Sil.
— burning, Amm-c. Bry. Calc. Lyc. Phosp-ac. Rhus. Sep. Sulph.
— horny, Ant.
— inflamed, Lyc. Sep. Sil.
— jerks, with, Sep. Sulph. Sulph-ac.
— painful, Ant. Arn. Bar-c. Bry. Calc. Caust. Hep. Igt. Lach. *Lyc.* Ntr-m. Nitr-ac. Nux. Phosp. Puls. Ran-sc. Rhus. Sep. *Sil.* Spig. Sulph.
— — as if ulcerated, Amm-c. Borax.
— pressing, Ant. *Bry.* Caust. *Lyc.* Sep. Sil. *Sulph.*
— sore, smarting, Ambr. Ant. Bry. Hep. Igt. Lyc. Nux. Rhus. Sep.
— stinging, Alum. Amm-c. Ant. Bar-c. Bov. Bry. *Calc.* Chenop. Hep. Igt. Kali-c. Lyc. Ntr-c. Ntr-m. Petr. Phosp. Phosp-ac. Puls. Ran-sc. Rhod. Rhus. Rumex. Sep. Sil. Staph. *Sulph.* Sulph-ac.
— — and boring, Ntr-m.
— — — and drawing, Ntr-c.
— — burning, Bar-c.
— tearing, Amm-c. Arn. Bry. Cocc. *Lyc.* Sep. *Sil.* Sulph. Sulph-ac.
Cutting, Bell. Calc. Mur-ac. Ntr-c. Viol-tr.
Cystic tumors, Acon. Agar. Bar-c. *Calc. Graph.* Hep. Kali-c. Nitr-ac. Sabin. Sil. Spong. Sulph.
Dermatitis, inflammation of the skin, Acon. Ars. Asa-f. Bar-m. Calc. *Cham.* Clem. Hep. *Merc.* Nitr-ac. *Puls.* Rhus. Staph. *Sil.* Sulph.
Desquamation of the skin, Ars. *Amm-c.* Amm-m. Arum-trif. Ars. Aur. *Bell.*

33. SKIN.

Bov. Coloc. Croton. Dulc. Ferr. Graph.
Hell. Laur. Mgn-c. Merc. *Mez.* Oleand.
Op. Phosp. Phosp-ac. Puls. Sec-c. Sep.
Sil. Staph. Verat.
Desquamation, sensation of, Agar. Amm-c.
Bar-c. Lach. Phosp. Phosp-ac.
— of whole body, Coloc. Dig. Hell. Mez.
Phosp. Sec-c.
— palms of hands, Amm-c.
— after scratching, Dros.
— of hardened pieces, Sep.
— — parts affected, Acon.
Dropsy, (compare, Sect. 34.)
Dry skin, Acon. Ambr. Amm-c. Arn. Ars.
Bell. Bism. Bry. *Calc.* Camph. Cannab.
Cham. Chin. Coff. *Colch.* Coloc. *Dulc.*
Graph. Hyosc. Iod. Ip. Kali-b. *Kali-c.*
Kalm. Lach. Led. *Lyc.* Mgn-c. Merc.
Mosch. Murex. *Ntr-c.* Nitr-ac. *Nux-m.*
Oleand. Op. *Phosp.* Phosp-ac. Phyt. Plat.
Puls. Rhus. Sabad. Scill. *Sec-c. Seneg.*
Sep. *Sil.* Spong. Staph. *Sulph. Verb.*
Viol-od.
— — with heat, dry burning of skin, *Acon.*
Arn. *Ars.* Bell. *Bry.* Calc. Cocc.
Coff. Dulc. Hell. Kali-c. *Lach.* Led.
Lyc. Merc. *Nux.* Op. *Phosp.* Phosp-ac.
Puls. Rhus. Samb. Scill. Sec-c. Sep.
Sil. Stann. Sulph.
— — alternating with night sweats, Apis.
Ntr-c.
— — and brittle, Hyosc.
— — and rough, Iod. Merc. Ntr-c.
— — chronic, *Graph.*
— — when exercising, Calc.
— — parched, Calc. Hyosc. Iod.
— — parchment like, Ars. Chin. Lyc. Sil.
Dryness sense of, Ars. Camph. Sabad.
Ecchymosis, *Arn.* Bry. Calc. Con. Hep.
Nux. Puls. Rhus. Ruta. Sulph. *Sulph-ac.*
Elasticity, want of, Bov. Cupr. Rhus.
Verat.
Elevations, small, colorless, Op.
Eruptions, Acon. Agar. *Amm-c.* Ant.
Ars. Bar-c. Bell. Bov. Bry. Calc.
Carb-an. Carb-veg. *Caust.* Cham. Cic.
Clem. *Con.* Cop. *Creos.* Cupr. Cycl. Dig.
Dulc. Euph. Graph. Guaj. Hell. Ign. Ip.
Jatr. Kali-b. Kali-c. Lach. *Lyc.* Merc.
Ntr-m. Nitr-ac. Oleand. Petr. Phosp.
Phosp-ac. Ran-b. Ran-sc. *Rhus.* Sass.
Sep. Sil. Staph. *Sulph.* Tart. Thuj.
Viol-tr.
— biting, Amm-m. Bry. Calc. Caust.
Colch. *Euph.* Ip. Lach. *Led. Lyc.*
Merc. Mez. Oleand. Plat. *Puls.*
— blackish, Ars. Bell. Bry. Lach. Rhus.
Sec-c.
— — pock shaped, Ars. Rhus.
— bleeding, Alum. Lyc. Merc. Par. Tart.
— blue, dark, Lach. *Ran-b.*
— brownish, Nitr-ac.
— burning, Ambr. Amm-c. Ant. Apis.

Arg. *Ars.* Bell. Bry. Calad. Calc.
Carb-an. Carb-veg. *Caust.* Cic. Cocc.
Con. Hep. Lyc. *Merc.* Mez. *Oleand.*
Nitr. Nux. Phosp-ac. Puls. *Ran-b.*
Rhus. Scill. Sil. Staph. Stront. Sulph.
Verat. Viol-od.
— — better when scratched, *Nitr.*
— — when touched, Canth.
— chapped, Calc. Cycl. Hep. Lach. *Puls.*
Rhus. *Sep. Sulph.*
— chronic, Amm-c. Bar-c. Borax. *Calc.*
Cham. Clem. Con. Creos. *Euph. Graph.*
Hep. Ntr-c. Nitr-ac. *Petr. Sil.* Staph.
Sulph. Zinc.
— clustery, Agar. Calc. Phosp-ac. Rhus.
Staph.
— confluent, Cic. Hyosc. Phosp-ac. Tart.
Valer.
— copper-colored, Ars. Carb-an. Creos.
Mez. Rhus. Verat.
— covered parts on, Led. Thuj.
— corroding, Bar-c. Borax. Calc. *Cham.*
Clem. Con. *Graph.* Hep. Ntr-c. Nitr-ac.
Petr. Rhus. Scill. Sep. *Sil.* Staph.
Viol-od. (compare corroding.)
— — with hair, Merc. Ntr-m. Rhus.
— crusty, (compare scurfy).
— cutting, Lyc.
— dense, Agar. Calc.
— dry, *Bar-c.* Bov. Bry. *Calc.* Carb-veg.
Cupr. Dulc. *Evon.* Fluor-ac. Graph.
Hyosc. Lach. *Led.* Merc. Petr. Phosp.
Sass. *Sep. Sil.* Staph. *Verat.* Viol-tr.
— eating, Bar-c. Bov. Calc. Cham. Clem.
Con. Graph. Grat. Hep. Ntr-c.
Nitr-ac. Petr. Rhus. Scill. Sep. Sil. Staph.
Viol-od. (compare eating.)
— excoriated, as if, Graph.
— fiery red, Acon. Bell. Stram. Sulph.
— flat, Amm-c. Ant. Ars. Asa-f. Bell.
Lach. Lyc. Ntr-c. Phosp-ac. Selen. Sep.
Sil.
— fluid, containing, an acrid, *Calc.* Graph.
Ran-sc.
— — excoriating, Clem. Merc. *Rhus.*
Scill.
— — greenish, *Rhus.*
— — ichorous, Clem. Ran-sc. *Rhus.*
Tart.
— granular, Ars. Carb-veg. Hep.
— grape shaped, Calc.
— hard, Ant. Ran-b.
— herpetic, An c. Clem. Dulc. Merc.
Ntr-c. *Rhus.* Staph (compare Herpes).
— — alternating with affections of the
chest and dysenteric stools, Rhus.
— horny, Ant. Ran-b.
— inflamed, Ars. Calc.
— itch, Ant. Ars. *Carb-veg. Caust.* Coloc.
Con. Creos. Cupr. Dulc. Grat. Lach.
Mang. Merc. Ol-an. Phosp-ac. Scill.
Selen. Sep. Sulph. Verat. Zinc.
— itching, Acon. Agar. Amm-c. Ant. Ars.

33. SKIN.

Arum-trif. Bov. Bry. Calad. Calc.
Canth. *Caust.* Cham. Cic. Clem. Con.
Creos. Igt. Kali-c. Lach. Led Lyc.
Merc. Mez. Ntr-m. Ntr-s. Nitr-ac. Nux.
O.eand. Par. Petr. Puls. Ran-b. *Rhus*.
Scill. Selen. *Sep.* Sil. *Staph.* Stront.
Sulph. Tabac. Tart. Thuj. Verat.
Viol-tr.

- Eruptions, itching in bed, Ant. Merc. M tr-ac. Puls. *Rhus.* Verat.
- — — evening, Creos. Mgn-m. Staph.
- — — at night, Ant. Creos. *Merc. Rhus.* Tart. Verat.
- — in warmth, Cocc. Sass. Verat.
- knotty, tuberculous, Agar. Alum. Ant. Bry. Calc. Caust. Cocc. Dulc. Hep. Lach. Led. Lyc. Mgn-c. Mang. Mez. Ntr-m. Op. Petr. Puls. Rhus. Sec-c. Sep. Sil. Staph. Thuj. Verat.
- miliary, (compare Malaria).
- millet-like, Agar. Cocc. Led. Par.
- minute, Carb-veg. Hep. Phosp-ac.
- moist, Alum. Bov. Calc. *Carb-veg* Cic. Clem. Creos. *Graph.* Grat. Hep. Kali-c. Lach. Lyc. Merc. Mez. Ntr-c. Nitr-ac. Oleand. Petr. *Rhus.* Selen. Sep. Staph. Sulph.
- painful, *Arn.* Ars. Asa-f. *Bell.* Chin. Clem. Con. Cupr. Dulc. Hep. Lach. Lyc. Mgn-c. Mgn-m. Merc Nux. Petr. Phosp. Phosp-ac. Puls. Sep. Sil. Spig. Verat.
- painless, Ambr. Anac. Cocc Con. Hell. Hyosc. *Lyc.* Oleand. Phosp-ac. Sec-c. Stram. Sulph.
- pale. colorless, Ars.
- peeling, Acon. *Amm-c.* Amm-m. *Bell.* Clem. Led. Mez. Phosp. *Sep.* Sil Staph. Thuj.
- pimples, Acon. Ant. Ars. Bell. Bry. Canth. *Caust.* Cham. Cocc. Con. Dulc. Merc. Ntr-m. *Nitr-ac.* Phosp. Phosp-ac. Puls. Rhus. Scill. *Sep.* Spong. Staph. Sulph. Tart. Thuj. Zinc.
- purulent, Ant. Cic. Dulc. Lyc. *Merc.* *Ntr-c.* Rhus. Sep. Staph. Zinc.
- pustules, Ant. Ars. Hyosc. Kali-b. Hyosc. Merc. Puls. *Rhus.* Staph. Sulph. *Tart.*
- pustulous, Amm-m. Ant. *Ars.* Bell Bry. Canth. Carb-an. Caust. Clem. Creos. Croton. Dulc. Graph. Hell. Hep. Kali-c. *Lach.* Ntr-c. Nitr. *Phosp. Ran-s* Ran-sc. *Rhus.* Sabin. Sec-c Sep. Sulph
- — — containing blood, Ars. Sec-c.
- — — blue, Ars. Lach. *Ran-b.*
- — — on chilblains, Rhus.
- — — with erysipelas, Ars. Bell. Graph. Kali-b. Lach. *Rhus.* Sep.
- — — gangrenous, Ars. Camph. Ran-b. Sabin. Sec-c.
- — — around ulcers, Lach. Rhus.
- — red, Acon. Agar. Amm-c. Ant. Arn. Ars. Aur. Bell. Berb. Bruc. Calc.

Cham. Cic. Clem. Cocc Con. Croton.
Cycl. Dulc. Fluor-ac. Graph. Kali c.
Lach. Mgn-c. Merc. Nitr-ac. Ox-ac.
Phosp. Phosp-ac. Rhus. Sabad. Sass.
Sep. Sil. Spig. Stram. Sulph. Sulph-ac.
Thuj Tilia. Valer.

- — bright or dark colored, elevated, itching, Cop.
- — spotted, Merc. Verat.
- — areola, Anac. Borax. Cocc. Tabac. Tart.
- — scarlet, or rose colored irregular broad shape, Cop.
- — rough, Anac. Dulc. Phosp. Sep.
- — sandy, Ars.
- — scaly, Amm-m. Aur. Cic. Clem. Hep. Led. Mgn-c. Merc. Oleand. Phosp. Sulph.
- — like fish scales. Ars.
- — scratched, when, burning, Merc. Ntr-s. Staph. Stront. Verat.
- — scrofulous, Mur-ac.
- — scurfy, *Alum.* Amm-c. Amm-m. Ant. *Ars.* Aur. Aur-m. *Bar-c.* Bell. Bov. Bry. *Calc.* Carb-an. Carb-veg. *Cic.* Clem. Coloc. *Con.* Dulc. *Graph.* Hell. Hep. Kali-c Lach. Led. Lyc. Merc. Mur-ac. Ntr-m. Oleand. Petr. Phosp. Phusp-ac. Puls. Ran-b. *Rhus.* Sabad. *Sass.* Sep. Sil. Staph. Sulph. Thuj. Verat. Viol-tr.
- — over whole body, Dulc. Psor.
- — black, Bell.
- — bleeding, Merc.
- — brown, Ant.
- — burning, Amm-c. Calc. Cic. Puls. Sass.
- — dry, Aur. Aur-m. Bar-c. Calc. Sulph.
- — fall off and are renewed in one night, Croton
- — fetid, Merc. Sulph.
- — gnawing, Mang.
- — gray. Ars, Merc.
- — brown, Croton.
- — greenish, Calc
- — heavy, which fall off, leaving a brown-ish yellow appearance under, Petr.
- — herpetic, Bov. Calc. Ran-b. Sep.
- — honey colored, Carb-veg.
- — horny, Ant. Graph. Ran-b.
- — humid, Alum. *Ars. Bar-c.* Calc. Cic. Clem. Graph. *Hell.* Hep. *Lyc. Merc.* Mez. Oleand. Rhus. Ruta. Sil. *Staph. Sulph.*
- — inflamed, Lyc.
- — itching, Rhus
- — jerking and painful, Staph.
- — livid, Chilin.
- — painful, Mgn-m.
- — — as if sore, Sil.
- — raised, Sabin.
- — red-brown, Amm-m.
- — smarting, Puls.
- — suppurating, Ars. Sulph. (compare,

33. SKIN.

Eruptions, scurfy tensive, Amm-m.
— — yellow, Ant. Cic.
— shining through, Merc.
— smarting, Bry. Colch. Euph. Ips. Lach. Led. Merc. Mez. Oleand. Plat. Puls. Spong.
— sore, Alum. *Arg.* Aur. Bry. Calc. Colch. Dros. *Graph.* Merc. Ntr-m. Nitr-ac. Par. Petr. Phosp-ac Puls. Rhus. Scill. *Sep* Sulph. Verat. Viol-tr.
— — when touched, *Hep.* Spig.
— stinging, Ant Apis. Ars. Bar-c. Bell. Berb. Bry. Clem. Cycl. Dros. Euph. Hep. Lach Mgn-c. Merc. Ntr-m. *Nitr-ac.* Plat. *Puls.* Ran-b. Rhus Sabin. Scill. Sep. Sil. Staph. Sulph. Viol-tr.
— suppressed, Ars. Bell. Bry. Caust Ip. Lach. Lyc. Merc. Phosp-ac. Psor. Puls. Rhus. Sep. Sil. Staph Stram. Sulph.
— — and from it, fever, Millef.
— — signs of effusion developed, pupils dilated, eyes converge or diverge, Zinc.
— suppurating, Cic. Graph. Lyc. Merc. Rhus. Sec-c. Sep. Sil. Spig. Staph. Verat. (compare Moist and purulent.)
— swelling, with, Bell. Kali. *Merc.* Puls. *Rhus.* Sep Sulph. Thuj.
— tearing, pain, with, Calc. Kali. *Lyc.* Sep. Sil Staph. Sulph.
— tensive, Arn. *Caust.* Phosp. *Rhus.* Stront.
— twitching, painful, Caust. Puls. Rhus. Staph.
— ulcerous pain, Amm-m. Mang. Phosp. Puls. Rhus. Sep. *Sil.* Staph.
— vaccination, as after, Sulph.
— varicella like, Led.
— vesicles, drying up and forming itching scabs, Rhus.
— whitish, Agar. Ars. Bov. Bry. Ip. Phosp. Puls. Sulph. Valer.
— — on margins, Bell.
— yellow, Agar. Cic. Euph. Lach. Merc. Ntr-c. Nitr ac. Sep.
— zona, Ars. Graph. *Merc.* Puls. *Rhus.* Sil.
— after abuse of belladonna, Hep. Hyosc.
— cold, after a. appearing, Dulc.
— — in, air. appearing, Dulc.
— — — disappearing, Calc.
— suppressed gonorrhœa, after Clem. Thuj.
— heat of bed, Clem.
— hot weather, in, Kali-b.
— night, at, Ant.
— open air, in the, appearing, Nitr-ac.
— overheated, from being, Con.
— pork, from, Cycl. *Puls.*
— slow to appear, or not well developed, or go back before coming well out, Bry.
— touch relieves, Thuj.
— — aggravates, Mes.

— washing from, Clem.
— with difficult dentition, Calc.
— — glandular swelling, Amm-c. Dulc.
— — hair within eruption falls out, Ars.
— — swelling of parts affected, Bell. Clem. Kali-c. Merc. Puls. Rhus. Samb. Sep. Sulph. Thuj.
— alternating with dysenteric stools, Rhus.
— — — tightness of chest, Calad. Kalm Rhus.
Erysipelas, *Acon.* Amm-c. Ant. Apis. Ars. *Bell.* Borax. Bry. Calc. Camph. Canth. Carb-an. Cham. Chin. Clem. Crotal. Dulc. Euph. Gels. *Graph.* Hep. Hydrast. Iod. Lach. Lyc. *Merc.* Mur-ac Nitr-ac. Phosp. Phosp-ac. Puls. *Rhus.* Ruta. Sabad. Samb. Sil. Sulph. Thuj. Verat.
— boring, Euph.
— burning, Rhus.
— creeping, Rhus.
— digging, Euph.
— gangrenous, Ars. Bell. Camph. Sabin. Sec-c.
— gnawing, Euph.
— hard, Sulph.
— — red and hot, Bell.
— inflamed, *Acon. Bell.* Borax. *Bry. Cham. Hep. Lach. Merc.* Petr. *Phosp. Puls. Rhus. Sulph.*
— itching, Rhus.
— peeling off, with, Dulc. Puls. Rhus.
— pustules, with, Ars. Bell. Graph. Lach. *Rhus.*
— right side, Amm-c. Bell.
— — — then left, Apis.
— left side, Arn. Graph. Lach.
— — — then right, Rhus.
— scarlet color, *Amm-c.* Ars. *Bell.* Bry. Croc Hyosc. *Merc.* Sulph.
— in stripes, Graph.
— swollen, Acon. Arn. Ars. Bell. Calc. Chin. Hep. Kali-c. Lyc. *Merc. Rhus.* Sulph. Thuj. Zinc.
— tensive, Rhus.
— with throbbing and stinging, Sulph.
— vesicular, Ars. Bell. Euph. Graph. Lach. Puls. Ran-sc. Rhus. Sol-m.
— zone shaped, Ars Graph. Nux. Puls.
— similar to that caused by rhus poisoning, with oppressed breathing, Kalm.
Excresences, Ant. *Ars.* Aur. *Bell. Calc. Carb-an. Carb-veg. Caust. Clem.* Cocc. *Graph.* Hep. Iod. Lach. *Lyc.* Ntr m. *Nitr-ac.* Nux. Phosp. Plb. Puls. Ran-b. Rhus. Sabin. *Sil. Staph. Sulph.* Tart. *Thuj.*
— comedones, Ntr-c. Selen.
— disorganization of skin, Ant.
— fleshy, *Staph. Thuj.*
— fungus, Ant. Con. Creos. Lach. Sang. Sil. Staph.
— — hamatodes, *Ars.* Carb-an. Carb-veg.

Lach. Lyc. Merc. Nitra-c. *Phosp. Sil.* Sulph.
Excrescences, fungus, medullaris, Carb-an. Phosp. Thuj.
— hang-nails, Calc. Merc. *Ntr-m.* Rhus. Stann. Sulph.
— horny, Ant. Ran-b. Sulph.
— humid, Nitr-ac.
— moles, Calc. Sulph.
— nodi, arthritici, Ant. Aur. Bry. *Calc.* Caust. Cic. Dig. Graph. Led. *Lyc.* Rhod. Rhus. Staph.
— painfully, Spig.
— polypus, Aur. *Calc.* Con. Hep. Lyc. Merc. Mez. *Phosp.* Sang. Sil. *Staph.* Teucr. Thuj.
— red, Thuj.
— smooth, Thuj.
— spongy, Ars. *Carb-an.* Clem. *Lach.* Phosp. Sep. *Sil.* Staph. Sulph. Thuj.
— sycotic, Cinnab. Euph. Lyc. Nitr-ac. Nux. Phosp-ac. Psor. Sabin. Staph. Thuj.
— — bleeding, Thuj.
— — burning, Thuj.
— — horny, Thuj.
— — pedunculated, Lyc.
— — suppurating, Thuj.
— wens, Amm-c. Calc. Phosp. Sil.
Exudations bloody, Calc. Crotal. Lach. Nux.
Filthy skin, appearance of, Bry. Ferr. Iod. Merc. Phosp. Sec-c.
Flaccidity of skin, *Calc.* Caps. Chin. Cocc. Iod. Lyc. Sec-c. Verat.
Formication, tingling, creeping, crawling, Acon. Alum. Bar-c. Carb-veg. Cist. Euphr. Ferr. Led. Lyc. Mgn-c. Mur-ac. Ntr-c. Oleand. Ol-an. Phosp. *Phosp-ac.* Pallad. *Plat. Rhod.* Sabad. *Sec-c.* Selen. Sil. Staph. Stram. Sulph. Verat. Zinc.
— under skin, Ntr-c.
— between skin and flesh, Zinc.
— with numbness of parts, Euphr.
— in many places, as if frostbitten, when weather changes, Colch.
— at night, Bar-c. Sulph.
Freckles, *Amm-c.* Ant. Calc. Con. Dros. Dulc. Graph. Kali-c. *Lyc.* Merc. *Ntr-c.* Nitr-ac. Nux-m. Petr. *Phosp.* Puls. Sep. Sil. *Sulph.* Verat.
Gangrene, Acon. *Ars.* Bell. Camph. Carb-veg. *Chin. Creos.* Crotal. Euph. Lach. Ran-b. Sabin. Scill. *Sil.* Sulph. Sulph-ac.
— hot, Acon. Bell.
— humid, Chin. Euph. Hell. Scill.
— cold, Ars. Asa-f. Euph. Lach. Plb. Scill. Sec-c. Sil.
Gangrenous spots and vesicles on skin, Hyosc.
Gnawing, Agar. *Agn.* Alum. Ant. Bar-c. Bism. Canth. Caps. Cycl. Dig. Dros. Kali-c. **Led** *Lyc.* Meny. *Oleand.* Par.

Phosp. *Plat.* Puls. Ran-sc. Rhus. Ruta. Spong. *Staph.* Verat.
Gray color of skin, Carb-veg.
— livid, sallow, *Ars.* Borax. Bry. Canth. Carb-veg. *Chin.* Creos. Cre-c. Ign. Ip. Lach. Lyc. *Merc.* Nux. Samb. Sep. Sil.
Greasiness, Bry. Chin. Merc. Ntr-m.
Green color, Ars. Carb-veg. Verat.
Hang-nails, Calc. Ntr-m. Merc. Rhus. Stann. Sulph.
Hardness of skin, *Ant.* Ars. Dulc. Graph. Lyc. Ran-b. *Rhus. Sep.* Sil. Thuj.
— — like parchment. Ars. Lyc. Sil.
Harsh skin, Hyosc. Sec-c.
Healing of skin, difficult, Alum. *Bar-c.* Borax. Calc. *Carb-veg. Cham.* Con. Cicc. *Graph. Hep.* Lach. Lyc. Mang. Merc. Nitr-ac. *Petr. Rhus.* Selen. Sep. Sil. Staph. Sulph.
Heat of skin, Acon. Aloe. Arn. Ars. Bell. Borax. Bry. Chin. Cocc. Coloc. Dulc. Hep. Hyosc. Iod. Kali-b. Lach. Mgn-c. Mur-ac. Nux. Phosp. Puls. Rhus. Sang. Sep. Sil. Sulph. (compare External heat in Fever, Sect. 32.)
— — when exercising, Calc.
Herpes, Alum. Ambr. *Ars.* Borax. *Bov. Bry.* Calc. Carb-veg. Caust. Chin. *Clem.* Con. *Dulc. Graph.* Kali-c. Led. *Lyc. Merc.* Ntr-c. Ntr-m. Nitr-ac. Nux. Petr. Phosp-ac. Ran-b. *Rhus.* Sass. *Sep.* Sil. Sol-m. Spong. Staph. *Sulph.* Zinc.
— bleeding, Dulc. Lyc.
— — when scratched, Dulc.
— brown, Dulc.
— burning, Ambr. *Ars.* Bov. Bry. Calad. Calc. Carb-veg. *Caust.* Con. Kali-c. Led. Lyc. *Merc.* Mosch. Nux. *Rhus.* Sass. Sep. Sil. Sulph.
— — at night, Ars. Caust. Merc. Rhus. Staph.
— — in open air, Led.
— — when scratched, Staph.
— all over the body, Dulc. *Psor. Ran-b.*
— change of moon, during, Clem.
— chronic, Clem. Con. Lach. Sacch. Staph.
— circinnatus, Ntr-c. Sep. Tellur.
— clustery, Dulc.
— cold water, to sensitive, Dulc.
— cracked, Calc. Lyc. Puls. Rhus. Sep. Sulph.
— dry, Bar-c. Bov. Calc. Creos. Dulc. Kali-jod. Led. Merc. Phosp. Phosp-ac. Psor. Rhus. *Sep. Sil.* Staph. Sulph. Verat.
— dysentery, alternating with, Rhus.
— eating, corroding, Calc. Clem. Con. *Graph.* Merc. Petr. Rhus. Sep. *Sil.*
— gonorrhoeal, Zinc.
— grayish yellow, Sulph.
— humid, *Bov. Calc.* Carb-veg. Caust. Clem. Con. Creos. *Dulc. Graph.* Hep.

33. SKIN.

Lyc. Merc. Ntr-c. Phosp-ac. Psor. *Rhus*. Sep. Sil. Sulph.
Herpes impetiginous, Merc.
— indolent, Lyc. Mgn-c. Psor.
— inflamed, Graph.
— itching, Ambr. Amm-c. Ars. Bov. Bry. Caust. *Clem*. Con. Graph. Kali-c. Kali-jod. Led. Lyc. Mang. Merc. Ntr-m. Nicc. Nitr-ac. Petr. Psor. *Rhus. Sep*. Sil. Staph. Sulph.
— — scabby, Graph. Rhus. Sep. Thuj.
— — with thick crust, Clem.
— — when moon changes, Clem.
— — in evening, Alum. Graph. Staph.
— — at night, Ars. Graph. Staph.
— — in warmth of bed, Clem.
— jerking, *Rhus*. Staph.
— mealy, furfuraceous, Amm-c. *Ars*. Bov. Bry. Calc. Cic. Creos. Dulc. Led. Lyc. Merc. Phosp. Sep. *Sil*. Sulph. Verat.
— mercurial, Aur. Mosch. Nitr-ac.
— painful, Dulc.
— painless, Mgn c.
— pale, when moon is waning, Clem.
— pale red, Clem. Dulc.
— peeling off of skin, with, Dulc. Merc.
— pricking, *Ars. Clem*. Merc. Nitr-ac. Puls. Rhus. *Sep*. Sil. Sulph.
— pustules, Creos.
— raised, Merc.
— red, Amm-c. Ars. Clem. Dulc. Lach. Lyc. Mgn-c. Mgn-s. Merc.
— — pimples, Bov.
— — areola, Dulc.
— rough, Bov. Oleand.
— round, Dulc.
— scaly, Ars. *Clem*. Cupr. Dulc. Led. Lyc. Mgn-c. Merc. Phosp. Sulph.
— scrofulous, Aur.
— scratched, when, burning, Staph.
— scurfy, Bov. Calc. Clem. Con. Dulc. *Graph*. Lach. Lyc. Merc. Ran-b. *Rhus*. Sep. Sil. *Sulph*.
— — whitish, Graph. Lyc.
— shrunk and cleft, Lyc.
— small, Dulc. Lach. Mgn-c.
— smarting, biting, Alum.
— smooth, Mgn-c.
— spreading, Alum. Merc.
— stinging, Anac.
— suppressed, Alum. Ambr. Calc. Lach. Lyc. Psor. Sulph.
— suppuration, Ars. Dulc. Kali-c. Lyc. Merc. Ntr-c. Rhus. Sep. Sil.
— syphilitic. Merc. Nitr-ac. Thuj.
— tearing, Calc. *Lyc*. Sep. Sil. Sulph.
— ulcerated, Zinc.
— vesicles, with, burning at night, coverings like fish scales, Ars.
— vesicular, Sulph.
— watery vesicles, with, Sulph.
— white. Ars. Graph. Lyc. Zinc.
— — scaly, dry, mealy, Ars. Calc. Dulc.

Lyc. Sep. Sil. Thuj.
— wrinkled and cracked, Lyc.
— yellow, Dulc. Lyc. Merc. Sulph.
— — brown, Dulc. Lyc. Ntr-c.
— — scaly, Cupr. Sulph.
— zoster, Graph. Rhus. Thuj.
Herpetic, Anac. Rhus.
— blisters, Nitr-ac.
— scurfs, Bov. Calc. Ran-b. Sep.
— spots, Hyosc. Merc. Nitr-m. Sep.
Inactivity of skin. *Anac*. Ars. Bry. *Con*. Dulc. Ip. *Kali-c*. Laur. *Lyc*. Nitr-ac. Oleand. *Phosp-ac*. Sec-c. Sil. Sulph.
Inflamed, skin inclined to be, Asa-f. Bar-c. Borax. *Cham*. Hep. Merc. Nitr-ac. Puls. *Sil*. Sulph.
Inflammation, (compare Dermatitis.)
Insensibility, numbness, of skin. Ambr. *Anac*. Con. Lyc. Oleand. Phosp-ac. Puls. *Sec-c*. Sulph.
Insect stings, Arn. Bell. Calad. Led. Seneg.
Itch, scabies, Ant. Ars. *Carb-veg*. Caust. Creos. Cupr. Dulc. Lach. Mang. Merc. Ntr-c. Phosp. *Selen. Sep. Sulph*. Verat. Zinc.
— bleeding, Calc. Merc. Sulph.
— dry, Carb-veg. Caust. Creos. Merc. Ntr-c. Sep. Sulph. Verat.
— fat, Caust. Creos. Merc. Sep. Sulph.
— humid, Carb-veg. Caust. Creos. Graph. Lyc. Sep. Sulph.
— millet like, dry, Merc. Sep. Sil.
— purulent, Creos. Merc. Scill.
— rash-like. Carb-veg. Merc. Sulph.
— suppressed, Ambr. Ars. Carb-veg. Caust. Selen. Sep. Sulph.
— — with mercury and sulphur, *Caust*. Chin. Puls. Selen. *Sep*. Staph.
Itch-like, eruption, Ambr. Ant. *Ars. Calc*. Carb-an. *Carb-veg. Caust*. Cupr. Dulc. Lach. Mang. *Merc*. Merc-cor. Mez. *Ntr-c. Phosp-ac*. Scill. Selen. Sep. Sil. Staph. *Sulph*. Sulph-ac. Tart. *Verat*.
Itching, Acon. Agn. Amm-c. Amm-m. Ant. Berb. Bov. Bry. Calad. Canth. Carb-an. Chelid. Chin. Cic. Cocc. Con. Creos. Croton. Dolich. Dros. Ferr. Graph. Igt. Ip. Kali-b. Kali-c. Lach. Laur. Led. Lyc. Mgn-c. *Merc*. Mez. Nicc. Nitr-ac. Nux. Oleand. Op. Par. Phosp. Plat. Plb. Psor. *Puls*. Ran-b. *Rhus*. Ruta. Sabad. Sabin. Sass. Scill. Selen. *Sil*. Spig. *Spong*. Staph. *Sulph*. Sulph-ac. Tart. Thuj. Verat. Viol-tr.
— on parts affected, Acon.
— as from ants, Puls.
— biting, *Agn*. Amm-c. Berb. Bry. Calc. Caust. Chin. Colch. *Euph*. Lach. Lact. *Led*. Lyc. Merc. Mez. Nux. Oleand. Ol-an. Phell. *Puls*. Sil. Spong.
— burning, Acon. Agar. Ambr. Anac. Arg. Ars. Bell. Bry. Calad. Calc. Caps.

33. SKIN.

Caust. Chin. Cic. Colch. Croton. Dig. Euph. Hep. Igt. Kali-c. *Lach.* Lyc. Merc. Mez. Nux. O. an. Phell Phosp. Plat. Puls. Ran-b. Rhus. Scill. Sep. *Sil.* Spig. Stann. Sulph.
Itching, burning terminating, with, Ambr. Con. Graph. Lyc Mgn-c. Merc. Op. Puls. Rhus. Sep. Sil.
— — redness, as if frostbitten, Agar.
— crawling, Bar-c. Lyc. Oleand. Pallad. Plat. R-od. Rhus. Sabad. Sec-c. Sil. Spong. *Staph.* Sulph.
— gnawing, *Agn.* Bar-c. Led. *Lyc. Oleand. Plat.* Spong. *Staph.*
— intolerable, Merc. Sil.
— jerking, Lyc. Staph.
— as of lice, Arg. Canth. Mgn-m. Plat. Zinc.
— as from mosquito-bites, Rhus-ver.
— — of nettles, Colch. Lupulus,
— pinching, Mosch.
— p easant, Merc.
— prickling, Cina. Plat. Zinc.
— sore, Arg. Berb. Cannab. Graph. Led. Mez. *Plat.* Ruta Staph. Sulph. Zinc.
— stinging, Agn. Arg. Arn. Asa f. *Bar-c. Bry.* Caust. Cocc. Con Cycl. Dig. Dros. Graph. Igt. *Kali-c* Led. Merc. Mur-ac. Ntr-m. Nux. O eand. Plat. *Puls. Rhus.* Ruta. Sabad. Sabin. Scill. Sep. Sil. Spig. *Spong.* Stann. Staph. Sulph. Tabac. Teucr. Thuj. Verat. *Viol-tr.* Zinc.
— tearing, Bell. Bry. Staph.
— tickling, *Acon.* Agar. *Arn.* Bar-c. Caust. *Colch.* Evon. Kali-c. Merc. Mur-ac. Nux. *Plat. Puls.* Ran-b. Rhod. *Rhus.* Sabad. Sec-c. Selen. *Sep.* Sil. *Spig.* Staph. *Sulph.*
— titillating, Ambr. Arg. Bell. Chelid. Coin. Merc. Plat. Puls. Rhod. *Sabad.* Scill. *Sil.* Spig. Sulph. Teucr.
— troublesome, Coloc. Op. Stram.
— violent, Agar. Dros. Dulc. Ip. Lach. Op.
— voluptuous, Anac. Merc. Mur-ac. Sep. Sil. Sulph.
— wandering, Cham. Graph. Kali-c. Mgn-m. Mez. Rat. Rhus-ver. Spong. Staph. Zinc.
— of wounds, Chin. Tart.
— — drunkards, Carb-veg.
— as from fleas, not relieved by scratching, followed by vesicles, Nicc.
— on hairy parts, Rhus.
— in March, Fluor-ac.
— with nausea, Ip.
— before nausea, Sang.
— followed by perspiration, Coloc.
— on spots which perspire most, Tellur.
— begins when pains cease, Stront.
— in bed, *Bov.* Carb-an. Carb-veg. Clem. Cocc. Cycl. Coloc. Kali-b. Kali-c Kobalt. **Lyc. Merc. Mez. Mur-ac. Nux. Psor.**

Puls. Sass. *Sulph.* Thuj. Zinc.
Itching in in bed evening, Carb-an. Carb-veg. Coloc Cycl. *Merc.* Nux. *Puls.* Sass. Thuj. Zinc.
— — at night, Cocc. Kali-b. *Merc. Sulph.*
— — in morning, Rhus. Sulph.
— in cold air, Spong. Sep.
— — evening, Carb-an. Carb-veg. Cocc. Coloc. Creos. Cycl. Lyc. *Merc.* Mez Nux. Oleand. *Puls.* Sass. Selen. Sil. Thuj. Zinc.
— — — whenun dressing. Ars. Cocc. Dros. Mez. Nux. Oleand. Sil. Siann.
— in morning, Sass Staph. Sulph.
— — — in bed, Sulph.
— — — when rising. Sass.
— at night, Amm-c. Amm-m. Bar-c. Berb. Caust. Cocc. Creos. Croc. Lachn *Merc. Mez.* Nux. Sass. *Sulph.* Thuj.
— when overheating in the day time, Igt. *Lyc.*
— — body is warm, not relieved by scratching, Bov.
— after scratching, relieved, Ambr. Amm-c. Anac. Arn. *Asa-f.* Bry. *Calc.* Canth. Caps. Cycl. Dros. Dulc. Guaj. Igt. Mang. Merc. Mur-ac. Ntr c. Phosp. Plb. Rhus. Ruta. Sabin. Spig. Sulph. Sulph-ac. Zinc.
— changing the place by scratching, Anac. Calc. Chelid. Con. Cycl. Igt. Mgn-c. Mez. Nitr-ac Sang. Spong. Staph. Sulph-ac. Zinc.
— unchanged by scratching, Ang. Arg. Arn. Bov. Cham. Chelid. Cupr. Euph. Ip. Mgn-m. Merc. Nicc. Puls. Ran-sc. Sil. Spig. Spong. Sulph. Sulph-ac.
— after scratching, worse, *Anac.* Bism. Calad. Caps. Caust. Con. Croton. Dolich. Guaj. Lachn. *Led.* Mez. Puls. Sil. Spong. Stront.
— after scratching, biting, Amm-m. Caust. Euph. *Lach.* Led. Lyc. Mez. *Oleand.* Puls. Spong. Sulph.
— — bleeding, Ars. Chin. Cocc. Dulc. Kali-c. Merc. Nitr-ac. Psor. Sulph.
— — blisters, Amm-c. Amm-m. Ant. Caust. Chin. Cycl. Hep. *Lach.* Mang. Ntr-c. Ntr-m. Nitr. Phosp. Ran-b. *Rhus.* Sass. Spong.
— — blotches, Lach. Lyc. Merc. Ntr-c. Nitr-ac. Op. Rhus. Spig. Verat. Zinc.
— — bumps, Calc. Caust. *Dulc.* Hep. *Lach.* Lyc. *Mez.* Petr. *Rhus.* Staph.
— — burning, Amm-c. Ars. Bell. Bry. Caps. *Caust.* Croton. Creos. Dulc. Euph. Evon. Grat. Hep. *Lach.* Led. Lyc. Mgn-m. Mgn-s. Merc. Mez. Ntr-s. Oleand. Phosp. *Rhus.* Scill. Seneg. Sep. *Sil.* Staph. *Sulph.* Thuj. Tilia.
— — blisters, Amm-c.

33. SKIN. 273

Itching, after scratching, eruption, *Amm-c.* Amm-m. Ars. Bar-c. *Caust.* Creos. Cycl. Hep. Kali-c. *Lyc.* Merc. Oeand. Petr. Puls. *Rhus.* Sass. Sep. Sil. Staph. Stront. *Sulph.*
— — erysipelas, Amm-c. Bell. Graph. Hep. Lach. Lyc. *Merc. Rhus.* Sulph.
— — gnawing, Lyc. *Oleand.* Staph.
— — heat, Spong. Sulph.
— — herpes, Dulc.
— — miliary eruption, Lach. Merc. Rhus. Spong. Sulph.
— — moistness, Carb-veg. Creos. Dulc. Graph. Kali-c. *Lach. Lyc.* Oleand. Petr. *Rhus.* Selen. Staph.
— — nodules, white, Ars.
— — numbness of skin, Anac. Lach. Lyc. Oleand. Sulph.
— — peeling off of skin, Dros.
— — pimples, Amm-m. Ant. Bov. Bry. Caust. Cnin. Cycl. Graph. Grat. Lach. Laur. Mgn-c. Merc. Mosch. Ntr-m. Nitr-ac. Phosp. Puls. Rhus. Sabin. Sass. *Sep.* Spong. Sulph. Verat. Zinc.
— — pricking, *Bar-c.* Bry. Caust. Cycl. Graph. Merc. Puls. *Rhus.* Sabad. Spong. Sulph. Viol-tr.
— — pustules, Rhus. Sulph.
— — rash, Amm-c. Caust. Lach. Merc. Rhus. Selen. Sulph. Verat.
— — red skin, Agar. Arn. Bell. Bov. Graph. Lyc. Merc. Ntr-m. Nux. Oleand. Phosp-ac. Puls. Rhus. Spong. Tar. Teucr.
— — red streaks, Carb-veg. Euph. Phosp-ac. Sabad.
— — scurf, Bar-c. Calc. Con. Dulc. Graph. Hep. *Lyc.* Merc. *Rhus.* Sabad. Staph. *Sulph.*
— — — bloody, Dulc. Lach *Merc.* Par. *Sulph.*
— — simple, indefinite pain, *Bar-c.* Petr. Sulph.
— — smarting, Bry. Carb-an. Hell. *Sulph.* Zinc.
— — soreness, as if raw, Hep. Mez. *Oleand.* Petr. Rhus. Sabin. *Sep. Sulph.*
— — spots, Amm-c. Phosp. Rhus. Sabad. Sulph.
— — sweating blood, Lach. Lyc.
— — swelling, *Lach.* Lyc. Puls. Rhus. Sulph.
— — tearing, Lyc. *Sulph.*
— — tension, Lach. Stront.
— — thickened skin, Lach.
— — tickling, Merc. Sabad. Sil.
— — ulcers, Ars Asa-f. Caust. Hep. *Lach.* Lyc. Merc. Petr. Rhus. Sil. *Sulph.*
— — — pain as from, *Amm-m.* Graph. Puls *Rhus.*
— — — aching as from internal, Arn. Graph. Phosp. Puls. Rhus. *Sil.* Sulph.

Itching, after scratching voluptuous, tickling, Sil.
— — when sitting. Cycl.
— — touched, Euph.
— — — relieved, *Thuj.* Zinc.
— — becoming warm in bed, Bov. Clem. Carb veg. Cocc Kobalt. *Merc.* Psor. Puls. Spong. Sulph.
— — walking in open air, Igt.
— with restlessness, Coloc.
Measels, Acon. Ant. Ars. Bell. Bry. Calc. Coff. Cop. Dros Dulc. Gels. Iod. Ip. Kali-b. Phosp. *Puls.* Rhus. Sulph.
— suppressed, Phosp. Puls. Rhus.
Measel shaped, eruption, Acon. Ars. Bell. Bry. Carb-veg Merc. Phosp Puls. Rhus. Sulph.
Miliaria, *Acon.* Agar. Alum. Amm-c Amm-m. Ant. Ars. *Bell.* Bov. Bry. *Calad.* Calc. Carb-veg. Caust. *Cham.* Cupr. Euph. Hell. Hep. *Ip* Lach. Led. *Merc.* Mez. Ntr-m. Nux. *Phosp-ac.* Puls. Rhus. Sass. Sec-c. Selen. Spong. Staph. *Sulph.* Tart. Verat. Viol-tr.
— after abuse of belladonna, Hyosc.
— with burning and itching, Agar.
— in children, Acon. *Bry. Cham.* Ip. Sulph.
— chronic, Amm-c. Clem. Mez. *Staph.*
— close, white, with burning, Agar. Bry. Nux.
— — — — and itching, Agar. Bry. Calad. Sulph.
— in cold air, Dulc Sass. Sep.
— with excoriated skin, *Sulph.*
— in lying-in women, *Bry.* Ip.
— purple colored, Acon. Bell. Coff.
— scarlet colored, Acon. Amm-c. Bell. Bry. Calc. Ip. Merc. Zinc.
— stinging, biting, Viol-tr.
— suppressed, Ip.
— with tightness of chest, asthma alternating, *Calad.*
— on coming into warm room from the open air, Sass.
— white, Agar. Ars. Bov. Bry. Ip. Phosp. Sulph. Va'er.
— — in open air, Sass.
— — — room, Clem.
Moon, change of, new and full, aggravation, Alum.
Moles, Calc. Sulph.
— itching and stinging in. Graph.
Nails, complaints of, Alum. Ant. Ars. Borax. Calc. Caust. Con. *Graph.* Hell. Hep. Lach. Merc. Ntr-m. Nitr-ac. Nux. Puls. Ran-b. Rhus. Sabad. Scill. Sep. Sil. Sulph. Sulph-ac.
— beating, Amm-m.
— bleeding, Crotal.
— blue, Aur. Chelid. Chin. Dig. Ntr-m. Nux. Sil.
— boring, Colch.
— breaking off, Graph. Merc. Sil. Sulph.

33. SKIN.

Nails, brittle, Alum. Graph. Sil. Sulph.
— burning, Caust.
— dirty, discolored, Ant. Ars. Graph. Nitr-ac.
— distorted, Graph. Sabad. Sep. Sil. Sulph.
— falling off, Graph. Merc. Scill. Sec-c. Thuj.
— furrowed, Sabad. Sil.
— gnawing, Alum.
— growing into flesh, Sil. Sulph. Teucr.
—, — slowly, Ant.
— hang-nails, Calc. Rhus. Sulph.
— harsh, Ant.
— inflammation, Con. Hell. Kali-c. Lyc. Ntr-m. Phosp-ac. Teucr.
— itching, Hep.
— jerking pain, Graph. Puls.
— pain, Ant. Caust. Graph. Hep. Merc. Nitr-ac. Scill. Sil. Sulph.
— — as if contused, Nitr.
— — — — ulcerated, Amm-m. Ars. Bell. Graph. Hep. Kali c. Merc. Nitr-ac. Puls. Rhus. Sil. Sulph. Sulph-ac.
— pressure, Calc. Caust. Sass. Sulph.
— roughness, Sabad. Sil.
— sensitive, Nux. Sil.
— sore, Alum. Graph. Hep. Kali-c. Merc. Mez. Ntr-m. Nux. Puls. Sep. Sulph.
— splinter, pain as from, Nitr-ac. Sil. Sulph.
— splitting, Scill. Sil.
— spotted, Nitr-ac. Sep. Sil.
— stinging, Kali-c. Nitr-ac. Nitr. Sil. Sulph.
— suppuration, Calc. Kali-c. Phosp-ac. Sep.
— swelling around, Ntr-m.
— tearing around, Carb-veg. Colch.
— thickened, Graph. Sabad. Sil. Sulph.
— yellow, Con. Merc. Nitr-ac. Nux. Sep. Sil. Sulph.
Nettle-rash, urticaria, Acon. Aloe. Alnus. Ant. Apis. Ars. Bell. Bry. Calc. Carb-veg. Caust. Con. Cop. Creos. Dulc. Hep. Ign. Kali-c. Lyc. Mgn-s. Merc. Mez. Ntr-m. Nitr-ac. Nux. Petr. Phosp. Puls. Rhus. Sass. Sep. Sulph. Urt-ur. Verat.
— before the nausea, Sang.
— after exercise, Con. Ntr-m.
— — — violent, itching, Con. Nitr-ac.
— — open cool air, Nitr-ac.
— — — — disappearing, Calc.
— in open air, itching, Nitr-ac.
— with eruptions on head, Psor.
— pale, red, or bright red, Cop.
— after poisoning by mussels, Cop.
— if ague is suppressed, urticaria break out, Elat.
Network of small veins, red, Carb-veg. Caust. Lyc. Plat. Thuj.
Paleness of skin, Ars. Bell. Calc. Camph. Chin Cocc. Con. Crotal. Ferr. Graph. Hell. Kali c. Lach. Lyc. Ntr-m. Nitr-ac.

Nux. Phosp. Plat. Plb. Puls. Sec-c. Sep. Spig. Sulph.
Panaritia, All-cep. Alum. Amm-m. Apis. Ars. Bar-c. Bov. Bufo. Calc. Caust. Con. Crotal. Diosc. Fluor-ac. Graph. Hep. Iod. Kali-c. Lach. Led. Lyc. Merc. Ntr-m. Ntr-s. Nitr-ac. Phosp. Puls. Rhus. Sep. Sil. Sulph. Teucr.
— tendency to, Ntr-s.
Parchment like, hard, skin, Ars. Chin. Lyc. Sil.
Peeling off, sensation of, Agar. Bar-c. Lach. Phosp. Phosp-ac.
Petechia, Arn. Ars. Bell. Bry. Con. Hyosc. Lach. Led. Nux. Phell. Phosp. Rhus. Sec-c. Sil. Sulph-ac.
— in putrid fevers, Ars. Hyosc.
— — old people, Con.
Phagadenic blisters, Bar-c. Borax. Calc. Caust. Cham. Clem. Con. Graph. Hep. Kali-c. Mgn-c. Ntr-c. Nitr-ac. Petr. Rhus. Scill. Sep. Sil. Staph. Sulph.
— — on covered parts only, Led Thuj.
Pimples, Acon. Ant. Arg. Ars. Bell. Bov. Bry. Canth. Caust. Cham. Cic. Cocc. Con. Dulc. Hep. Kali-jod. Merc. Mur-ac. Ntr-m. Nitr-ac. Nux. Phosp. Phosp-ac. Puls. Rhus. Sass. Scill. Sep. Spong. Staph. Stront. Sulph. Tabac. Tart. Thuj. Tilia. Verat. Zinc.
— acne shaped, Bell. Carb-veg.
— acuminated, Ant. Ars. Tart.
— black, Carb-veg. Spig.
— bleeding, Stront. Thuj.
— boil shaped, Ntr-c.
— brown, Verat.
— burning, Ars. Canth. Caust. Graph. Kali. Merc-acet. Phosp-ac. Scill. Staph. Stront. Sulph.
— close together, Cham. Verat.
— confluent, Mur-ac. Phosp-ac.
— containing blood, Ars.
— cracked, Merc-acet.
— cutting, Rhus.
— drawing, Con. Mgn-m. Staph.
— as in drunkards, Creos. Led.
— dry, Bov. Creos.
— fine, Kali-c.
— flat, Ant.
— gnawing, itching, Ant. Caust. Mang. Nitr-ac. Tar.
— greasy, Creos.
— green crusts, Calc.
— hard, Bov. Sabin. Verat.
— — red, like flea bites, Agar.
— humid, Calc. Graph Kali-c. Ntr-s. Ol-an. Puls. Sil. Sulph. Thuj. Zinc.
— inflamed, Agar. Berb. Petr.
— as from insects, Ant. Ars.
— itching, Acon. Ambr. Amm-c. Ant. Bar-c. Bry. Calc. Carb-an. Caus. Cham. Con. Hep. Kali-c. Laur. Lyc. Merc. Merc-acet. Ntr-c. Ntr-m. Nu— Nitr-ac.

33. SKIN.

Phosp-ac. Puls. Selen. Sep. Sil. Staph.
Pimples itching, when exposed to heat, Sass.
— itch-like, Ant. Bar-m. Bry. Creos. Rhus. Scill. Ta t.
— miliary, Agar. Amm-c. Ant. Ars. Cocc. Creos. Grat. Kali c.
— painful, Ant. Arg. Arn. Cocc. Con. Graph. Kali-c. Kali-chl. Kali-jod. Lach. Mur-ac. Ntr-c. Nitr-ac. Nux. Phosp. Plb. Puls. Scill. Seneg. Spong. Sulph. Verat.
— — as if ulcerated, Dulc. Staph.
— painless, Alum. Sulph.
— pale, pale red, Bell.
— peeling off, with, Thuj.
— pock-shaped, Ant. Arn. Petr. Tart.
— pressure, with, Stann.
— pus filled with, *Ant*. Berb. Sass. *Tart.*
— rash like, Bov. Kali-chl. Rhus. Sass.
— red, Ant. Berb. Bov. Lach. Mgn-c. Phosp-ac. Scill. Staph. Stront. Thuj.
— — areola, Anac. Canth. Cycl. Samb. Tar.
— rough, Alum.
— scaly, Dros. Merc.
— scars old, upon, Iod.
— scattered, Berb. Crotal. Kali-chl.
— scurfy, Bell. *Calc.* Carb-an. Chan. Hep. Mur-ac *Oleand.* Petr. Sabin. Staph.
— sensitive to touch, Berb.
— small, followed by desquamation, Elaps.
— smarting, Agar. Bell. Calc. Cham. Coloc. D g Kali-c. Lyc. Merc. Nitr. Teucr. Verat.
— sore, as if excoriated, Alum. Arg. Bell. Bov. Calc. Clem. Guaj. *Hep.* Hyosc. Lam. Mez. Phosp-ac. *Rhus*. *Sabin*. Selen. Spig. Stann. Teucr. Verat. Zinc.
— sticking like a splinter, Arn.
— stinging, Alum. Ant. Arn. *Bell.* Calc-ph. *Canth.* Caps. Caust. Cocc. Creos. Hell. Kali-c. Ntr-c. Nitr. Petr. Scill. Staph.
— — itching in an old cicatrix, Iod.
— suppurating, Ars. Bell. *Cic.* Clem. *Dulc.* Merc Nitr-ac. Petr. Puls. *Rhus.* Staph. *Sulph. Tart.*
— tearing, Dulc.
— tensive, Ann. Bov. Con. Mang. Ntr-s.
— tick'ing, Canth.
— titillating, Bell. Caust. Mgn-m. Verat.
— touch, sensitive, to, Berb.
— transparent, Con.
— ulcers around, Sulph.
— ulcerated, *Merc.* Nitr-ac. Sabin. Sep.
— wart-shaped, Phell.
— water, full of, Coloc. Thuj.
— whitish, Ars. Bov. *Carb-veg.* Chelid. Coloc. Con. Cycl. Dros. *Kali-c.* Mgn-m Mang. Ntr-m. Petr. Phosp-ac. Staph. Sulph. Zinc.
— white tips, with, *Ant.* Puls. *Tart.*
— yellow, Ant. Grat. Mgn-m. Zinc.

Pocks, Acon. Ant. Arn. Ars. Bell. Bry. Clem. Cocc. Evon Hyosc. Kali-b. *Merc.* Millef. Psor. Puls. *Rhus.* Sil. Sol-m. Sulph. *Tart.* Thuj.
— black, *Ars.* Bell. Hyosc. Lach. Mur-ac. *Rhus.* Sec-c.
— burning, Ars. Lach. Merc.
— spurious, Acon. Bell. Puls. Rhus.
— suppurating, Bell. Merc. Sulph.
— whitish, Iod. Lyc.
Pores black, Graph. Ntr-c. Nitr-ac. Sabin. Sulph.
Prickling, Agar. Bar-m. Bell. Berb. Cannab. Cina. Croc. Dros. Ferr-m. Lyc. Mez. Mosch. *Plat.* Ran-sc. Sabad. Sep. Sulph. Tart. Zinc.
Pricking, stinging in skin, Acon. Arn. Ars. Asa-f. *Bar-c.* Bry. Calc. Caust. Chin. Cocc. Cycl. Dig. *Graph.* Merc. Nitr. Nitr-ac. Nux. Plat. Puls. Ran-b. Rhus. Sabad. Sep. Sil. *Spong.* Stann. Staph. Sulph. Tar. Teucr. *Thuj. Viol-tr.* Zinc.
— burning, Acon. *Asa-f.* Bar-c. Berb. Bry. Canth. Cocc. Merc. Mez. Nux. Puls. Rhus. Sabad. Sil. Staph. Sulph. Sulph-ac. *Thuj.*
— — succeeded by, *Nitr.*
— in evening in bed, Cycl. Thuj. Zinc.
— itching, Agn. Arn. Bar-c. *Bry.* Caust. Cocc. Con. Cycl. Dig. Dros. *Graph. Kali-c.* Merc. Mur-ac. Ntr-m. Nux. Plat. *Puls.* Rhus. Sep. Sil. Spig. *Spong.* Stann. Staph. Sulph Tabac. Tart. Teucr. *Thuj. Viol-tr.* Zinc.
— after mental affections, Bry.
— at night, Cannab. Merc. Thuj.
— tingling, Bar-c. Lact. Sabad.
Purple skin, Lach. Verat.
Purpura miliaris, *Acon.* Bell. *Coff.*
— hæmorragica, Kali-jod.
Pus in ulcers;
— black stain, leaving a, Chin. Sulph.
— bloody, Ars. Asa-f. Bell. Carb-veg. Caust. Con. Hep. Lyc. Merc. Nitr-ac. Puls. Sil.
— brownish, Ars. Bry. Carb-veg. Sil.
— cheesy, Merc.
— corrosive, acrid, Ars. Asa-f. *Carb-veg. Caust.* Clem. Con. Hep. Lyc. *Merc.* Mez. Nitr-ac. Ran-b. Ran-sc. *Rhus.* Scill. *Sil.* Sulph. Sulph-ac.
— foetid, (compare, Stinking.)
— filthy, Phosp-ac.
— gelatinous, Arg. Merc. Sep. Sil.
— gray, Ambr. Caust. Sil.
— greenish, Ars. Asa-f. Caust. Merc. Nux jug. Puls. Sil.
— ichorous, Amm-c. *Ars. Asa-f.* Bell. *Carb-veg.* Caust. Chin. Clem. Con. Lach. Lyc. *Merc. Nitr-ac.* Ran-sc. *Rhus.* Sang. Scill. Sep. Sil.
— maggoty, Sabad. Sil.
— pale red, Phosp. Plat. Puls. Rhod. Rhus.

33. SKIN.

Pus profuse, Ars. Asa-f. Calc. *Merc.* Ntr-c. Phosp. *Puls.* Rhus. *Sep.* Sil.
— salt, Ambr. Ars. Graph. *Lyc.* Ntr-c. Petr. Phosp. Puls. *Sep.* Sil.
— scanty, Bell. *Calc.* Cupr. Dulc. Hep. *Lach.* Merc. Nux. Plat. Sep. *Sil.*
— stinking, Amm-c. Ars. Asa-f. Bry. Calc. Carb-veg. Chin. Con. Graph. *Hep.* Lach. Lyc. Merc. *Phosp-ac.* Psor. Rhus. Sep. Sil. Staph. *Sulph.*
— — like herring brine, Ars. Calc. Graph.
— — old cheese, Hep. Merc. Sulph.
— — sour smell, Hep. Merc. Sulph.
— like tallow, Merc.
— tenacious, Bov. Con. Merc. Nux-jug.
— thin, Ars. *Asa-f.* Caust. *Merc.* Sil. Sulph.
— watery, Ars. Asa-f. Carb-veg. *Caust.* Merc. Nitr-ac. Ran-b. Ran-sc. Rhus. Scill. Sil. Staph. Sulph.
— whitish, milky, Calc. Lyc. Puls.
— yellow, Bry. Calc. Carb-veg. Caust. Cic. Clem. Creos. Merc. Nitr-ac. Phosp. *Puls.* Ruta. Sep. Sil. Staph.
Pustules, *Ars.* Aur. *Bell.* Cic. Clem. *Dulc.* Hydroc-ac. *Hyosc.* Kali-c. *Merc.* Nitr-ac. Petr. Puls. *Rhus.* Staph. Sulph. *Tart.*
— acuminated, Dulc. Thuj.
— black, Bry. Rhus.
— bleeding, Tart.
— brown, Tart.
— burning, Amm-c. Petr.
— — when touched, Canth.
— confluent, Cic. Merc. Tart.
— cowpox, like, Tart.
— cracked. Rhus.
— dry, Merc.
— greasy, Creos.
— hard, Anac. Crotal.
— humid, Bell.
— inflamed, Rhus. Stram.
— itching, Anthrok. Berb. Dulc. Graph. Hydroc-ac. Merc. Nux. Petr. Rhus. Sass. Sulph. Tart.
— itch like, Clem. Grat.
— lumpy, Anthrak. Cuam.
— mixed with vesicles, Tart.
— — — worse from scratching, from cold, Kali-b.
— painful, Ars. Berb. Stram. Tart.
— — as if sore, Bar-c.
— painless, Rhod.
— pale red, Ars.
— peeling off, Croton. Hyosc.
— pock shaped, Ant. Hyosc. Tart. Thuj.
— pustulous, Ant. Ars. Dulc. Hyosc. Merc. Petr. Puls. Rhus. Staph. Sulph. Tart.
— rose colored, Ars. Dulc.
— red, Anac. Ars. Berb. Caust. *Cic.* Crotal. Croton. Graph. Hydroc-ac. Kali-c. Mez. Nitr-ac. Tart.
— — areola, Anac. Borax. Lach. Nitr-ac. Par. Tart. Thuj.

Pustules scaly, Merc.
— scurfy, Ant. Bov. Croton. Dulc. Merc. Tart.
— small, Evon. Hydroc-ac. Nitr. Tart.
— sore, Merc.
— stinging, Amm-c. Berb. Dros. Rhus.
— tensive, Crotal. Mgn-s. Nitr. Tart.
— on the tetters, Creos.
— thin, which break, and send out an ichorous pus, which corrodes the skin and spreads, Tart.
— titillating, Mez.
— ulcerated, Ars. Dulc. Mgn-m. Merc. Sass. Sil. Tart.
— water, containing, Stram.
— white, Cycl.
— yellow, Carb-veg. Hyosc.
Redness of skin, Acon. Agar. Aloe. Apis. Arn. Ars. Asa-f. *Bell.* Bry. Canth. Cham. Chin. Cinnab. Clem. Dulc. Euph. *Graph.* Hep. Kali-b. Lach. Lyc. Mang. *Merc.* Nux. Op. Phosp. Phosp-ac. Puls. Rhod. *Rhus.* Ruta. Sec-c. Sep. Stram. Sulph. Sulph-ac.
— burning, Agar. Bell. Cicm.
— itching, Agar. Bell. Graph. Merc. Oleand. Rhus.
— scarlet, Amm-c. Bell. Cop. Croc. Croton. Euph. Phosp-ac. Tereb. (compare Erysipelas.)
— bluish, Lach.
— brown, Nitr-ac. Phosp. Thuj.
— hot, swollen, shining, painful, Acon.
— smooth, even, shining redness, with dryness of skin, Acon. Bell. Bry. Lach. Lyc. Nux. Op. Phosp. Puls. Rhus.
Rhagades, Aloe. Alum. Arn. Aur. *Calc.* Cham. Creos. Cycl. *Hep.* Lach. *Lyc. Mang.* Merc. Nitr-ac. Nux Petr. Phosp. *Puls.* Rhus *Sass. Sep. Sulph.* Zinc.
— in bends of joints, Mang.
— bleeding, Merc. Petr. Sulph.
— burning, Zinc.
— deep, bloody, Merc. Sass.
— yellow, Merc.
— ulcerated, Bry. *Merc.*
— itching, Merc.
— mercurial Hep. Sulph.
— humid, Aloe.
— after washing, Ant. *Calc.* Hep. Graph. Puls. *Sep. Sulph.*
— painful, Graph. Mang. Zinc.
Rings, yellow, on skin, Nitr-m. Sep.
Ringworms. Dulc. Hell. Ntr-c. Phosp. Sep. Tellur.
Roughness of skin, Bell. *Calc.* Graph. Iod. Merc. Ntr-c. Rhus. Sec-c. *Sep.* Sulph.
Scarlatina, Acon. Ailanth. Amm-c. Amm-m. Apis. Ars. Arum-trif. *Bell.* Bry. Calc. Carb-an. Cop. Cr-c. Cupr-acet. Euph. Gels. Graph. Hep. Hyosc. Iod. Lach. Lyc. *Merc.* Mur-ac. Nitr-ac. Nux. Phosp. *Phosp-ac.* Rhus. Stram. Sulph. Tereb. Thuj.

33. SKIN.

Scarlatina smooth, (genuine) Amm-c. Bell. Merc.
— gangrenous, Amm-c. Ars. Lach.
— suppressed, Phosp.
Sensitiveness of skin, Agar. Arn. *Bell.* Calc. Camph. *Chin.* Coff. Con. Creos. Ferr. Graph. Hep. Igt. Ip. Led. Mgn-c. Mosch. Ntr-m. Nux-m. Nux. *Petr.* Phosp-ac. Rhus. Scill. Selen. Sep. *Sil.* Spig. Thuj. Verat.
— — when shaving, Ox-ac.
Shrivelled, wrinkled, skin, Ant. Calc. Cupr. Lyc. Sass. Sec-c. Sep. Verat.
Soreness of skin, (by long lying) decubitus, (compare Chafing.)
— sensation of, Alum. Bry. Calc. Cic. Graph. *Hep.* Igt. Ntr-m. Nux. Petr. Plat. Puls. Rhus. *Sep.* Sulph. *Zinc.*
Spots, black, Ars. Crotal. Lach. Rhus.
— — in old people, Con.
— blue, Ant. Ars. Bar-c. Bry. Cic. Ferr. Led. Op. Plat. Sulph. Sulph-ac.
— — red, Ferr-m. Lach. Phosp.
— brown, Ant. Ars. Carb-veg. Con. Dulc. Hyosc. *Lyc. Merc.* Mez. Ntr-c. *Nitr-ac.* Petr. Phosp. Plb. *Sep. Sulph.*
— — red. Nitr-ac. Phosp. Thuj.
— — white, Ars. Phosp. Sep. Sil. Thuj.
— burning, Amm-c. Ars. Berb. Chelid. Ip. Kali-c. Merc. Mez. *Phosp-ac.* Rhus. Sep. Sulph-ac. Tabac.
— burnt, as if, Ars. Caust. Cycl.
— chronic, Con.
— claret colored, Cocc. Sep.
— close together, Calc.
— in the cold, appearing, Sabad.
— confluent, Bell. Cic. Hyosc. Valer.
— coppery, Ars. Carb-veg. Creos. Lach. Mez. Nitr-ac. Phosp. Rhus. Verat.
— coral colored, Cor-r.
— dark colored, Aur. Calc. Cor-r. Crotal. Phosp. Plb. Tart.
— dirty, Berb. Sabin. Sec-c.
— dry, Bar-c. Kali-jod.
— excoriated, Lach. Merc.
— fiery red, Ferr-m.
— flea bites, like, Acon. Bell. Dulc. Graph. Kali-b. Mez. Puls. Sec-c. Stram. Tart.
— freckles, Amm-c. Ant. Calc. Con. Dros. Dulc. Graph. Kali-c. Merc. Ntr-c. Nitr-ac. Nux-m. Petr. *Phosp.* Puls. Sep. *Suplh.*
— gangrenous, Cycl. Hyosc. Sec-c.
— gnawing, itching, Phosp.
— gray, Nitr-ac.
— green, Arn. *Con.*
— hepatic, Ant. Laur. Lyc. *Sulph.*
— herpetic, Hyosc. Merc. Ntr-m. Phosp. *Sep.*
— humid, Hell. Sil. Sulph.
— — after scratching, Kali-c.
— inflamed. Ars. Hell.
— — red, Kalm.

Spots irregular, Cocc. Sulph.
— itching, Arn. Berb. Con. Euph. Graph. Iod. Kali-c. Lach. Led. Lyc. Merc. Mez. Ntr-m. Nitr-ac. Sep. Sil. Spong. Sulph-ac. Zinc.
— large, Lyc. Phosp-ac. Tart.
— leprous, Ntr-c.
— livid, Crotal. Lach. Sep.
— marbled, Berb. Carb-veg. Caust. Ntr-m. Thuj.
— measel shaped, Ars.
— miliary, Thuj.
— moles, like, Calc. Carb-veg. Graph. Petr. Phosp-ac. Sil. Sulph. Sulph-ac. *Thuj.*
— mottled, Ox-ac.
— nettle rash, like, Berb.
— painful, Con.
— as if sore, Ferr. Hep. Phosp-ac. Verat.
— — as if contused, Berb.
— painless, Graph. Led. Phosp-ac. Sep. Stann.
— pale, Lach.
— turning, in the cold, Sabad.
— — — under pressure of finger, Bry. Ferr-m.
— red, Cannab. Carb-an. Carb-veg. Rhod. Sass. Thuj. Vipr-red.
— peeling off, Amm-c. Sep.
— petechiae, Ars. Berb. *Bry.* Hyosc. Lach. Nux. Phosp. Rhus. Sec-c.
— — as if ecchymosed, Arn. Bry. Calc. Con. Hep. Nux. Puls. Sulph. Sulph-ac.
— purple, Lach.
— rash, like, Mez.
— recurring yearly, Crotal.
— red, Alum. Ambr. *Amm-c.* Aur. Ars. *Bell.* Berb. Bry. Calad. Calc. Carb-veg. Cocc. Con. Cor-r. Crotal. Cycl. Dros. Dulc. Ferr. Graph Iod. Ip. Kali-c. Lach. Lyc. Mgn-c. Mgn-m Merc. Ntr-c. Ntr-m. Petr. *Phosp.* Phosp-ac. Plb. Rhus. *Sabad.* Samb. Sass. Scill. Sep. Sil. Spong. Stann. Stram. Sulph. Sulph-ac. Tabac. Vipra-red. Vipra-torv. Zinc.
— — in the cold, Sabad.
— — — increase of the moon. Clem.
— checkered, Carb-veg. Caust. Ntr-m. Thuj
— — pale, Sacch.
— — blue, Bell. Phosp.
— rose red (tubercles), Ntr-c. *Sil.*
— rough, Merc Sass. Zinc.
— round, Merc.
— scarlet colored, Amm-c. Ars. Bell. Bry. Croc. Euph. Hep. Hyosc. Merc. Phosp. Phosp-ac Stram. Sulph. Tereb.
— scaly, Kali-c. Merc.
— scorbutic, Merc-cor. Nitr-ac.
— scurfy, Merc. Nitr-ac.
— shining, Phosp.

33. SKIN.

Spots, small, Bry. Lach. Led. Lyc. Merc. Op. Rat. Scill. *Sulph-ac.* Tart. Vipr-torv.
— smarting, Puls.
— smooth, Carb-an. Carb-veg. Cor-r. Lach. Mgn-c. Petr.
— sore, Bry. Calc. Carb-veg. Ferr. Led. Sulph.
— as from stings of insects, Lyc.
— stinging, Canth. Chelid. Lach. Merc. *Nitr-ac.* Puls.
— star shaped, Stram.
— syphilitic, *Merc.* Nitr-ac.
— tuberculous, Alum. Nitr-c. *Sil.*
— turning yellow and green, Con. Crotal.
— ulcerated, Merc. Sabin.
— violet colored, Phosp. Verat.
— white, Alum. *Ars.* Merc. Nitr-c. Phosp. Sep. Sil. Sulph.
— — brown, Ars. Phosp. Sep. Sil. Thuj.
— yellow, *Arn.* Con. *Ferr.* Kali-c. Lyc. Nitr-c. Petr. *Phosp.* Ruta. Sabab. *Sep. Sulph.*
— — rings, Nitr c. Nitr-m.
Stinging, Bar-c. Bry. Graph. Puls. Rhus. Spong. Viol-tr. (compare Pricking.)
Streaks, brown red, Carb-veg.
— red, *Sabad.*
— scarlet colored, Euph.
Suppurations, Am. Ars. Asa-f. Aur. Bell. Bry. Calc. Calc-ph. Canth. Carb-veg. Cham. Cist. Con. Creos. Dulc. *Hep.* Lach. Lyc. Mang. *Merc.* Mez. Nitr-ac. Phosp. Phosp-ac. *Puls.* Rhus. Sep. *Sil.* Staph. Sulph.
— after previous inflammations, Bell. Hep. Lach. Lyc. Merc. Mez. Puls. Sil.
— benign, Calc. Cham. Hep. Lach. Merc. Puls. Sil. Sulph.
— checked, Ars. Bell. Calc. Cupr. Dulc. Hep. Lach. Merc. Sep. Sil. Verat.
— malignant, Ars. Asa-f. Calc. Creos. Hep. Lach. Merc. Phosp. Rhus. Sil. Sulph. Vipr-torv.
— of bruised parts, Croc.
— — cellular tissue, Carb-veg.
— in membranous parts, Sil.
Tension of skin, Acon. Ant. Arn. Bar-c. Bell. Bry. Carb-an. Carb-veg. Caust. Coloc. Con. Kali-c. Lach. Mez. Nux. Oleand. Par. Phosp. Phosp-ac. Plat. Puls. Rhus. Ruta. Sabin. Sep. Spig. Spong. Staph. Stront. Sulph. Thuj. Viol-od.
— in evening, in bed, Stront.
Tightness of skin, Acon. Caust. Croton. *Nitr-ac.* Nux. *Phosp.* Plat. Sep. Stront.
Touch, by the, cutaneous affections, relieved, *Thuj.*
Tubercles, Agar. Alum. Amm-m. Ang. Ant. Apis. Ars. Bar-c. *Bry. Calc* Carb-an. Carb-veg. *Caust.* Cic. Cocc. Con. Dulc. Graph. Hell. Hep. Kali-c. *Lach.* Led. Lyc. Mgn-c. Mgn-m. Mgn-s.

Mang. Merc. *Mez.* Mur-ac *Nitr-c.* Nitr-m. Nitr. Nux. Oleand. Petr. Phosp. Puls. *Rhus.* Ruta. Sec-c. Selen. Sep Sil. Spig. Staph. Sulph. Tar. Thuj. Valer. Verat. Zinc.
— burning, Amm-c. Amm-m. Calc. Carb-an. Cocc. Dulc. Kali-jod. Mgn-m. Mgn-s. Merc. Mur-ac. Nicc. Nitr-ac. Phosp. Staph.
— suppurating, Amm-c. Bov. Nitr-ac.
— inflamed, Amm-m. Rhus.
— raised, Oleand. Rhus-ver. Valer.
— gnawing, Rhus.
— yellow, Ant. Rhus.
— smooth, Phosp-ac.
— scurfy, Sulph.
— hard, *Bry.* Lach. Mgn-c. Mgn-s.
— miliary, Nitr-m.
— itching, Aur. Canth. Carb-an. Cham. Cocc. Dulc. Graph. Kali-c. Lach. Lyc. Mgn-c. Mgn-s. Mur-ac. Nitr-m. Nitr-ac. Nitr. Op. Rhus. Staph. Stram. Stront Zinc.
— tuberous, Nitr-c. Phosp. Sil.
— leprous, Nitr-c. Phosp. Sil.
— humid, Nitr. Selen.
— tearing, Cham. Con.
— erysipelatous, Nit-c. Phosp. Sil.
— red, Amm-m. Hep. Lach. Led.
— — areola, Cocc. Dulc. Phosp-ac.
— painful, Amm-c. Ars. Bell. Bov. Lach. Lyc. Phosp-ac. Zinc.
— painless, Am. Bell. Graph. Ign. Led. Oleand. Scill. Verat.
— tensive, Caust. Mur-ac.
— stinging, Calc. Caust. Dulc. Kali-jod. Led. Mgn-c. Phosp. Rhus. Scill. Stram.
— stab-wound, after, Sep.
— tuberculous, Lach.
— malignant, Ars.
— wart shaped, Lyc.
— watery, Graph. Mgn-c.
— soft, Bell. Crotal. Lach.
— white, Dulc. Sep. Valer.
— sore, Sep.
— — painful as if, Ant. Caust. Phosp-ac.
— drawing, painful, Cham.
Ulcers, Ant. Ars. *Asa-f.* Aur. Bell. Bry. Calc. Calc-ph Carb-veg. Cham. Chelid. Chin. Cist. Con. Cupr. Dulc. Euph. Gran. Hep *Lach.* Lyc. *Merc.* Nitr ac. Nux. Phosp. Phosp-ac. *Puls.* Rhus. Ruta. Sass. Sep. *Sil.* Staph. *Sulph.* Thuj. Zinc.
— aching, Camph. Carb-veg. Chin. *Graph.* Par. *Sil.*
— beaten, with pain as if, Ars. Con. *Hep.* Sulph.
— biting, Bry. Cham. Euph. Grat. Lach. Led. Lyc. *Puls.* Rhus. Staph.
— — at night, Rhus.
— black, becoming, *Ars.* Asa-f. Carb-veg. Con. Euph. Ip. Lach. Mur-ac. Plb. Sec-c. Sil. Sulph.

33. SKIN.

Ulcers, black on the base, *Ars.* Ip. Sil.
— — — edges, Ars. Con. Lach. Sil. Sulph.
— bleeding, *Ars.* Asa-f. Bell. *Carb-veg.* Con. *Hep.* Kali-c. Lach. *Lyc.* Merc. Mez. Nitr-ac. *Phosp.* Phosp-ac. Puls. Sil. *Sulph.*
— — on edges, *Ars.* Lyc. Merc. Sil.
— at night, Kali-c.
— blisters around, with, Ars. *Lach.* Rhus.
— bloody, crust, with, Bell.
— bluish, Ars. Asa-f. Aur. Con. Hep. *Lach.* Mang. Merc. Sil. Verat.
— — on edges, Asa-f.
— boring, Chin. Sil. Sulph.
— bubbling, (throbbing) Mur-ac.
— burning, Apis. *Ars.* Bell. Bov. Carb-veg. *Caust.* Cham. Chin. Clem. Coloc. Con. Graph. Hep. *Lyc. Merc.* Mez. Mur-ac. Ntr-c. Nitr-ac. Nux. Phosp. Plb. Puls. Ran-b. *Rhus.* Sep. *Sil.* Staph. Sulph.
— — on edges, *Ars.* Caust. Hep. Lyc. *Merc.* Mur-ac. *Sil.*
— — in circumference, Ars. Asa-f. Caust. Lyc. Merc. *Puls.* Rhus.
— — at night, Hep. Lyc. Rhus. Staph.
— — when touched, Ars. Bell. Carb-veg. Lach. Lyc. Merc. Mez. Puls. Rhus. Sil. Sulph.
— burnt, as if, *Ars.* Carb-veg. Cycl.
— cancerous, Ambr. *Ars.* Aur. Bell. Calc. Carb-an. Carb-veg. Chelid. Chinin. Clem. Con. Creos. Hep. Lach. Merc. Millef. Scill. Sep. *Sil. Sulph.*.
— chronic, Calc. Cham. Chelid. Con. Creos. Croc. Cupr. Euph. Grat. *Hep.* Lach. *Lyc.* Merc. Nitr-ac. Petr. Phosp-ac. Ran-b. Rhus. Sep. *Sil.* Staph. Sulph.
— cold feeling, with, Ars. *Bry.* Merc. Rhus. Sil.
— confluent, Tart.
— corroding, gnawing pain, Agn. Bar-c. Cham. Dros. Kali-c. Lyc. Merc. Phosp. Plat. Puls. Ran-sc. *Staph.* Sulph. Sulph-ac.
— crusty, scurfy, Ars. Bell. Bry. Calc. Cic. Con. Graph. Hep. Led. Lyc. Merc. Phosp-ac. Puls. Ran-b. Rhus. Sabin. Sep *Sil.* Staph. *Sulph.*
— cutting, *Bell.* Calc. Cham. Dros. Lyc. Ntr-c. Sil.
— deep, Ant. Asa-f. Aur. Bell. Bov. Calc. Carb-veg. Con. Dros. Hep. Lach. Lyc. Merc. Mur-ac. Nitr-ac. Petr. Phosp-ac. *Puls.* Sep. *Sil.* Sulph.
— digging, Asa-f. Sep.
— dirty, discolored, *Lach. Merc. Nitr-ac.* Sabin. Thuj.
— drawing, painful, Clem. Graph. Mez. Nitr. Nux. Staph. Sulph.
— dry oval, overhanging base, movable dark spot in centre, on healing cicatrix depressed, Kali-b.
— fat, Ars. *Hep. Merc.* Nitr-ac.

Ulcers, fat at base, Merc.
— fetid, Ammi-c. Ant. *Ars. Asa-f. Carb-veg.* Con. *Hep. Lyc.* Merc. Rhus. Sec-c. Sep. Sil. Staph.
— — putrid, Calc. Chin. *Hep. Mur-ac.* Phosp-ac. Rhus. *Sil.* Sulph.
— fistulous, Ant. Asa-f. Aur. Bell. *Calc.* Carb-veg. Caust. Con. Euph. Fluor-ac. Hep. Lach. *Lyc.* Millef Nitr-ac. Phosp. *Puls.* Ruta. Sep. *Sil.* Sulph.
— flat, Ant. Ars. Asa-f. Bell. Chin. *Lach.* Lyc. Merc. Nitr-ac. Petr. Phosp-ac. Puls. Ran-b Selen. Sep. Sil. Thuj.
— fringed at base, Phosp-ac.
— fungus, Lach. Merc. Sacch. Sil.
— gangrenous, *Ars.* Asa-f. Bell. Chin. Creos. Euph. Lach. *Plb.* Sabin. Scill. *Sec-c* Sil.
— gnawed, as if, Lach.
— gray, Ars. (compare Pus).
— greenish, Ars. Staph. (compare Pus).
— hard, *Ars. Bell.* Bry. Calc. Chin. Clem. Con. Hep. Lach. *Lyc.* Merc. *Puls.* Sil. Sulph.
— — on edges, Ars. *Asa-f.* Calc. Carb-veg. Caust. Hep. Lach. *Lyc. Merc.* Mez. Puls. *Sil.* Sulph.
— — in circumference, Ars. Asa-f. Bell. *Lach.* Lyc. *Puls.*
— — and high edges, *Ars.* Asa-f. Kali-b. *Lyc.* Merc. Puls. *Sil.*
— herpetic, Zinc.
— indolent, Ars. Carb-veg. Con. *Euph.* Lyc. Nitr-ac. Op. Phosp-ac. Sang. Sep. Sil. Sulph.
— inflamed, Acon. *Ars.* Bell. Bry. Calc. Cham. Colch. *Hep.* Lyc. *Merc.* Mez. Ntr-c. Nitr-ac. Petr. Phosp. Rhus. Ruta. Sep. *Sil.* Staph. Sulph.
— itching, Alum. Ambr. Ant. Ars. Bell. Bov. Calc. Canth. Caust. Cham. Chin. Clem. Coloc. Graph. *Hep. Lyc.* Phosp. Phosp-ac. Psor. Puls. Ran-b. Rhus. Sep. *Sil.* Staph. Sulph. Thuj.
— on margins, Ant. *Hep.* Lach. Lyc. *Puls* Sil.
— — at night, Lyc. Staph.
— jerking pain, Asa-f. Calc. *Caust.* Cham. Ntr-m. *Puls.* Rhus. *Sil.* Staph.
— lardaceous, Ars. Merc. Sabin.
— mercurial, Asa-f. Aur. Bell. Carb-veg. Euph. Hep. Lyc. Nitr-ac. Nux-jug. Op. Phosp-ac. Sep. Sil. Sulph. Thuj.
— movable base, Kali-b.
— painful, *Arn.* Ars. *Asa-f.* Bell. Calc. Carb-veg. Caust. Clem. Graph. *Hep.* Lach. Lyc. Merc. Mur-ac. Nux. Phosp-ac. Puls. Sabin. Sep. Sil.
— — on edges, Ars. *Asa-f. Hep.* Lach. Lyc *Merc. Sil.*
— — in circumference, Ars. Asa-f. Hep. *Lach. Puls.*
— — as if bruised, Ang. Arn. Cham.

33. SKIN.

Cocc. Con. Graph Hep. Hyosc. Ntr-m. Nux. Rhus. Ruta Sulph.
Ulcers painless, Ars. Bell. Carb-veg.Cocc. Con Hyosc. Lach. *Lyc.* Oleand. Op. Phosp. *Phosp-ac. Sep.* Stram.
— peeling off of skin, with, Merc.
— pimples around, *Carb-veg.* Caust. Lach. Puls. Sep. Sulph.
— pressing, Graph. *Sil.*
— proud flesh, with, *Ars.* Cham. Graph. Lach. Petr. Sacch. *Sep. Sil.* Sulph.
— prurient sensation, producing a, *Arn.* Clem. Con. *Rhus. Sep.*
— psoric, Psor.
— pustules, around, Calc. Clem. *Hep. Mur-ac.* Phosp-ac. Rhus. *Sil.* Sulph.
— putrid, *Ars.* Asa-f. Bell. Borax. Calc. Chin. Creos. Cycl. Graph. Hep. Lyc. *Merc. Mur-ac.* Nitr-ac. Phosp. Phosp-ac. Puls. Rhus. Sep. *Sil.* Sulph.
— pustulous, Sass. Tart.
— red areola, with, Acon. Ars. Asa-f. Calc. Cham. *Hep.* Kali-c. Lach Merc. Puls. Rhus. *Sil.* Staph. Sulph.
— salt rheum, like, Ambr. *Ars.* Graph. *Lyc.* Puls. *Sep.* Sil. Staph.
— sarcomatous, Ars. *Hep. Nitr-ac.* Sabin.
— scorbutic, Merc. Staph.
— scrofulous, Ars. Aur. Bell. Bov. Calc. Carb-an. Carb-veg. Caust. Cist. Graph. Hep. Lach. Lyc. Nux. Phosp. S.l. Sulph.
— shaggy, *Merc.* Phosp-ac.
— shining, Lac-can. Puls. Staph.
— shocks, jerks, with, Arn Clem. Ruta.
— smarting, Bell. Colch. Dig. Graph. Led. Lyc. Merc. Puls. Rhus. Sulph.
— — at night, Hep. Lyc. Rhus.
— sore pain, Ars. Bell. Graph. *Hep.* Igt. Merc. Mez. Phosp. Phosp-ac. *Puls.*Sep. Sil. Sulph.
— — when touched, Hep.
— spongy, Ant. *Ars.* Bell. *Carb-an.* Carb-veg. Clem. Lach. Merc. Petr. Phosp. Sep. *Sil.* Staph. Sulph. Thuj.
— — on edges, Ars. Carb-an. Lach. *Sil.*
— spotted, Arn. Ars. *Con.* Lach.
— — white, white spots, Ars. Con. *Lach.* Merc. Sil.
— spreading phagedœnic, Ars. Bell. Carb-veg. Caust. Cham. Chelid. Clem. Graph. Hep. Kali c. Lach. Lyc. Merc. Ntr-c. Nitr-ac. Petr. Puls. Ran-b. Ran-sc. Rhus. Scill. Sep. Sil. Sulph. Sulph-ac.
— stinging, Apis. Ars. Asa-f. Bell. Bry. Chin Clem. Graph. Hep Kali-b. Lam. Lyc. Merc. Mez. *Nitr-ac.* Nux. Petr. *Puls.* Ran-b. Rhus. Sep. *Sil.* Staph. *Sulph.*
— — on edges, Ars. Asa-f. Hep. Lyc.

Ulcers, stinging on edges when toched, Clem. *Merc.* Puls. *Sil* Sulph.
— — in circumference, Ars. Asa-f.*Merc.* Puls. *Sil.* Sulph.
— — at night, Rhus.
— — as from splinters, Nitr-ac.
— swollen, Ars. *Bell.* Bry Con. Hep. Kali-c. Lyc. *Merc.* Ntr-m. Nitr-ac. Petr. Phosp. *Puls.* Rhus. *Sep.* Sil. *Sulph.*
— — on edges, Ars. Hep. *Merc.* Puls. Sep. *Sil.* Sulph.
— — in circumference,Bell. Hep. Merc. Puls.
— — raised edges, Ars. Hep. Merc. Petr. Puls. Sep. Sil. Sulph.
— — and inflammatory redness of parts, Ntr-c.
— syphilitic, Cist Lac-can. *Merc.* Nitr-ac. Nux-jug. Thuj.
— tearing pain, Ars. Bell. Calc. Canth. Cycl. Graph. *Lyc.* Nux. Sep. Sil. Staph. *Sulph.*
— tensive, Asa-f. Bar-c. Caust. *Con.* Lach. Merc. Phosp. *Puls.* Rhus.Spong.Stront. *Sulph.*
— — in circumference, Asa-f. Lach. *Puls.* Stront. Sulph.
— throbbing, Asa-f. Bry. Calc.Chin.Clem. Hep. Kali-c. Lyc. *Merc* Sil. *Sulph.*
— tingling, Acon. Arn. Bell. Caust. Cham. Clem. Con. Hep. Lach. Phosp. *Rhus.* Sec-c. Sep. Sulph.
— — at night, Rhus.
— toothed edges, *Merc.* Phosp-ac. Thuj.
— to touch, tender, Asa-f. Bell. Cl.am. Clem. Cocc. Hep. Lach.
— ulcerated, as it, subcutaneously, Asa-f. Bry. Calc. Carb-veg. Con Graph.*Phosp. Puls.* Ran-b. Rhus. *Sil.* Sulph.
— varicose, Sec-c.
— wart shaped, Ars.
— yellow, Calc. Cor-r. Nitr-ac. Plb. Zinc. (compare Pus.)
Varicilla acuminata, Acon. *Ant.* Ars. Bry. Carb-veg. *Puls.* Rhus. Sep. *Tart.* Thuj.
— aquosa, *Bell* Puls. Rhus. Sil. *Tart.*
Vesicles, Amm-m. Ant. *Ars.* Bar-c. Bell. Bry. Calc. Canth. Carb-an. Carb-veg. Caust. Clem. Crotal. *Dulc.* Graph.Hell. Hep. *Lach.* Mgn-c. Ntr-c. *N'tr-m.* Nitr. Phosp. Ran-b. *Rhus.* Sabin. Sec-c. Sulph. Tabac.
— air, containing, Kali-c. Vipr-torr.
— black, Ars. Lach. Ntr-c.
— bleeding, Graph.
— blue, black blue, *Ars.Lach.* Ran-b. Rhus.
— brown, Vipr-red.
— burning, Amm-c. Amm m Aur. Bar-c. Bry. Graph. Merc. Mur-ac. Ntr-c.Ntr-m. Nitr-ac. Ran-b. Spig.
— burn, as from a, Ambr. Bell. Canth.

33. SKIN.

Carb-an. Clem. Lyc. Ntr-c. Phosp. Sep. Sulph.
— from burns, which are painless, Euph.
— bursting, and forming ulcers, Clem.
— close to each other, Ran-b. Rhus. Verat.
— confluent, Alum. Phell. Rhus.
— cracked, breaking, Bry. Crotal. Lach. Vipr-torv.
— cutting, Graph.
— drawing, painful, Clem.
— dry, Rhus.
— erysipelatous, *Ars. Bell. Graph. Hep. Lach. Rhus. Sep.*
— fistulous, Ca'c. Petr.
— gangrenous, Camph. Ran-b. Sec-c.
— — blood vesicle, Sil.
— grape shaped, Rhus.
— grouped, Rhus-ver. Sulph.
— hard, Lach. Phosp-ac Sil.
— heat of sun, as from, Clem.
— herpetic, Nitr-ac.
— humid, Hep. Merc. Rhus.
— inflamed, Amm-m. Bar-c. Bell. Nitr.
— itching, Amm-m. Bry. Calc. Canth. Caust. Lach. Mgn-c. Ntr-c. Sil. Sulph.
— itch-like, Lach Phosp-ac. Selen.
— painful, B-ll. Kali-c. Phosp.
— — as if ulcerated, Mez. Mur-ac.
— painless, Stront. Sulph.
— pale red, Rhus.
— peeling of, *Bry.* Puls. Rhus.
— pemphigus, Bell. Dulc Sep.
— penetrating deeply, Lach.
— phagedœnic, Ars. Cham. Clem. Graph. Hep Mgn-c. Nitr-ac. Sep. *Sil.*
— putrid, Vipr torv.
— raised, Merc. Selen. Sulph.
— red, Ant. Ntr-m.
— — round, elevated, blood vesicles, like little flesh warts, Fluor-ac.
— — areola, Cannab. Crotal. Kali-c. Kali-chl. Ntr-c. Sil. Sulph. Tabac. Vipr torv.
— — itching, Tart.
— sac-shaped, Kali-c.
— sanguineous, Ars. Fluor-ac. Ntr-c. Sec-c.
— scurfy, Hell. Kali-b. Ntr-c. Ran-b. Sil. Sulph.
— — white edges and œdematous swelling, Bell.
— serum, full of which becomes opaque, then large heavy scabs form, Kali-b.
— smarting, Graph. Mang. Phosp-ac. Plat. Rhod. Rhus. Staph.
— — sore, like a wound, Con. Hell. Mgn-c. Ntr-c. Phell. Rhus-ver. Sil. Staph. Thuj.
— spots, leaving, Caust.
— stinging, Amm-c. Calc. Cham. Sil. Spong Staph.
— stings of insects, as from, Ant.
— suppurating, Amm-m. Ntr-c.
— tensive, Amm-m. Mgn-c. Mgn-m.

Mur-ac. Ntr-c. Nitr.
Vesicles transparent, clear, Mgn-c. Ran-b.
— ulcers around, *Lach.* Rhus.
— ulcerated, Merc. Ntr-c. *Sulph.* Zinc.
— watery, Bell. Bov. Sulph.
— white, Hep. Lach. Merc. Ntr-c. Thuj.
— wound, around the, *Lach.* Rhus.
— yellowish, *Dulc.*
Warts. Amm-c. Arg-n. Ars. Bar-c. *Bell.* Bov. *Calc. Caust.* Dulc. Euph. Ferr-m. Hep. Kali-c. Lach. Lyc. Mgn-c. Ntr-c. Ntr-m. *Nitr-ac.* Ox-ac. Phosp. Phosp-at. Rhus. Ruta Sass. Sep. Sil. Staph. *Sulph.* Sulph-ac. *Thuj.*
— beating, Calc. Caust. Hep. Lyc. Sil.
— bleeding, Ntr-c. Nitr-ac Thuj.
— burning, Petr. Phosp. Rhus.
— flat, Dulc. Lach.
— hard, Dulc. Ran-b. Sulph.
— helved, Dulc. Lyc. Thuj.
— horny, Sulph. Thuj.
— indented, Phosp-ac. Rhus. Thuj.
— inflamed, Bell. Calc. Caust. Ntr-c. Nitr-ac. Sep. Sil. Sulph. Thuj.
— itching, Euphr Kali-c. Nitr-ac. Thuj.
— large, Caust. Dulc. Ntr-c. Nitr-ac. Sep. Thuj.
— — jagged, often pediculated, moist and often bleed, Caust. Lyc. Nitr-ac. Phosp-ac. Rhus. Staph. Thuj.
— old, Calc. Caust. Nitr-ac. Rhus. Sulph.
— painful, Caust. Ntr-c. Ntr-m. Nitr-ac. Sabin. Sulph. Thuj.
— — as if sore, Hep. Lach. Ntr-m. Ruta. Thuj.
— pedunculated. Lyc. Thuj.
— small, *Calc.* Rhus. Sass. Sep. Sulph *Thuj.*
— stinging, Calc. Hep. Lyc. Nitr-ac. Rhus. Sep. Sil.
— suppurating, Ars. Calc. Caust. Hep. Sil. Thuj.
— tickling, Sulph.
— toothed, Phosp-ac. Sabin. Thuj.
— ulcerated, Ars. Ntr-c.
White smelling, Ant. Ars. Bell. Bry. Calc. Chin. Creos. Hep. Iod. *Lyc.* Merc. Puls. Rhod. Rhus. Sabin. Sep. Sil. Sulph.
Wounds, Acon. *Arn.* Bell. Bry. Calc. Ca!end. Caust. Cham. Cic. Creos. Con. Diad. Euph. Glon. Merc. Millef. Ntr-c. Nitr-ac. Nux. Petr. Phosp. Puls. Rhus. Ruta. Seneg. Sil. Staph. Sulph. Sulph-ac. Zinc.
— beating, Bell. Cham. Hep. Merc. Puls. Sulph.
— bedsores, Arn. Carb-veg. Chin. Puls. Sulph-ac.
— bites, Arn. Sulph-ac.
— — poisonous, Amm-c. Ars. Bell. Caust. Lach. Seneg.
— bleeding profusely, Arn. Carb-veg. Chin. Cop. Creos. Diad. *Lach.* Merc.

33. SKIN.

Millef. Nitr-ac. *Phosp.* Sep. Sulph.
Wounds, small wounds bleed much, Lach.
Phosp.
— bruising, Arn. Cic. Con. Euphr. Iod.
Lach. Puls. Rhus. Ruta. Sulph.
Sulph-ac.
— burning, Acon. Ars. Carb-veg. Caust.
Ntr-c. Nitr-ac. Sulph. Sulph-ac.
— burns, Acon. Ars. Carb-veg. Caust.
Croc. Ham. Lach. Sapo Sec-c. Stram.
Urtica-urehs.
— cutting pain, Ntr-c.
— ecchymosed, Arn. Bry. Con. Dulc.
Hep. Lach. Nux. Puls. Rhus. Sulph-ac.
— fall, as from, or concussion, Arn. Bry.
Cic. Con. Puls. Rhus. Sulph-ac.
— gangrenous, Acon. Amm-c. Ars. Bell.
Carb veg. Chin. Lach. Sil.
— glandular, Arn. Cic. Con. Dulc. Iod.
Merc. Phosp. Puls. Rhus. Sil. Sulph.
— hernia, Acon. Cocc. Nux. Sulph.
— incised, Arn. Ntr-c. Plb. Sil. *Staph.*
Sulph. Sulph-ac.
— inflammation, with, Acon Ars. Calend.
Cham. Plb. Puls. Rhus. Sulph. Sulph-ac.
— injuries, of bones, Arn. Calc. Calend.
Phosp-ac. Puls. *Ruta.* Symph.
— inveterate, will not heal, Bar-c. Borax.
Calc. *Cham. Graph. Hep Lach.* Merc.
Nitr-ac. Petr. Rhus. *Sil.* Staph. *Sulph.*
— itching, Sulph.
— loss of substance, with, Calend. Croc.
— luxations, Arn. Ntr-ac. Rhus.
— muscular distortions, Arn. Ntr-c.
Rhus.
— operation for stone in bladder, after,
Millef
— painful, becoming again, Nitr-ac. Nux.
Sulph.

Wounds, as if sore, Amm-c. Bell. Hep.
Nux. *Phosp-ac. Sulph.*
— phthisis after, Ruta.
— from blow of sabre, Arn. Euphr. Lach.
Puls. Staph. Sulph. Sulph-ac.
— shot wounds, Arn. Euphr. Plb. Puls.
Ruta. Sulph. Sulph-ac.
— splinter, Acon. Arn. Carb-veg. Cic.
Hep. Nitr-ac. Sil.
— sprains or strains, Agn. Amm-m. Arn
Bry. Calc. Carb-an. Carb-veg. Igt. Lyc.
Ntr-c Nux. Petr. Phosp. Puls. Rhus.
Ruta. Sep. Sulph.
— stab wound, Arn. Carb-veg. Cic. Lach.
Nitr-ac. Sil.
— stinging, Acon. Arn. Bry. Caust. Merc.
Ntr-c. Nitr-ac. Sulph.
— straining or sprained, Arn. Bry. *Calc.*
Carb-an. Carc-veg. *Cocc.* Graph Kali-c.
Lyc. *N'tr-c.* Ntr-m. Nux. *Rhus.* Sep. *Sil.*
Sulph.
— — with hernia, Cocc. Nux. Sulph.
— — — prolapsus uteri. Bell. Nux. Sep.
— — suppurating, Asa-f. Bell. Borax.
Bufo. Calchd. Chin. Hep. *Merc.* Puls.
Sil. Sulph.
— swelling of affected part, with, Arn.
Bry. Puls. Rhus. Sulph.
— ulcerated, Cham. Graph. Hep. Lach.
Merc. Nitr-ac. Petr. Sil. Staph. Sulph.
Yellow color, Acon. Aur. Ars. Bell. Brom.
Bry. Bufo. Calc. Canth. Carb-veg.
Caust. Cham. *Chin. Con.* Cop. *Dig.*
Ferr. Hep. Igt. *Iod.* Lach. Laur. Lyc.
Mgn-m. *Merc.* Nitr-ac. *Nux.* Op. Phosp.
Plb. Puls. Rhus. Sang. *Sec-c.* Sep. Sulph.
Tar. Valer.
Zona, Ars. Graph. Iod. Merc. Ntr-c. Puls.
Rhus. Selen. Sep. Sil. Sulph.

34. Generalities.

AGGRAVATIONS AND AMELIORATIONS.

Abbreviations;—AGG., AGGRAVATION; AMEL., AMELIORATION,

Acids from, complaints, Acon. Aloe. Ant. Ars. Bell. Ferr. Hep. Lach. Ntr-m. Nux. Sep. Staph. Sulph.
Afternoon, in the, agg., *Anac. Alum. Amm-c. Ant. Asa-f.* Bell. Berb. Bism. Camph. *Canth. Chelid.*Coff.Colch. Coloc. Con. Igt. Ind. Iod. *Laur. Lyc. Mosch. Mur-ac.* Ntr c. *Nitr-ac.* Nux. Phosp. Plb. Puls. Ran-b. *Sass.* Selen. Seneg. Sil. Spong. Staph. Stront. Teucr. *Thuj.* Valer. Viol-tr. Zinc.
— every other, Lyc.
— periodically in the, Alum.
— 3–4, Apis.
— 4–3, A.M., Bell.
— 4–8, Hell. Lvc. Mgn-m.
— until 4, Merc-jod.
— 3–3 A.M., Thuj.
Alone when, agg , Ars. Dros Con. Kali-c. Lach. *Lyc.* Mez. Phosp. Sil.Stram.Verb. Zinc.
Alternation of contrary complaints, Bry. *Croc. Igt.* Kali-b. *Plat. Puls.* Rhus. Sep. Stront. Sulph.
— of mental and bodily symptoms.*Croc.Plat*
— constant change of symptoms, Sang.
Anger, from, agg. Acon. Alum. Ars. Bell. Bry. Cham. Chin. Cist. Cocc. *Coloc.* Hipp-m. Igt. Ip. Lach. Lyc. Mez. Ntr-m. Nux. Petr. Phosp. Plat. Puls. Sacch. Sep. *Staph.* Sulph. Verat.
— paralysis, one-sided, from, Staph.
Animal fluids, from loss of, Agar. Arg. Ars. Bell. Bov. Calad. *Calc.* Carb-veg. *Chin.*Cina. Ferr. Igt. Iod. Kali-c. Lyc. Merc. Ntr-c. Ntr-m. Nux. Petr. Phosp. Phosp-ac. Plb. *Puls.* Ran-b.Scill.Selen. *Sep.* Sil. Spig. *Staph.* Sulph. Zinc.
Anthrax, poison, from. Ars. Lach.
Anxiety, *Ars.* Bell. Bry. Calc. Canth. Carb-veg. *Cham.* Chin. Coff. Cupr. Lyc. Ntr-c. *Nux. Phosp-ac.* Puls. Rhod. Sec-c. Sep. Stann. Sulph. Tabac. Teucr. Verat.

Apoplexy, Acon. Anac. Ant. Apis. *Arn.* Aur. *Bar-c. Bell.* Camph. Carb-veg. Chin. *Colch. Coff.* Con. Dig. Ferr. Glon. *Hyosc. Ip. Lach. Laur. Lyc.* Ntr-m. Nux-m. Nux. *Op.* Phosp. Plb. *Puls.* R us. Sec-c. Sep. Sil. Stram. Sulph.
— from congestion of blood, Acon. *Bell. Coff.* Glon. *Ip.* Lyc. Merc. Nux.
— alternating with epileptic fits, Hyosc.
— gastric, Bry. Ign Ip. Nux.
— nervous, Arn. Bell. Chin. Coff. Hyosc. Phosp. Stram.
— serous, Arn. Dig. Ip. Merc.
— in old people, Apis. Con.
— — — with paralysis, Con. Laur.
— with sterterous breathing and snoring, Hyosc.
— — drowsiness, eyes open, congested, face, Bell.
— — — or from exposure to sun, Glon.
— preceded by profuse discharge of albuminous urine, Glon.
— with unconsciousness, involuntary urination, eyes wide open, lower jaw hanging down, Lyc.
— unconscious, eyes closed, loud stoterous breathing and snoring, Op.
Arsenic, poisoning from, Camph. Chin. Ferr. Graph. Iod. *Ip. Merc.* Nux. Samb. *Verat.*
Arthritic pains, Acon. *Agn.* Ant. *Art.*Arn. Ars. Asa-f. Bar-c. *Bell. Bry.* Calc. Canth. *Carb-an.* Carb-veg. *Caust.* Chelid. Chin. Cic. Cocc. *Colch.* Con. Dig. Dulc. Ferr. Graph. *Guaj.* Hep. Hyosc. Igt. *Kali-c. Led. Lyc.* Mang. *Meny.Merc.* Mez. Ntr-c. Ntr-m. Nux. Phosp. *Phosp-ac. Puls.* Ran-b. Ran-sc. *Rhod. Rhus. Sabin. Sass.* Sep. *Spig. Spong.* Stann. *Staph.* Stront. Sulph. Tart. *Thuj.* Zinc.
Arthritis with swelling, and heat, Acon. Ant. Ars. Bell. Chin. Coloc. Ferr. Hep. Nux. Puls. Sulph.

34. GENERALITIES.

Arthritic nodes Agar. Ant *Aur.* Benz-ac
Calc. Carb-veg. Caust. Cic. *Dig. Graph.*
Led. Lyc. Rhod. Rhus. *Sabin. Staph.*
Ascending, agg., Amm-c. Ang. *Ars.*
Bar-c. Borax. *Bry.* Calc. Cupr. Iod.
Merc. Nitr. Nux. Seneg. Sep. Spig.
Spong. Zinc.
— — an eminence. Ars. Aur. Bry. Spong.
Stann. Zinc.
— — a heighth, Calc. Oleand. Spig. Sulph.
— — steps, Acon. Alum. Ang. Calc.
Carb-veg. Nux. Plat. Plb. Rat.
Rhus. Stann. Sulph. Thuj.
— amel., Con. Ferr. Rhod. Valer
Asphyxia, Carb-veg Chin. Coff. Nitr-ac.
Op. Phosp- c. Tart.
Autumn, in, agg., Aur. Chin. Cic. Colch.
Merc. Nux. *Rhus.* Verat.
Awaking on, agg., *Ambr.* Amm-c.
Amm-m. Ant. Arn. *Ars. Calc.* Carb-an.
Carb-veg. *Caust.* Chin. Cocc. Dig.
Graph. *Hep.* Ign Ip. Kali-b. Kali-c.
Lach. Lyc. Merc. Ntr-m. *Nitr-ac.* Nux.
Phosp. Puls. Rhus. Samb. *Sep.* Sil.
Staph. *Sulph.*
— amel., Ars Calad. Colch. Nux. *Phosp.*
Sep.
Awkwardness, Ambr. Anac. Apis. Bov.
Caps. Ip. *Ntr-c. Ntr-m.* Nux. Sabin.
Sulph.
Ball. like a, in inner parts, *Ign.* Lach. Plb.
Sep.
Bathing, agg., from, Ant. Nitr-ac. Rhus.
— — cold water, Ant. Bell. Nitr-ac. Rhus.
— — convulsive twitches from, Rhus.
— — in the sea, Ars. Mgn-m. Rhus. Sep.
Xiphosura.
Beaten, pain as if, *Acon.* Alum. Arg. *Arn.*
Aur. Berb. Bry. Cic. *Cina. Colc.* Con.
Ntr-c. Nux-m. *Nux.* Oleand. Phosp.
Plat. *Ran-b.* Rhus. *Ruta.* Sulph. Verat.
— — pressing, Ntr nitr. Verat.
— — when touched, Hep Puls. Ruta.
— flesh as if from bones, Apis. Bry. Ign.
Lach Rhus. Sulph. Thuj.
Bed in, agg., Acon Ambr. Ars. Calc. Caust.
Daph. Graph. Hep. Ign. Kali-c. *Led.*
Lyc. Mgn-c. *Merc.* Nux. *Phosp.* Puls.
Rhod. Rhus. Sep. Sil. Staph Stront.
Sulph. Thuj. (compare lying in bed.)
— amel. Ars. Bry. Evon. Lyc. Merc. Scill.
Spong. Verat.
Bell ringing, from a agg., Ant.
Belladonna poisoning, from, Bell. Hyosc.
Beer, from, agg. Ars. Asa-f. Bell.
Coloc. Euph. Ferr. Kali-b. Lyc. Mez.
Nux. Puls. Rhus. Sep. Stann. Sulph.
Thuj. Verat.
— new, agg., Chin. Puls. Lyc. Teucr.
Bends of limbs, in, pain. Asa-f.
Bending down, agg., *Acon.* Alum. *Amm-c.*
Arg. Bar-c. *Bell.* Borax. *Bov. Calc.* Caps.
Carb-veg. Cham. Cic. Clem. Cocc.
Coloc. Croc. Diosc. Dros. Glon. Graph.
Hep. Ip. Kali-c. *Led. Lyc.* Mgn-m.
Mang. Meny. Merc. *Ntr-m.* Nitr. Nux-m.
Oleand. Petr Phosp. Plb. *Puls.* Rhod.
Rhus. Ruta. Seneg. *Sep. Sil. Spig.*
Stront. Sulph. Teucr. Thuj. *Valer.* Verat.
Bending, down after a long time, agg.,
Asar. Bov. Caust. Hep. Plat.
— amel., Bell. Cham. Chin. Puls. Scill. Thuj.
— or turning from left to right side, amel.,
Euph. Merc-jod. Thuj.
— backwards, amel., Bell. Cham. Lach.
Thuj.
— forwards, amel., Teucr.
— inwards, amel., Amm-m. *Bell.*
— sideway, amel., Meny. *Puls.*
— back the, shoulders, amel., *Calc.* Cycl.
— amel., (compare stooping).
Bent, keeping, amel., Puls. Rhus. *Scill.*
Bilious complaints, *Acon. Ant. Ars. Ars.*
Asar. *Asa-f.* Aur. Bell. Bry. *Cham.*
Chin. Colc. Dig. *Ign.* Ip. *Mgn-m. Merc.*
Ntr-c. Nux. Puls. Rhus. Sec-c. *Staph.*
Sulph. *Tar. Tart* Verat.
Biting from, amel. Cocc. *Staph.*
Biting-pricking, pain, Ambr. Canth.
Carb-veg. Clem. Dros. Hell. Ign. Ip.
Kali-c. Merc. Mez. *Nux.* Ran-b. *Ran-sc.*
Rhus. *Sep.* Staph. *Sulph.* Teucr. Zinc.
Black, the body turning, Acon. Ant. Arn.
Ars. Bell. Chin. Con. *Cupr.* Dig. Lach.
Merc. Nux. Op. Phosp-ac. Plb. Samb.
Sec-c. Verat.
Bleeding, after, of affected part, amel.,
Bov. Sass. Selen.
Bloatedness, scrofulous, body and face,
Ars. Asa-f. Bar-c. Bell. Calc. Hyosc.
Kali-c. Mez. Op. Phosp. Samb Sil. Spig.
Blood, abundance of, Plethora. Acon.
Aur. *Bell.* Bry. Calc. Chin. Dig. Ferr.
Hyosc. Kali-c. Lyc. Ntr-m. Nitr-ac. Nitr.
Nux. Phosp. *Puls.* Rhus. Sep. Stram.
Sulph.
— want of, anæmia, Ars. Bell. Bry. *Chin.*
Con. Ferr. Ign. Merc. Phosp-ac. *Puls.*
Rhus. *Scill.* Sep. *Staph.* Sulph.
— acrid, Amm-c. Canth. Kali-c. Nitr. Sass.
Sil.
— black, dark, Amm-c. Ant. Caust. Chin.
Croc. Merc-cor. Nitr-ac. Nitr. Nux.
Plat.
— brown, Bry. Calc. Carb-veg. Con. Puls.
Rhus.
— dark red, Cham Croc. Nux. Puls. Sep.
— — and not coaguable, Lach.
— clear bright, Acon. Arn. *Bell.* Calc.
Carb-veg. *Dulc.* Hyosc. Led. Merc.
Phosp. Rhus. Sabin. Zinc.
— coagulated, Arn. Bell. Caust. *Cham.*
Chin. Croc. Ferr. Hyosc. Ign. Ip. Merc.
Merc-cor. Nitr-ac. Nux. Phosp-ac. *Plat.*
Puls. *Rhus.* Sabin. Sec-c. Sep. Stram.
Stront. Zinc.

34. GENERALITIES.

Blood, decompose, tendency to Amm-c. Amm-m.
— offensive, Bell. Bry. Carb-an. Sabin.
— pale, Bell. Graph.
— thick, Arn. Croc. Cupr. Plat. Sulph.
— viscid, Croc. Cupr. Mgn-c. Sep.
— warm, Dulc.
— watery, Tart.
— — pale, Bell. Calc. Carb-veg. Cocc. Graph. Lyc. Nitr-ac. Plat. Puls. Sulph.
— congestion of the, Acon *Ambr.* Amm-m. *Arn. Aur.* Bell. Berb. B)v. Bry. *Calc.* Carb-an. Carb-veg. Caust. Chin. Con. Creos. Croc. *Ferr.* Glon. Hep. Iod. *Kali-c. Lyc. Merc.* Ntr-m. Nux. Op. *Petr. Phosp.* Phosp-ac. Puls. Samb. *Seneg. Sep.* Sil. Staph. *Sulph.* Tabac. *Thuj.*
— — in evening, Lyc. Samb. Thuj.
— — after lying down, Samb.
— — at night, Amm-c. Asar. Bar-c. Borax. Bry. Calc. Carb-an. Merc. Ntr-c. Ntr-m. Nux. Phosp. Puls. Ran-b. Rhus. Sabin. Senna. Sep. Sil.
— — — with palpitation of heart and pulsations, Sep.
— — after beer, Sulph.
— — slight exertion, Iod. Merc. Ntr-m. Thuj.
— — — motion, Ntr-m. Thuj.
— — in sitting, relieved, Thuj.
— — after vexation, Petr.
— — — walking in the open air, Ambr. Petr.
— — — drinking wine, Sil.
— sensation of stoppage of the, Acon. *Lyc.* Nux. Oleand. Rhod. *Sabad.*
— from loss of, consequences, Calc. Chin. Phosp-ac. Puls. Sep. Staph. Sulph.
— diminished circulation of, to parts most distant from heart, Camph.
Blood vessels, burning, Ars.
— — distended, Amm-c. Arn. Bar-c. *Bell. C un.* Croc. *Ferr. Hyosc.* Graph. Nux. Phosp. Puls. Sulph. *Thuj.*
— — nets in, like streaks in marble, Caust. Plat. Thuj.
— — inflamation of, Lach. *Tart.*
— — prickling in the, Merc.
— — pulsation, Acon. Ant. *Bell.* Carb-an. Creos. Graph. Hep. Iod. Kali-c. Merc. Nux. Phosp. Puls. Rhus. Sabin. Selen. Sep. Stront. Thuj. Zinc.
— — sensation of, cold in, Acon. Tart.
— — tremor, sense of, in, Vinca.
Blowing the nose, agg., Arn. *Aur.* Bell. Calc. Canth. Caust. Colch. *Hep.* Kali-c. *Merc.* Nux. Phosp-ac. *Puls.* Ran-b. Sep *Spig.* Staph. Sulph.
— — amel., Mang. Sil.
Bones, especially of the cylindrical,

Fluor-ac.
— caries. *Arg. Asa-f.* Aur. Calc. Chin. Cist. Con. Creos. Cupr. *Euph.* Graph. Guaj. Kali-b. Lach. *Lyc. Merc. Mez. Nitr-ac.* Op. Phosp. Phosp-ac. Puls. Rhus. Ruta. Sacch. Sec-c. Sep. *Sil.* Staph. Sulph.
— coldness, sensation of, Ars. Calc. Lyc. Sep. Zinc.
— curvature, Amm-c. *Asa-f.* Bell. *Calc.* Calc-ph. Hep. Iod. Lyc. *Merc.* Mez. Nitr-ac. Phosp. Phosp-ac. Plb. *Puls.* Rhus. Ruta. *Sil* Staph. Sulph.
— exostosis. Ang. Ars. *Asa-f.* Aur. Bry. *Calc.* Clem. Coloc. Creos. Daph. Dulc. Fluor-ac. Guaj. Hep. Lach. Lyc. Merc. *Mez. Phosp. Phosp-ac.* Puls. Rhus. Ruta. Sabin. Sep. Sil. Staph. Sulph.
— fractures, Arn. Calc. Lyc. Ruta. Sil. Sulph. Symph.
— looseness of flesh, sensation of, Bry. Igt. Nitr-ac. Rhus. Sulph. Thuj.
— from mercury, abuse of, Asa-f. Aur. Lyc. Nitr-ac.
— when moving rapidly, amel, Sabad.
— necrosis, Ars. Ang. Asa-f. Merc. Phosp. Plb. Sabin. Sec-c. Sil. Thuj.
— ostitis. inflammation, Acon. Ars. *Asa-f. Aur.* Bell. Bry. Calc. Chin. Clem. Con. Hep. *Lyc. Mang. Merc. Mez. Nitr-ac.* Phosp. Phosp-ac. Puls. Rhus. Sep. *Sil. Stap* . Sulph.
— — periosteum, Asa-f. Merc. Merc-cor. Phosp-ac. Sil.
— — of petrous bone, tender to touch. Caps.
— softness of, Asa-f. Bell. Calc. Dulc. Hep. Guaj. Lyc. Merc. Mez. Nitr-ac. Phosp. Puls. Ruta. Sep. Sil. Staph. Sulph.
— pains in general, Arg. *Asa-f.* Aur. Bar-c. Calc. Camph. Chin. Con. *Cupr. Diad.* Hep. Lyc. *Mang. Merc.* Mez. Mur-ac. *Nitr-ac.* Phosp. Phosp-ac. *Plb.* Puls. Rhod. Rhus. Ruta. Sep. Sil. Staph. Sulph.
— — as of a band around, Alum. Nitr-ac. Puls. Sulph.
— — — if beaten, *Bell.* Bry. Cocc. Hep. Igt. Ip. Led. Nitr-ac. Phosp. Puls. Rhus. *Ruta.* Sulph. Verat.
— — boring (piercing), Asa-f. Bell. Calc. Hell. Merc. Puls. Sep. Sil.
— — burning, Asa-f. Carb-veg. Euph. Phosp-ac. Rhus. Ruta. Sabin. Sulph.
— — in cool air, increased, Hell.
— — contraction, Nitr-ac, Puls. Sulph.
— — digging. *Diad. Mang.*
— — disabling, Cocc.
— — drawing, Agar. Amm-m. *Arg.* Aur. Bar-c. Bell. Bry. Cannab. Carb-veg. Caust. *Chin. Cocc. Colch.* Cupr. Cycl. Dros. *Kali-c.* Lyc. Mgn-c. *Merc.*

34. GENERALITIES.

Nitr. Phosp. Phosp-ac. *Rhod.* Rhus. Ruta. Sabad. Sabin. Spig. Staph. Stront. Valer. Zinc.
Bones, pain after drinking, Hell.
— — as from excoriating, Daph.
— — gnawing, Dros. Mang. Ruta. Sulph.
— — jerking, *Asa-f.* Calc. *Chin. Colch.* Ntr-m. Puls. Valer.
— — lacerating, Arg Bell. Bism. Caust. Chin. Cocc. Cycl. Phosp-ac. Plb. Stront. Zinc.
— — after paroxysms of madness, Cupr.
— — — meals, Hell.
— — nocturnal, Amm-m. Anac. Aur. Daph. Iod. Lach. *Lyc. Mang. Merc.* Phosp-ac.
— — pressure, Arg. Bell. Bism. Cupr. Cycl. Guaj. Kali-c. Oleand. Rhus. Sabin. Staph.
— — rending, tearing. Agar. Amm-m. Arg. Aur. Bar-c. Bell. Bism. Cannab. Carb-veg Caust. *Chin.* Cocc. Cupr. Cycl. Dros. Kali-c. Lyc. Mgn-c. Merc. Nitr-ac. Phosp. Phosp-ac. Plb Rhod. Ruta. Sabin. Staph. Stront. Teucr. Zinc.
— — — jerking, Chin.
— — — by jerks, Plb.
— — — paralytic, Cocc.
— — scraping, Asa-f. Berb. Chin. *Phosp-ac.* Rhus. *Sabad.* Spig.
— — — in interior of bones, Sabad.
— — smarting, Phosp-ac.
— — stinging, Bell. *Calc. Caust* Chin. *Con.* Dros. *Hell.* Lach. *Merc.* Puls. Ran-sc. Ruta. Sabin. *Sass. Sep.*
— — — burning, Ars. Euph. Zinc.
— — — pressing, Anac. Ruta.
— — — tearing (drawing), Acon. *Ars.* Chelid. Merc. Phosp. Thuj.
— — tingling, Plb. Rhus. Sep.
— soreness in wounds of, Hep. Phosp-ac. Symph.
— syphilitic pains in, Asa-f. Merc.
— throbbing in, Asa-f. Calc. Merc. Sulph
— when touched, agg, Sabad.
— warmth, amel., from, Caust.
Boots, on taking off the, agg, Calc. Graph.
Boring, piercing, pains, Agar. Arg. Aur. *Bell. Bism.* Calc. Caust. Cina. Dulc. Hell. Hep. Kali-c. Mgn-m. Merc. Mez Ntr-c. Ntr-m. *Ran-sc.* Rhod. Seneg. Sep. Sil. *Spig.* Tar. Thuj. Zinc.
— in the evening, Ran-sc.
— from inner parts, Bism. Dulc. Staph.
— — outer parts, Kali-c.
Boring with the finger in ear or nose, amel., Bar-c. *Calc.* Chelid. Croc. Igt. *Iod.* Lach. Plat. Ran-b. Sabad. Sep. Spig. *Staph.* Tar. Verb.
Bread, from eating, agg., Bry. Caust. Chin. Kali-c, Merc. Ntr-m. Nitr-ac. Phosp.

Phosp ac. *Puls.* Sass. Sep. Staph. Sulph.
Breakfast, before, agg., Bar-c. Calc. Chelid *Croc.* Igt. *Iod.* Lach. Plat. Ran-b. Sabad. Sep. Spig. *Staph.* Tar. Verb.
— amel., Bry. Caust. *Cham.* Chin. *Con.* Dig. Kali-c. *Ntr-m.* Nux-m. Phosp-ac. Sil. Zinc.
— after. agg., Amm-m. Bry. Calc. Caust. *Cham.* Con. Dig. Graph. Kali-b. Kali-c. Ntr-c. Ntr-m. Nitr. *Nux. Phosp.* Sep. Sulph.
— amel, *Calc.* Chelid. Croc. Igt. *Iod.* Lach. Plat. Ran-b. Sabad. Sep. Spig. *Staph.* Verb.
Breath, drawing a, agg., Acon. Amm-m. Anac. Bell. *Bry.* Calc. Cannab. Caps. Cina. *Colch.* Hep. Kali-c. Mgn-c. Mur-ac. Ntr m. Nitr-ac. Puls. Rhus. Sabad. Selen. *Sep. Spig.* Sulph.
— exhaling. agg., *Colch.* Dig. Dros. Igt. Iod. Oleand. *Puls.* Sep. *Spig.* Staph. Viol-od. Viol-tr.
— amel., Acon. Borax. *Bry. Rhus. Sabin.* Scill.
— inspiring. agg., *Acon.* Agar. Anac. Arg. Arn. Asar. Borax. *Bry.* Calc. Caps. Cham Chelid. Creos. Guaj Ip. Kali-c. *Bry.* Calc. Caps. Cham. Chelid. Creos. Guaj. Ip Kali c. Lyc. Meny. Merc. Nitr. Ran-b. *Rhus.* Sabad. *Sabin.* Scill. Selen. Seneg. Spong. Valer.
— amel., Chin *Colch.* Cupr. Dig. *Igt.* Lach. Oleand. Puls. *Spig.* Stann.
— holding one's breath, amel., Bell.
— — agg., Nitr. Spig.
— taking a deep. agg., *Acon.* Aloe. Arn. Borax. *Bry* Cycl. Graph. Hell. Kali-c. Kobalt. Lyc. Merc. Nitr. Ol. and. Ran-sc. *Rhus.* Sabad. *Sabin.* Scill. Sil.
— — amel., *Colch.* Cupr. Igt. Lach. Ox-ac. Spig. Stann.
— pains take away the, Diosc.
Broken, pain as if, Cupr. Hyper. Par. Ruta.
Bruised (beaten) pain, Agar. Aloe. Alum. Ang. Arg. *Arn.* Asar Aur. Berb. Bry. Calc. Caust. *Carb-veg.* Cham. Chenop. Chin. *Cic.* Cinnab. Cocc. Colch. Cor-r. Creos. Croc. Croton. *Cupr.* Daph. *Dros.* Dulc. Eupat. Ferr. Gels. Grat. *Guaj.* Hep. Igt. Ip. Kobalt. Lact. Lith. Mgn-c. Mgn-m. Mgn-s. Merc. Mez. Ntr-c. *Ntr-m. Ntr-s. Nux.* Oleand. Pallad. Phosp. Phosp-ac. *Plat.* Puls. Ran-b. Rhus. *Ruta.* Sep. Sil. Spig. Spong. Stann. *Staph.* Sulph. Sulph-ac. Tart. Tart-ac. Thuj. Valer. *Verat.* Zinc.
— when ascending steps, Calc.
— in evening, Amm-c. Bry. Phosp-ac. Sil.
— — extensors, Bruc.

34. GENERALITIES.

Bruised pain, lower extremities Berb.
— — morning, *Carb-veg.* Mosch. Ntr-c. *Ntr-m. Nux.* Phosp-ac. Viol-od.
— — — in bed, Mosch. *Nux.*
— — — after rising, *Carb-veg.* Ntr-m.
— when moving, *Agar.* Arn. Calc. Croc. Staph.
— at night, Creos.
— in open air, Amm-c. Cor-r.
— when at rest, Aur. Con. Ntr-m.
— — — relieved, Staph.
— in sitting, after a short walk, Ruta.
— when touched, Bry. *H p.* Puls. Ruta.
— — pressing on part affected, Plat.
— — uncovering, *Aur.*
Brunettes, for, suitable, Acon. Anac. Arn. Ars. Bry. Kali-c. Ntr-m. *Nitr-ac.* Nux. Phosp. *Plat.* Puls. Sep. Staph. Sulph.
Bubbling. Am'br. Ant. Asa-f. Bell. Colch. Lyc. Nux. Puls *Rheum. Scill.* Spig. Tar.
— sensation in muscles, Rheum.
Burning pains, Acon. Arn. *Ars.* Asa-f. Berb. Borax. Bry. Carb-an. *Carb-veg. Caust.* Chelid. Coloc. Cop. Creos. Cycl. Euph. Igt. Kali-c. Lyc. Merc. Mez. Mur-ac. Ntr-c. *Nux.* Phosp. *Phosp-ac.* Plb. Puls. *Rhus.* Sabin. Sec-c. Sep Spig. *Stann.* Staph. Stram. *Sulph.* Tar. Zinc.
— through lower half of body, extremities cold to touch, Phosp-ac.
— by friction increased, Berb.
— of interior parts, *Acon.* Arn. Ars. *Bell.* Berb. *Bry.* Calc. *Canth.* Carb-veg. Caust. Chelid. Chin. Cic. Cupr. Dulc. Euph. Graph. Laur. Lyc. *Merc.* Mez. Ntr-c. Nux. *Phosp.* Phosp-ac. Ran-b. Rhus. *Sabad.* Sec-c. *Sep.* Sil. *Sulph.* Verat.
— prickling, *Plat.*
— stinging, Apis. Bar-c. Bell. Cina. Dig. Gum-gut. *Plat.* Puls.
— when touched, Sabin.
— on small spots, Fluor-ac.
— throbbing as from a boil, Amm-m.
Burnt, pain as from being, Bar-c. Igt. Mgn-m. Plat. Puls. Sabad. Sep.
Bursting, pain as from, Asar. *Bell.* Bry. *Calc.* Caps. *Caust.* Con. Euph. *Igt.* Kali-c. Par. *Ran-b.* Sabin. *Sep.* Sil. *Spig* Stront.
Caresses, agg., by, Bell. Calc. Chin. Igt. Plat.
Carphologia, (picking the bed clothes), Arn. Ars. Bell. Cham. Chin. Cocc. .Colch. Hep. Hydroc-ac. Hyosc. Iod. Lyc. Mur-ac. Op. Phosp. Phosp-ac. Psor. Rhus. Stram. Sulph. Zinc.
Carried on the arm, child amel., when, Bell. Cham. Kali-c. Merc. Tart.
Catalepsy, Acon. Amm-c. Ang. Ars. *Bell.* Camph. Cham. *Cic.* Cupr. Hyosc. Igt. Ip. Lyc. Merc. *Mosch.* Op. Petr. *Plat.* Sec-c. Sep. *Stram.* Verat.

— bent backwards, *Ang.* Bell. Cham. *Igt.* Stann.
— rigor in, Acon. Stram.
— syncope, like, Verat.
Catarrh, agg., during, Amm-m. *Ars.* Calc. Carb-veg. *Cham.* Graph. Lach. Lyc. *Merc. Nux.* Puls. Sabad. Sep. Spig.
— suppressed, agg, from a, *Bry. Calc.* Chin. Dulc. Nitr-ac. *Nux.* Puls. Sep. Sil.
Cellars, in, cough agg., Sep. Stram. Tart.
Chamomilla, from abuse of, Acon. Alum. Borax. *Cocc.* Coff. Coloc. Igt. Nux. Puls. Zinc.
Changing position, agg., *Caps.* Carb-veg. Con. *Euph. Ferr.* Lach. Lyc. Phosp. *Puls.* Samb. (compare Beginning to move.)
— — amel., Igt. Valer.
Charcoal vapors, from, Arn. Bov.
Chewing motion, Acon. Cham. Lach.
— when, agg., Alum. *Amm-c.* Amm-m. Bry. Chin. Euphr. Guaj. *Hep.* Hyosc. Igt. *Meny.* Ntr-m. Oleand. Phosp. Phosp-ac. Puls. *Rhus.* Sabin. Sep. Staph. Thuj. Verb. Zinc.
— amel., Bry. Seneg.
— after, agg., Sabin. Staph.
Chills, attending paroxysms of pain, Ars. Bar-c. Bov. Bry. Coloc. Dulc. Euph. Graph. Igt. Kali-c. Led Lyc. Mez. Ntr-m. Nitr. Puls Rhus. Scill. Sep.
— at night, during, agg., Hep. Igt.
Chlorosis, Alum. Ars. *Bell. Calc.* Chin. *Cocc. Con.* Dig. *Ferr.* Graph. Hell. Kali-c. *Lyc.* Merc. Ntr-m. *Nitr-ac.* Nux. Phosp. *Plat.* Plb. *Puls.* Sep. Spig. Staph. *Sulph.* Valer. Zinc.
— after, anger, Sacch.
— with dropsy, Sacch.
Cholera, Acon. Ars. *Camph.* Carb-veg. Coloc. Cupr. Dulc. *Ip.* Jatr. Nux. Op. *Phosp. Phosp-ac. Sec-c. Verat.*
— infantum, Aeth. Ant. Ars. Bell. Benz-ac. Bry. Calc. Camph. Carb-veg. Chin. Croton. Dulc. Erecthiles. Grat. Ip. Laur. Merc. Nux. Phosp. Phosp-ac. Pod. Sec-c. Sulph. Verat.
— sporadic, Ars. Ip. Phosp. Phosp-ac. Sec-c. Verat.
Choleric, temperaments, for, Ars. Bry. Cham. Cocc. Lach. Nitr-ac. Nux. Phosp.
Cinchona (quinine) abuse of, *Arn. Ars. Bell* Calc. Caps. Carb-veg. Cina. *Ferr. Ip.* Lach. Meny. Merc. Ntr-c. *Ntr-m.* Nux. Phosp-ac. *Puls.* Sep. Sulph. *Tart. Verat.*
— — cough, Arn. Ferr.
Coffee, from, Ars. Cainca. *Canth. Caust. Cham.* Cist. Cocc. Hep. *Igt.* Merc. Merc-sulph. Millef. *Nux.* Puls. Rhus. Sulph.

Coffee, from amel., Ars. *Cham.* Coloc. Op.
— smell of, agg., Sulph-ac.
- Coition, during, agg., Graph. Kali-c. Selen.
— after, agg., *Agar.* Bov. Calad. *Calc.* Chin. *Kali-c.* Ntr-c. Petr. Selen. *Sep.* Spig.
Clothes, feeling uneasy and encumbered by, Amm-c. Calc. Caust. Hep. Lyc. *Nux.* Ran-b. Sass. Sep. Spong.
Cold, to take, disposition, *Acon. Anac. Bar-c. Bell. Bry. Calc. Carb-veg. Cham.* Chin. *Coff* Con. *Dulc.* Graph. Hep. Hyosc. *Kali-c. Lyc.* Mgn-m. Merc. Merc-cor. *Ntr-c.* Ntr-m. *Nitr-ac. Nux-m. Nux.* Petr. Phosp. Plat. Puls. Rhus. *Sep. Sil. Sulph.*
— — after overheating, Kali-c.
— — when uncovering the feet, Sil.
Cold, after a. affections, *Acon.* Bar-c. *Bell.* Calc. Carb-veg. *Cham.* Chin. *Coff.* Coloc. Con. *Dulc.* Graph. Hyosc. *Ip.* Lyc. *Mang.* Ntr-c. Ntr-m. *Nitr-ac. Nux-m.* Phosp. Puls. Sass. Sil. Sulph.
— — in dry weather, Nux.
— — wet weather, Borax.
— — from cold water, (internally, and externally), Ars. *Puls.*
— in stomach, Ars. Puls.
— — general, agg., Acon. Agar. Amm-c. *Ars.* Aur. Bar-c. Bell. Borax. *Camph.* Caps. *Caust.* Cic. Cocc. Con. *Dulc.* Hell. Hep. Hyosc. Igt. *Kali-c.* Mgn-c. M.ing. *Mosch.* Nux-m. *Nux.* Petr. Ran-b. Rhod. *Rhus. Sabad.* Sil. *Stront.*
— — amel., Dros. *Iod.* Led. *Puls.* Sec-c. Seneg. Tart.
— place, on getting into a, agg., *Ars.* Nux. *Ran-b.* Verb.
— air, agg., Acon. Agar. Alum. Amm-c. Apis. *Ars. Aur.* Bar-c. Bell. Bry. Calc. *Camph.* Caps. Carb-an. Carb-veg. *Caust.* Chin. Cist. Colch. Con. Daph. *Dulc. Hell. Hep.* Igt. Kali-b. *Kali-c.* Lyc Mang. Merc. Mez. *Mosch. Nux-m. Nux.* Petr. Phosp. Rhod. *Rhus. Sabad.* Sep. *Stront.* Verat.
— — amel., Ant. *Asar.* Colch. *Iod.* Lyc. *Puls.* Sulph.
— — and dry, agg., Acon. *Asar.* Bry. *Caust. Hep.* Ip. *Nux.* Sabad. Spong.
— — wet, agg., *Amm-c.* Borax. *Calc.* Colch. *Dulc.* Lach. Lyc. Mang. Merc. *Nux-m. Rhus.* Stront. Sulph. Thuj. Verat.
— on becoming, agg., Agar. Amm-c. Arn. *Ars.* Asar. *Aur.* Bar-c. Bry. Calc. Camph. Canth. Caps. Caust. Dulc. Graph. Hep. Hyosc. *Kali-c.* Lyc. Merc. *Mosch.* Nux-m. Nitr-ac. *Nux.* Phosp. Rhus. *Sabad.* Sep. Stront. Sulph.
— — amel., Apis. Bry. Cham. Dros.

Iod. Led. *Lyc.* Merc. *Puls.* Sabin. Sec-c. Sulph. Thuj. Verat.
— — the head, becoming, agg., *Bell.* Led. Puls. *Sep.*
— — feet becoming, agg., Cham. Puls. *Sil.*
— change of and warmth, agg., Ars. Carb-veg. Ran-b. Verb.
Coldness of body with paroxysms of pain, Ars. Bry.
— part affected, Bell. Caust. Merc. Mosch. Rhus. Sec-c. Verat.
— on isolated spots as from cold metal or drops of water, Acon. Berb. Cannab. Thuj.
Comfortable feeling, Coff. Op.
Company, in, agg., Bar-c. Lyc. Mgn-c. Plb. *Sep.*
— — amel., Ars. Dros. *Lyc. Stram.*
Concussions, *Arn.* Bell. Cocc. *Led.* Ntr-m. Nux. Rhus. Spig.
— agg., from, *Arn.* Bell. Bry. *Cic.* Hep. Hyper. Symph.
Concussive pain, Amm-c. Cupr. Mang. *Valer.*
Congestion of blood, *Acon.* Aloe. Apis. Arn. *Aur. Bell.* Bry. Cact. Calc. Cham. *Chin. Ferr.* Glon. Graph. Hyosc. Lyc. Merc. Ntr-m. Nitr-ac. *Nux. Phosp. Puls.* Rhus. Seneg. Sep. Sil. Spong. Stram. *Sulph.* Viol-od.
— active, Acon. Bry.
— passive, Nux. Puls. Sec-c.
Constricting, pains, *Alum.* Cocc. *Igt. Plat.* Plb.
Consumption, wasting, Arn. Ars. Bar-c. Bry. Calc. Chin. Con. Creos. Cupr. Dros. Dulc. Ferr. Graph. Guaj. Hep. *Iod.* Ip. *Kali-c.* Lach. *Laur.* Led. *Lyc.* Ntr-m. Nitr-ac. Nux-m. *Nux. Phosp. Puls.* Sec-c. Sep. Sil. *Stann.* Staph. Sulph.
— with acute laryngial phthisis, Dros.
— in children, Ars. Bar-c. Bell. Calc. Cham. Chin. Cina. Lyc. Mgn-c. Nux. Petr. Phosp. Puls. Rhus. Sulph.
Continence from, sexual diseases, Bell. Con. Hyosc. Stram.
Contortions of limbs, *Bell.* Cham. Cupr. Hyosc. Op. *Plat.* Sec-c. *Stram.*
Contracting pains, Coloc. Gels. Lith. Mgn-m.
— in injured parts, Arn.
Contraction, sensation of, Anac. Asar. Bism. Chin. Cocc. *Graph.* Lyc. Nitr-ac. *Nux.* Plat. *Rhus. Sep.* Stann. Stront.
Contraction of all the limbs, Amm-c. Bry. Caps. Caust. Coloc. Guaj. Rhus. Sil. Sulph.
— — single parts alternating with extension, Lyc.
— — flexors, Amm-c. Amm-m. Caust. Coloc. Graph. Guaj. Lach. Lyc.

34. GENERALITIES.

Ntr-c. Ntr-m. Puls. Rat. Rhus. Sep. Sol-n. Sulph.
Contradiction from, agg., Aur. Oleand.
Contusions, Arg. *Arn.* Cic. Con. Dros. Oleand. Ruta. Sulph-ac.
Contusion, pain as if, Arg. *Arn.* Caust. Cic. *Dros.* Nux-m. Oleand. Plat. Rhus. *Ruta.* Sulph ac.
Copper, vapors of, agg., Ip. Merc. Puls.
Corroding, pain, Ars. *Merc.* Sil. Sulph.
Coughing, before, agg., Cina.
— when, agg., Acon. Arg. Arn. Ars. Bell. *Bry.* Calc. Caps. Carb-veg. Chin. Cina. *Dros.* Hep. *Ip.* Lac-can. Ntr-m. *Nux. Phosp. Puls. Rhus.* Scill. *Sep.* Sulph. Verat.
— after, agg., Cina. Phosp. Sep.
— — and expectoration, agg., Calad. Sep.
Crackling, sensation of, Acon. Calc. *Rheum.* Spig.
Cramping, pain, inner parts, *Ang.* Cina. Petr. *Plat.*
Creeping like a mouse, sensation of, Alum. Laur. Nux.
— — — — — in limbs, Bell. *Calc.* Nitr-ac. Sep. *Sulph.*
Crookedness of limbs, Calc. Caust. Chin. *Coloc.* Ferr. Graph. Guaj. Hyosc. Lyc. Merc. Plb. *Sec-c.* Sil. Stram.
Crossing the limbs, agg., Asa-f. Dig.
Cutaneous eruptions, suppressed, agg., from, Ars. Bell. *Bry.* Caust. Cham. Hep. Ip. Lyc. Ntr-m. Nux-c. *Phosp-ac.* Puls. Rhus. Sep Staph. Sulph. Zinc.
Cutting pain, outer parts, Alum. Ambr. Ang. *Bell. Calc. Dros.* Graph. Hyosc. Ign. Lyc. Merc jod. Merc-ac. *Ntr-c.* Phosp-ac. Rhus. Samb. Sep. Sil. Sulph-ac.
— — inner parts, Ang. Arn. Bell. Calad. *Calc. Canth.* Chin. Cina. Con. *Kali-c.* Lyc. *Merc.* Mur-ac Nitr. Nux. Par. Phosp. Puls. Rheum. Sep. Stann. Staph. Stront *Sulph.*
— — where bones are least covered with flesh, not in joints, on touch pain goes to another part, Sang.
— — tearing, Hyosc.
— — when at rest, Mur-ac.
Cyanosis, Acon. Arn. Ars. Bell. Calc. Carb-veg. Chin. Con. *Cupr.* Dig. Lach. Laur. *Op.* Phosp. Samb. Sec-c. Sulph. Verat.
Cystic tumors, Calc. Graph. Hep. Sil. Sulph.
Dancing, from, amel., Ign. *Sep.*
Dark, in the, agg., Amm-m. Calc. Carb-an. Caust. Valer.
— — — amel., Acon. Ant. Bar-c. Bell. *Calc.* Chin. Con. Croc. Dros. *Euph. Graph.* Hep. Ign. Lyc. Merc. Ntr-c. Nux. *Phosp.* Phosp-ac. Puls. Sep. Sil. Stram. Sulph.

Deadness, torpor, coldness and whiteness of limbs, Ars. *Calc.* Caust. *Chelid.* Cic. Con. Creos. Lyc. Nux. Phosp. Puls. Sec-c. Sulph. Tart. *Thuj.* Zinc.
— sensation of, in injured parts, Arn.
Debauches, from, diseases, Ip.
Delirium, caused by paroxysms of pain, Ars. Dulc. Verat.
Dentition, during, Ars. Bell. Borax. *Calc.* Calc-ph. *Cham.* Cina. Coff. *Ign.* Mgn-c. Mgn-m. *Nux.* Pod. Rheum. Sil. Stann. Sulph.
Despair, accompanying pains, Ars. Carb-veg. Cham. Colch. Lil-tigr. Nux.
Diagonal pains, Agar. Calc. Eupat. Hyper. Lach. Mang. Nitr-ac. Nitr. Nux-m. Sang. Sil. Valer.
Diet, disorders from small excesses in, Ntr-c.
Digging pains, Ars. Cadm. Cocc. Cycl. Graph. Hyosc. Kali-c. Lach. Nux. Puls. Rhus. Verat.
— drawing, *Colch.* Ind. Puls.
— pressing, *Nux-m.*
Disabling, laming pains, Aloe. Arn. Ars. Aur. Bar-c. *Cannab.* Carb-veg. *Cham.* Chelid. *Chin.* Cina. *Cocc.* Colch. Dros. Hep. Mgn-m. Meph. Ntr-c. Ntr-m. Nitr. Sass. Sil. Stram. Sulph. Valer. Verat.
— in walking, Verat.
— after a walk, Valer.
Disability of limbs, *Amm-c.* Bar-m. Carb-veg. Chelid. *Chin.* Cina. Cocc. Colch. Dros. Mez. Ntr-c. Nitr. *Plat. Puls. Rhod.* Rhus. *Sil.* Valer.
— in evening, Bry. Sil.
— of parts affected, Cham. Chin. Colch. Plb.
— after sprains, Ruta.
Dislocations, Iasy, Agn. Bry. Calc. Lyc. Ntr-c Ntr-m. Phosp. Rhus.
— — from, agg., *Agn.* Amm-c. Arn. Bry. *Calc.* Carb-an. Ign. *Lyc.* Merc. Ntr-c. Ntr-m. Nitr-ac. Nitr. Nux. Petr; *Phosp.* Puls. *Rhus.* Ruta. Sulph.
Distention, sense of in body, Cinnab.
Distortions, *Agn.* Amm-c. Arn. Bry. *Calc.* Carb-an. Cina. Graph. Ign. *Lyc.* Merc. Ntr-c. Ntr-m. Nitr-ac. Nitr. Nux. *Petr. Phosp.* Puls. *Rhus.* Ruta. Sec-c. Sol-nig. Sulph.
Downwards, moving pains, Agar. Bar-c. Bry. *Kalm.* Phosp-ac. Sabin. Sass. *Valer.* Verat. Zinc.
Draft of air, agg., Anac. *Bell.* Benz-ac. Cadm. *Calc.* Caps. Carb-an. Caust. *Chin.* Graph. Hep. Hipp. Kali-c. Ntr-c. Ntr-m. Phosp. Rat. Selen. Sep. *Sil.* Sulph.
Drawing sensation through whole body, Ambr. Amm-c. Bar-c. *Bry.* Calc. *Graph. Merc-cor.* Mez. Nux. Puls. *Rhus.* Sep.

34. GENERALITIES.

Drawing sensation, as before intermittents, Calc. Nux. *Puls.* Sep.
— — on surface of body, in sitting, Samb.
Drawing pains, Ambr Ang. *Ant.* Arg. Arn. Ars. Bar-c. Bell. *Bry.* Caps. *Carb-veg. Caust. Cham.* Chin. *Cina.* Cinnab. Clem. Cocc. Cycl. Dulc.Graph. *Hell. Hep.* Hyosc. Iod. *Kali-c.* Lach. Lam. *Lyc.* Mgn-m. *Mang. Merc.* Mez. Mosch. *Mur-ac.* Ntr-c. Ntr-m. Nitr-ac. *Nitr.* Nux-m. *Nux.* Ol-an. Petr. Phosp-ac. *Plat. Plb. Puls.* Ran-sc.*Rhod. Rhus.* Ruta. *Sabad.* Sabin. Sec-c. Sep, Sil. *Stann. Staph. Stram.* Sulph. Sulph-ac. *Tart. Tereb.* Valer. Verat. Viol-od.
— in periosteum, or where skin covers the bones, Cycl.
— every other afternoon, *Lyc.*
— after a cold, *Nitr-ac.*
— digging, Colch. Ind. Puls.
— disabling, Arn. Bar-c. Carb-veg. *Cham. Chelid. Cina.* Cocc. Hep. Mgn-m. Mez. Ntr-c. Nitr.
— jerking, Colch. Ind. Puls.
— when moving, *Bry.* Cannab. Caps.
— at night, Cham. Plb.
— in parts affected, Bry.
— pressing, *Anac.* Ang. Arg.Cannab.Cycl. Ntr-m. Ruta *Stann.*
— rending, tearing, *Cham.* Colch. Hell. Igt. Lam. *Merc. Plb.* Puls. *Rhod. Rhus.* Sec-c. Staph.
— when at rest, *Mur-ac.* Nux-m. *Rhod. Rhus.*
— — — relieved, *Sabad.*
— by rubbing, relieved, Plb.
— — shocks, *Cocc. Colch.*
— in sitting, Staph.
— spasmodic, cramping, Asar.Cina. Ntr-c. Ol-an. Ruta.
— stinging, Borax. *Colch.* Dulc. *Merc.*
— in walking, Verat.
— — the abdomen, when amel., Igt. Sahin.
— — shoulders, when agg., Calc. Cycl.
— back of soft parts, *Ang.* Bell. *Merc.*
— in soft parts, Calad. Dros. Mosch. *Plb.*
— — sensation of, Hep. Plb. Verb.
— — of cold air, agg., from, All-cep. Ars. Aur. Bell. Bry. Calc. *Caust.* Hep. *Hyosc.* Kali-c. *Merc.* Nux-m. *Nux.* Rhod. Rhus. *Sabad.* Sep. Stront.
Drinking, while, agg., *Bell.* Bry. *Canth.* Cina. Hyosc. Iod. Lach. Phosp. Stram.
— after, agg., Acon. *Arn. Ars.* Aur. Bry. Cimex. *Chin. Cocc.* Coloc. *Con.* Croc. Croton. Ferr. Hell. Hep. Hipp. Hyosc. Lob Lyc. *Ntr-c. N'tr-m.* Nitr-ac *Nux.* Puls. *Rhus.* Sep. *Sil.* Staph. Sulph. Tar. Tart. Teucr. *Verat.*
— — cold liquids, agg., Alum. Ars. Bell. Calc.*Canth.* Croc. Dig.Elaps.Graph.Igt. Kali-b. Lachn. Lyc. Mur-ac. *Ntr-c.*

Ntr-m. *Nux.* Rhod. *Rhus.* Spig. Staph. Sulph. Thuj.
— — amel., Aloe. Apis. Asar. Camph. *Caust.* Coff. Cupr. *Phosp.* Puls. *Sep.*
— — warm liquids, Anac. Bry. *Cham.* Carb-veg. Dros. Euph. Hell. Kali-c. Lach. *Merc.* Mez. Phosp. Phosp-ac. Phyt. Puls.
— — amel., Alum. Ars. Lyc. Nux. Rhus. Sulph. Verat.
— — amel., Bry. Caust.Cinnab.Cist.Cupr. Phosp. Sil. Tellur.
— — quickly, agg., Ars. *Nitr-ac.* Nux. *Sil.*
Driving one about, pains which, w.th restlessness, Ars.
— — at night, Mgn-c.
Dropsy, Acon. Agn. *Ant.* Apis. Apocyn. *Ars. Aur.* Bell. Bism. Bry. Buto. Calc. Cannab. Canth. Caps. *Chin.Coloc.*Colch. Con. *Dig. Dulc.* Euphr. Ferr. *Graph. Hell.* Iod. Kali c. Lach. Lact. Led. *Lyc.* Meny Merc. Mur-ac. Ntr-c. Nitr-ac. *Nitr.*Nux-m.*Oleand.Op.Plb.* Prun. Psor. Puls. Rhod. Ruta. Sacch. Sabin. Samb. Sass. *Scill.* Seneg. Sep. Sol-m. *Sulph.* Tereb. Verat. Verb.
— pale, sudden, Hell. Nitr. Samb.
— of drunkards, Fluor-ac.
— with thirstlessness, Apis.
— upper parts discharge first, last of all the swelling in the limbs, Sacch.
— in old people, Kali-c.
— after purpura miliaris, Hell.
— — scarlet fever, Apis. Arn. Ars. Bell. Bry. Dig. Hell. Phosp-ac. Sacch. Samb. Seneg. Sulph.
— of inner parts, Arg. Arn. *Ars. Bell. Bry.* Calad. Calc. *Chin. Colch.* Cun. *Dig. Dulc. Hell.* Iod. Kali-c. *Led.* Lyc. Merc. Merc-sulph. Rhus.Scill.Seneg. Sep. *Sulph.*
Dry weather, agg., Acon. *Asar.* Bell. Bry. *Caust. Hep.* Ip. *Nux.* Sabad. Sep.Spong.
— — amel., Anim-c. *Calc. Dulc.* Lach.Lyc. Mang. Merc. *Nux-m. Rhus.* Ruta. Stront Sulph. Verat.
Drying up, of palms of hands and soles of feet, Bism.
Dryness of inner parts, usually moist, Acon. Ars *B.ll.* Bry. *Calad. Calc.*Cham. Graph. Hyosc. Lyc. Mang. Merc. Nitr-ac. Nux. *Phosp.* Puls. Rhod. Rhus. Seneg. Sil. Stram. Stront. *Sulph.* Verat.
— sensation of, Acon. Asa-f. Asar. Bry. Calad. Calc. Camph. *Nux-m.* Phosp. Phosp-ac. Puls. *Rhus.* Seneg. Stram. Sulph. Verat.
Dull pain, *Agar.* Ant. Chin. Creos. Dulc. Hell. *Hyosc.* Igt. Laur.
Dust, like, in inner parts, Amm-c. Bell. *Calc.* Igt.
Dysentery, Acon. Aloe. Ars. Bell. Canth. Carb-veg. Caps. Cinnab. Colch. Coloc.

34. GENERALITIES.

Ip. Kali-b. Mgn-c. Mgn-m. Merc. Merc-cor. Nux. Rhus. Sang. Staph. Sulph. Thromb.
Dwarfish. Bar-c.
East wind, from, agg., (compare Wind).
Easy feeling, Coff. Op. Stram.
Eating, before, agg., Ambr. Bov. Calc. Cannab. Chelid. Chin. Croc. Ferr. Graph. Igt. *Iod.* Lach. *Laur. Ntr-c. Phosp.* Plb. Puls. Rhus. Sabad. Sep. Stront. Sulph. Tar.
— while, agg., *Amm*-c. Arg. Arn. Bar-c. Borax. Bry. Calc. *Carb-an.* Caust. Cham. Cic. *Cocc. Con.* Graph. Hep. *Kali-c.* Lyc. Mgn-m. Merc. Ntr-c. *Ntr-m. Nitr-ac. Phosp.* Puls. Sabin. Sec-c. Sep. Teucr.
— — amel., Alum. Ambr. *Anac.* Aur. Benz ac. Caps. Chelid. Cannab. *Igt.* Lach. Mez. Spig. Tellur. *Zinc.*
— after agg., Alum. Amm-m. Anac. Ant. Arn. Arg. Borax. *Bry.* Cact. *Calc.* Cannab. Carb-an. Carb-veg. *Caust.* Chelid. Chin Cocc. *Con.* Croton. Cycl. Evon. Graph. Grat. Hyosc. Igt Kali-c. *Kali-c.* Lith. Lyc. Ntr-c. *Ntr-m.* Nitr-ac. *Nux.* Petr. *Phosp.* Phosp-ac. Puls. Ran-b. Rhus. *Sep. Sil.* Sulph. Valer. *Zinc.*
— — amel., Alum Bov. Cannab. Chelid. Cinnab. Ferr. Igt. *Iod.* Laur. Ntr-c. Ntr-m. Phosp. Sabad Stront.
— after dinner, agg.. Alum. Ars. Igt. Nux. Phosp. Valer. Zinc.
— and having satisfied the appetite, agg., Calc. *Lyc.* Sulph.
— — amel., Iod. Phosp.
— cold food, agg., *Ars.* Cast. Con. Creos. Graph. Hell. *Hep.* Kali-c. Kali-jod. Lyc. Mang. *Merc.* Nux-m. *Nux.* Par. Plb. Rhod. *Phosp.* Spig. Staph. Sulph. Thuj.
— warm food, agg., Ambr. Bar-c. Bell. Bry. Calc. Carb-veg. Cham. Euph Graph. Hell. Kali c. Merc. Mez. *Phosp.* Phosp-ac. *Puls* Sep. Sil. Sulph-ac.
Eclampsia, Bell. Caust. Cham. Cic. *Cina.* Igt. Mgn-c. Nux-m. Nux. Phosp. Plat. *Stram.*
— of children. Cina. Nux-m.
Eggs, smell of, agg., Colch.
Emaciation, Ambr. *Amm-c.* Anac. *Ant.* Apis. Arn. *Ars. Bar-c.* Bell. Borax. Bry. *Calc.* Carb-veg. Clem Cham. *Chin.* Cina. Cocc. Cupr. Dig. Dros. Dulc. *Ferr. Graph.* Guaj. Hep. Igt. *Iod.* Ip. Kali-b. Lach. *Lyc.* Mgn-c. Merc. Mez. Ntr-c. *Ntr-m. Nitr-ac.* Nux-m. *Nux.* Op. *Petr* Phosp. *Phosp-ac.* Raph. Plb. *Puls.* Samb. *Sass. Sec-c.* Selen. Sep. Sil. *Stann.* Staph. Stront. *Sulph. Tabac.* Thuj. *Verat.*
— of single parts, Mez. Selen.
— — parts affected, Carb-veg. Graph. Led.

Mez. Plb. Puls.
— in children, Bar-c. Calc. Cham. *Chin.* Hep. Iod. *Lyc.* Mgn c. *Nux.* Petr. Phosp. Puls. Rhus. Sulph.
— with good appetite, Iod. Sacch. Staph.
— — — — and swollen abdomen, Calc. Iod. Staph.
— bloated face and swollen abdomen, Bar-c.
— of face, thighs and hands, Selen.
— and deadness of parts, Ars. Carb-veg. Graph. Mez. Plb. Selen. Thuj.
Emissions, nocturnal, agg., Alum. Chin. Iod. *Kali-c. Nux.* Sep. Staph. (compare Animal fluids, loss of).
Emptiness, sensation of, Calad. Cocc. *Igt.* Kali-c. Mur-ac. Oleand. *Puls.* Sass. *Sep. Stann.*
Enlargement, sensation of, *Alum.* Asar. Bell. Bism. Bov. Bry. Caps. Diad. Kali-c. Laur. Merc. Nitr. *Par. Puls. Rhus. Spig.* Stann. Verat.
Epilepsy, Actea-r Aeth. *Agar.* Ang. Arg. Arg-n *Ars.* Ars-calc. Artem *Bell.* Bufo. *Calc.* Camph. Canth. *Caust.* Cauloph. Cham. *Cic. Cina.* Cocc. Con. *Cupr.* Dig. Dros. Dulc. Gels. Glon Grat. Hep. *Hyosc.* Hyper. *Igt.* Iod. Ip. Kali-c. Lach. Laur. Lyc. *Mgn-c.* Merc. Millef. Mosch. Ntr-m. Nitr ac. Nux-m. Nux. *Op. Petr. Phosp.* Phosp-ac. *Plat.* Plb. Puls. Ran-b. Ran-sc. Sec-c. Sep. Sil. *Sol-m. Stann. Stram. Sulph.* Tabac. Tar. Tart. Tarantula. Tong.
— with catalepsy, Ang. Asa-f. Camph. Cic. Coloc. Dios. Igt. *Ip.* Laur. Merc. *Mosch. Op.* Petr. *Plat.* Verat.
— consciousness, Canth. *Cina.* Kali-c. Mgn-m. Nux-m. Nux. Plat. *Stram.*
— without consciousness, Ars-calc. Bell. *Calc.* Camph. *Canth.* Cic. Cocc. Cupr. *Hyosc. Plb.* Sep. Sil. Sulph.
— in children, Bell. *Igt.* Stann.
— during dentition, Igt. Stann.
— in evening, Stann,
— at night. Calc. Caust. Cina. Cupr. Kali-c. Phosp.
— after grief, Igt.
— — fright, Arg-n. Bufo. Igt. Tarantula.
— with great exertions of strength, Agar.
— — delirium, Hyosc.
— — rigidity of body, Cina.
— — suffocative paroxysms, Op.
— — ending with deep heavy sleep, Hyosc.
— — hœmoptisis, Dros.
— — headache, Cupr.
— headache, before and after, Cina.
— during full moon, with hallooing and shouting, Calc.
— — sleep, Caust.
— from suppressed menses, Millef. Puls.
Ergotism, Cic. Sol-n.

34. GENERALITIES.

Eructations, agg., from, Agar. Cannab. Cham. Cocc. Lach. Phosp. Rhus. Sep. Verb. Zinc.
— amel., Aur. Bar-c. Bry. Canth. *Carb-veg.* Cocc. *Graph. Igt. Kali-c* Lyc. Ntr-c. Nitr-ac. Nux. Plat. Sil. Sulph. *Tart.*
Evacuation, amel., after. Amm-m. Bora\. *Bry. Colch.* Con. Puls. *Rhus.* Spig. Sulph.
Evening, in the, agg., *Acon.* Agn. Aloe. Alum. *Ambr. Amm-c.* Amm-m. Anac. *Ant.* Apis. *Arn.* Ars. *Asa-f.* Asar. *Bell.* Bufo. Calad. Calc. *Caps.* Carb-an. Carb-veg. *Caust.* Cham. Cinnab Cist. Cocc. *Colch.* Coloc. *Cycl.* Daph. Dulc. *Euphr.*Eugen. *Guaj.Hell.Hyosc.* Igt. Ind. Ip. Iris. *Kali-c.* Kalm. *Lach.* Laur. Led. Lyc. *Mgn-c.* Mgn-m. Mang. *Meny.* *Merc.* Merc-cor.*Mez.* Ntr c. Ntr-m.Ntr-s *Nitr-ac. Nitr.* Nux-m. Ol-an. Par. Petr. *Phosp.* Phosp-ac. *Plat.* Plb. *Puls.* *Ran-b. Ran-sc.* Rhod. Rhus. Sabin. Sang. Seneg. *Sep.* Sil. Spig. *Stann Stront. Sulph.* Sulph-ac. *Tart.* Teucr. Thuj. Tilia. Valer. *Zinc.*
— 9 P. M., Bry.
— 3 to 5 P. M., Clem.
— 6 P. M. to 6 A. M., Creos.
— 5 P. M., Coloc.
— 6 P. M. to 7 P. M., Hep.
— 4 P. M. to 10 P. M., Plat.
— and do not diminish until day-break, pains, Colch.
— amel., Arn. Bruc. Lyc.
— after lying down, agg., Ars. *Igt.* Led. *Phosp.* Stront. *Sulph.* Thuj.
— — amel., Nitr.
Evening air, agg., Carb-veg. Merc. Sulph.
Excitement, nervous, Acon. Ambr. Ang *Bell.* Cham. Chin. *Coff.* Creos. Ferr. Iod. *Nux.* Petr. Phosp-ac. Sep. Teucr. Valer.
Extending of limbs, Alum. Clem.
Extending the part, agg., Alum. Calc. Coloc. Rhus. Sep. Staph. Sulph. Thuj.
Extension involuntarily of muscles and limbs, Lyc. Stram. Sulph.
Extensors, in the, pain, Verat.
Exertion of body, agg., from, Ambr. *Arn.* Ars. Aur. *Bry.* Calc. Cannab. Carb-veg. Caust. *Cocc.* Colch. Croc. Hell. Kali-b. Kali-c. *Lyc.* Merc. Ntr-c. Ntr-m. Nux. Ox-ac. Phosp. Phosp-ac. Puls. Rheum. *Rhus.* Ruta. Sabin. Sep. Sil. Spig. Staph. *Sulph. Verat.* Zinc.
— amel., Igt. *Sep.*
— — mind., agg., Anac. Aur. Bell. *Calc.* Cist. Cocc. Colch. *Igt.* Kali-b. Lach. Lyc. Ntr-c. Ntr-m. *Nux.* Oleand. Plat. Puls. *Sep.* Sil. Sulph.
— — amel., Croc. Ntr-c.
Eyes, opening the, agg., Bry. Calc. Clem. Croc. Igt. Lyc. Nux. Spig.

— — amel., *Bell.* Bry. Chin. Clem. Hell. Mgn-m. Puls.
— shutting the, agg., *Bell. Bry.* Chin. Clem. Hell. Led. Mgn-m. Puls. Therid.
— turning the, agg., Sil. Spig.
Fainting, *Acon.* Arn. *Ars.* Bar-m. **Bell.** Bry. Bufo. Calad.Calc. Camph. Cannab. Carb-veg. *Cham. Chin.* Cocc. Coff. Coloc. Con. Creos. *Croc.* Cupr. *Dig.* Dros. Ferr. Gels. Hell. *Hep.* Hyosc. Igt. Ip. Kali-c. Lach. Laur. Led. Lyc. Mgn-m. Merc. Mosch. *Nux-m.* Nux. *Oleand.* Ol-an. Op. Petr. Phosp. Phosp-ac. Plb. Puls. Ran-b. Ran-sc. Rhus. Sacch. Sass. Sec-c. *Seneg. Sep.* Sil. Spig. Staph. *Stram.* Sulph. Tabac. *Tart.* Verat.
— with agitation of chest, Acon. Bell.
— from anemia, Mosch.
— with asthma, Berb. Creos. Lach.
— cheeks, paleness of, which were red when lying, Acon. Lach.
— — coldness of limbs, Acon. Calc. Coloc.
— with convulsions, Lach.
— in a crowd, Plb.
— with epistaxis, Croc. Lach.
— in evening, Calc. Hep. Lyc. Mosch. Ntr-m. Nux.
— from exercise, Nux.
— with face pale, Acon. Berb. Lach. Ntr-m. Nux.
— with formication and tremor of feet, Borax.
— — heat, Berb. Nux. Petr.
— from heat of room, Creos. Spig.
— hours, at certain, in the day, Lyc.
— hysteric, Ars. Cham. Cocc. Igt. *Mosch.* Ntr-m. Nux-m. Nux.
— after lying down, Calad.
— when lying on the side, Lyc. Sil.
— in morning, Carb-veg. Creos. Ntr-m. Nux.
— — when rising too early, Creos.
— — after eating, Nux.
— at night, Mosch. Nux-m.
— with numb limbs, Ntr-m.
— pressure on heart, Act. Petr.
— pain in heart, Lach.
— after every afterpain, Nux.
— with palpitation of heart, followed by sleep, Nux-m.
— — perspiration, Dig.
— — cold, Lach.
— from riding in a carriage, Berb.
— when rising, Bry. Op. Thromb.
— after rising up from lying, Acon. Calad.
— by slight pains produced, Cocc. Hep. Nux-m.
— (sinking) spells in consumptives, Gels.
— stomach, from pains in, Ran-sc.
— with sterterous breathing, Stram.
— — thirst, Acon.

34. GENERALITIES.

Fainting, with trembling, Nux. Petr.
— with vomiting, Kali-c. Lach. Sulph.
— from walking in open air, Ferr. Kali-c Seneg.
— as from weakness, relieved by perspiration, Oleand.
— from weakness, with scarcely perceptible pulse, Ars.
— after writing, Calad.
— after, agg., writing Mosch. Op.
Falling down, with consciousness, Ang Ars. Bell. Camph. Canth. Cina. Hell Mgn-c. Ntr-m. Nitr-ac. Nux-m. Phosp Plat. Puls. Sulph.
— — without consciousness, Glon.
Falling out of inner parts, sensation of. Bell. Nux. Plat. Sulph.
— to pieces, sensation of, Bapt.
Fanned, wants to be, hard, Carb-veg.
False step, making a, Bry. Lyc. Puls.
Fasting, amel., Nux-m.
Fat food, from agg., Ant. Ars. Asa-f Carb-veg. Coich. Cycl. Dros. Ferr. Hell Mgn-m. Ntr-m. Nitr-ac. Puls. Sep. Spong. Sulph. Tar. Thuj.
Fatigue, Alum. Arn. Ars. Bar-c. Benz-ac. Calc. Camph. Cannab. Carb-veg. Caust. Coff. Colch. Con. Corn-c. Croc Graph. Hep. Ip. Iris. Lach. Mgn-c. Merc. Ntr-c. Nux. Par. Plat. Puls. Rheum. Rhod. Rhus. Sec-c. Sep. Sil. Stann. Staph. Sulph. Tabac. Tart. Verat.
— nervous, Calc. (compare Weakness).
— from night study, Colch.
— — speaking, Alum. Ambr. Amm-c Calc. Cannab. Ferr. Ntr-m. Stann. Sulph.
— — hearing others talk, Alum. Amm-c. Ars. Verat.
— — a thunder storm, Caust. Ntr-c. Nitr-ac. Petr. Phosp. Rhod. Sil.
— — walking, Cannab. Carb-an. Kali-c.
— — — in open air, Coff. Con. Ferr. Kali-c. Verat.
— — writing, Cannab. Sil.
— after paroxysms of cough, Dig. Spong.
— from, agg., Arn Coff. Rhus.
Fear from, Acon. Bell. Bufo. Caust. Coff. Cupr. Gels. Glon. Hyosc. Igt. Merc. Nux. Op. Plat. Puls.
Festering pain, Bry. Cycl. Phosp. Puls. Ran-b.
Fever, before the, agg., Arn. Ars. Calc. Carb-veg. Chin. Cina. Ip. Puls. Rhus.
— during the, agg., Ant. Ars. Bry. Calc. Cham. Chin. Ferr. Ip. Kali-c. Lyc. Ntr-m. Nux. Op. Phosp. Puls. Rhus. Sep. Sulph.
— after the agg., Ars. Bell. Chin. Hep Nux.
Fire, glare of, agg., Ant. Euph Zinc.
Flabbiness in limbs, Ars. Camph. Euph. Mgn-c. Ntr-c.
Flexing or turning, agg., Amm-c. Cic. Igt. Kali-c. Lyc. Nux. Puls.

Flatus, amel., by discharge of, Carb-veg. Cham. Chin. Cocc. Coloc. Igt. Lyc. Nux. Plb Puls. Rhod. Stach. Verat.
Fluids, animal, loss of, agg., Ars. Calad. Calc. Carb-veg. Chin. Cina. Con. Iod. Kali-c. Merc. Nux. Phosp. Phosp-ac. Puls. Scill. Sep. Sil. Staph. Sulph.
Forenoon, in the, agg., Cact. Cannab. Carb-veg. Grat. Guaj. Hep. Laur. Mang. Ntr-c. Ntr-m. Nux. Phosp. Phosp-ac. Sabad. Sass. Sep. Sil. Staph. Sulph-ac. Valer. Viol-tr.
— 12, Arg. Carb-veg.
— 11, Gels.
— 12, Kali-b.
— amel., Alum.
Fretfulness accompanying pains, Chin. Coff. Nux. Phosp.
Fright, agg., from, Acon. Arg-n. Bell. Calc. Caust. Chin. Coff. Igt. Gels. Glon. Igt. Lach. Lyc. Merc. Nux. Op. Petr. Phosp. Plat. Puls. Ruta. Samb. Sec-c. Stann. Stram. Sulph. Tarant. Verat.
— followed by diarrhœa, Gels. Op. Puls.
Frostbitten, from being agg., Agar. Ars. Carb-veg. Colch. Nitr-ac. Phosp. Puls.
— itching burning, as if, Agar.
Fruits, agg., from, Ars. Bry. Borax. Carb-veg. Chin. Mgn-m. Merc. Ntr-c. Puls. Rhod. Selen. Sep. Verat.
Fulness, sensation of, in outer parts, Ars. Caust. Phosp.
— — inner parts, Acon. Arn. Asa-f. Asar. Bar-c. Bell. Canth. Carb-veg. Cham. Chin. Cycl. Ferr. Hell. Kali-c. Lyc. Mosch. Nux-m. Phosp. Puls. Ran-sc. Rhus. Ruta. Sabin. Sep. Sulph. Valer.
Fur, as if in inner parts. Phosp. Puls.
Ganglia. Amm-c. Phosp. Phosp-ac. Plb. Sil. Zinc.
Gargling, from, agg., Carb-veg.
Gastric troubles, Acon. Ant. Ars. Asa-f. Asar. Aur. Bell. Bry. Calc. Cham. Chin. Cocc. Coff. Colch. Cup. Cor-r. Cupr. Cycl. Dig. Igt. Ip. Lyc. Ntr-m. Nux. Phosp. Plb. Puls. Rheum. Scill. Sec-c. Staph. Sulph. Tabac. Tar. Tart. Therid. Verat. Zinc.
Glands, Amm-c. Asa-f. Aur. Bar-c. Bell. Bry. Calend. Calc. Carb-an Carb-veg. Cham. Cist. Clem. Cocc. Con. Dulc. Graph. Hep. Iod. Kali-c. Lyc. Merc. Ntr-c. Ntr-m. Nitr-ac. Petr. Phosp. Phosp-ac. Rhus. Sep. Sil. Spig. Spong. Staph. Sulph. Thuj.
— air, as if. went through, Spong.
— by a blow or confusion produced, Con. Dulc Iod. Kali c. Petr. Phosp.
— excitement of glandular system, Iod.
— flabby, Cham. Con. Iod. Nitr-ac. Sec-c.
— heaviness, Bell. Phosp.
— induration, Bar-c. Bell. Bry. Calc. Carb-an. Carb-veg. Chin. Clem. Cocc.

Con. Dig. Dulc. Graph. Iod. Kali-c. Lyc.
Mgn-m. Nux. Petr. Phosp. Puls. Ran-b.
Raus. Sil. Spo.g. Sulph.
Glands, inflammation, Acon. Bar-c. Bell.
Camph. Carb-an. Carb-veg. Cham. Con.
Dulc. Hep. Kali-c. Merc. Nitr-ac. Nux.
Petr. Phosp. Phyt. Puls. Rhus. Sass.
Sil. Sulph. Sulph-ac.
— — lymphatic, Merc-cor.
— as of something alive in, Spong.
— pains, A um. Amm-c. Arn. Bell. Calc.
Cannab. Carb-an. Caust. Coloc. Con. Iod.
Lyc. Merc. Mez. Nitr-ac. Phosp. Puls.
Rhus. Sil. Spig. Staph. Sulph. Thuj.
— — boring. Bell. Lyc. Puls. Sabad.
— — burning, Ars. Bell. Cannab. Carb-veg.
Hep. Merc. Phosp.
— — contracting, Igt. Iod. Mang. Nitr-ac.
Nux.
— — contusion, as of a, Arn. Carb-an. Cic.
Con. Kali-c. Petr. Ruta. Sep.
— — cramping. Ang. Plat.
— — cutting, Bell. Lyc. Sep.
— — drawing, Bell. Chin. Seneg.
— — gnawing, Plat. Spong.
— — itching, Anac. Carb-an. Carb-veg.
Caust. Con. Kali-c. Mgn-c. Phosp.
Sep. Sil. Spong.
— — jerking, Calc Clem. Ntr-m. Puls.
— — numb, Plat.
— — piercing, Bell.
— — pinching, Calc. Rhod.
— — pressing, Aur. Bell. Calc. Lyc. Mang.
Merc. Phosp-ac. Spong. Staun. Staph.
Sulph.
— — — inwards, Merc. Spong.
— — — outwards, Calc. Staph.
— — prickling, Amm-m. Asa-f. Bell. Bry.
Calc. Cocc. Con. Igt. Merc. Ntr-m.
Phosp. Puls. Ran-sc. Sep. Sulph.
— — pulsation, Amm-m. Calc. Clem
Kali-c. Merc. Phosp. Sabad. Sil.
Sulph.
— — rending, tearing, Arn. Bell. Bry.
Chin. Kali-c. Lyc. Sil. Sulph.
— — soreness, as of, Con. Igt. Sep. Zinc.
— — stinging, Bell Cocc. Con. Merc.
Ntr-m (compare Prickling)
— — tension, Bar-c. Bry. Caust. Con.
Graph. Phosp. Puls. Rhus. Spong.
Sulph.
— — tickling, Arn. Con. Merc. Plat. Rhus.
Spong.
— — ulcerous, Amm-m. Phosp. Puls. Rhus.
— secretion of, more profuse, Iod.
— sensitiveness of, Aur. Cham. Cist. Con.
Kali-jod. Lyc. Nitr-ac. Phosp. Sep.
— swelling of, Alum. Amm-c. Arn. Ars.
Asa-f. Bar-c. Bell. Bov. Brom. Bry.
B fo. Calc. Carb-an. Carb-veg. Caust.
Cham. Cist. Clem. Cocc. Con. Dulc.
Graph. Hep. Iod. Kali-c. Lyc. Mgn-c.
Mgn-m. Merc. Mez. Mur-ac. Ntr-c.

Ntr-m. Nitr-ac. Nux jug. Nux. Phosp.
Phosp-ac. Puls. Rhus. Sass. Sep. Sil.
Spo. g. Staun. Staph. Sulph. Sulph-ac.
Thuj. Zinc.
— — blu sh, Carb-an. Lach.
— — cold, Arn. Cocc. Con.
— — hard, Bry. Con. Phosp. Puls. Rhus.
Sulph.
— — hot, Acon. Bell. Bry. Calc. Merc. Phosp.
Sulph.
— — inflammatory, Acon. Arn. Bell. Bry.
Carb-an. Hep. Lyc. Merc. Phosp.
Rhus. Thuj.
— — knotty, like ropes. Dulc. Iod.
— — engorged, like small nodes under
skin. Bry.
— — painful, Arn. Bell. Chin. Puls. Sil.
— — painless, Con. Igt. Phosp-ac. Sep.
Sil.
— — suppuration, Bar-c. Bell Calc. Carb-veg.
Cist. Coloc. Dulc. Hep. Kali-jod. Lach.
Lyc. Merc. Nitr-ac. Petr. Phosp. Rhus.
Sep. Sil. Sulph.
— — ulceration, Ambr. Ars. Bell. Canth. Con.
Hep. Lach. Phosp. Sil. Sulph.
— — cancerous, Ars. Bell. Con. Creos.
Hep. Sep. Sil. Sulph.
— — spongy, Carb-an. Lach. Merc. Sil.
Sulph. Thuj.
— — withering of, Cham. Con. Iod. Nitr-ac.
Sec.
Gnawing, pain, Herb. Dros. Mez.
Going down, descending, agg. from, Con.
Ferr. Rhod. Verat.
— — — amel., Amm-c. Ang. Ars. Bar-c.
Borax. Bry. Calc. Cupr. Merc.
Nitr. Nux. Seneg. Sep. Spig.
Spong. Zinc.
— up, ascending, amel., Con. Ferr. Rhod.
Valer.
Gonorrhœa, suppressed, from, Agn-c. Aur.
Benz-ac. Brom. Clem. Daph. Merc.
Mez. Nitr-ac. Puls. Sass. Tussilago.
Verat. Zinc.
Grief, from, Cocc. Coloc. Igt. Lyc.
Phosp-ac. Staph.
— — with indignation. Coloc. Nux. Staph.
— — — vehemence, Acon. Bry. Cham. Coff.
Nux.
Hemmorhages, Acon. Ant. Arn. Ars. Asa-f.
Bar-c. Bell. Bry. Cact. Calc. Canth. Caps.
Carb-veg. Cl am. Chin. Cinnam. Cocc.
Cop. Creos. Crotal. Croc. Crotal. Cupr.
Dros. Dind Ferr. Ham. Hyosc. Iod. Ip.
Lach. Led. Lyc. Merc. Millef. Nitr-ac.
Nux. Phosp. Puls. Rat. Rhus. Sabin.
Seb. Sil. Stram. Sulph.
— from every orifice of the body, Crotal.
Ip.
Hœmmorhoidal disposition, Aloe. Ambr.
Kali-chl. Nux.
Hair. as if pulled by the, Acon. Laur. Nux.
— from combing the, agg., Bry. Selen.

34. GENERALITIES.

Hair, from cutting, agg., *Bell.* Glon. Sep.
— putting back, the agg., Puls. Rhus.
— tying up the, amel., Nitr.
— dark, persons with, Acon. Caust. Nitr-ac. Nux. Phosp. Plat. Sep.
Hammering, Phosp.
Hands, from working with the, agg., Amm-m. Bov. Lach. *Ntr-m.* Sil. Verat.
— on putting on the, from, amel., Bell. Croc. Meny. (compare, Touching and pressure.)
Hang down, from letting the limb, agg., Alum. Amm-c. Calc. Sabin.
— — amel., Arn. Bar-c. Bell. Ferr. Kali-c. Led. Rhus. Sil.
Hanging loose, as if skin were, *Phosp.* Sabad.
Hat, pressure of, agg., Carb-veg. Nitr-ac. Sil. Valer.
Head, bending backwards, agg., Cic. Puls. Sep.
— — — amel., Cham. Hep. Led.
— — forward, agg., Viol-od.
— — sideways, agg., Spong.
— — — amel., Puls.
— leaning on something, amel., Bell Merc.
— resting on a table, amel., Ferr. Sabad.
— shaking, agg., Arn. *Bell.* Bry. Colch. Glon. Hep. Led. Nux-m. *Nux.* Spig.
— — amel., Lach.
— turning, agg., Arn. Bell. Bry. *Calc.* Cic. Hep. Igt. Kali. Lyc. Ntr-c. *Ntr-m.* Nux. Puls. Rhus. Selen. Sep. *Spong.*
— uncovering, agg., Aur. Bell. Colch. Con. *Hep.* Hyosc. Nux-m. *Nux. Rhus.* Samb. Scill. *Sil.* Stront.
— — amel., Acon. Borax. Calc. Ferr. Iod. *Lyc.* Puls. Spig. Verat.
Heat during the pains, Carb-veg.
— and redness of one cheek, during the pains, Cham.
— of parts affected, *Acon.* Bry. Sulph.
Heated, agg., from getting, *Ant.* Bell. *Bry.* Carb-veg. Dig. *Kali-c. Op.* Thuj. Zinc.
— near a fire, agg., Ant. Euph. Zinc.
Heaviness. Agar. Alum. Ant. Ant. Asa-f. Bar-c. *Bell.* Camph. Carb-veg. Chin. Creos. Croc. Ferr-m. Hipp. Igt. Led. Merc. Mez. Mosch Ntr-c. Nti-m. *Nux.* Par. Petr. *Phosp.* Plb. *Puls.* Rheum. Rhod. *Rhus.* Ruta. Sabad. Sec-c. Sep. Spig. Spong. *Stann.* Staph. Stram. Sulph. Tereb. Thuj. Verat.
— inner parts, *Acon.* Amm-c. Amm-m. Bar-c Bell. *Bism.* Borax. Bov Bry. Calc. Carb-an. Carb-veg. Chin. Graph. Hell. Kali-c. Laur. Lyc. Mgn-c. Mgn m. Merc. Mur-ac. Ntr-m. Nux-m. *Nux.* Oleand. *Op.* Plb. *Rhus.* Sabad. Sabin. Sep. *Sil.* Stann Staph. *Sulph.*
— alternating with sensation of lightness, Nux.

— in forenoon, *Sabad.*
— — morning on awaking, *Zinc.*
— on movement, Ammonica. Calc. Kali-c. Mez. Ntr-c. Nti-m. Sep. Sil. Spong. Stram.
— from playing the piano, Anac.
— when rising from a seat, Spig.
— on sitting, Ruta.
— after sleep at noon, Staph.
Hoop or band, sensation of, around parts, Anac. Asar. Aur. Con. Graph. Ntr-m. Nitr-ac. Plat. Puls. Sulph.
Humming in body, Caust. Creos. Nux-m. *Nux. Oleand.* Puls. Rhus. Sep. *Spig. Sulph.*
Hungry, on being, agg., Iod. Kali-c. Spig.
Hydrophobia, *bell. Canth.* Hydroph. *Hyosc.* Lach. Phosp. *Stram.*
Hypochondriacal, Asa-f. Aur. Bell. Cham. Chin. Con. *Graf.* Hell. Mgn-m. Mosch. Mez. *Ntr-c. Nux. Phosp.* Phosp-ac. Plb. Puls. Sacch. *Stann. Staph. Sulph.* Valer. *Verat. Viol-od.* Zinc. (compare Sect. 1.)
Hysterical, Actea-r. Agn. Anac. Arn. Ars. Asa-f. Aur. Bell. *Bry.* Calc. Cannab. Caust. Cham. Chin. Cic. *Coce.* Coff. Con. Cycl. Euphr. Gels. Graph. *Grat.* Hell. Hyosc. Igt. Iod. Ip. Lach. Lyc. *Men-m.* Merc. Mez. *Mosch. Ntr-c. Nitr-ac. Nux-m. Nux.* Pallad. *Phosp.* Plat. *Plb.* Puls. Rheum. Sabad. Sabin. Sep. Sil. *Stann.* Staph. *Stram. Sulph.* Valer. Verat. *Viol-od.* Znc.
— laughing and crying alternately, Alum.
— with constant weeping, Viol-od.
— — weight at uterus and vagina, after every attack. Elaps.
— at puberty or climacteric, with headache, Therid.
— spasms, with full consciousness, at break of day, Plat.
— with pain at abdomen and diaphragm, Stann.
— after sexual excesses, Anac. Con.
Ill, sensation of being, *Acon.* Alum. Ars. Chelid. Con. Mez. *Nux.* Spong. Sulph. Tart.
Illusions of feeling, Alum. Asa-f. Bell. Calc. Croc. Igt. Lach Par. Plb. Puls. *Rhus.* Spig. Stram. Sulph.
Impressions, deep, of instruments, Bov.
Increasing pains, then gradually decreasing, *Plat.* Stann. Stront.
— — suddenly disappear, Sulph-ac.
— suddenly, decreasing suddenly, Nitr-ac.
Incurvation crooking, spasmodic, of single parts. Ambr. *Calc.* Carb-veg. Caust. Chin. Cina. Colch. *Coloc.* Con. Euph. Ferr. *Graph.* Guaj. *Hyosc.* Kali-c. Kali-jod. *Lyc.* Meny. *Merc.* Nux. Phosp. Plb. Rhus. *Sec-c. Sil.* Stram. Sulph. Tart.

Indignation, from, agg., *Coloc.* Ip. Nux. Plat. Staph.
— — ill-treatment, *Coloc.* Staph.
Induration after inflammations, Agn. *Bell.* Bry. Calc. *Carb-an. Carb-veg. Chin. Clem.* Con. Dulc. Graph. *Iod.* Kali-c. Lyc. *Mgn-m.* Nux. Plb. Puls. Ran-b. Rhus. Spong. *Sulph.*
— of cellular tissue, Bell
Infants, for, Acon. Ambr. Bar-c. *Bell.* Borax. *Calc. Caps. Cham.* Chin. Cocc. Croc. *Hyosc.* Igt. Iod. Ip. Lyc. Mgn-c. *Merc. Nux-m. Aux.* Puls. *Rheum. Sil.* Spong Stann. Staph. Sulph.
Inflammation of external parts, Acon. *Ars.* Bell. Calc. Cham. Euphr. Hep. Lyc. Merc. Nitr-ac. Nitr. Phosp. *Puls.* Rhus. *Sil.* Spig. *Staph.* Sulph.
— inner parts, *Acon.* Ars. *Bell. Bry.* Cannab. *Canth.* Cham, Cop. Dig. Dros. Hyosc. Kali-c. Laur. Lyc. *Merc.* Mez. Nitr-ac. Nitr. *Aux. Phosp. Puls.* Rhus. Sabad. Scill. Seneg. Sep. Spong. Sulph. Verat.
— of mucus membrane, *Acon.* Agar. Apis. *Ars. Bell.* Borax. Bry. Calc. Canth. Cham. Dros. Igt. *Merc.* Ntr-m. *Nux.* Par. Phosp. Puls. Scill. Sep. Sil. *Sulph.*
— with burning pains, Ars. Canth. Euph. Mez.
— — dry heat, Acon. Bell. Bry.
— nervous, Bell. Bry. *Ll osc.* Lyc. *Rhus.*
— with disposition to suppurate, Asa-f. Bell. *Hep. Lyc. Merc. Puls.* Sil. Sulph.
— — perspiration and weakness, *Merc.* Phosp-ac.
Inflation, feeling of, Par. Ran-b.
Inflexibility of joints of limbs, Bell. Caps. Carb-an. Caust. Cocc. Coloc. Graph. Kali-c.Lyc.*Petr.*Puls. Rhus. *Sep.* Sulph.
Influenza, Acon. Ars. Bell. Bry. *Camph.* Carb-veg. Caust. *Lyc. Merc.* Nux. Phosp. *Rhus.* Sabad. Spig.
Infuriating pains, Ars. Verat.
Injuries, agg. from,*Arn.Co .*Dulc.*Hep.*Iod. Lach. Phosp. *Puls Rhus.* Ruta Staph *Sulph-ac* (compare Mechanical injuries).
— profusely bleeding, Arn. Carb-veg. *Lach.* Phosp. Sulph.
— bruises, Arn. Con. Ruta. Sulph-ac.
— cuts, Arn. *Staph.* Sulph-ac.
— stabs, Carb-veg. Nitr-ac.
— with sugillation. Arn. Con. Hep. Puls. Sulph. *Sulph-ac.*
— of soft parts, Arn. Con. Puls. Sulph-ac.
— — glands, Arn. *Con.* Dulc. Iod. Phosp.
— — bones, Phosp-ac. *Ruta.*
Intermittents, after suppressed. Arn. Ars. Bell. *Calc. Caps.* Carb-veg. Cina. Ferr. *Ip.* Meny. Merc. *Ntr-m. Puls.* Sep. Sulph. *Verat.*
Intermit, pains, in severity, Cinnab.
— — every third day, Plb.

Interrupted, jerking, pains, Asa-f. *Plat.* Rhod. *Valer.*
Intolerable, pa.ns seeming, Acon. All-cep. Ars. *Cham. Coff.* Lach. Verat.
Intoxication from, agg., Amm-m. Bry. Cadm. Carb-veg. Cocc. *Coff.* Ip. Laur. *Nux. Op.* Puls. Spong. Stram.
Inwards. moving, pains, Anac Arn. Calc. Canth. Igt. Kali-c. *Oleand.* Plat. Spig. Staph. Zinc.
Iron, as if a hot, were forced in, Alum.
Irritability of body, excessive, Asar. Aur. *Canth.* Cham. Chin. Cocc. *Coff.* Ferr. *Merc. Nux.* Phosp. Puls. Sil. Staph. Teucr. Verat.
— — diminished, Anac. Ars. Calc. Camph. Carb-an. Carb-veg. *Con.* Dulc. Iod. Ip. Laur. Lyc. Nitr-ac. *Oleand,* Op. *Phosp-ac.* Rhod. Sep. Stram. Sulph.
Itching, inner parts, *Ambr.* Ferr. *Iod. Nux. Phosp.* Stann.
Jactitation, tossing about, caused by the pains, *Acon.* Alum. *Ars. Bell. Calc. Cham. Chin.* Cina. *Coff. Hell.* Lach. Lyc. *Mgn-c.* Mang. Op. Phosp. *Puls.* Rhus. Sep. *Sulph.* Tabac. Tart.
Jaundice, *Acon.* Ambr. Ars. Bell. Bry. Calc. Canth. Carb-veg. *Chin. Con.* Cup. Cupr. *Dig.* Dolich. Ferr. Igt. Iod. Lach. Lyc. *Merc. Nitr-ac. Aux.* Plb. Pod. Puls. Ran-b. Rhus. Sang. Sec-c. *Sep.* Spig. *Sulph.* Sulph-ac.
Jerks, convulsive, Acon. Agar. *Alum.* Ambr. Ang. Arn. Ars. Asa-f. Bar-c. Bell.Bry. *Calc.*Cannab.Carb-veg. Caust. Cham. Cic. *Cina.* Cocc. Colch. Con. Cupr. Euphr. Graph. *Hyosc. Iod.* Kali c. Lach. Lact. *Laur.* Lob. *Lyc.* Mgn-m. Mosch. *Ntr-c. Ntr-m.* Nux-m. Nux. Op *Petr.* Plat. Plb. Puls. Ran-sc. Scill. *Sec-c.* Sep. Sil. *Sol-nig.* Spig. Spong. Stann. *Stram.* Sulph. Tabac. Tart. Thuj. Valer.
Jerking pain, Alum. Anac. Arn. *Asa-f.* Asar. Aur. *Bell.* Bry. *Calc. Caust.* Chin. Cina. Clem Cocc. Colch. Graph. Ind. Mgn-c. Mang. *Meny.* Merc. Mez. Mosch. Nitr-c. *Nitr-m.* Nitr-ac. *Nux.* Petr. Phosp-ac. Plat. *Puls.* Rat. *Rhus.* Sep. Sil. *Tar.* Valer.
— — inner parts, in, Calc. *Chin.* Igt. *Kali-c. Nitr-ac.* Puls. Sep. *Sil.* Valer.
— in blood vessels, Sabin.
— disabling, *Chin.* Cina. Colch.
— drawing Colch. Ind. Puls.
— in evening, Ntr-s.
— at night, Ntr-s.
— rending, tearing, *Amm-m.* Asar. *Chin.* Cocc. Cupr. Ntr-s Phosp-ac Puls.
Jests, rediculous or foolish, Bell. *Cic.* Hyosc. *Stram.* Tanec. *Verat.*
Joints, arthritic complaints of, *Agn.* Amm-c. Arg. Arn. Asa-f. Aur. Bar-c.

34. GENERALITIES. 297

Bell. Bry. Calc. *Carb-an.* Caust. Chin. Cocc. *Colch. Dig.* Ferr. Graph. Hyosc. Igt. Kali-b. *Kali-c. Led. Lyc. Mang.* Meny. *Merc.* Mez. Ntr-c. Ntr-m. *Petr.* Phosp. *Puls.* Rhod. *Rhus. Sabin.* Sep. *Spong* Stann. *Staph.* Stront. *Sulph.* Thuj. Zinc.

Joints, arthritic pains, chronic, pains at night, without swelling, Iod.
— in bed, warmth of, Sulph.
— coldness. Cinnab. Petr.
— contraction, *Anac. Aur.* Graph. *Ntr-m. Nitr-ac.* Petr Stront.
— cracking, Acon. Ang. Ant. Calc. Camph *Caps.* Carb-an. Cham. Cocc. Croc. Ferr. *Led.* Merc. Ntr-m. *Nitr-ac.* Nux. *Petr.* Phosp. Sabad. Sulph. Thuj.
— cramping, Anac. Ang. Bell. *Calc. Plat.* Sec-c. Sulph.
— creeping, tingling, Arn. Ip. Sec-c.
— disjointed, sensation as if. Stram.
— dislocation, easy, Carb-an. Croc. Sil.
— dryness, sensation of, Canth. *Nux. Puls.*
— eruption, Sep.
— erysipelatous inflammation, Bry. Rhod.
— excoriation, Bell. Caust. Lyc. *Mang. Ol-an.* Petr. *Sep.* Sulph.
— fungus at, Ant.
— heaviness, Phosp-ac.
— herpes, Dulc. Staph.
— inflammation, Bry.
— itching, Merc. Sep. Zinc.
— — at night, Merc.
— jerks, Sulph-ac. Verat.
— looseness, sense of, Croc.
— numbness, sense of, Ip. Lyc. Plat.
— paralytic, Acon. Arn. Croc. Rhus. Sulph.
— on one side, Mang.
— vesicles around, Phosp.
— pains, Acon. Bar-c. Caps. Cocc. Colch. Guaj. Igt. Iod. *Jatr.* Led. Lyc. Mang. *Merc.* Ntr-m. Nux. *Puls. Rheum.* Staph. Sulph.
— — in bed, Sulph.
— — beaten, bruised, Agar. Ang. *Arg. Arn. Aur. Bell.* Bov Carb-an. Caust. Chin. Con. *Cupr.* Dig. Dros. Ferr. Mez. Mur-ac. Ntr-m. Ntr-nitr. Nitr-ac. Nux. Par. Phosp. Phosp-ac. *Puls. Ruta.* Sep. Spig. Verat. Viol-od.
— — blow, as from a, Cupr.
— — boring, Arg.
— — burning, Ntr-c. Ntr-nitr.
— — cold, after a. Mang. *Nux-m.*
— — cutting, Hyosc.
— — digging, *Mang.* Rhod.
— — drawing, (compare Rending.)
— — in evening, Ntr c. Stront.
— — fatigued, as if, Dig.
— — jerking, Mang. Ntr-c. Plat. Sulph-ac. Verat.

— — in morning, Aur. Staph. Viol-od.
— — motion, by, agg., Acon. Arn. Bry. Led Par. *Rheum.* Staph.
— — at night, *Carb-an. Mang.* Ntr-c. Sil. Stront.
— — paralytic, Amm-c. Arn. Asar. Aur. Bov. Caps. Carb-veg. Chin. Croc. Dros. Euph. Kali-c. Led. Mez. Ntr-c. Par. Plb. Puls. Sabin. *Sass.* Seneg. *Staph.* Stram. Valer.
— — penetrating, Dig.
— — position, in a wrong, Staph.
— — pressing, Agn. Kali-c. Led.
— — perspiration, around, Amm-c. Lyc.
— — rasping, Mang.
— — rending, tearing, Agn. Aloe. Ambr. Amm-c. *Arg. Aur.* Bov. Bry. Calc. Caust. Chin. Cist. Creos. *Graph. Hyosc. Iod. Kali-c. Led. Lyc. Merc.* Mez. Ntr-c. Ntr-m. Nitr. Nux. Petr. *Plat. Phosh.* Phosp-ac. Puls. Rhod. *Rhus. Sabin. Sass. Sec-c. Sep. Staph. Stram. Stront. Sulph.* Teucr. Zinc.
— — rest, when at, Aur. Dros.
— — rheumatic, Agn. Arg. Bell. Bry. Colch. Guaj. Kali-c. Led. Merc. Rhus. Sabin. Sep. Spong. Staph.
— — spasmodic cramping, *Par. Plat. Stram.*
— — spraining, pain, Amm-c. Arn. Caps. Igt. Lach. Par. Phosp. Puls Rhus. Ruta. Sulph.
— stinging, stitches, Agn. Arn. Bar-c. Bell. Bov. Bry. *Calc.* Caust. Cocc. Colch. Con. Creos. Dros Graph. *Hell.* Hep. Igt. *Kali-c. Led.* Mgn-m. *Mang.* Meny. *Merc.* Ntr-m. Nitr. Phosp. Puls. Rhod. *Rhus. Sabin.* Sass. Sep. *Sil.* Spig. Stann. Staph. Stront. *Sulph.* Sulph-ac. *Tar. Thuj.* Zinc.
— — at night, Sil.
— — throbbing, Led.
— stiffness, Ars. Bell. Bry. Canth. *Caps. Carb-an.* Caust. Cocc. Colch Graph. Kali-c. *Lyc.* Nux. *Petr.* Puls. Rhus. *Sep.* Staph. Sulph.
— in morning, Staph.
— swelling of, Acon. Agn. Led. *Mang.* Ntr-m. *Rhod.* Sabin. *Sil. Sulph.*
— tension, Arg. Bov. *Bry. Caust.* Croc. Kali-c. Lyc. Mgn-m. Mang. Mez. *Ntr-m.* Nitr-ac. *Puls* Rhod. *Seneg. Sep.* Stann. *Sulph.* Teucr. Verat.
— tension, straining, Amm-c. Amm-m. Mang. Rhus. Sulph.
— — as from shortening of muscles, Amm-m.
— tremor, Mang.
— weakness, *Acon.* Aloe. *Arn.* Borax. *Bov.* Bry. *Calc.* Carb an. Carb-veg. Caust. Chin. Euph. *Kali c.* Led. *Lyc.* Mang. Merc. Mez. Ntr-m. Nitr-ac. Nux. Petr. Phosp. Puls. Rhod. *Rhus. Sep.* Sil. Staph. *Sulph.* Verat.

Joy, from excessive, agg., Coff. Puls.
Jumping, like something alive, Croc. Mosch.
Kind hearted persons, for suitable, Puls.
Kneeling, agg., Ant. Cocc. Sep.
Knitting, amel., from, Lyc.
Labor like pains, *Acon.* Asa-f. *Bell.* Carb-an. *Cham.* Cina. Coff. Creos. Ferr. Hyosc. Igt. Kali-c. Nux. Op. Plat. *Puls.* Rhus *Sabin.* Sec c.
Lacing, forcing, together of apertures, Bell. Hyosc. Plb. Staph. Verat.
Lactation, during, *Bell. Bry. Ca'c.* Carb-an. Cham. Chin. Croton. Dulc. *Graph. Ip. Lyc. Nux.* Phosp. Phosp-ac. *Puls. Sip.* Staph. *Sulph.* Zinc.
Lassitude, bod ly and mental, Alum. Ant. Arum. Bism. Calc. Carb-veg. *Caust. Chin.* Cocc. Colch. Coloc. *Con.* Diad. Lact. Laur. Lyc. Ntr-c. *Ntr-m.* Op. Phosp. *Phosp-ac. Seneg. Spong.* Stann. Teucr. Valer. Viol-tr.
— with convulsive laughing, Calc. Con.
— in the evening, *Caust.* Stront.
— after exertion, Ntr-m.
— in the morning Lact. Nitr. Stront.
— at noon, Carb veg.
— with thirst, Diad.
Laughing, agg., from, Ars. Bell. *Borax.* Carb-veg. Chin. Mang. *Phos.* Plb. Stann.
Laying on a hard place, as from, Arn.
Lead poisoning. Alum. Bell. Cham. Hyosc. Nux. *Op. Plat.* Stram.
Lean or aged people, Ambr.
Leaning against something, agg., Nitr-ac. *Sulph.*
— — amel., Carb-veg. Ferr. (compare Pressure).
Left side, Acon. Arn. Asa-f. Asar. Bar c. Calc. Caust. Chin. Colch. Coloc. Croc. Cupr. Elaps Iod. Lach. Merc. Nitr-ac. Nitr. Petr. Phosp. Rhod. Selen. Spig. Sulph. Sulph-ac. Tart. Thuj. Tilia. (compare one sided complaints).
Lepra, *Alum. Ars.* Carb-veg. Caust Graph. Ntr-c. Petr. *Sep. Sil. Sulph.*
Lid, or valve, sensation in throat, of, Iod. *Spong.*
Lifting, from, agg., Arn. Borax. Bry. *Calc. Carb-an. Carb-veg.* Con. *Graph.* Kali-c. *Lyc.* Merc. Ntr-c. Ntr-m. Phosp. Phosp-ac. *Rhus.* Sep. Sil. Sulph.
— raising the arm, agg., Acon. Bar-c. Bell. Con. Cupr. Ferr. Led.
— raising the part affected, agg., Arn. Bar-c. Bell. Con. Ferr. Kali-c. Led. Rhss. Sil.
Light, from, agg., Acon. Ant. Bar-c. Bell. Cact. *Calc.* Chin. *Con.* Croc. Dros Euphr. *Graph.* Hep. Igt. Lyc. Merc. Ntr-c. Nux. *Phosp.* Phosp-ac. Puls. Sang. Sep. Sil. Stram. Sulph.
— of a candle, agg., Bar-c. Bell. *Calc.* Caust. Colch. *Con.* Cor-r. Croc. Dros.

Graph. Hep. Igt. *Lyc. Merc. Phosp.* Phosp-ac. Sep. Sil.
— of day, agg., Ant. Calc. *Con.* Dros. Euphr. *Graph. Hep.* Kali-c. Nux. *Phosp.* Sep. *Sil.* Thuj.
— of sun. agg., Agar. Ant. Calc. Chin. Con. Euphr. Graph. Hep. Igt. Ntr-c. Nux. Phosp. Phosp-ac. Puls. Sil. Sulph.
— amel., Carb-an. Carb-veg Plat. *Stront.*
— bright, amel., Amm-m. Calc. Carb-an. Plat. *Stront.* Valer.
— desire for, Acon. Amm-c. Bell. Calc. Stram.
Light haired people, suitable for, Ang. Bell. Borax. Brom Bry. Calc. Caps. Cham. Clem. Cocc. Con. Dig. Graph. Hep. Hyosc. Iod. Kali-b. Lach Lyc. Merc. Mez. Petr. Phosp. Rhus. Selen. Seneg. Sil. Spig. Spong. Sulph. Sulph-ac. Thuj.
Lightness, sensation of in body, Asar. Coff. Lact. Ntr-m. Petr. Stram.
— — when walking. Chin. Lac-can. Ntr-m. Nux. Op. Rhus. Spig Thuj.
— — alternating with langor, Ntr-m.
Limbs as if separated from body, Stram.
Lively temperaments, for, Acon. Ars. Cham. Nitr-ac. Nux.
Liver grown, in children, Cham.
Living, as of something, in inner parts, *Croc.* Igt.
Loathing, attending the paroxysms, *Ip.*
Locomotor ataxia, Alum. Calc. Kali-c. Rhus.
Looking at a distance, agg , Ruta.
— down, agg., Calc. Oleand. Spig.
— — amel., Sabad.
— straight forward, agg., Oleand.
— — amel., Bell.
— fixedly, at an object, agg., Asa-f. Aur. *Calc.* Carb-veg. Caust. Cic. *Cina.* Croc. Graph. *Kali-c. Lyc.* Ntr-c. *Ntr-m.* Phosp. *Rhod. Ruta.* Sass. *Seneg.* Sep. Sil. Spig. Spong.
— amel., Ntr-c.
— towards the light, agg., Bry. Calc. Mgn-m. Merc. Phosp.
— long at an object, agg., Ruta. Spig.
— at shining objects, *Bell.* Hyosc. Stram.
— sideways, agg , Bell. Gels.
— — amel., Oleand.
— upwards, agg., *Calc.* Puls. Sabad. Selen. Thuj.
— at running water, agg., Bell. Ferr. Hyosc.
— around, Cic. *Con.*
Looseness of flesh, sensation of, Bry. Nitr-ac. Rhus. Sulph. (compare Beaten, pain as if).
Loosening the clothes, amel., Bry. *Calc.* Caps. Carb-veg. Caust. Hep. *Lyc. Nux.* Sass. Sep. Stann.
Love, unhappy, from, Coff. *Hyosc. Igt.* Phosp-ac. Staph.

34. GENERALITIES

Love, unhappy with jealousy, *hjesc. Igt.*
— — — silent, grief, *Igt. Phosp-ac.*
Lukewarm water, agg., from, Ang.
Lie down, inclination to, *Acon.* Alum. *Ars Bar-c.* Bry. *Calad.* Canth. *Cham.* Chelid. Clem. Coff. Cycl. Daph. Dig. Grat. Guaj. Hipp. Igt Led. *Lyc.* Nitr-ac. *Nux.* Pallad. *Rhus. Selen.* Sep. Spong. Staph. Stram. Tar. Tart. *Thea.*
Lying down, agg., when, Ambr. Amm-m. Arg. *Ars.* Asa-f. *Aur.* Benz-ac. Cadm. Calc. Carb-veg. *Caps.* Caust. *Cham.* Cist. Con. Cycl. Dig. *Dros.* Dulc. *Euph.* Euphr. *Ferr.* Hyosc. Igt. Lith. *Lyc.* Mgn-m. *Meny.* Mosch. Mur-ac. Ntr-c. Nux-m. Nux. Phosp-ac. *Plat. Puls.* Rhod. *Rhus.* Ruta. Sabad. Samb. Sep. *Sil.* Stront. Sulph. *Tar.* Thuj. Valer. Verb. Viol-tr.
— — amel, Alum. Amm-c. Arn. Asar. Bell. *Bry.* Calc. Canth. Carb-an. Colch. Cupr. Glon. Hipp-m. Kalm. Mgn-c. Merc. Ntr-m. Nitr-ac. *Nux.* Pallad. Phell. Sang. Scill. Staph. Verat.
— in bed, agg., *Ambr.* Amm-c. Arg. *Ars.* Aur. Borax. *Calc.* Caust. Coloc. Dros. Euph. Ferr. Graph. *Igt. Iod.* Kali c. *Led. Lyc.* Mang. Mgn-c. Nux. Phosp. Plat. *Puls. Rhod.* Rhus. Selen. *Sep.* Sil. Spig. Staph. Tart. Verat.
— — cough, Anac. Cocc-c. Creos. Dros. Euph. Hep. Igt. Mgn-c. Mgn-m. Meph. Ntr-m. Rhus. Samb. Sang. Sep. Scill. Staph. Tart. Thuj. Verb.
— — amel., Ars. *Bry.* Canth. Cic. Cocc. Con. Evon. Hep. Lach. Lyc. *Nux.* Psor. Rhus. Sabad. *Scill.* Sil. Staph. Stram.
— on painful side, agg. Acon. Amm-c. Ars. *Bar-c.* Bell. Calad. Calc. Chin. Dros. Graph. *Hep.* Igt. *Iod.* Lyc. Mgn-c. Mgn-m Mosch. Mur-ac. Nitr-ac. *Nux-m.* Nux. Par. Phosp. Phosp-ac. Puls. Rheum. *Ruta.* Sabad. *Sil.* Spong.
— — painful side, amel., Ambr. *Bry. Calc.* Caust. *Cham. Coloc.* Igt. Kali-c. *Puls.* Rhus. Sep. Stram. Viol-tr.
— on back, agg., Amm-m. Ars. Caust. Cham. Coloc. Cupr. Iod. Nitr. *Nux. Phosp.* Puls. Rhus. Sep. Sil.
— — — amel., Acon. Anac. Apis. *Bry.* Calc. Carb-an. Igt. Iod. Kali-c. Lyc. Ntr-m. Puls. Stann. Tellur.
— on side, agg., *Acon. Anac.* Ars. Bar-c. *Bry.* Calad. *Calc. Carb-an.* Cina. Con. Creos. Ferr. Graph. Hep. Igt. *Kali-c.* Lyc. Merc. Par. Puls. Sabad. Seneg. Sil. *Stann.* Sulph.
— — — amel., *Nux.* Phosp.
— on left side, agg., *Acon.* Agar. Amm-c. Arg. Arn. Bar-c. Bell. Calc. Canth. Eupat. Graph. Kali-c. *Lyc.* Merc.

Ntr-c. Ntr-m. Nux. Par. *Phosp. Puls.* Seneg. Sep. Sulph. Tabac. Thuj.
— on right side, agg., Ammi m. Ars. Borax. Calc. Carb-an. Euph. Mgn-m. Merc. Nux. Seneg. Sep. Spig. Spong. Stann. Tar.
— with the head low, agg., Arg. Ars. Chin. Colch. Hep. Nitr. *Puls.* Spig. Tart.
— on something hard amel., Bell. Ntr-m. Rhus.
— horizontally, amel., Arn. Spong.
— crooked, amel., Colch. *Coloc.* Rheum.
— on stomach, amel., Aloe. Alum. Amm-c. Calc. Pho-p. Pod. Rhus.
After lying down, agg., *Ambr.* Amm-c. *Ars.* Asa-f. *Aur.* Bry. Calc. Clem. Con. Cycl. *Dulc.* Euph. Euphr. Ferr. Hyosc. Ip. Kali-c. *Lyc.* Mgn-c. Mgn-m. Meny. Mosch. Ntr-m. *Nux.* Ol-an. Petr. *Phosp-ac. Plat.* Plb. *Puls. Rhus.* Sabad. *Samb.* Sep. *Stront.* Sulph. Sulph-ac. Tar. Verat.
— — — amel., Bell. Bry. Calc. Carb-veg. Cina. Croc. Graph. Hep. Iod. *Ntr-m. Nux.* Oleand. *Scill.* Spig. Staph Stram.
From lying on a limb, agg., Arn. Bell. Con. Kali-c. Rhus. Sil.
Male sex, for the, Nux. Phosp.
Mania á potu, Ars. Bell. Calc.Cannab-ind. Coff. Dig. Hyosc. Lach. Nux. Op. Sep. Stram. Sulph.
Meals, after, (compare, Eating.)
Measels, during the, agg., *Acon.* Ant. Bell. Bry. Ip. Kali-b. *Puls.* Rhus.
— after the, agg., Arn. Bell. Camph. Carb-veg· Con. Dulc. *Puls* Rhus.
— suppressed, agg., Acon. Bry. Dros. Dulc. *Puls.* Rhus.
Mechanical injuries, Arg. *Arn.* Calend. Caust. Cic. *Con.* Dulc. Glon. *Hep.* Hyper. Iod. Kali-c. Lach. Phosp. Phosp-ac. Plat. *Puls. Rhus.* Ruta. Staph. Sulph. *Sulph-ac.* Symph.
— — bloatedness and dark red swelling after, Samb.
— — from a fall from a height, Millef.
— — sprains, Agn. Bry. Lyc. Nitr-c. Petr. Phosp. Rhus.
Menstruation before, agg., Bar-c. *Calc.* Carb-veg. Con. Creos *Cupr. Lyc.* Merc. Ntr-m. Phosp. Phesp-ac. Plat. *Puls.* Sep. *Sulph.* Verat.
— commencement of agg., Acon. Caust. Cham. Hyosc. Lyc. Phosp. Plat. Puls. Sep.
— during, agg., *Amm-c.* Amm-m. Calc. *Cham.* Cocc. Coff. Creos. *Graph. Hyosc.* Igt. *Kali-c.* Lyc. Mgn-c. Mgn-m. Nux. Phosp. *Puls.* Sep. Sulph.
— after, agg., *Borax. Creos.* Graph. Lyc. Ntr-m. *Nux.* Phosp. Stram.
— suppressed, agg., Acon. Amm-c. Bar-c. Calc. Caust. Cham. Cocc. *Con.* Cupr.

34. GENERALITIES.

Dulc. Ferr. Graph. Kali-c. Lyc. Ntr-m.
Phosp. Puls. Sabad. Sep. Sil. Staph.
Sulph. Valer.
Mercury, abuse of, Ant. Arg. Ars. Asa-f.
Aur. Bell. Calc. Carb-veg. Caust. Chin.
Clem. Colch. Cupr. Daph. Dulc. Euph.
Grat. Hep. Iod. Lach. Led. Lyc. Mez.
Nitr-ac. Op. Phosp-ac. Phyt. Puls.
Sang. Sass. Sep. Sil. Spig. Staph Stront.
Sulph. Thuj. Valer.
Mercurial vapors, agg., Chin. Stram.
Mesmerized, desire to be, Calc. Phosp.
Mesmerism, amel., from, Bell. Cupr. Lyc.
Nux. Phosp. Sil. Teucr.
Midnight, before, agg., Ang. Arn. Bell.
Brom. Bry. Carb-veg Caust. Cham. Graph.
Hep. Lach. Led. Lyc. Mang. Merc. Mez.
Mur-ac. Petr. Phosp. Puls. Ran-b.
Ran-sc. Rhus. Sabad. Spig. Spong. Stann.
Staph. Stront. Tart. Valer.
— after, Acon. Amm-c. Ars. Bell. Calc.
Cannab. Canth. Caps. Caust. Coff. Croc.
Dros. Dulc. Ferr. Graph. Hep. Igt. Iod.
Kali-c. Mgn-c. Mang. Merc. Ntr-c.
Nitr. Nux. Plat. Ran-sc. Rhus. Samb.
Scill. Sulph-ac. Tart. Thuj.
— — 1 A. M., Ars.
— — 2 A. M., Benz-ac. Lachn.
— — 3 A. M., Calc. Euphr. Kali-c. Pariera.
Staph. Thuj.
— — to noon, Ars. Cist.
Mild though distinctly perceptible pains,
Viol-od.
Milk, agg., from, Alum. Ambr. Ang. Arg.
Ars. Brom. Bry. Calc. Carb-veg. Cham.
Chelid. Chin. Cic. Con. Cupr. Kali-c.
Lyc. Ntr-m. Ntr-m. Nitr-ac. Nux. Phosp.
Sep. Stram. Sulph. Valer. Zinc.
— amel., Chelid. Iod. Verat.
Moaning and lamenting from the pains,
Canth. Cham.
Mobility too great, Bell. Stram.
Moon, when declining, agg., Dulc.
— — increasing agg., Alum. Thuj.
— full, during, agg., Alum. Graph.
Sulph.
— new, during, agg., Alum. Amm-c. Calc.
Caust. Cupr. Daph. Sep. Sil.
Moonshine, in agg., Ant. Bell. Thuj.
Morning, agg., Acon. Agar Ambr. Amm-c.
Amm-m. Anac. Ant. Apis. Arn. Aur.
Bar-c. Bell. Bov. Bry. Bufo. Cadm.
Calc. Carb-an. Carb-veg. Caust. Chelid.
Chin. Cina. Cist. Clem. Coff. Con.
Creos. Croc. Cupr. Daph. Dig. Dros.
Dulc. Euph. Euphr. Ferr. Graph. Guaj.
Hell. Hep. Igt. Kali-c. Mgn-m. Meph.
Mez. Ntr-c. Ntr-m. Ntr-s. Nitr-ac. Nitr.
Nux. Op. Petr. Phosp. Phosp-ac. Pod.
Ran-b. Rheum Rhod. Rhus. Sabin.
Scill. Sep. Stann. Staph. Stram. Sulph.
Sulph-ac. Tar. Tart. Thuj. Valer. Verat.
Viol-od.

— in bed, Hep. Phosp.
— after rising up, Guaj. Kali-b. Igt.
— increasing until noon, diminishing as
sun declines, Acon. Glon. Kali-ferr-cyn.
Spig. Stram.
Motion difficult, Ang. Ars. Bell. Bry. Calc.
Camph. Carb-an. Caust. Cham. Chelid.
Cic. Cocc. Coloc. Graph Igt. Kali-c.
Lyc. Ntr-m. Nux. Petr. Rhus. Sep.
Sil. Spig. Stapu. Sulph. Tereb. Thuj.
Verat.
— extraordinary, Bell. Coff. Op. Stram.
Tanac. Tarant.
— convulsive, Bell. Camph. Canth.
Cham. Cic. Cocc. Cupr. Glon. Hell.
Hyosc. Igt. Iod. Ip. Nux. Op. Plb.
Rheum Ruta. Scill. Sec-c. Stann. Stram.
Verat.
— involuntary, Cocc. Cupr. Hyosc. Igt.
Lach. Op. Stram.
Mouth, opening the, agg., Ang. Merc.
Phosp. Sabad.
— closing the, agg., Mez.
Move, on beginning to, agg., Bry. Caps.
Carb-veg. Caust. Ccn. Euph. Ferr.
Fluor-ac. Lyc. Phosp. Puls. Rhus.
Sabad. Samb. Sil.
Movement wrong, on, agg., Bry. Lyc.
Moving, aversion to, Acon. Amm-c. Ars.
Bar-c. Caps. Chelid. Cocc. Cycl.
Dig. Guaj. Igt. Lyc. Mez. Mur ac.
Ntr-m. Nux. Pallad. Thea. Thuj. Zinc.
— inclination to, Arn. Cham. Chin. Ferr.
Rhus.
— sensation of, Bell. Croc. Igt. Rhod.
Rhus. Sep. Sil Sulph.
— — up and down, Lach Spong.
Moving, on, agg., Acon. Agn. Aloe. Apis.
Arn. Ars. Asar. Bell. Berb. Bry. Calad.
Calc. Camph. Cannab. Caps. Carb-an.
Chelid. Chin. Cic. Cina Cist. Cocc.
Cocc-c. Coff. Colch. Coloc. Ccn. Cupr.
Dig. Elaps Graph. Hell. Hep. Igt.
Iod. Ip. Iris. Kalm. Laur. Led. Merc.
Mez. Ntr-m. Nitr-ac. Nux. Ol-an.
Ox-ac. Pallad. Phosp. Plb. Puls. Ran-b.
Rheum. Sang. Sass. Scill. Selen. Spig.
Stann. Staph. Tilia. Verat. Zinc.
— outwards, agg., Caps. Caust. (compare
Turning).
— inwards, agg., Igt. Staph.
— backwards, agg., Calc. Kali-c. Puls.
Sep. Sulph.
— sideways, agg., Bell. Ntr-m.
— forwards, agg., Coff. Thuj.
— extending the part, agg., Alum. Calc.
Coloc. Rhus. Sep. Staph. Sulph. Thuj.
— flexing or turning, agg, Amm-m. Cic.
Igt. Kali-c. Lyc. Nux. Puls. Spig.
Spong.
— of rocking, agg., Borax. Carb-veg.
— slow, amel., Ambr. Caps. Con. Euph.
Ferr. Puls. Samb.

34. GENERALITIES. 301

— amel., from, Agar. Ambr. Amm-m.Arn. Ars. *Asa-f.* *Aur.* Bar-c. Bism. Brom. Calc. *Caps.* Coloc.*Con.* Cub.*Cycl.* Diosc. Dros. *Dulc.* *Euph.* *Ferr.* Glon. Grat. Ind. Kali-c. Kali-jod. Lith. *Lyc.* Mgn-c. Mgn-m. Meny. *Mosch.* *Mur-ac.* *Ntr-c.* Ntr-s. Op. Phell. Phosp-ac. Plat. *Puls.* Rhod. *Rhus.* Ruta. *Sabad.* *Samb.* *Seneg.* *Sp.*Sulph. *Tar.*Tilia. *Valer.*Verat. Verb. Viol-tr.
— of arms, agg., Acon. Anac. Ang. Dig. Lach. Led. Ran-b. Rhus.
— — eyes, agg., Bell.*Bry* Caps.Cham.Hep. Nux. Op. Sil. Spig. Sulph. Valer.
— — eyelids, agg., Coloc.
— — head, agg., Arn. Bell. Bry. Calc. Caps. Cupr. Lyc. Sep. Spig.
— part affected, agg., Arn. Bell. Bry. Cannab. Caps. Cham. Chin. Cocc. Led. Merc. Nux. Puls. Spig.
— — — amel., Amm-m. Ars. Aur. *Caps.* Chin. Con. *Dulc.* Euph. *Ferr.* Lyc. Mgn-m. Mosch. Phosp-ac. *Puls.* Rhod. *Rhus.* Sabad. Samb. Sep. Tar.
— after, agg., *Agar.* Anac. *Ars. Cannab.* Carb-veg. Caust. Croc. Hyosc. Kali-c. Nitr-ac. Phosp. *Puls. Rhus.* Ruta. Sep. Spig. Spong. *Stann.* Stram. *Valer.* Zinc.
— continuous, amel., Ambr. Amm-m. *Caps. Con.* Cycl. Dros. *Euph. Ferr.* Lyc. Puls. Sabad. *Samb.* Sil. Valer. Verat.
Mucus membranes, Acon. *Alum.* Apis. Arg. *Ars.* Asa-f. *Bell.* Bry. *Calc. Caps. Carb-veg. Caust.* Chin. *Dulc. Euph.* Ferr. Fluor-ac. Hep. *Ip.* Lac-can. Lyc. *Merc.* Mez. Nitr-ac. *Nux.* *Phosp.* Plb. Puls. Rheum. *Seneg.* *Stann.* *Sulph.* *Tart.*
Mucus, secretion increased, Alum. Apis. Bell. Borax. *Calc.* Cham. Chin. Dulc. Graph. Hyosc.*Merc.* *Nux.* Par. *Phosp.* Puls. Seneg. Stann. *Sulph.*
Muscles, cramping pain in, *Anac.* Arn. Ars. Asa-f. *Bell. Calc.* Cannab. Caust. *Cina.* Cocc Coloc. Con. Dulc. Euphr. Mag. Daph. Igt. Kali-c. *Lyc.* Mgn-m. Meny. *Merc.* Mur-ac. Nitr-ac. Petr. *Plat.* Rhus. *Sep.* Sil. Spig. Spong. Stann. Sulph. Thuj.
— convulsive motions,subsultus tendinum, Arg. Asa-f. Clem. Coloc. Cupr. Graph. *Iod. Kali-c.* Meny. *Mez.* Ntr-c. Plat. Sec-c. (compare Twitching).
— induration of, Caust. Lyc.
— jerk, Anac. *Cic.* Colch. Nux. Phosp Plat. Puls. Rhus. *Sep.* Spig. Stann. *Sulph. Sulph-ac.*
— laxness, relaxation of, Agar. Bar-m. *Calc. Caps.* Cham. Clem. *Cocc.*Con.Croc. Cupr. Ferr-m. Hell. Hyosc. Iod. Lyc. Merc. *Nux.* Seneg. Spong. Sulph. Verat. Viol-od.
— — sudden in walking, Con.

— pressure in, Anac. Asa-f. Asar. Caps. Carb-an. Cupr. *Lyc.* Igt. Led. Mosch. *Nux-m.* Oleand. Phosp. Phosp-ac. *Ruta.* Sabad. Staph. Sulph-ac. Tar. Teucr. Valer.
— rigidity, of, Acon. Ntr-ac. Phosp. Plat.
— shortness, contraction of, Amm-c. *Amm-m.* Ars. Bar-c. Caust. *Coloc. Graph.* Lach. Lyc. Ntr-c. *Ntr-m.*Nux.Rhus.Sep.
— — general, all over the body, Caust. Coloc.
— stinging in, Alum. Amm-m. Arn. *Asa-f. Bell.* Bry. *Calc.* Caust. *Chin.* Cocc. Con. Dros. Graph. Hell. Igt. Kali-c. Laur. Meny. *Merc.* Mur-ac. Ntr-c. Ntr-m. Nitr-ac. Par. Phosp. *Puls.* Ran-sc. *Rhus.* Sabad. Sabin. Sass. Sep. *Sil. Spig.* Spong. Stann. *Staph. Sulph.* Tar. Thuj. Viol-tr. Zinc.
— — burning, in, Alum. Arg. *Asa-f. Cocc. Mez. Nux.* Oleand. Rhus.Sabad. Staph. *Sulph-ac. Thuj.*
— — pressing, in, Asa-f. Mur-ac. *Sass.* Thuj. Zinc.
— — tearing in, Anac. Ars. *Calc.* Camph. Chin. Guaj. Mang. *Puls.* Sass. *Thuj.*
— tension, in, Amm-c. Ang. Ant. Arn. Bar-c. *Bry.* Coloc. *Euph.* Mang. *Mez.* Nux. Plat *Rhus.*
— — when exercising, Bry.
— — at rest, *Rhus.*
— — when walking, Ang.
— tightness, *Acon.* Amm-c. *Amm-m.* Bar-c. Carb-an. Caust. Graph. Guaj. Mang. Mosch. *Nitr-ac.* Nux. Ol-an. *Phosp.* Plat. Puls. Rhus. Sep. Sulph.
— tearing in, Ambr. Amm-m. Arg. Ars. Asa-f Aur. Bell. Bism. Borax. Bry.*Calc.* Canth. Carb-an. *Carb-veg. Caust.*Chelid. China. Cina. Colch. Dulc. Graph. Hep. *Kali-c. Lyc.* Mang.Mgn-m. *Merc.*Mur-ac. Ntr-c. Ntr-m. Nitr. *Nitr-ac.* Phosp. Puls. *Rhod.* Ruta. Sabin. *Sep. Sil.* Stann. *Staph. Stront. Sulph.* Teucr. Zinc.
— — burning in, Carb-veg. Nitr-ac.
— — crampy, in, *Anac.* Calc. Chin. Meny. *Mur-ac. Ntr-c.* Petr. *Plat.*
— — jerking, in, *Chin.* Puls. Staph.
— — paralytic, Chin. Cina. Hell. Kali-c. Sabin. Sass.
— — pressing, in, Carb-veg. Kali-c. Stann. Staph.
— — pricking, Colch. Euph. *Zinc.*
— twitching of, Alum. Ambr. Ang. Arn. Ars. Asa-f. *Bar-c.* Bell. Bry. Bufo. Caust. Cham. Chin. Cina. Clem. Cocc. Coff. Coloc. Cupr. Graph. Hell. Hyosc. Igt. Iod. Ip. Kali-c. Lach. Laur. Lyc. Mgn-c. Meny. Merc. Merc-cor. *Mez. Ntr-c.* Ntr-m. Plat. Ran-b. Ran-sc. Rat. Rhus. Sec-c. Sep. Sil. Spig. Stram. Sulph. Sulph-ac. Tar. Tart. Thuj. Viol-tr.

34. GENERALITIES.

Muscles, twitching, general, Bar-c.
— — at night, Bar-c.
— — when at rest, Meny.
— — of one side of body, while the other is paralyzed, Apis.
— upper part of body, Ntr-m. Nitr-ac. Sep. Thuj.
— spasmodic, Ang.
— increased excitability of voluntary, less of involuntary, Op.
— movements of subject to will, are easier, Stram.
— motions, involuntary of, Alum.
— increased ability to exercise, without fatigue, Fluor-ac.
— weak, and will not obey the will, Gels.
— refuse, if not governed by the will, Hell.
Music, from, agg., Acon. Calc. Cham. Coff. Kali-c. Lyc. *Ntr-c.* Nux. Phosp-ac. *Sep.* Stann. Tabac. Viol-od. Zinc.
— lively, causes weeping, Creos. Ntr-s. Thuj.
Narcotic medicines, from, *Bell. Cham. Coff.* Dig. Graph. Hyosc. Ip. *Lach. Lyc.* Merc. Mur-ac. *Nux. Op.* Puls. Sep. Valer.
Nervous debility, Ars. Asar. *Bar-c.* Bell. *Calc. Chin.* Cocc. Coff. Con. Cupr. Dig. Hep. Igt. Iod. *Laur.* Merc. *Nux. Phosp. Phosp-ac.* Plat. *Puls. Sil.* Stann. Sulph. Valer. Viol-od.
— pains, *Acon. Arn.* Ars. Bell. Caust. Cham. Chin. Cocc. *Coff.* Con. Hep. *Igt. Merc. Nux.* Phosp. Puls. Rhus. Sep. Staph. Sulph. Verat.
Night, at, agg., *Acon.* Amm-m. Ant. Apis. Arn. Ars. Aur. *Bar-c.* Bell. Bism. Bry. Cact. Calc. Camph. Cannab. Canth. Caps. *Carb-an.* Carb-veg. *Caust.* Cham. Chin. Cina. Cinnab. Cist. Clem. Coff. *Colch. Con.* Croc. Cupr. Dig. Dros. *Dulc.* Eugen. Euphr. *Ferr. Graph. Grat.* Guaj. Hell. *Hep.* Hyosc. Igt. *Iod.* Kali-c. Lach. Led. *Lyc. Mgn-c. Mgn-m. Mgn-s. Mang. Merc.* Mez. Mur-ac. Ntr-c. Ntr-m. Nicc. *Nitr-ac.* Oleand. Ol-an. Op. Par. Phosp. *Plb.* Puls. Ran-b. Rheum. Rhus. Sabad. Samb. *Sec-c.* Selen. Sep. *Sil.* Spig. *Spong.* Staph. *Stront. Sulph. Sulph-ac.* Tart. *Thuj.*
— — in bed, Acon. Mgn-m. Merc. Rhus.
— — with chills, Hep.
— — hemiplagia, Ntr-m.
— — dyspnoea, Ntr-m.
— — cough, agg., Acon. Bell. Dros. Merc. Nux. Puls. Rumex. Sang. Sticta.
Night study, or watching at, agg., Cocc. Colch. Laur. Nux. Puls. Selen.
Noise, from, agg., Ang. Arn. Bell. Cact. Calc. Cannab-ind. Cham. *Coff.* Colch. Con. Igt. Kali-b. Lyc. Mang. Ntr-c. *Nux.* Phosp-ac. Plat. Sang. Sep. Sil.

Spig. Zinc.
Noon, at, Alum. *Arg.* Ars. Carb-veg. Cic. Kali-b. *Nux.* Phosp. *Stram.* Valer. *Zinc.*
Numbness, Ambr. Apis. Arg. Bar-c. Calc. Caps. *Carb-an.* Carb-veg. Chin. *Cocc.* Croc. Graph. Gauj. *Igt. Kali-c.* Led. Lyc. Mgn-m. Merc. Ntr-m. *Nux.* Petr. Phosp. Phosp-ac. Puls. *Rheum. Rhod.* Rhus. Sep. *Sil. Sulph. Thuj. Verat.*
— as if made of wood, Nitr. Plb. Rhus. Thuj.
— after previous tingling and twitching, Rhus.
— even if not lying on the part, Fluor-ac.
— on side on which he lies, Bry. Chin. Kali-c. Lyc. Mez. Phell. Puls. Rheum. Rhod. Rhus. Sil.
— of lower half of body, Spong.
— with coldness, Plat.
— after manual labor, Sep.
— at night, *Croc.* Thuj.
— when at rest, Puls.
— in sitting, Merc.
— of whole surface of body in morning, Ambr.
Nursing infants, for, Arn. *Bell.* Borax. Bry. Calc. Cham. Cina. Igt. *Ip.* Lyc. Merc. Nux. *Rheum.* Rhus. *Sil. Sulph.* Sulph-ac.
Obstruction of breath, caused by the pains, Diosc. Ntr-m. *Puls.*
Old age, for, Ambr. Ant-cr. Aur. Caust. Con. Fluor-ac. Kali-c. Led. Millef Op. Pothos. Sec-c.
Onanism, from, Arg. Aur. Bell. *Calc.* Carb-veg. *Chin.* Cina. Con. Iod. Lyc. Merc. Mosch. Ntr-m. Nux-m. Nux. Phosp. *Phosp-ac.* Plat. Puls. Selen. *Sep.* Spig. *Staph. Sulph.*
One sided complaints, Agar. *Alum.* Ambr. Amm-c. *Anac.* Arg. *Asa-f.* Bar-c. Bell. Calc. *Canth.* Cina. Cocc. Cycl. Dulc. Guaj. *Kali-c.* Lach. Mang. *Mez.* Mur-ac. Oleand. Par. Phosp. *Phosp-ac. Puls.* Rhus. Sabad. Sabin. *Sass.* Spig. Staph. Stront. *Sulph-ac.* Thuj. *Verb.* Zinc.
— right side, Agar. Alum. Amm-c. Amm-m. Canth. Caust. Dros. Hep. Igt. Lyc. Mosch. Plb. Ran-b. Ruta. Sabad. Sabin. Sang. Tei cr.
— left side, Arn. Asa-f. Asar. Calc. Chin. Colch. Coloc. Croc. Cupr. Iod. Lach. Merc. Nitr-ac. Rhod. Selen. Spig. Sulph. Tar.
— — first right then left and vice versa, Lac-can.
— on the side on which one lies, Acon. Amm-c. Ars. Bar-c. Bell. Calad. Calc. Carb-an. Caust. Chin. Dros. Graph. Hep. Igt. Iod. Kali-c. Kali-jod. Lyc. Mgn-c. Mgn-m. Mosch. Nitr-ac. Nux. Par. Phosp. Phosp-ac. Rheum. Ruta. Sabad. Sep. Spig. Spong. Stann. Tart.

34. GENERALITIES.

On the side one does not lie, Ambr. Bry. Calc. Caust. Cham. Coloc. Igt. Phell. Puls. Rhus. Verb.
Onions, agg., from, Lyc. Puls. Thuj.
Open air, in the, agg., Agar. Amm-c. Arn. Ars. Benz-ac. *Bry. Calc. Camph.* Cannab. Caps. Carb-an. Carb-veg. *Caust.* Cham. Chelid. Chin. Cic. *Cocc. Coff. Con.* Creos. Ferr. Graph. Grat. *Guaj.* Hep. *Igt. Ip. Kali-c.* Lach. Led. *Lyc.* Mang. Merc. Mosch. Ntr-c. Nitr-ac. *Nux-m. Nux.* Petr. Rhus. Sabad. Sabin. *Seneg.* Sep. *Sil.* Spig. Staph. *Stram. Sulph.* Sulph-ac. Tabac. Teucr. Thuj. *Valer. Verat.* Viol-tr. Zinc.
— — amel., Acon. Agn. Aeth. *Alum. Ambr.* Amm-c. Anac.Ant. Arg. Asa-f. Asar. *Aur.* Bar-c. Brom. Cic. *Croc. Graph.* Hell. Kali-jod. *Mgn-c.* Mgn-m. Mang. Mez. Ntr-s. Ol-an. Op. Phell. Phosp. Plat. *Puls.* Ran-sc. *Rhod. Sabin* Sass. Seneg. Sep. Spong. Stann. Stront. Sulph-ac. Tabac. Tart-ac.
— — desire for, Alum. Aur. Croc. Kali-jod. Phosp. Puls. Tellur.
— — aversion to, Camph. Chin. Cina. Lach. Merc. Nitr-ac. Nux-m.
Opisthotonos, Ang. Bell. Cham. Cic. Cina. Cupr. Igt. *Ip.* Op. Rhus. Stann. Stram. Zinc.
Oppressing pain, Bell. Con. Mgn-c. Mosch.
Outwards moving, pain, Arg. Asa-f. Bell. Bry. Chin. Con. Ntr-m. Rhus. Samb. Spong. Thuj.
Overheating, slight, Alcohol, Bell. Bry. Carb-an. Kali-c. Op.
— — — complaints from, Carb-veg. Sil. Thuj. Zinc.
Over-irritation, nervous, Asar. *Cham.* Chin. *Coff.* Cupr. Igt. Ind. Iod. *Merc.* Nux. Puls. Rhus. Stann. Teucr. *Valer.*
— — from calomel, *Hep. Nitr-ac.*
— — in lying-in women, *Coff.*
Over-sensitiveness of the body, Acon. Agar. Arn. Ars. *Asar. Aur.* Bar-c. Bell. Calc. *Canth.* Caust. *Cham.* Chin. Cocc. *Coff.* Colch. *Con.* Cupr. Hep. Hyosc. *Lyc.* Mgn-c. Merc. Ntr-c. *Nux.* Petr. *Phosp.* Puls. *Sep.* Sil. Spig. Staph. Sulph. Valer.
— — to heat and cold, Ip. Lach.
— — — external impressions, Arn. Cocc. Coff. Nux.
— — of parts affected. Coff.
Pains begin when itching ceases and vice versa, Stront.
— appear on small longitudinal spots, Ox-ac.
Painlessness, insensibility of body, Bell. Chelid. *Cocc.* Con. Hell. *Hyosc.*Igt.Laur. *Lyc.* Mosch. *Oleand.*Op.Phosp.*Phosp-ac.*

Puls. Rhus. Sec-c. *Stram.*
— of inner parts, Ars. Bell. Bov. Hyosc. *Op. Plat.* Spig.
— — parts affected, Anac. Asa-f. Cocc. Con. Lyc. Oleand. *Plat.* Puls. Rhus.
— with all complaints, Cocc. Laur. Lyc. Oleand. Op. Stram.
Paralysis, lameness, Acon.Aloe.*Anac.*Ang. Arg-n. Ars. Bell. Bry. Calc. Carb-veg. *Caust.* Chelid.*Cocc.*Con.Dulc.Ferr.Gels. Hyosc. Hydroc-ac. Kali-c. Kali-jod. Lach. Laur. Lyc. Millef. Merc cor. *Ntr-m. Nux. Oleand. Op. Phosp.* Plb. *Rhus.* Ruta. Sec-c. Sep. *Sil. Stann.* Stront. Stram. *Sulph.* Verat. Zinc.
— one sided (hemiplagia) Alum. Anac. Arg-n. Caust. Cocc. Kali-c. Lach. Ntr-c. Phosp ac. Rhus. Sass. Staph. Stront. Sulph-ac.
— — in the evening, Sil. Stront.
— — caused by the pains, Ntr-m.
— — right side, Arn. Bell. Calc. Caust. Ntr-c. Op. Phosp. Plb. Sil. Stront. Sulph.
— left side, Acon. Anac. Arn. Bapt. Bell. Caust. Lach. Lyc. Nitr-ac. Ox-ac. Petr. Stann. Stram. Sulph.
— — from anger, Staph.
— painless, Anac. *Cocc.* Con. Hyosc. Lyc. *Oleand. Rhus.*
— of the organs of special sense, Acon. Anac. *Bell.* Bry. Calc. Caust. Cocc. *Dulc. Hyosc.* Laur. Lyc. Nitr-ac. Nux. Oleand. *Op.* Phosp. Plb. *Puls.* Rhus. Ruta. *Sec-c. Sil.* Stram. Sulph. Verat.
— — inner parts, Acon. Ars. Bell. Cocc. Dulc. Hyosc. Nux-m. Nux. Puls. Rhus.
— after apoplexy, Anac. Bar-c. Bell. Con. Laur. Nux. Stann. Stram. Zinc.
— of aged persons, Bar-c. Con. Kali-c.
— with coldness of parts, Nux.
— of different single parts, Dulc.
— — flexors, Caust.
— one side twitches, the other is paralyzed, Apis.
— first of lower then upper limbs, Hydroc-ac.
Paralyzed pain, Aur. Bell. Bism. Cham. Chin. *Cina. Cocc. Cycl.* Mez. Ntr-m. *Nux.* Rhus. *Sabin.* Sil. Staph. Verat.
— sensation as if, in inner parts, Lyc.
Pastry rich, from agg., Ars. Carb-veg. Cycl. *Puls.*
Peeling off, as if skin were, sensation, Agar. Bar-c. Lach. Phosp. Phosp-ac.
Periodical complaints, *Alum. Anac.* Ant. Arn. *Ars.* Aur. Bar-c. Bell. Calc. *Canth.* Caps. Carb-veg. *Chin.* Con. *Cupr.* Diad. Ferr. Ferr-m. *Igt. Ip.* Hyosc. Lach. Lyc. Merc. *Ntr-m. Nux.* Par. Plb. Puls. Ran-sc. Rhod. Rhus. Sabad. Sec-c. Sep. Sil.Staph.Sulph.Tarant.Thuj.*Valer.*Verat.

34. GENERALITIES.

Periodical complaints, daily, Ars. Chin. Lach. Lyc. Mgn-c. Nux. Thuj.
— alternate days, Alum. Phosp.
— every seven days, Canth. Croc. Sacch. Sil. Sulph.
— — fortnight, Lach. Nicc.
— — third week, Mgn-c.
— — two or three months, Valer.
— — three months, Kali-b.
— — spring, Lach.
— — year, Ars. Kali-b. Nicc. Thuj.
Perspiration on head attending pains, Cham.
— of parts affected, Cocc. Fluor-ac. Merc. Sil. Stront. *Tart.*
— by, pains accompanied, *Merc. Ntr-c.* Op. Tabac. Tart. Tilia. Verat.
— during, agg., Acon. *Ars. Bry. Caust.* *Cham.* Igt. Ip. *Merc.* Ntr-c. Nitr-ac. *Nux. Op.* Phosp. Puls. *Rhus.* Sabad. *Sep. Stram. Sulph.* Tart. *Verat.*
— — amel., Bov. Calad. Cupr. Elat. *Lyc.*
— — cold, amel., Nux.
— after agg., Calc. *Chin.* Kali-c. Merc. *Phosp-ac.* Puls. *Sep.* Staph. Sulph.
— — amel., Bry. Calad. Canth. Cham. Cocc-c. Gels. Glon. Graph. Hep. Ntr-m. Oleand. Rhus. Stront. Thuj.
Phlegmatic temperament, Bar-c. Caps. Cocc. Croc. Igt. Lyc. *Puls.* Seneg. Sil.
Phthisis, Ars. Bar-c. Calc. Carb-an. Carb-veg. Chin. Con. Cupr. Dulc. Graph. Hep. Iod. Kali-c. Lyc. Ntr-m. Nux-m. Nitr-ac. Nux. Phosp. Sep. Sil. Spong. Stann. Staph. Sulph. (compare Consumption).
— or drunkards, Chin.
Pinching in outer parts, Calc. Hyosc. Ip. Meny. Mur-ac. *Rhod.* Rhus. *Sabad. Stann.* Sulph.
— — inner parts, Amm-c. Bell. Bry. *Calc.* Cannab. Canth. Carb-veg. *Chelid.* Chin. *Cocc.* Dulc. Graph. Hell. *Igt.* Kali-c. *Lyc.* Meny. Merc. Mur-ac. Ntr-c. Ntr-m. Par. Petr. Phosp. Plat. Puls. Ran-b. *Ran-sc.* Rhod. Rhus. Ruta. Sabad. Sep. Spig. Spong. Staun. Staph. Thuj. Verat. Verb. Zinc.
— together, Cocc.
Playing on piano, agg., from, Anac. Calc. Kali-c. *Ntr-c.* Sep. Zinc.
Plethoric habit, *Acon.* Arn. Aur. *Bell.* Bry Calc. Chin. Cocc. Dig. *Ferr. Hep. Hyosc.* Kali-c. *Lyc.* Merc. Ntr-m. Nitr-ac. Nitr. Nux. Phosp. *Puls.* Rhus. Seneg. Sep. Stram. Sulph.
Plug, pain as from, Anac. Ant. Arn. Asa-f. Hep. Igt. Lith. Nux. Plat. Ruta. Spong. Sulph. Sulph-ac.
Polypus. *Calc.* Caust. Con. Merc. Phosp. Sang. Staph. Teucr.
Polysarcia, excessive corpulency, Ant. *Calc. Caps.* Cupr. *Ferr.* Lyc. Puls. Sulph.

Pork, agg., from, *Carb-veg.* Colch. Ip. Ntr-c. Ntr-m. *Puls. Sep.* Thuj.
— — smell of, Colch.
Posture, agg., from change of, Caps. Caust. Carb-veg. Con. Euph. Ferr. Lach. Nitr-ac. *Puls.* Ran-b. Samb.
— amel., from change of, Cham. *Igt.* Nux. Phosp-ac. Valer. Zinc.
Potatoes, agg., from, Alum. Sep. Verat.
Poultices, from wet, agg., Amm-c. Ant. Bell. *Calc.* Canth. Carb-veg. Cham. *Clem.* Lyc. Merc. Nitr. *Rhus.* Sep. Spig. Stront. *Sulph.*
— — — amel., (compare Wetting).
Pox small, having the, agg., when, Ant. Bell. *Merc.* Puls. *Rhus.* Sulph. *Tart.*
Pregnancy, during, Acon. Alum. Bar-c. *Bell.* Bry. *Calc.* Caps. Caust. Cham. Cic. *Cocc. Coff. Con. Croc.* Dulc. Gels. Graph. Hyosc. *Ip.* Lyc. Mgn-c. Ntr-m. Nux-m. *Nux.* Petr. Phosp. Plat. Psor. *Puls.* Rhus. *Sabin.* Sec-c. *Sep.* Stram. Sulph. Verat.
Pressing pains, outer parts, Anac. Arg. Bell. Calc. Carb-veg. *Caust.* Cycl. Lyc. Oleand. Phosp-ac. Ruta Sass. *Stann. Staph.* Sulph. Tar. Verat. Zinc.
— — inner parts, Acon. Alum. Ambr. *Anac.* Ang. Arg. Arn. Ars *Asa-f.* Aur. *Bell.* Bism. Borax. *Calc.* Camph. Cannab. Caps. Carb-an. Carb-veg. Caust. *Chin.* Cina. Cocc. Con. *Cupr.* Cycl. Dig. Dros. Euph. Graph. *Igt.* Led. *Lyc.* Mgn-c. Merc. Mez. Mur-ac. Ntr-m. Nux. *Oleand.* Petr. Phosp. Plat. Ran-sc. Ruta. Seneg. Sep. Stann. Staph. Sulph. Sulph-ac. Tar. *Valer.* Verat. Zinc.
— from outward parts, *Anac.* Calc. Cocc. Creos. Dulc. Hell. Nitr-ac. Oleand. Plat. Staph. Zinc.
— — inner parts, Acon. *Asa-f.* Dros. Igt. Merc. Mur-ac. Nux. Par. Phosp. Phosp-ac. Rhus. Spig. Spong. Teucr. Verb.
— as from a heavy load, *Acon.* Amm-m. Bar-c. Creos. Cupr. Ntr-c. Nux. Op. Par. Puls. Rhus. Samb. Sec-c. *Sep.* Spig. Sulph.
— together, *Alum.* Anac. Arn. *Asar.* Bell. Bov. Cannab. Canth. *Cocc.* Dros. Hell. Ip. Mosch Ntr-m. *Plat.* Sass. Spong. Stann. Sulph. Sulph-ac. Verat.
— asunder, Igt.
— burning, Amm-m.
— constructing, Cannab.
— digging, Nux-m.
— drawing, *Anac.* Ang. Arg. Cannab. Cycl. Ntr-m. Ruta. Stann.
— squeezing, *Oleand.* Plat. Phosp-ac.
— stinging, *Asa-f.* Canth. Cina. Dros. Euph. Igt. *Mur-ac.* Plat. Sabad. *Sulph-ac.* Thuj.

34. GENERALITIES.

Pressing, tearing, rending, Arg. Bell. Bism. Cannab. Cupr. Cycl. Led. Ruta. Sass. Stann.
— by touch increased, *Cupr.*
Pressure outwards, agg., from, *Agar.* Ang. *Bar-c.* Bell. Bry. Calad. Cannab. Caps. Carb-veg. *Cina.* Guaj. *Hep.* Igt. *Iod.* Lach. *Lyc.* Mgn-c. Merc. Mez. Mosch Ntr-c. Nitr-ac Nux. Oleand. Plat. Phosp. Ran-b. Ran-sc. Ruta. Selen. Sep. *Sil.* Spong. Staph. Tarantula. Teucr. Verb. Zinc.
— — amel., Agn. Alum. Amm-c. Amm-m. Apis. Aur. Borax. Chelid. Chin. Clem. Cocc. *Con.* Dulc. Graph. Ind. Kali-c. *Mgn-m.* Mang. Mur-ac. *Ntr-c.* Par. Phosp. Phosp-ac. Plb. *Puls.* Rhus. Stann. Tong.
— — — of nightly pains, Phosp-ac.
— on painless side, agg., Ambr. Amm-c. *Bry.* Calc. Caust. Cham. Coff. Coloc. *Con.* Hep. *Igt.* Kali-c. *Nux.* Puls. Rhus. Sep. Spong. Stann. Viol-tr.
Prickling, Ferr-m. Mosch. Plat.
Pride, wounded and non-approval of others, agg., from, Pallad.
Pulsation, Ambr. Amm-m. Arn. Carb-veg. Clem. Creos. Glon. *Graph.* Kali-c. *Iod.* Ntr-m. Plb. *Puls.* Sabad. *Sabin.* Sec-c. Sep. Sil. Stront. Tabac. Tart. Thuj Zinc.
— outer parts, Acon. Agar. Arg. Asa-f. Igt. Kali-c. Ntr-m. *Oleand.* Plat Tar.
— inner parts, *Alum.* Asa-f. *Calc.* Iod. Merc. Oleand. Phosp. Plb. *Puls.* Spig. Spong. *Tart.* Thuj.
— in evening, Thuj.
— when at rest, Creos.
— from exertion and slight motion, Graph. *Iod.* Ntr-m. Puls. Thuj.
Pupurea miliaris, after, Acon. Coff. *Hell.*
Putrefaction of the flesh, Lach.
Quivering in external parts. Agar. *Asa-f.* Bell. Calc. *Kali-c.* Mez. *Ntr-c.* Nux. Sil. Spong. Sann. Stront.
— internal parts, Cannab.
Raising the limb, amel., Alum. *Calc.* Sabin.
Rawness, sense of. Ang. Canth.
Reaction, want of, Camph. Carb-veg. Cocc. *Laur.* Mosch. Nitr-ac. Op. *Sulph.*
Reading, from, agg., Agn. Asa-f. Bell *Calc.* Chin. Cina. *Cocc.* Con. Dulc Graph. Hep. Kali-c. Lyc. *Ntr-m.* Nux. Oleand. Phosp. Puls. Rhod. Ruta. *Sil.* Sulph. Sulph-ac. Verb.
— — aloud, agg., Carb-veg. Par. Phosp. Verb. (compare Talking.)
— amel., from, Ntr c.
Recline the head, inclination to, Carb-veg.
Redness of the cheeks, pain attended with, Cham.

Rending, tearing, pains, Aeth. *Agar.* Alum. Ambr. Amm-c. *Amm-m.* Arg. Arn. Ars. Asa-f. *Aur.* Bar-c. Bell. Berb. Bism. Borax. Bruc. *Bry.* Cannab. Calc. Canth. Carb-an Carb-veg. *Caust.* Cham. Chelid. *Chin.* Cina. Cocc. Colch. Coloc. Cupr. *Dulc.* Euph. Ferr. Graph. Grat. Guaj. *Hell.* Hep. Hyosc. Igt. Iod. *Kali-c.* Kali-jod. Lam. Laur. *Led.* Lyc. Mgn-c. Mgn-m. Mgn-s. Mang. *Merc. Mez. Mur-ac.* Ntr-c. Ntr-m. Ntr-s. *Nitr-ac. Nitr. Nux.* Ol-an. Petr. *Phosp. Phosp-ac. Plb. Puls.* Ran-b. Rat. *Rhod. Rhus.* Ruta. Sabin. *Sass. Sec-c. Sep. Sil. Spig.* Stann. *Staph. Stront. Sulph.* Sulph-ac. Tart. Teucr. Thuj. Tong. *Valer.* Verat. Verb. *Zinc.*
— outer parts, Acon. Alum. Ambr. Anac. *Arn.* Asa-f. Bell. *Bry.* Calc. Carb-veg. Caust. Cham. *Chin.* Dulc. Ferr. *Kali-c. Lyc.* Merc. Ntr-c. Nux. Puls. Rhed. Rhus. Sep. *Sil.* Stront. *Sulph.* Valer. *Zinc.*
— inner parts, Ambr. Arg. Aur. *Bell.* Bry. Caps. Cham. *Con.* Igt. *Lyc.* Merc. Ntr-m. *Nux.* Phosp. *Puls.* Rhod. *Sil.* Spig. Tar. Zinc.
— upwards, Anac. Ars. *Bell.* Con. Dulc. Ntr-c. Nitr-ac. Nux. Stront.
— downwards. Acon. Agar. Agn. Bar-c. Bry. *Caps.* Carb-veg. Chin. Ferr. Graph. Kali-c. *Lyc.* Merc. Ntr-c. Nux. Puls. Rhus. Sep. Sulph. Verat. Verb.
— in bed., Phosp. Stront. Sulph.
— after a cold, Dulc. Nitr-ac. Phosp.
— day and night, Nitr.
— in evening. Ntr-s. Stront. Sulph.
— — extensors, Verat.
— when moving, *Bry.* Chin. Zinc.
— — — relieved, Valer.
— at night, Lyc. Merc. Ntr-s. Phosp. *Plb.* Stront. *Sulph.*
— outwards, Asa-f.
— alter overheating, Zinc.
— by pressure upon, relieved, Tong.
— when at rest, Agar. Kali-c. Lyc. Mur-ac. Rhod. Rhus. Valer.
— by rubbing, relieved, Plb.
— when sitting. Agar. Cina. Staph. Verat.
— after sitting, when rising, *Puls.*
— in standing, *Agar.*
— with swelling of the parts, Kali-c.
— when touched, Chin.
— crampy, *Anac.* Calc. Chin. Meny. Mur-ac. *Ntr-c.* Petr. *Plat.*
— cutting, Hyosc.
— disabling, paralytic, *Aur.* Cham. Chin. Cina. *Cocc. Colch. Kali-c.* Mgn-m. Mez. Ntr-c. Sabin. Sass.
— drawing, *Cham.* Hell. Lam. Lyc. *Merc. Plb. Rhod. Rhus. Sec-c.* Staph.
— jerking, *Amm-m.* Asar. *Chin. Cocc.* Cupr. Ntr-s. Phosp-ac. *Puls.* Staph.
— pressing, Arg. Bell. Bism. Cannab.

34. GENERALITIES.

Carb-veg. Cupr. Cycl. Kali-c. Led. Ruta. Sass. *Stann.* Staph.
Rending, tearing, squeezing, cramping, Cina. Ntr-c. *Ruta.*
— stinging, *Cannab.* Canth. Colch. *Coloc.* Dig. Euph. *Guaj. Merc.* Thuj. Zinc.
— sensation, Plb. *Rhus.*
— pain as from, *Coff.* Ntr-m. *Nux.* Staph. Teucr.
Rest, inclination to, Carb-veg. (compare, Lie down; and sit down.)
— by, agg., *Agar.* Amm-c. Amm-m. *Asa-f. Aur.* Benz-ac. Brom. *Caps.* Coloc. *Con. Cycl.* Dros. *Dulc. Euph. Ferr.* Glon. Kali-c. Kali-jod. *Lyc. Mgn-c.* Mgn-m. Meny. *Mosch. Mur-ac.* Ntr-s. Op. Phell. *Phosp-ac. Plat. Puls. Rhod. Rhus.* Ruta. *Sabad. Samb. Seneg. Sep. Sil.* Stann. *Sulph. Tar.* Tong. *Valer.* Verb. *Viol-od.* Zinc.
— — cough, agg., Ambr. Ars. Dros. Dulc. Euphr. Ferr. Hyosc. Mgn-c. Mgn-m. Phosp-ac. Puls. Rhus. Sabad. Samb. Seneg. Sep. Sil. Stann. Sulph. Verb. Zinc.
— amel., by, Acon. Agn. Ant. Arn. Asar. Bar-c. *Bell. Bry.* Calad. Camph. Cannab. Carb-an. Chelid. Cocc. Coff. *Colch.* Coloc. Croc. Cupr. Dig. Graph Hell. Hep. Igt. Iod. Ip. Kali-c. Laur. *Led.* Merc. Nitr-ac. Nitr. *Nux.* Ol-an. Phosp. Ran-b. Rheum. Sabad. Sass. Scill. Selen. Spig. Spong. Stram. Verat.
Resting limb on something, amel., Amm-c. Calc. Puls. Staph.
— knees, amel., Euph.
Restlessness, Acon. Ambr. *Anac.* Apis. *Ars.* Asar. *Bell.* Borax. Bry. Calc. Carb-veg. Caust. Cham. Chin. Croc. Ferr. *Hyosc.* Igt. Iod. *Merc.* Lam. Nux-m. *Nux.* Op. Phosp-ac. Plat. *Puls. Rhus.* Samb. Scill. *Sep. Sil. Staph. Stram. Sulph.* Tabac. *Valer.*
— at 3 A. M., everything feels, sore, must walk about, Nicc.
— in bed, Mgn-m.
— — children, Borax. *Cham. Jalap.* Rheum. Tart.
— — — by being carried, relieved, *Cham.* Kali-c. Tart.
— by close thinking, Borax.
— in evening, *Alum. Amm-c. Caust.* Lyc. Mgn-c. Mgn-m. *Merc.* Ntr-c.
— — 4 to 6 P. M., Carb-veg.
— — open air, Plat.
— with the pains, Ars. *Cham. Coff. Mgn-c.* Mang. Tabac.
— in parts affected, Arn. Chin. Ferr.
— when at rest, Cros. Plat.
— after siting, Caust. Mgn-c. Ntr-m. *Sil.* Sulph.
— — talking and walking, Ambr.
— — with nausea, Borax.

— when lying long in one position, changing is painful, Ntr-s.
— from sensation as if everything in abdomen was constricted, Mosch.
— with dyspnoea, Prun.
— — pulsations, Borax.
— — vomiting, colic and suppressed menses, Nicc.
Rhacitic affections, *Asa-f. Bell.* Calc. *Lyc. Merc.* Mez. Nitr-ac. Petr. Phosp. Phosp-ac. Puls. *Sil. Staph. Sulph.*
Rheumatic affections, *Acon. Ant. Arn. Ars. Bell. Bry.* Calc. Camph. Cannab. *Carb-veg. Caust. Cham. Chin. Colch.* Cupr. Dulc. Euph. Gels. *Igt.* Kalm. Kali-chl. Led. Mgn-c. Mgn-s. Meph. *Merc.* Merc-sulph Mez. Mur-ac. Nitr-ac Nux-m. *Nux.* Ol-an. Pallad. Psor. Puls. *Ran-b.* Rhod. *Rhus.* Sacch. Sang. Scill. Sil. Stann. Tart. Teucr. *Valer.* Verat.
— — after a cold, Dulc. Nitr ac.
— — — suppressed gonorrhoea, Cop. Daph. Sass.
— — upper arms and lower part of legs, Kalm.
— — go from upper to lower parts, Kalm.
— — — lower to upper parts, Led.
— — commence on left side, Elaps.
— — with decreased secretion of urine, Sass.
— — — profuse secretion of urine, Led.
— — in warm weather, stitches in cold, Colch.
— — on places least covered by flesh, (not joints), Sang.
— — with diseases of urinary organs, Berb.
— — gastric symptoms alternate with, Kali-b.
Rhus, poisoning, from, Cop. Kalm. Sang.
Riding in a carriage, agg., Ars. Bry. Borax. Carb-veg. *Cocc.* Graph. Hep. Hyosc. Igt. Lach. Mgn-c. Meph. Ntr-m. Nux-m. Op. Petr. Phosp. Rhus. Selen. *Sep.* Sil. Sulph.
— amel., Ars. Graph. *Nitr-ac.* Phosp.
— on horseback, agg , Ntr-c. *Sep.* Sulph-ac.
— — amel., Brom. Kali-c.
Rigid, skin and muscles, Acon.
Right side, (compare One-sided.)
Rising, on, agg., *Acon.* Amm-m. Arn. Ars. *Bell. Bry.* Cannab. Cham. Cic. Cocc. Con. Ferr. Igt. Lyc. Mur-ac. Ntr-m. Nitr-ac. *Nux. Op.* Phosp. Puls. *Rhus.* Scill. *Sulph.* Viol-tr.
— amel., *Amm-c.* Ars. Borax. *Calc.* Cham. Dig. Hyosc. Igt. Kali-c. Puls. Sabin. *Samb. Sep.* Sil. Tart.
— from bed, agg., Acon. Apis. Bell. *Bry.* Calc. Caps. *Carb-veg.* Cham. Cina. Cocc. *Con.* Graph. Guaj. Hep. *Igt.* Kali-b. *Lach.* Lyc. Ntr-m. Nux. Oleand.

34. GENERALITIES.

Phosp. Phosp-ac. Rhod. Rhus. Sabin.
Samb. Selen. Sil. Spig. Staph. Thuj.
Valer. Verat.
Rising from bed, amel., Ars. Aur. Caps.
Dulc. Ferr. Igt Led Lyc. Plat. Puls. Rhus.
Samb. Sep. Verat.
— after, from bed, agg., Amm-m. Calc.
Carb veg. Cham. Graph. Guaj. Hell.
Igt. Kali-b. Lach. Ntr-m. Nux. Oleand.
Phosp. Puls. Ran-b. Rhus. Spig. Staph.
Sulph. Verat.
— — — — amel., Ambr. Amm-c. Arg.
Ars. Aur. Bell. Borax. Carb-an.
Coloc. Dros. Euph. Ferr. Igt.
Iod Kali-c. Led. Lyc. Mgn-c.
Merc. Nux. Phosp. Plat. Puls.
Rhod. Rhus. Selen. Sep. Spig.
Stront. Sulph. Tart. Verat.
— from a seat, agg., Acon. Apis. Bar-c.
Bell. Bry. Caps. Carb-veg. Caust. Chin.
Con. Euph. Ferr. Fluor-ac. Laur. Led.
Lyc. Ntr-m. Nitr-ac. Nux. Oleand. Petr.
Phosp. Phosp-ac. Puls. Rhus. Ruta. Sep.
Spig. Staph. Sulph. Tart. Thuj. Verat.
— — — amel., Aur. Dulc. Igt. Mgn-c.
Nux-m. Puls. Sep. Verat.
— after from a seat, agg., (compare Beginning to move).
— — — amel., Agar. Ambr. Ang. Arg.
Asa-f. Bar-c. Caps. Cina. Con.
Cycl. Dros. Dulc. Euph. Ferr.
Lach. Lyc. Mgn-m. Meny. Mosch.
Mur-ac. Ntr-c. Phosp-ac. Plat.
Puls. Rhod. Rhus. Ruta. Sabad.
Seneg. Sep. Tar. Valer. Verb.
Viol-tr.
Rocked all the time, the child wants to be, Cina.
—agg., from being, Borax. Carb-veg.
Room, in a, agg., Acon. Aeth. Agn. Alum.
Ambr. Anac. Ant. Arg. Asa-f. Asar.
Aur. Croc. Dig. Graph. Hell. Hep.
Mgn-c. Mgn-m. Mang. Mez. Ntr-m.
Nux. Op. Phosp. Phosp-ac. Plat. Puls.
Ran-sc. Rhod. Rhus Sabin. Sep. Spong.
Sulph.
— — — amel., Agar. Arn. Bry. Camph.
Carb-an. Carb-veg. Caust. Cham.
Chelid. Chin. Cocc. Coff.
Con. Creos. Ferr. Guaj. Lach.
Mang. Mosch. Nux-m. Nux. Petr.
Sang. Sass. Selen. Sil. Spig.
Stann. Stram. Teucr. Tilia. Valer.
— — full of people, agg., Hell. Lyc.
Mgn-c. Phosp. Puls. Sep. Sulph.
— warm, agg., Acon. Agn. All-cep. Alum.
Ambr. Anac Ant. Apis. Asar. Brom.
Croc. Hipp. Iod. Puls. Sabin. Seneg.
Roughness, sensation of, in inner parts,
Alum. Calc. Carb-veg. Caust. Cocc.
Dig. Dros. Laur. Mgn-c. Nux. Par.
Phosp. Phosp-ac. Puls. Rhus. Sass.
Seneg. Stann. Stront. Sulph. Sulph-ac.

Zinc.
Rubbing, agg., from, Anac. Bism. Calad.
Caps. Caust. Coff. Con. Led. Mez. Puls.
Sep. Sil. Stront.
— amel., Alum. Arn. Asa-f. Calc. Canth.
Cycl. Dros. Guaj. Ind. Igt. Merc.
Mur-ac. Ntr-c. Phosp. Plb. Ruta.'Sulph.
Thuj. Zinc.
Running, agg., from, Ang. Arn. Ars. Bell.
Bry. Cannab. Caust. Cupr. Igt. Kali-c.
Led. Lyc. Merc. Ntr-m. Nux. Oleand.
Rhod. Rhus. Seneg. Sil. Spig. Sulph.
— amel., Igt. Sep.
— in limbs like a mouse, Bell. Calc. Sep.
Sulph.
Salt food, agg., from, Carb-veg. Dros.
Scarlet fever, suppressed, from, Amm-c.
Apis. Bell. Bry. Cham. Ferr. Hep.
Kali-c. Lach. Merc.
Sciatica, Curare. Gnaphel. Iris. Kali-b.
Lach. Lyc. Phyt. Plantago-maj.
Tellur.
— right side, Tellur.
— worse from least motion, must lie still, Lach.
Scraping pain, Chin. Lyc. Puls.
Scratching, agg., from, Anac. Bism. Calad.
Caps. Caust. Con. Led. Led. Mez. Puls.
Sil. Stront.
— amel., Arn. Asa-f. Bry. Calc. Canth.
Cycl. Dros. Guaj. Igt. Mang. Mur-ac.
Ntr-c. Phosp. Plb. Ruta. Sulph. Thuj.
Zinc.
— on linen, agg., Asar.
Scrofulous, complaints, Ambr. Ars. Asa-f.
Aur. Bar-c. Bell. Bov. Bry. Calc. Chin.
Cina. Cocc. Con. Dulc. Ferr. Hep. Igt.
Lyc Mgn-c. Merc. Mez. Mur-ac. Ntr-c.
Ntr-m. Nux. Phosp. Puls. Ran-b. Rhus.
Sep. Sil. Staph. Sulph. Verat.
— incipient, Ars. Bell. Calc. Chin. Cina.
Ferr. Mgn-c. Puls. Rheum. Sep. Sulph.
— with glandular swelling, Bar-c. Calc.
Cist. Con. Dulc. Graph. Hep. Lyc.
Mgn-c. Ntr-c. Nitr-ac. Phosp. Rhus.
Sep. Sil. Spong. Staph. Sulph.
— in the fully developed stage, Ars. Asa-f.
Bar-c. Bell. Calc. Con. Cupr. Igt. Mez.
Op. Sil.
Scurvy, Ars. Canth. Carb-an. Carb-veg.
Caust. Merc. Mur-ac. Ntr-m. Nitr-ac.
Nux. Staph. Sulph.
Sea-sickness, Cocc. Colch. Ferr. Hyosc.
Kali-b. Ntr-m. Nux. Op. Petr. Sec-c.
Sep. Sil. Tabac. Therid.
Sedentary life, from a, Acon. Aloe. Alum.
Ars. Aur. Bry. Croc. Lyc. Mgn-c.
Mgn-m. Nux. Op. Phosp. Puls. Rhus.
Sulph.
Sensation, loss of, Acon. Anac. Arn. Ars.
Bell. Calc. Caust. Chin. Cic. Cocc.
Hell. Laur. Lyc. Merc. Mosch. Nux.
Oleand. Op. Phosp. Phosp-ac. Plat. Plb.

34. GENERALITIES.

Puls. Rhus. Sec-c. Sep. Stram. *Sulph.* Zinc.
Sensitiveness, to cold air, Agar. Amm-c. Anac. Ant. *Aur. Calc. Camph.* Carb-an. *Caust.* Cist. *Cocc. Coff.* Ip. Lyc. Mez. Mosch. Ntr-c. Nux. Petr. *Phosp.* Rhod. Rhus. *Sabad. Sep.* Spig. Sulph.
— — damp, Amm-c. Calc. Carb-veg. Dulc. Mur-ac. Nux-m. Rhod. Rhus. Sep. Sulph.
— — draft, of air, *Acon.* Anac. Bell. *Calc.* Camph. Carb-an. *Caust. Cham.* Chin. Cocc. Coff. Graph. *Hep. Ign.* Kali-c. *Lach. Lyc.* Merc. Ntr-c. Ntr-m. Nitr-ac. *Nux-m. Nux.* Petr. Puls. Selen. *Sil.* Stram. Sulph. Verat.
— evening air, Carb-an. Carb-veg. Sulph.
— open air, Bell. Calc. *Carb-an.* Caust. *Cham.* Cocc. *Coff.* Graph. Guaj. Ign. Kali-c. Lyc. Merc-cor. Mosch. Ntr-c. Nux-m. Nux. Petr. Phosp. Plb. Puls. Rhus. Sep. Sil.
— warm air, Aur. Calc. *Cocc.* Ign. Rhus. Sep.
— to pain, Acon. Agar. Arn. Asar. *Aur.* Bar-c. Bell. Cantn. *Cham.* Chin. Cina. Cocc. *Coff.* Colch. Con. Cupr. *Lyc.* Mgn-c. Ntr-c. Nux. Petr. *Phosp. Sep* Spig.
— — touch, *Acon. Agar.* Ant. *Bell. Bry.* Camph. Cina. Cocc. Colch. Mez. Nux-m. *Tart.*
— — wind, *Cham.* Sulph.
— — north wind, Sep.
Sewing agg., from, Lach. *Ntr-m.*
Sexual excesses, agg., from, Agar. Anac. Bov. *Calc.* Carb-veg. Chin. *Con.* Iod. Kali-c. Merc. *Mosch.* Ntr-c. Ntr-m. Nux. *Phosp. Phosp-ac.* Puls. *Sep.* Sil. Spig. *Staph.* Sulph.
— instinct, suppression of, agg., Con.
Shocks, Acon. *Ambr.* Anac. Ang. *Arn.* Bar-c. Bell. Cannab. Cic. *Cina.* Cocc. Colch. Croc. Cupr. Dulc. Hell. *Lyc.* Mez. Mur-ac. Nux-m. Nux. Oleand. *Plat.* Ran-b. *Ruta.* Spig. *Sulph. Sulph-ac.* Zinc.
Shuddering, pains accompanied by, Ars. Bar-c. Euph. Mez. Ran-b. Sep.
— on parts affected, Ars.
Singing, when, agg., Amm-c. *Carb-veg.* Dros. *Phosp.* Stann. Sulph.
— after, agg., Hep.
Sit, inclination to, Agar. Amm-m. Ars. *Bar-c.* Bell. Cannab. Carb-veg. Chelid. *Chin.* Cocc. *Con.* Euphr. *Graph.* Guaj. Iod. Mur-ac. Ntr-m. Nitr-ac. *Nux. Phosp.* Phosp-ac. Ran-sc. *Scill.* Sec-c. Sep. Sulph. Tar. Teucr. Zinc.
Sitting, while agg., *Acon.* Agar. Aloe. Alum. Ambr. *Anac.* Ang. *Ars.* Asa-f. Bar-c. Bell. Brom. Cadm. Calc. *Caps.* Caust. *Chin.* Cic. Cina. *Con.* Cycl. Dig.

Dros. *Dulc. Euph.* Euphr. Ferr Glon. Graph. Grat. *Guaj.* Kali-c. Kobalt. Lach. *Lyc.* Mgn-c. Mgn m. Meny. Merc. Mosch. Mur-ac. Ntr-c. *Ntr-m.* Op. Phell. Phosp-ac. *Plat. Puls.* Rhod. *Rhus.* Ruta. Sabad. Seneg. *Sep.* Sil. Staph. *Sulph.* Sulph-ac. Tar. *Tart.* Tong. Valer. Verat. *Verb. Viol-tr.*
— amel., Aur. *Bry.* Calad. Calc. Carb-an. Coff. *Colch.* Mang. Ntr-m. *Nux.* Petr. Phosp-ac. Rheum. Scill. Staph. Verat.
— after, agg., Ang. Caps. Con. Euph. Ferr. Lyc. Nitr-ac. Nux. Puls. Sep. Sil.
— crooked, agg., Acon. Ang. Amm-m. Ars. Brom. Cic. *Dig.* Phosp. Rhus. Sabin. Samb. Sang. Scill. Sulph. *Tart.*
— amel., Bell. Colch. Coloc Con. Ign. *Kali-c.* Lyc. Merc. Mez. Rheum.
— down, on, agg., Agn. Chelid. Coff. Hell. Ip. Mgn-c. Samb. Spong. Valer.
— amel., Bar-c. Bell. *Caps.* Carb-veg. Caust. Con. Euph. Ferr. Laur. Led. Ntr-m. Nux. Oleand. Petr. Phosp. Sep. Spig. Sulph.
Skin and flesh, between, pains seem to be, Zinc.
Sleepiness, by, pains attended, Apis. Nux-m.
Sleep, in, pains perceptible, *Ars.* Carb-veg. Chin. Graph. Hep. *Nitr-ac.* Sil. Sulph. Sulph-ac.
— —, pains disturbing, *Cham. Coff.*
— — during, cough, agg., Acon. Arn. Calc. Carb-an. Cham. Hyosc. Lach. Merc. Samb. Sep. Stram Verb.
— in first part, agg., *Ars. Bry.* Calc. Carb-an. Carb-veg. Graph. Lyc. Merc. Phosp. *Puls.* Rhus. *Sep.*
— during, agg., Acon. *Ars.* Bar-c. *Bell.* Borax. *Bry. Cham.* Chin. Con. *Hep.* Hyosc. Ign. Kali-c. Lyc. Merc. Mur-ac. *Op.* Phosp. Phosp-ac. *Puls.* Rheum. Samb. Sep. *Sil.* Stram. *Sulph.*
— before falling in, Merc.
— on falling in, pains return, Lil-tigr.
— after, agg., Acon. Anac. Apis. Arn. Camph. Carb-veg. Caust. Cina. *Cocc.* Con. Euphr. Ferr. Graph. Hep. Lac-can. Lach. Lyc. Mur-ac. *Op.* Puls. Rheum. Sabad. Stann. Staph. *Stram. Sulph.* Thuj. Verat.
— — amel., Ars. Calad. Colch. Nux. *Phosp.* Sep.
— after a long, agg., Calc. Caust. Con. Euphr. Graph. Hep. Nux. Stram. *Sulph.*
— in the afternoon, agg., Lach. Phosp. Puls. *Staph.* Sulph.
— in a state of half, amel., Selen.
Sluggishness of body, Amm-m. Anac. Ars. Calc. Camph. Carb-an. Carb-veg. Chelid. Cinnab. Con. Dulc. Guaj. Iod. Ip. Kali-c. Laur. Lyc. Mgn-m. Merc. Mez. Mur-ac. Ntr-c. Ntr-m. Nitr-ac.

34. GENERALITIES.

Nux. Oleand. Op. Petr. Phosp. Phosp-ac. Plb. Puls. Rhod. Sec-c. Sep. Stann. Stram. Sulph. Verb.
Sluggishness, in morning, Carb-an. Chelid. Ntr-c. Ntr-m. Verb.
— — sttting, Chelid.
Small, spot to a, pains confined, Fluor-ac.
Smaller, sensation of becoming, Calc.
Smells, strong, agg., from, Acon. *Aur. Bell.* Cham. Chin. *Coff.* Colch. Graph. *Igt.* Lyc. *Nux. Phosp.* Sulph.
— — of camphor, agg., Nitr.
Smoke, agg., from, Euphr. Sep. Spig.
Sneezing, agg., from, Amm-m. Ars. Bell. Borax. Carb-veg. Cham. Dros. Lyc. Merc. Nux. Puls. Rhus. Sabad. Sep. Spig.
— while, amel., Mgn-m.
Snowy air, agg., from, Calc. *Con.* Lyc. Phosp-ac. Puls. *Sep.* Sil. Sulph.
Sobbing, hiccoughing, agg., from, *Amm-m.* Bry. Cycl. Hyosc. Igt. Nux. Teucr.
Soft, hard parts feeling, Merc. Nitr-ac.
Solitude, agg., (compare Alone).
— amel., from, Bar-c. Lyc. Plb. *Sep.*
Sore pains, (as of excoriation,) Acon. Alum. Amm-m. Ant. Arg. Arn. Berb. Bry. Calc. *Canth.* Caust. Cic. Colch. *Graph. Hep. Igt.* Merc. Mez. Ntr-m. *Nux.* Phosp. Phyt. *Plat.* Puls. Rat. Rhus. Staph. Sulph. Sulph-ac. Zinc.
— — inner parts, Alum. Arg. Bry. Calc *Canth.* Chin. *Igt.* Lyc. Mez. Nitr-m Nitr-ac. *Nux.* Phosp. Phosp-ac. Puls. Ran-b. *Sep.* Stann. Zinc.
— — of mucus membranes, *Mez.*
— — — parts affected, *Canth.* Hep. *Puls.*
— — — — on which he lies Ruta.
— — when touched, *Hep.* Mang. *Puls.*
— — under the ribs, Apis.
Spasms, Aeth. Alum. *Ambr.* Ang. Arn. *Ars. Asa-f.* Aur. Bar-c. *Bell.* Bry. Calc *Camph. Canth.* Carb-veg. Caust. *Cham.* Cic. Cina. Cocc. *Coff.* Coloc. *Con.* Croc. Cupr. Dig. Ferr. Hell. *Hyosc. Igt. Ip.* Jatr. Kali-c. Lach. *Laur.* Lyc. *Mosch.* Ntr-s. Nitr. *Nux-m.* Nux. *Op.* Phosp. Plat. *Plb.* Puls. Ran-sc. Rhus. Sabad. *Scill.* Sec-c. Sep. Sil. Sol-nig. Spig. Stann. *Stram. Sulph.* Tabac. Tanac. Tart. Thuj. *Verat.*
— body stretched out stiff and becomes rigid, Cina. Ip.
— by bright light produced, Bell. Stram.
— cataleptic, Acon. Ars. Bell. Cham. Cic. Cupr. Merc. Plat. Stram. Verat.
— clonic, Agar. Arn. *Ars.* Asa-f. Bar-c. *Bell.* Bry. Calc. *Camph. Canth.* Caust. *Cham.* Cic. Cina. Cocc. *Coff.* Con. Croc. *Cupr.* Dig. Hell. *Hyosc. Igt. Ip.* Jatr. Kali-c. *Laur.* Lyc. Merc. Mez. *Mosch.* Ntr-m *Nux-m. Nux. Op.* Phosp. Plat *Plb.* Ran-sc. Sabad. *Scill.* Sec-c. Sep.

Spig. *Stann.* Stram. Sulph. Tabac. *Tanac. Tart.* Verat.
Spasms, from cockle seed, Camph.
— with coldness, Camph. Caust. Cic. Hyosc. Mosch. Op. Verat.
— — of limbs, Cham. Coff.
— commences in fingers and toes, Cupr.
— — — face, Dulc.
— with convulsive laughing, *Alum.* Apis. Aur. Calc. Con. Croc. Igt. Phosp.
— — weeping. Alum. Aur. Caust. Cupr. Stram.
— from congestions to head, fingers spread apart and stretched out, Glon.
— with cries, piercing, Cupr.
— — sudden shrill, Apis. Op.
— — in dentition, Bell. Calc. *Cham.* Chin. Cupr. Dolich. *Igt.* Stann. Stram.
— delirium, followed by, Kali-chl.
— with watery diarrhœa, Hyosc.
— after drinking, Hyosc.
— when eruptions are driven in, Cupr.
— falls senseless, rigid, eyes turned up and open during attack; after, confusion of mind and no recollection of paroxysm, Tarantula.
— with foam at mouth, Op.
— from fright, Hyosc. Igt. Op. *Sec-c. Stram.* Sulph. Zinc.
— with gnashing of teeth, Acon. Caust. Coff. Hyosc. Sulph.
— hiccough, preceded by, Cupr.
— hysteric, Alum. Asa f. *Aur.* Bell. *Bry.* Calc. Caust. *Cocc. Con. Igt.* Iod. Ip. *Mgn-m.* Millef. Mosch. Nux-m. *Plat.* Sec-c. *Sep. Stann. Stram.* Sulph. Valer.
— — with full consciousness, at break of day, Plat.
— inner parts, Alum. Asa-f. Bell. Bism. Bry. Calc. Carb an. Carb-veg. *Caust.* Cham. *Cocc.* Coff *Coloc.* Con. *Croc.* Cupr. Euphr. Ferr. Graph. *Hyosc. Igt.* Ip. Kali-c. Lyc. Mgn-m. Merc. Mosch. Ntr-m. *Nux.* Phosp. *Plb. Puls.* Sec-c. Sep. *Stann* Staph. Valer. Zinc.
— inveterate, chronic, Cupr.
— from lukewarm water, Ang.
— in lying-in women, Cham. Cic. Hyosc. Op.
— with suppressed menstruation, Gels.
— from mercurial vapors, Stram.
— at night, Calc. Cina. Cupr. Hyosc. Kali-c. Lyc. Sec-c. Sil. Sulph.
— — midnight, Cocc.
— by noise excited, Ang. Arn. Igt.
— from obstinacy, Bell.
— one sided with speechlessness, Dulc.
— with opisthotonous, Ang. Arg. Bell. Cham. Cic. Cina. Cupr. Igt. Nux. Op. Rhus. Stann. Stram.
— — — and distorted face, Stram.
— by oppression of chest followed, Bell.
— — — — alternating with, Igt.

34. GENERALITIES.

Spasms, palms of hands and soles of feet spasmodically turned inwards, Verat.
— by paralysis followed, Plb.
— on paralysed side, Phosp.
— periodically returning, Bar-m. Sec-c. Str..m.
— with profuse perspiration, followed by sleep, Stram.
— cold, perspiration, Ferr.
— in pregnant women, *Cham.* Cic. *Hyosc.* Millef.
— in sleep, at night, *Cupr.* Kali-c. Sil.
— with deep, heavy, sleep, Hyosc.
— by smiling preceded, Bell.
— — stretching out the parts, amel., Sec-c.
— from swallowing liquids, Bell. Hyosc. Stram.
— with thirst, Cic.
— tonic, *Alum. Ambr. Ang.* Ars. Aur. *Bell.* C*amph.* Caust. *Cham.* Cic. Cina. *Cocc. Coloc.* Con. Croc. Cupr. Hell. *Hyosc.* Igt. *Ip.* Kali-c. *Laur. Lyc.* Meny. Merc. *Mosch.* Nitr. *Nux-m. Nux.* Op. Petr. *Plat.* Plb. Ran-b. Sabad. Scill. *Sec-c. Sep. Sol-nig.* Stann. *Stram.* Sulph. *Tabac. Tart.* Verat.
— by touch excited, *Ang. Bell.* Cocc. *Stram* Tart.
— from an ulcer originating, Cocc.
— with vomiting and colic, Camph. Cupr. Ip. Lach. Lyc. Ntr-m. Nux. Puls.
— from worms, Cic. Hyosc. Merc. Sulph.
Spasmodic pains, *Coloc. Con.* Gels. Mgn-m.
Spamodic (cramping), drawing in limbs. Ambr. Amm-c. Asar. *Calc.* Camph. *Caps.* Cocc. Coff. Coloc. Con. Ferr *Graph.* Hyosc. Kali-c. Lyc. Nitr-ac. *Nux.* Phosp. Plat. Rhus. Sil. Staph. Stram. *Sulph.* Sulph-ac. Zinc.
— — in muscles, Agar. *Ambr. Anac. Ang. Asa-f.* Asar. Calc. Chelid. Cina. *Coloc. Con. Graph.* Lyc. Merc. Mosch. Ntr-c. *Oleand. Plat.* Ruta. Sec-c. Sep. Stram.
— curvature of limbs, Ambr. *Calc.* Carb-an. Caust. Chin. Cina. Colch. *Coloc.* Con. Euph. Ferr. *Graph.* Guaj. *Hyosc.* Kali-c. Kali-jod. *Lyc.* Meny. *Merc.* Nux. Phosp. Plb. Rhus. *Sec-c. Sil.* Stram. Sulph.
— jerking, Anac. Asa-f. Mosch.
— pressing, Bar-c. *Oleand. Plat.*
— rending, tearing, Cina. Ntr-c. *Ruta.*
— in sitting, Agar.
Spirituous liquors, agg., from, Agar. Ant. Ars. Bell. Bov. Calc. Carb-veg. Chelid. Chin. Coff. Con. Igt. *Lach.* Led. Lyc. Ntr-c. Ntr-m. Nux-m. *Nux. Op.* Puls *Ran-b.* Rhod. Rhus. Ruta. Sacch. Selen. Sil. Spig. Stram. Verat. Zinc.
Spitting, agg., from, Led. Nux.
Splinters, as from, pain, Carb-veg. Cham. Chin. Lac-can. Nitr-ac. Sil.
Spraining, disposition to, Agn. Carb-an. Con. Lyc. *Ntr-c.* Ntr-m. Nitr-ac. Nux.

Petr. Phosp. *Rhus.* Ruta Sulph.
— easy, Ntr-c. Ntr-m. Rhus. Sep.
— spontaneous, Bry. Calc. Lyc. Nitr-ac. Petr. Phosp. Sulph. Zinc.
— violent, Amm-c. *Arn. Rhus. Ruta.*
— pains, Agn. Ambr. *Amm-c. Arn.* Asar. Bar-c. Bell. Berb. Bry. Calc. *Carb-veg. Caust.* Dios. Igt. Mez. *N'tr-m.* Oleand. Petr. Phosp. Puls. Rhod. *Rhus.* Sep.
Spig. Stann. *Sulph.* Thuj. Zinc.
— — at night, in lying, Mosch.
— — inner parts, Lyc.
Spring, sensation like a, Rheum.
Spring in the, agg., Ambr. *Aur.* Bell. Calc. Carb-veg. Lyc. Ntr-m. Rhus. *Verat.*
Squeezing pains, outer parts, Anac. *Ang.* Bell. Calc. Carb-veg. Cina. Nitr *Plat.*
— — inner parts, Acon. *Ambr.* Ang. Calc. Carb-veg. Cocc. Colch. Coloc. *Igt.* Kali-c. Mez. Nux. *Phosp-ac. Plat.* Staph. Zinc.
Staggering when walking, Acon. Agar. Arg-n. Asar. *Bell. Bry.* Camph. *Cannab.* Caps. Caust. Cocc. Coff. Con. Hyosc. Igt. Iod. Lact. Laur. Mez. Mur-ac. Ntr-c. Ntr m. Nux-m. *Nux.* Oleand. *Op.* Phosp-ac. Rhus. *Ruta.* Sec-c. Sil. *Stram. Sulph.* Teucr. Thuj. *Verat.* Verb.
Standing, agg., when, Acon. Agar. Aloe. Amm-c. Aur. Bry. Caps. Cic. Cocc. Con. *Cycl.* Euph. Euphr. Ferr. Mgn-c. Mang. Nitr-ac. Nux-m. Pallad. Petr. Phosp. Phosp-ac. Plat. Puls. Rhus. Sabad. Samb. Sep. Sulph. Tar. *Valer.* Verat. Verb. Zinc.
— cough, agg., Euph. Sep. Sulph. Zinc.
— erect, cough, agg., Ntr-m.
— still during a walk, cough, agg., Igt.
— amel., when, *Ars.* Asar. *Bell.* Calad. Calc. Cannab. Colch. Iod. Ip. Led. Mur-ac. Nux. Phosp. Ran-b. Scill. Selen.
Startings, Acon. Ars. *Bell.* Bism. *Bry.* Caust. Chin. Colch. Hep. Igt. Kali-c. Merc. *Nux.* Rhus. *Stront.* Sulph.
Stepping heavily on ground, agg., from, Anac. Ang. Ant. Arn. Asar. Bell. *Bry.* Calc. Caust. Chin. *Con.* Graph. Hell. Led. Lyc. Mgn-m. Ntr-c. Ntr-m. Nitr-ac. Nux. Phosp. Ran-b. *Rhus.* Sabad. Sep. *Sil.* Sulph.
— — amel., Caps.
Stiffness of limbs, Acon. Aeth. Agar. Ang. Arn. Bar-m. *Bell.* Berb. Bry. *Caps.* Carb-an Caust. Cham. Cocc. Coloc. Cupr. Graph. Kali-c. Lach. Led. Lith. Lyc. Nux. Ol-an. *Petr. Plat.* Plb. Puls. *Rhus.* Sass. Sep. Stram. *Sulph. Tereb.* Thuj. Verat.
— — convulsive, Sang.
— — after exertion, Arn.

34. GENERALITIES.

Stiffness of limbs in morning, amel., by walking in openair, Amm-m.
— — with coldness, Plat.
— — on right side, as if paralyzed, Stront.
— — immovable, as if paralyzed, Sass.
— — painless, Oleand.
— — spasmodic, without loss of consciousness, with spasmodic yawning and trismus and speechlessness, Plat.
— — in evening, after sitting, Ang.
— — — forenoon, Verat.
— — when moving the part after rest, Rhus.
— — after walking, Verat.
Stinging, stitches, *Acon.* Aeth. All-cep. Alum. *Amm-c. Amm-m.* Ant. Arn. *Asa-f.* Aur. *Bell.* Borax. *Bry.* Calc. Camph. *Cannab.* Canth. Caust. Chin. Cocc. Colch. Con. Daph. Dig. Dios. Dulc. Euph. Evon. Ferr. Graph. Guaj. *Hell.* Igt. Ind. Kali-c. Laur. *Lyc.* Mang. Meny. *Merc.* Mosch Mur-ac. Ntr-c. Ntr-m. Ntr-s. Nicc. Nitr-ac. Nitr. *Nux.* Par. Phosp. Puls. *Ran-b. Ran-sc.* Rat. *Rhus.* Sabad. Sabin. *Sass. Sep.* Sil. *Spig* Spong. Stann. *Staph. Sulph.* Tar. *Thuj.* Verat. Viol-tr. Zinc.
— boring, Hell.
— burning, Alum. Apis. Arg. *Asa-f.* Bar-c Bell. Berb. Cina. *Cocc.* Dig. *Mez.* Nux. Oleand. *Plat.* Puls. Rhus. Sabad. *Staph. Sulph-ac. Thuj.*
— — ending with a stitch, Lith.
— after a cold, Dulc.
— concussive, Nux.
— crosswise, Sep.
— downwards, *Carb-veg.* Caust. *Ferr.* Puls.
— drawing, Borax. Calc. Dulc. Merc.
— in evening, Ntr-s. Ran-sc.
— gnawing, *Dros.*
— jerking, Calc. *Cina.* Lyc. *Mang. Nux.*
— inward, Alum. Arg. *Asa-f.* Bell. Calc. Canth. *Chin.* Con. Dulc. Lyc. Mez. Ntr-c. Rhus. Sabad. Sil. *Spig. Spong.* Stann. Staph. *Sulph.* Tar. *Valer.*
— inner parts, Acon. Alum. Arn. *Asa-f.* Bell. Bov. *Bry.* Calc. *Canth.* Caust. *Chelid. Chin.* Creos. *Igt.* Kali-c. Laur. Lyc. Mgn-c. Mgn-m. Ntr-c. Nitr-ac. *Phosp.* Phosp-ac. Plb. *Puls.* Rhus. Sabad. Sass. *Sep. Spig.* Staph. Sulph. Tar. *Verb.* Zinc.
— lengthwise, *Coloc.*
— when moving, Arn. Bry.
— at night, Ntr-s. Sulph.
— outwards, *Arn.* Calc. *Canth.* Igt. Laur. Plb. Sabin.
— in parts injured, Arn.
— pressing, *Asa-f.* Canth. Chin. Dros. *Euph. Igt.* Mur-ac Plat. Sabad. *Sass. Sulph-ac.* Thuj. Zinc.
— rending, tearing, *Anac.* Ars. *Calc.*

Camph. *Cannab.* Canth. Chin. *Coloc.* Dig. Euph. *Guaj. Mang. Merc.* Plat. *Puls.* Sabad. Sass. *Sulph-ac. Thuj.* Zinc.
— shaking, Nux.
— sudden, Berb.
— tensive, Asa-f. Calc. Spig. Staph.
— throbbing, Sabad.
— tingling, Ntr-c.
— when touched, Bry. Nitr-ac.
— upwards, *Bell.* Caust. Cham. Chin.
— in warmth of bed, *Sulph.*
Stomach, derangement of, agg., from, Acon. *Ant.* Ars. *Bry.* Carb-veg. *Coff.* Euph. Ntr-c. *Ip. Nux.* Puls. Staph. Tart.
Stone-cutters, for, *Calc.* Lyc. Puls. *Sil.*
Stool, before the, agg., Ant. Bar-c. Borax. Bry. Caps. Caust. Cham. Dulc. Kali-c. *Merc.* Mez. Op. Phosp. Puls. Rhus. Sabad. Spig. *Verat.*
— during the, agg., Ant. *Ars.* Calc. Caps. Carb-veg. *Cham.* Chin. Coloc. Dulc. Ferr. Hep. Ip. *Merc.* Ntr-m. Nitr-ac. Nux. Phosp. *Puls.* Rhus. Sep. Spig. Staph. *Sulph. Verat.*
— after the, agg., Ars. Calc. Canth. Carb-veg. *Caust.* Chin. Kali-c. Lach. Mgn-m. Merc. Mez. Nitr-ac. *Nux. Phosp.* Rheum. *Selen.* Staph. Sulph. Verat.
Stooping, agg., when, (compare Bending down).
— — cough, Arn. Bar-c. Caust. Kali-c. Laur. Lyc. Seneg. Sil. Spong. Staph. Verat.
— amel., when, Cannab. Cocc-c. *Colch.* Con. *Hyosc.* Kali-c. Ran-b. Tart. Viol-tr.
— — diarrhœa, Aloe. Bell. Cast. Chin. Coloc. Cop. Iris. Lach. Petr. Pod. Rheum. Rhus. Sulph.
Stories, exciting, agg., from, Calc. Teucr.
Strangers, among, agg., Sep. Stram.
Stretching of limbs, Acon. *Alum.* Ang. *Bell.* Calc. Cham. *Cina.* Igt. Ip.
— and extending, *Alum.* Amm-c. Bell. Bruc. Bry. Calc. Canth. Caust. Graph. Guaj. Led. Meph. Mez. Mur-ac. Ntr-s. Nux. Oleand. Ol-an. Petr. Plat. Puls. Ruta. Sabad. Sec-c Seneg. Sep. Spong. Staph. *Sulph.* Tart-ac. Verb.
— agg., from, Amm-c. *Ran-b.* Rhus.
— and twisting, amel., from, Guaj.
— the limb, agg., from, Alum. Ant. Bry. *Calc.* Chin. Hep. Mang. Ruta. *Sep. Sulph.* Thuj.
— — amel., from, *Rhus. Sec-c.* Tart.
— colic, agg., of, Bell.
— pain in stomach, agg., of, Nitr-ac.
Stunning pain, Calc. Cina. Mez. *Oleand.* Puls. Rheum. *Sabad.* Verat. *Verb.*
Sucking the gums, agg., from, Nux-m. Sil.
Sulphur, from abuse of, Chin. *Merc.* Nux. *Puls.* Sep. Sil. Thuj.

34. GENERALITIES.

Sulphur vapors, abuse of, Puls.
Summer, in, agg.. Bell. Bry. Carb-veg. Kali-b. Kalm. Ntr-c. Ntr-m. Puls.
Sun, in the, ag. . Agar. *Ant cr.* Bell. Bry. Camph. Eu ,n. Glon. Hyosc. Lach. *Ntr-c.* Puls. Selen. Therid. Valer.
Sun-light, in th.., agg., Acon. Agar. Ant. Bell. *Calc.* Camph. Chin. *Con.* Euphr Glon. *Graph.* Igt. Ntr-c. Phosp-ac. Sulph.
— amel., Plat. Stram. Stront.
Sunrise, after, agg., Cham. Nux.
Sunset, after, agg., Puls.
Supporting the body, difficulty in, Arn. Asar. Cic. Cocc. Kali-c. Ntr-m. Nux. Sil. Staph. Tar. *V rat.*
Suppurating, pain as if, Bry. Cycl. *Phosp. Puls. Kan-o.*
Swallowing, agg , when, Bar-c. *Bry.* Cocc. Croc. *Hep.* Merc. Nitr-ac. Nux. Petr. Phosp. Phyt. Puls. Rhus. Sep. Sulph. Thuj.
— amel., from, Ambr. Arn. Caps. *Igt.* Kali-b. Lach. Led. Spong.
— fluids, agg., when, Apis. *Bell.* Canth. Iod. Merc. *Phosp.*
— food, agg., when, Bar-c. Bry. Dros. *Hep.* Nitr-ac. Nux. Petr. Phosp. Rhus. Sep. *Sulph.*
— saliva, agg , when, Bry. *Cocc.* Hep. Lach. Merc Puls. Rhus.
Swallowed, after having, the food, agg.. Ambr. Bry. *Nux.* Phosp. Puls. Rhus. Sulph. Zinc.
Swelling, Acon. Amm-c. Arn. Ant. *Ars.* Asa-f. Bar-c *Bell.* Bov. *Bry.* Calc. Canth Caust. Cham. Chin. Dulc Hep. Kali-c. Led. Lyc. *Merc.* Merc-cor. Ntr-c Nitr-ac. *Nux.* Phosp. Phosp-ac. Plb. *Pu s.* Rhus Sal in Samb. Sep. Si. S,ig. Stann. Stram. Sulph. Thuj
— of affected parts, *Bell.* Bry. Calc. Canth. Caust. Hep. *Kali-c.* Lyc. *Merc.* Ntr-m. Nitr-ac. Phosp. *Puls. Rhus.* Samb. *Sep.* Sil. Spong. *Sulph.*
— aching, Merc.
— arthritic, Acon. *Ant.* Arn. Ars. Asa-f. Bell. Bry. Chin. Cocc. *Colch.* Creos Hep. Kali-c. *Led. Lyc.* Mang. *Merc* Ntr-m. *Puls. Rhus.* Sabin. *Sulph.* Thuj.
— black, Arn. Ars. Bell. Dig. Lach. Merc. Op. Puls. Verat.
— bleeding, Nux. Sulph.
— blue black, Ars. Bell. Carb-veg. Dig Lach. Merc. Op. Puls. Verat.
— blue-red, Arn. Ars. Bell. Cham Kali-c. Lach. Sil.
— burning, Ars. Carb-veg. Caust. Lyc Phosp. Puls. *Rhus.* Sulph.
— cold, Ars. *Asa-f.* Bell. Calc. Cocc. Con Dulc. Merc. Rhod. Spig.
— after a cold, Mang.
— contusion, after a, Arn. Con.

— cystic tumors, *Calc.* Graph. Hep. *Sil.* Sulph.
— dropsical, Ant. Apis. *Ars. Aur.* Bell. Bry. *Chin.* Colch. *Con.* Dig. *Dulc.* Ferr. *Hell. Iod.* Kali-c. Led. *Lyc.* Merc. Mur-ac. Nitr. Op. Plb. Prun. Puls. Sabin. Samb. Scill. *Seneg.* Sep. *Sulph.* Tereb.
— — with asthmatic complaints, Lact.
— — elastic, Ars. Dig.
— — sudden, Hell. Nitr.
— in the evening, Cocc. Phosp.
— exuding, Lyc.
— hard, *Arn. Ars.* Bry. Chin. Graph. Lach. *Led.* Phosp. Puls. Rhus. Sep. Sulph. Tabac. Thuj.
— hot, *Ant.* Arn. Asa-f. Borax. Bry. Canth. Cocc. Hep. Led. Merc. Petr. Puls. Rhus. *Sulph.*
— humid, Sulph.
— indolent, painless, Ars. Cocc. Merc. Rhus.
— inflammatory, *Acon.* Agn. Ant. *Arn.* Asa-f. *Aur. Bell.* Bry. *Calc. Canth.* Carb-an. Cocc. Colch. Dulc. Euph. *Kali-c.* Lyc. Mang. *Merc.* Ntr-m. Nitr-ac. *Puls. Rhus.* Seneg. *Sep.* Sil. *Sulph. Thuj.*
— lymphatic, Berb. Carb-veg. Hep. Sep. Sil.
— at night, Dig Phosp.
— in nodes, Alum.
— painful, Aloe. Amm-c. Arn. Ars. Bell. Caust. Cham. Chin. Con. Daph. Ferr. Hep. Lach. Led. Lyc. Merc. Merc-cor. Nitr-ac. Nux. Phosp. Phosp-ac. Puls. Rhus. Sep. Sil. Sulph. Thuj.
— pale, Arn. Bov. *Bry.* Iod. Lach. Lyc. Rhus. *Sulph.*
— of parts maimed, Plb.
— red, Ant. Apis *Arn.* Asa-f. *Aur. Bell. Bry.* Canth. Chin. Hep. Mang. *Merc. Puls. Rhus. Sabin.* Sep. Sulph. Thuj.
— red, spotted, Sep.
— rending, tearing painful, Ars. Led.
— scarlet colored, Bell.
— shining, Arn. Ars. Bell. Bry. Mang. Merc. Rhus. Sabin. Sulph.
— soft, Ars. Lach. Sil.
— sore, painful, Borax. Graph. Hep. Rhus. Sil.
— stinging, Acon. Ant. Apis. Bry. Caust. Cocc. Ferr. Graph. Mang. *Puls. Rhus.* Sep. Sulph. Thuj.
— steatoma, Ant. Bar-c. Sabin.
— suppurating, *Calc.* Graph. Hep. Mang. *Sil. Staph.* Sulph.
— tense, Ant *Bell.* Bry. Dig. Led. *Rhus. Sulph.* Thuj.
— throbbing, Sulph.
— white, Ant. Ars. Bry. Calc. Euph. Graph. Iod. Lyc. Merc. Puls. Rhus. Sabin. Sep. Sulph.

34. GENERALITIES.

Swelling, white of whole body, Dig.
— yellow, Canth.
— sensation of, Bell. Berb. Bism. Bry. Caps. Guaj. Kali-b. Laur. Par. Puls. Rhus. Spig.
Sycosis, Cham. Cinnab. Euph. Lyc. Nitr-ac. Nux. Phosp. Phosp-ac. Psor. Sabin. Staph. Thuj.
Syphilis, Asa-f. Aur. Fluor-ac. Hep Jac-cor. Kali-b. Lac-can. Merc. Mez Nitr-ac. Phyt. Sass.
Tabes dorsalis, Nux-m. Phosp.
Taking hold of something, agg., from, Anac. Amm-c. Calc. Carb-veg. Caust. Cham. Lyc. Puls. Sil.
Talking, from, agg., Alum. Ambr. Amm-c. Anac. Arn. Ars. Aur. Bell. Bry. Calc. Cannab. Carb-veg. Cham. Chin. Cocc Dros. Dulc. Ferr. Graph. Hep. Iod. Kali-c. Lach. Mgn-c. Mgn-m. Mang. Mez. Ntr-c. Ntr-m. Nux. Phosp Phosp-ac. Plat. Rhus. Sass. Selen. Sep. Sil. Spig. Stann. Sulph. Verat.
— — amel., Dulc. Eupat. Ferr.
— — unpleasant things, agg., Calc. Teucr.
— — of other people, agg., Amm-c. Ars. Ntr-c. Nux. Sep. Teucr. Verat
Tea, from abuse of, Chin. Ferr. Selen. Thuj.
Teeth, from cleaning the, agg., Staph.
— — pressing together the, agg., Amm-c Guaj. Hep. Ip. Rhus. Sep. Verb.
Temperature, on changing the, agg., Ars. Carb-veg. Puls. Ran-b. Sabin. Verb.
Tenesmus, pain like, Arn. Ars. Bell. Calc. Caps. Cham. Colch. Euph. Laur. Merc. Mez. Nux. Phosp. Plat. Puls. Rheum. Rhus. Sabad. Spong. Sulph.
Tendinum, subsultus, Ang. Asa-f. Bell. Clem. Coloc. Con. Cupr. Graph. H osc. Iod. Meny. Ntr-c. Plat. Puls. Rhus. Sec-c. Spong. Sulph-ac.
Tendons inflamed, Ant.
Tension, Alum. Arn. Asa-f. Bar-c. Bell Bry. Carb an. Caust. Coloc. Con. Kali-c. Mez. Nux. Oleand. Phosp. Plat. Puls. Rhus. Sabin. Sep. Spig. Spong. Staph. Stront. Sulph. Thuj. Verb. Viol-od. Zinc.
— inner parts, Ars. Asa-f. Bell. Calc. Cannab. Caust. Dulc. Graph. Lyc. Merc. Mosch. Nitr. Nux. Puls. Rheum. Stann. Staph. Stront. Sulph. Tart. Verat.
Tetanus, Ang. Bell. Bry. Camph. Cannab Canth. Cham. Cic. Grat. Hyper. Igt. Ip. Laur. Millef. Mosch. Op. Plat. Rhus. Sec-c. Stram.
— hysterical, Bry. Plat.
— from lukewarm water, swallowed, Ang.
— — noise. Ang.
— — touch, Ang. Bell.
— while vomiting, Camph.
— of upper limbs and trunk, Cannab

Thin persons, for, Ambr. Bry. Chin. Lach. Nitr-ac. Nux. Phosp. Puls. Sulph.
Thinking of the pains, agg., when, Bar-c. Lach. Ox-ac. Phosp. Ran-b.
— — — amel., Camph. Hell.
Thirst with the pains, Acon. Cham. Diad.
Thirstlessness with the pains, Lyc. Puls.
Throbbing pains, Amm-m. Ars. Bry. Calc. Carb-an. Carb-veg. Cham. Hep. Kali-c. Lach. Led. Lyc. Merc. Plat. Puls. Rheum. Sil. Thuj. Zinc.
Thrusting pains, Cannab. Cupr. Plat.
Thunderstorm, during a, agg., Bry. Caust. Lach. Ntr-c. Ntr-m. Nitr-ac. Petr. Phosp. Rhod. Sil. Thuj.
— just before a, agg., Agar. Lach. Ntr-c. Phosp. Rhod. Sil.
Tingling, creeping, on limbs, Acon. Amm-c. Arn. Bell. Caps. Carb-veg. Chin. Cic. Colch. Croc. Euphr. Glon. Igt. Kali-c. Mgn-m. Merc. Ntr-c. Ol-an. Par. Phosp Phosp-ac. Plat. Plb. Puls. Ran-sc. Rhod. Rhus. Sabad. Sec-c. Sep. Sol-nig. Spig. Stram. Sulph. Tabac. Verat.
— — internal parts, Acon. Colch. Plat. Rhus.
— formicating, as from ants, Carb-veg. Mgn-m. Ol-an. Phosp-ac. Plat. Rhod. Sabad. Sec-c. Staph. Zinc.
— when moved, Merc.
— in parts affected, Arn. Rhus.
— — maimed, Rhus.
— stinging, Ntr-c.
Tired easily, Anac. Ars. Calad. Calc. Cupr. Diad. Hydroc-ac. Mgn-c. Murex. Sep.
— feeling in all the limbs, especially when lying on left side, Euph. Merc-jod. Thuj.
Tobacco, agg., from, Ant. Calc. Clem. Cocc. Coloc. Cycl. Euphr. Gels. Hell. Igt. Ip. Lach. Ntr-m. Nux. Par. Petr. Phosp. Puls. Ruta. Sass. Selen. Sep. Sil. Spong. Stann. Staph. Sulph-ac. Tar. Thuj.
— amel., Coloc. Diad. Hep. Merc. Ntr-c. Sep.
Torn out, sensation as of something, Calc. Cocc. Rhus. Sil. Spig.
Torpidity, Bell. Cic. Dros. Hyosc. Led. Plat. Puls. Sec-c. Stram.
— sensation of, Ang. Arg. Asa-f. Cocc. Plat.
Touch, agg., from, Acon. Agar. Agn. Ang. Ant. Arn. Ars. Bad. Bell. Bry. Cannab. Caps. Carb-veg. Cham. Chin. Cina. Cocc. Colch. Coloc. Crocus. Cupr. Dig. Dros. Euph. Hell. Hep. Hyosc. Igt. Led. Lyc. Mgn c. Mgn-m. Mang Merc. Mez. Ntr-c. Ntr-m. Nitr-ac. Nux-m. Nux. Phosp. Phosp-ac. Ran-b. Rhod. Rhus. Sabin. Scill. Sec-c. Sep. Sil. Spig.

34. GENERALITIES.

Staph. Stram. Stront. *Sulph.* Tar. Tart. Verat.
Touch amel., *Asa-f.* Bism. *Calc. Cycl.* Grat. Mang. Meny. *Mur-ac.* Ntr-c. Ol-an. Phosp. Plb. Thuj.
— — pains disappear on touch, but re-appear in another part, Sang.
— but softly, agg., from, *Bell. Chin. Nux.* Phosp. Stann.
Touching, on, anything, agg., Calc. Cannab. Carb-veg. Caust. Cham. Puls.
— — — amel., Spig.
— anything cold, agg , Hep. Ntr-m.
— the hair, agg., Bell. Ferr. Nux. Puls. *Selen.*
Travelling on foot, ailments from, ' Ferr-m.
Trembling, tremor, Agar. Alum. Ambr. Anac. Arn. *Ars.* Bar-m. *Bell.* Berb. Brom. Bry. Calc. Carb-veg. Caust. Chin. *Cic. Cocc.* Con. Croc. Cupr. Euphr. Ferr. Ferr-m. Graph. Hyosc. Hyper. Igt. *Iod.* Kali-c. Lach. Lam. Lyc. Mgn-s. *Merc.* Merc-cor. Ntr-c. Ntr-m. Nicc. Nitr-ac. Nux. Oleand. *Op.* Ox-ac. Petr. *Phosp.* Plat. *Plb.* Puls. Ran-b. *Rhus.* Sabad. Sass. Sec-c. Seneg Sep. Stann. *Stram.* Stront. *Sulph.* Sulph-ac. *Tabac.* Tart. Teucr. *Therid.* Thuj. Verat. Viol-od. *Zinc.*
— inner parts, *Calc.* Caust. Graph. *Iod.* Kali-c. Lyc. Ntr-m. Phosp. Puls. *Rhus* Sabad. Spig. *Staph.* Stront. Sulph-ac. Teucr.
— anxious, Ferr. *Puls.* Samb.
— with coldness and twitching, Op.
— convulsive, Bar-m.
— evening, in, Lyc.
— after slight exertion, Merc. Phosp. Rhus.
— from mental affections, Zinc.
— morning, in, Sil.
— open air, in, Calc. Kali-c. Laur. Plat.
— with the pains, Ntr-c. Plat.
— — palpitation of heart, Benz-ac.
— of part affected, with remitting pains, Bry.
— from piano playing, Ntr-c.
— when at rest, Plat.
— — raising up, Bry.
— from talking, Ambr. Borax.
— when thinking closely, Borax.
— after vexation, with dyspnoea, Ran-b.
— during and after a walk, Kali-c. Laur.
— with weakness, Calc. Caust. Hyper. Kali-b. Ox-ac.
Tremulous sensation, Graph. Samb. Sulph-ac.
— — in evening in bed, Samb.
Tugging, Coloc. Nux. Petr. *Puls.*
Turning, twisting, Igt. Merc. Nux. Plat. Rhus. Sabad. *Sil.*
— while. agg., Amm-m. Bell Bry. Chin. Hep. Ntr-m. Rhus. Selen. Spong. Stann.

— — amel , (compare Bending).
— — part affected, agg., Amm-m. Bell. Bry. *Calc.* Chelid. Chin. Cic. Coff. *Igt.* Kali-c. Lyc. Mgn-c. Ntr-m. Nux. Puls. Rhus. Selen. Sep. Spig. Spong.
— — outwards, agg., Caps. Caust.
— — inwards, agg., Igt. Staph.
— — backwards. agg., Anac. Bar-c. Calc. Con. Igt. Kali-c. Nitr-ac. Plat. Puls. *Sep.* Sulph.
— — backward and forward, agg., Chelid. Coff.
— — forward, Chelid. Coff. Thuj.
— — to the right, agg., Carb an. Spig.
— — sideways, agg., Bell. Calc. Kali-c. Ntr-m.
— — round, agg., Calc. Ip. Kali-c. Par.
— — in bed, agg., Acon. Borax. Bry. Cannab. Caps. Carb-veg. Con. Euph. Ferr. Hep. Lyc. Ntr-m. Nux. *Puls.* Sil. Staph. Sulph.
Twilight, in the, agg., Amm-m. Ars. Calc. *Puls.*
— — amel., Bry. Phosp.
Ulcerous pain, Anac. Amm-c. *Amm-m.* Bry. Caust. Cham. Cic. Creos. Graph. *Igt. Kali-c. Lach. Mang. Merc. Mur-ac. Ntr-m. Puls. Rhus.* Sil. Zinc.
— — inner parts, Amm-c. Bry. Cannab. *Lach.* Merc. Millef. Nux. *Puls.* Rhus.
Uncleanliness, agg., from, *Caps.* Chin. Sulph.
Uncomfortable, Bry. Calc. Camph. Chelid. Creos. Croton. Guaj. Mgn-m. Mang. Petr. Puls. Sulph.
— in the evening, Calc.
— inexpressible, bodily, and mental, Hyosc.
Uncovering the body, agg., from, Ars. Aur. Cic. Clem. Cocc. Colch. Con. *Hep.* Merc. Nux-m. Nux. *Rhus. Samb. Scill. Sil. Stront.*
— — cough, Nux. Sil.
— — amel., Acon. Apis. Borax. Calc. Ferr. Iod. *Lyc.* Spig. Verat.
Undressing, after, agg., *Ars.* Cocc. *Dros.* Mur-ac. *Nux.* Oleand. Plat. Puls. *Rhus.* Spong.
Undulating pains, Anac. Asa-f. Cocc.
Undulation, Graph. Nux. Sep.
Unwieldiness of body, Asa-f. Camph. Canth. Ntr-c. Ntr-m. Rheum. Sep. Stann.
Urinating, before, agg., Arn. *Borax.* Bry. *Coloc.* Creos. Dig. *Nux.* Phosp-ac. *Puls.* Rhus. Sulph. Tart.
— beginning to, agg., Canth. Clem. Merc.
— while, agg., Acon. *Alum.* Calc. *Cannab. Canth.* Clem. Colch. Con. *Hep.* Ip. *Lyc. Merc.* Nitr-ac. Nux. Phosp. *Phosp-ac. Puls.* Sass. Sep. Sil. Sulph. *Thuj.* Verat.
— on stopping, agg., Canth. Sulph.

34. GENERALITIES 315

Urinating, after, agg., Amm-m. Anac Arn.
Bell Bov Calc *Cannab.Canth.*Caps.Chin.
Coloc. Con. Dig. *Hep.* Merc. Ntr-c.
Ntr-m. Nicc. Nux. Par. Puls. Ruta. Sep.
Staph. Sulph. *Thuj* Zinc.
Varices, Ambr. *Arn.* Ars. Berb. Calc.
Carb-veg. *Caust.* Creos. *Ferr.* Graph.
Lach. *Lyc.* Ntr-m. *Puls.* Spig. Sulph.
Tart. Zinc.
— blue, Carb-veg.
— hard, Carb-veg. Ham. Lyc.
— inflamed, Arn. *Ars.* Calc. Creos. Lyc.
Puls. Sil. Spig. Sulph. Zinc.
— itching, Graph.
— painful, Caust. Puls.
— painless of, pregnant women, Millef.
— of pregnant women, *Lyc.* Puls.
— soreness of, Graph.
— stinging, Apis. Graph. Tart.
— suppurating, Ars. Lach. Lyc. Puls. Sil.
Vaulted places, agg., in, (churches, cellars), *Ars.* Bry. Carb-an. *Puls.* Sep. Stram.
Veal, agg., from, Calc. Caust. *Ip. Nitr.* Sep. Zinc.
Veins, small, marbled red, Carb-veg. Caust. Lyc. Plat. Thuj.
— swelling of, Tart.
Vexation, agg., from, *Acon.* Alum. Ars. Bell. *Bry. Cham.* Chin. Cocc. Coff. *Coloc. Igt.* Lyc. Mgn-c. *Ntr-m.* Nux. Op. Petr. Phosp. Phosp-ac. *Plat.* Puls. Ran-b. Sep. *Staph.* Sulph.
Vibration through the body, Amm-c. Arn. Bell. Clem. Meph. Nitr-ac. Oleand. Op. *Sep. Sulph.*
— after lying down, Clem.
— when stepping, Arn.
Vigor, sensation of, Coff. *Op.*
St. Vitus' dance, chorea, Actea-r. *Agar.* Apis. Ars. Asa-f. *Bell.* Bry. Calc.Caust. *Cham.* Chin. Cic. Coff. Con. *Croc. Cupr.* Dulc. *Hyosc.* Igt. Iod. Ip. Kali-c. Laur. Merc. *Mez.* Ntr-m. Nux. *Op.* Plat. Puls. Rhus. Sabin. Sec-c. *Sep.* Sil. Stann. *Stram.* Stront. Sulph. Tanec. Tarantula. Verat-viridi.
Voluptuous pains, Lach.
Vomiting, agg., from, *Ars.* Asar. Bry. Calc. Colch. *Cupr.* Dros. *Ip.* Lyc. Nux. Phosp. Plb. *Puls.* Sass. Sep. *Sulph.* Verat.
— after, amel., Dig. Hipp. Sang. Sec-c.
Waking during the night, agg., Cocc. Colch. *Nux.* Selen.
Walk, to, is learned with difficulty by children, Bell. *Calc.* Nux. Sil. Sulph.
Walking awkward, Sabad. Sil.
— bent, Mez. *Sulph.* Tereb.
— difficult, Chin. Oleand. Tereb.
— slow, Tereb.
— staggering, (compare Staggering.)

Walking, unsteady, Caust. Gels. Glon. Mgn-c. Ntr-c. Ol-an. Phosp. Sulph.
— when feet turn inwards, Cic.
— — drags the feet, Nux.
— wavering from weakness of thighs, Mur-ac.
Walk, when beginning to, agg., Bry. *Caps.* Carb-veg. Caust. *Con. Euph. Ferr. Lyc.* Phosp. *Puls.* Rhus. Ruta. Sabad. Samb. Sil. Thuj.
— while, agg., Agn. Arg. *Arn.* Asar. *Bell.* Bry. Calad. *Calc.* Camph. Cannab. Carb-an. *Carb-veg.* Chelid. Chin. Cina. Cocc. Coff. *Colch.* Con. Cor-r. Croc. Dig. Dros. Graph. Hell. Hep. Iod. Ip. *Led.* Mgn-m. Merc. Ntr-m. Nitr-ac. Nux. Ol-an. Phosp. Ran-b. Rheum. Sabad Sass. Scill. Selen. Sep. Spig. Staph. *Sulph.* Sulph-ac. *Verat.*
— amel., Agar. Aloe.Alum.Ambr.Amm-c. Amm-m. Apis. Ars. *Aur. Caps.Con.Cycl.* Dros. *Dulc. Euph. Ferr.* Graph. Kali-c. Lyc. Mgn-c. Mgn-m. Meny. *Mosch. Mur-ac.* Ntr-c. Phosp-ac. *Plat. Puls.* Rhod. *Rhus. Sabad. Samb.* Sep. Stann. Sulph. *Tar. Valer. Verat.* Verb. Viol-tr.
— in open air, agg., Ambr. Ars. Bell. Bry. Calc. *Camph.* Carb-an. Carb-veg. Caust. Chelid. Chin. *Cocc. Coff.* Colch. *Con.* Croc. Euph. Ferr. Guaj. Hep. Ip. Kali-c. *Led.* Lyc. Merc. Nux-m. *Nux.* Petr. Phosp. *Puls.* Selen. Sil. *Spig.* Stann. *Stram. Sulph.* Sulph-ac. *Verat.*
— — amel., *Alum.* Ambr. Asa-f. Aur. Caps Con. Dulc. Graph. Kali-b. Kali-jod. Lyc. Mgn-c. Mgn m. Mez. *Nux.* Op. *Puls.* Rhus.Sabin. Seneg. Sep. Stann. Tar.
— bent, agg., when, Bry.
— — amel., *Con.* Hyosc. Lyc.Rhus.Viol-tr.
— quickly, agg., when, Ang. Arn. *Ars.* Aur. Bell. Bry. Cannab. Caust. Cupr. Igt. *Iod.* Kali-c. Led. Lyc. Merc. Ntr-m. Nux. Oleand. Rhod. Rhus. Seneg. Sil. Spig. *Sulph.*
— — amel., Igt. *Sep.* Sil.
— along or across a river, agg., Ferr. Sulph.
— on stone pavements, agg., Con.
— in the wind, agg., Asar. *Bell. Nux.* Phosp.
— sideways, agg., Caust.
— after, agg., Ambr. Anac.
Wandering pains, Ant. Arn. Bell. Benz-ac. Daph. Ev. n. Gels. Kali-b. Lac-can. Lact. Mang. Meph. Nux-m. Plb. *Puls.* Rhod. Sacch. Sass. Sulph. Zinc.
Warmth, deficiency of, Alum. Ang. Calc. Caps. Chelid. Con. Euph. Ferr. Hydroc-ac. Ip. Laur. *Led. Lyc. Ntr-m.* Nux. Oleand. Op. Phosp. Sass. *Sep.* Teucr.
— sensation of, Alum. Asar. *Cannab. Coff.*

34. GENERALITIES.

Iod. Laur. Nux-m. Nux. Sabad. Seneg. Sulph-ac. Verat.

Warmth, sensation, transient, Berb. Glon.
— is intolerable, Acon. Apis. Croc. Iod. Puls Sabin. Sec-c. Tilia.
— agg., from, Ambr. Apis. Arg-n. Arn. Ant. Aur. Brom. Bry. Bufo. Calc. Cannab. Dros. Iod. Kali-c. Laur. Led. Lyc. Puls. Sec-c. Seneg. Sep. Thuj.
— — cough, All-cep. Dros. Laur. Puls. Seneg. Verat.
— amel., Acon. Agar. Amm-c. Ars. Aur. Bar-c. Bell. Borax. Camph. Caust. Cic. Cocc. Coloc. Con. Dulc. Hell. Hep. Hyosc. Igt. Kali-b. Kali-c. Lyc. Mgn-c. Mang. Merc. Mosch. Nux-m. Nux. Petr. Phosp. Ran-b. Rhod. Rhus. Sabad. Sil. Stront. Sulph.
— of bed, agg., from, Carb-veg. Caust Cham. Cina. Chin. Clem. Cocc. Dros. Glon. Graph. Hell. Iod. Kali-c. Led. Lyc. Merc. Mur-ac. Nux-m. Phosp-ac. Puls. Sabin. Sec-c. Spong. Sulph. Thuj. Verat.
— — cough, Brom. Led. Merc. Ntr-m. Nux-m. Puls. Tart. Verat.
— — amel., Amm m. Ars. Bar-c. Bry. Caust. Clem. Kali-c. Lyc. Nux. Sabad.
— applied externally, amel., from, Ars. Aur. Cham. Chin. Cic. Clem. Cocc. Colch. Con. Cor-r. Hell. Hep. Nux-m. Nux. Rhod. Rhus. Samb. Scill. Sep. Sil. Stront. Sulph.
— — to head and face, amel., Lach. Rhus. Thuj.

Warm air, agg., in the, Asar. Aur. Brom. Calc. Carb-veg. Colch. Igt. Iod. Lyc. Op. Puls. Selen. Sep. Sulph.
— — cough, Ant. Iod.
— amel., Acon. Agar. Amm-c. Ars. Aur. Bar-c. Bell. Bry. Calc. amph Caps. Carb-veg. Faust. Cocc. Con. Dulc. Hell. Hep. Hyosc. Igt. Kali-c. Lyc. Mang. Merc. Mosch. Nux-m. Nux. Petr. Phosp. Rhod. Rhus. Rumex. Sabad. Sep. Stront. Verat.
— when getting, in the open air, agg., Bry. Dulc. Iod. Lyc. Puls. Sabad. Spig. Tilia.
— stove, near the, amel., Ars. Igt. Nux. Rhus. Stront.

Washing, aversion to, Amm-c. Ant. Bell. Borax. Bry. Calc. Canth. Carb-veg. Cham. Clem. Laur. Mez. Ntr. Puls. Rhus. Sass. Sep. Spig. Staph. Stront. Sus. inc.
— and working in water, agg., from, Amm-c. Ambr. Ant. B ll. Calc. Canth. Carb-veg. Cham. Chin. Clem. Diad.. Elaps. Kobalt. Lyc. Merc. Mez. Nitr-ac. Nitr. Nux-m. Puls. Rhus. Sass. Sep. Spig. Stann. Str nt. Sulph.
— — cough, Ant. Calc. Zinc.

Washing and water bathing, Ant.
— — twitches from cold, Rhus.
— — amel., Amm-m. Asar. Caust. Chelid. Euph. P-L. Spig.
— — lukewarm, in, agg., Ang.
— — the face, amel., Asar.

Watery eyes, with, pains accompanied, Sabad.

Weakness, debility, langor, lassitude, Agar Alum. Ambr. Amm-c. Amm-m. Anac. Arg-n. Ars. Bar-c. Bell. Benz-ac. Berb. Bism. Borax. Bov. Brom. Bruc. Bry. Cact. Calc. Camph. Cannab. Canth. Carb-veg Caust. Cham. Chin. Cinnab. Clem. Cocc. Colch. Con. Croc. Cupr. Diad. Dig. Dulc. Ferr. Ferr-m. Hyosc. Igt. Iod. Ip. Iris. Jatr. Kali-b. Kali-c. Lach. Laur. Lept. Lyc. Mgn-c. Mgn-m. Merc. Mez Mosch. Mur-ac Ntr-c. Ntr-m. Nitr-ac. Nitr Nux-m. Nux. Oleand. Ol-an. Petr. Phosp. Phosp-ac. Plat. Pod. Psor Puls. Ran-b. Raph. Rheum. Rhod. Rumex. Rhus. Ruta. Sang. S.c-c. Seneg. Sep. Spig. Stann. Sulph. Sulph-ac. Tabac. Tar. Thea. Therid. Thuj. Valer. Verat. Zinc.
— as if from abdomen rising, Ferr-m. Mgn-m.
— — chest, Seneg.
— he had worked hard, Apis.
— the marrow of the bone was stiff, Ang.
— as of approaching death, Oleand.
— when ascending steps, Anac.
— with aversion to occupation and indifference, Rumex.
— when awaking in the morning, Ambr. Ant. Bry. Chelid. Con. Lact. Lyc. Nux. Phosp. Sep. Zinc.
— in bed, Ambr. Carb-veg. Con. Ntr-m. Phosp.
— benumbing, Phosp-ac.
— after breakfast, Brom. Dig. Nux.
— in children, Bar-c. Bell. Calc. Lach. Lyc. Nux. Sil. Sulph.
— chronic, Ars. Chin. Cupr. Hep. Ntr-c. Nitr-ac. Phosp-ac. Verat.
— after delivery, Kali-c.
— with the complaints, Ars. Cham. Ip. Sec-c. Verat.
— in the evening, Amm-c. Asar. Caust. Cycl. Nicc. Petr. Stront. Tabac.
— 3 to 5 P. M., Clem.
— excessive, Ars. Chin. Hyosc. Iod. Jatr. Laur. Ntr-m. Nitr-ac. Oleand. Op. Phosp. Phosp-ac. Plat. Plb. Rhus. Sil. Stann. Stram. Tart. Therid. Verat.
— after slight exercise, Alum. Anac. Berb. Calc. Cannab. Carb-veg. Cocc. Kali-c. Mgn-m. Merc. Nux-m. Petr. Plb. Psor. Sep. Spig. Stann. Staph. Verat.
— — amel., Nitr.

34. GENERALITIES.

Weakness after slight exertion, Anac. Berb. Calc. Carb-veg. Cocc. Ferr. Mgn-c. Nux-m. Petr. Sep. Sulph.
— — relaxation of bodily powers, Ntr-m.
— with pale face, Hipp.
— from loss of animal fluids, Carb-veg. Chin. Hep. Kali-c. Ntr-c. Ntr-m. Nux. Phosp-ac. Psor. Sulph. Verat.
— in forenoon, Sabad.
— hysteric, Ars. Cham. Ign. Mosch. Ntr-m. Nux. Phosp. Sep. Sulph.
— in lying, agg., Alum. Carb-veg. Croc. Cycl. Ntr-c. Ntr-m. Nitr-ac. Nux. Petr. Puls.
— — amel., Ars.
— in the morning, Ambr. Bry. Calc. Carb-an. Carb-veg. Chelid. Con. Croc. Dig. Lach. Lyc. Ntr-c. Ntr-m. Nitr-ac. Ntr. Nux. Petr. Phosp. Puls. Staph. Stront.
— nervous, Ars. Asar. Bar-c. Bell. Calc. Chin. Cocc. Con. Dig. Hep. Ign. Iod. Laur. Merc. Ntr-c. Nux. Phosp. Phosp-ac. Plat. Puls. Sil. Stann. Sulph. Teucr.
— at night, Ambr. Ant. Creos.
— noon, Carb-veg. Teucr.
— in old age, Ambr. Aur. Bar-c. Con. Op. Phosp. Sec-c.
— in the open air, Ambr. Amm-c. Bry. Calc. Coff. Coloc. Con. Ferr. Kali-c. Mgn-c. Nux. Plat. Sang. Spig. Verat.
— painful, Tabac.
— without pain, must groan, Graph.
— after the pains, Carb-veg.
— of parts affected, Arn. Cham. Chin.
— with palpitation of heart, Sang.
— perspiration, Dig.
— as if paralyzed, disabling, Amm-c. Anac. Caust. Cham. Chin. Colch. Euph. Oleand. Phosp. Phosp-ac. Puls. Rhod. Rhus. Tabac. Verat.
— by rest, agg. Lyc. Mosch. Plat.
— — amel., Ars. Staph.
— from riding in a carriage, Cocc. Petr. Sep.
— in sitting, Mgn-c. Ntr-m. Nitr. Plb. Ruta.
— with sleepiness, Merc-sulph. Mez. Nitr-ac.
— sudden, Acon. Ars. Camph. Carb-veg. Cham. Con. Dig. Graph. Ip. Lach. Laur. Nux. Phosp. Ran-b. Sec-c. Verat.
— — as soon as an eruption comes out, Ars.
— from talking, Alum. Ambr. Amm-c. Calc. Cannab. Ferr. Iod. Ntr-m. Stann. Sulph.
— — — of people, Alum. Amm-c. Ars. Verat.
— during a thunder storm, Caust. Ntr-c. Nitr-ac. Petr. Rhod. Sil.

— from tobacco smoking, Hep.
— with the vomiting, Ars. Ip. Tart. Verat.
— after vomiting, with weak pulse, Aloe.
— from walking, Alum. Anac. Berb. Calc. Carb-an. Carb-veg. Con. Fluor-ac. Hep. Kali-c. Meny. Ntr-c. Ntr-m. Phosp. Phosp-ac. Psor. Sep. Stann. Sulph. Zinc.
— when commencing to walk, Carb-veg.
— by waking, amel., Sulph.
— — in open air, Ambr. Amm-c. Bry. Calc. Coloc Hep. Kali-c. Mgn-c. Nux. Sang. Spig.
— from a short walk, in openair, Alum. Cocc. Kali-c. Ntr-m. Puls.
— from want of sleep, Carb-veg. Cocc. Colch. Glon. Nux. Puls.
— — excessive cold or warm weather, Lach.
— — writing, Cannab. Sil.
Weather changing, agg., Bry. Calc. Colch. Graph. Merc. Mang. Merc. Mosch. Nitr-ac. Nux-m. Nux. Phosp. Phyt. Rhod. Rhus. Sil. Sulph. Verat.
— — cold to warm, agg., Ntr-m.
— excessive heat or cold does not affect much, Fluor-ac.
— — — — does affect, Ip. Lach.
— less chilliness, in cold weather, Meph.
— in clear, fine, agg., Acon. Asar. Bry. Caust. Hep. Nux. Sabad. Spong.
— — foggy, agg., Cham. Chin. Mang. Nux-m. Rhus. Sep.
— — snowy, agg., Calc. Con. Lyc. Phosp. Phosp-ac. Puls. Rhod. Rhus. Sep. Sil. Sulph.
— in wet, agg., Amm-c. Borax. Calc. Carb-veg. Dulc. Lach. Lyc. Mang. Merc. Nux-m. Rhod. Rhus. Ruta. Sep. Stront. Sulph. Verat.
— — amel., Acon. Asar. Caust. Hep. Ip. Nux. Sabad. Spong.
— — and cold, agg., Amm-c. Borax. Calc. Dulc. Nux-m. Rhod. Ruta. Thuj.
— — windy, stormy, agg., Cham. Chin. Lach. Mur-ac. Nux-m. Nux. Phosp. Puls. Rhod.
— dry, (compare Dry).
Weeping, from, agg., Arn. Bell. Croc. Cupr. Hep. Stann. Teucr. Verat.
Wet, from getting, agg., All-cep. Bell. Bry. Calc. Colch. Daph. Dulc. Hep. Ip. Lyc. Nux-m. Puls. Rhus. Sass. Sep. Sil. Sulph.
— — cough, Calc. Dulc. Lach. Nitr-ac. Rhus. Sep.
— — while perspiring, agg., Acon. Dulc. Rhus. Sep.
— — the feet, agg., All-cep. Puls. Sep. Sil.
— — — head, agg., Bell. Puls.

34. GENERALITIES.

Wetting the affected parts, amel., Acon. Amm-m. *Asar*. Euphr. Fluor-ac. *Puls*. Spig.
— — agg., Sil.
White, red parts becoming, Borax. *Hell. Merc.* Nitr-ac. Nux. Staph. Sulph.
Wind, in the, agg., Ars. Aur. Bell. Carb-veg. Cham. Chin. Con. Euphr. Graph. Lach. *Lyc. Nux. Phosp.* Plat. Puls. Sulph. Thuj.
— — cough, Cham. Euph. Lyc. Stram.
— east, agg., Asar. Carb-veg. Caust. *Hep.* Nux. *Spong.*
— north, agg., Asar. Caust. Hep. Nux. *Spong.*
— — cough, Acon. Cham. Cupr. Hep. Samb. Spong.
— south, Euphr.
Wine, from, agg., Ant. Arn. *Ars.* Bell. Cact. *Calc.* Carb-an. *Carb-veg. Coff.* Con. Lach. *Lyc.* Ntr-c. Ntr-m. Nux-m. *Nux. Op.* Ox-ac. Petr. Puls. *Ran-b.* Rhod. Sabad. Selen. *Sil.* Stront. Thuj Zinc.
— — containing lead, agg., Bell. Op. Sulph.
— sour, agg, Ant. Ars.
— sulphurated, Merc. *Puls.*
— amel., Acon. Con. Op.
Winter, in, agg, Acon. Amm-c. Apis. Ars. *Aur.* Bry. Camph. Caust. Dulc. Hell. Hep. Kali-c. Mosch. Nux-m. Nux. Petr. Puls. *Rhus.* Sabad. Sep. Stront. Sulph. Verat.
Women, for, *Bell.* Bry. Calc. Caps. *Cham*,

Chin. Cic. Cocc. Con. Croc. Hyosc. Ign. Mang. Millef. *Nux-m. Plat. Puls.* Rhus. Sabin. Sec-c. Selen. *Sep. Valer.*
Worms, from, agg., *Calc.* Chin. *Cina.* Graph. Nux. Plat. Sabad. *Sil.* Spig. *Sulph.*
— ascarides, agg., Asar. *Calc.* Chin. *Cina. Ferr. Ign.* Nux. Plat. Scill. Sil. Spig. Spong. *Sulph. Teucr.*
— lumbrici, agg., Acon. Anac. Cham. Cina. Graph. Ntr-m. Ruta. *Sabad.* Sec-c. *Sil. Spig. Sulph.*
— tape-worm, agg., Calc. Carb-veg. Graph. Nux. Petr. Phosp. *Plat. Puls. Sabad. Sil. Sulph.*
Wrapping oneself up warmly, agg., from, Acon. Asar. Borax. Calc. Ferr. Iod. *Lyc.* Spig. Verat.
— — — amel., (compare Warmth external).
Writing, while, agg., Asa-f. Bry. *Calc.* Cannab. Cina. Cocc. *Kali-c.* Lyc. *Ntr-m.* Nux. Oleand. Rhod. Ruta. Sabin. Sep. *Sil.* Zinc.
— from amel., Ferr.
Wrong positions, when in, agg., Ars. Bry. Lyc. Tar.
Yawning, agg, from, Arn. Caust. Chelid. Cina. Creos. Graph. *Ign.* Mgn-c. Meny. Mur-ac. *Nux.* Oleand. Phosp. *Rhus.* Sabad. *Sass.* Staph.
— after, agg., Amm-m. Nux.
— — amel., Staph.

LIST OF REMEDIES.

Acetic acid,	Acet-ac.	Bufo,	Bufo.
Aconite,	Acon.	Cactus grand,	Cact.
Actea racemosa,	Actea-r.	Cadmium,	Cad.
Actea spicata,	Actea-s.	Cainca,	Cainca.
Aesculus hippocastanum,	Aesc-hip.	Caladium,	Calad.
Aethusa cynapium,	Aeth.	Calcarea carb.,	Calc.
Agaricus,	Agar.	Calcarea caustica,	Calc-caust.
Agave americana,	Agave americ.	Calcarea oxalata,	Calc-ox.
Agnus castus,	Agn.	Calcarea-phosporica,	Calc-ph.
Ailanthus gland,	Ailanth.	Calendula,	Calend.
Alcohol,	Alc.	Camphor,	Camph.
Aletris farinosa,	Alet.	Cannabis ind,	Cannab-ind.
Allium cepa,	All-cep.	Cannabis sativa,	Cannab.
Alnus rubra,	Alnus.	Cantharis,	Canth.
Aloes,	Aloe.	Capsicum,	Caps.
Alumina,	Alum.	Carbo animalis,	Carb-an.
Ambra grisea,	Ambr.	Carbo vegetabilis,	Carb veg.
Ammon. carb.,	Amm-c.	Cascarilla,	Casc.
Ammon. mur.,	Amm-m.	Castor equorum,	Cast-eq.
Anacardium,	Anac.	Caulophyllum,	Cauloph.
Angustura,	Ang.	Causticum,	Caust.
Angusturia spuria,	Bruc.	Chamomilla,	Cham.
Anthrakokali,	Anthrak.	Chelidoneum majus,	Chel.d.
Antimonium crudum.,	Ant.	Chenopodium,	Chenop.
Apis mel.,	Apis.	China officinalis,	Chin.
Apocynum cannabis,	Apoc.	Chininum sulph,	Chin-sulph.
Argentum,	Arg.	Cicuta virosa,	Cic.
Argentum nitricum,	Arg-n.	Cina,	Cina.
Arnica montana,	Arn.	Cinnabaris,	Cinnab.
Arsenicum,	Ars.	Cinnamomum,	Cinnam.
Artemesia vulgaris,	Artem.	Cistus canad,	Cist.
Arum maculatum,	Arum.	Citric acid,	Citr-ac.
Arum tryph,	Arum-tryph.	Clematis erecta,	Clem.
Asafoetida,	Asa-f.	Cocculus,	Cocc.
Asarum,	Asar.	Coccus cacti,	Cocc-c.
Asparagus officinalis,	Aspar.	Cochlearia armoracia,	Cochlear.
Asterias rubrens,	Aster.	Coffea,	Coff.
Aurum,	Aur.	Colchicum autumale,	Colch.
Badiaga,	Bad.	Collinsonia,	Collin.
Baptisia,	Bapt.	Colocynthus,	Coloc.
Baryta carb.,	Bar-c.	Conium maculatum,	Con.
Baryta mur.,	Bar-m.	Copaivæ,	Cop.
Belladonna,	Bell.	Cornus cir,	Corn-c.
Benzoic ac.,	Benz-ac.	Corallium rubrum,	Cor-r.
Berberis,	Berb.	Creosotum,	Creos.
Bismuth,	Bism.	Crocus sativus,	Croc.
Borax,	Borax.	Crotalus,	Crotal.
Bovista,	Bov.	Croton tigl,	Croton.
Bromine,	Brom.	Cubebs,	Cub.
Bryonia,	Bry.	Cuprum,	Cupr.

REMEDIES.

Cuprum acet,	Cupr-acet.	Lac caninum,	Lac-can.
Cuprum carb,	Cupr-carb.	Lachesis,	Lach.
Cyclamen europ,	Cycl.	Lacernanthes,	Lachn.
Daphne indica,	Daph.	Lamium album,	Lam.
Diadema,	Diad.	Laurocerasus,	Laur.
Dictamnus,	Dict.	Ledum,	Led.
Digitalis,	Dig.	Leptandria	Lept.
Dioscorea villosa,	Diosc.	Linum tigr,	Lil-tigr.
Dolichos,	Dolich.	Lobelia inflata,	Lob.
Doryanthes,	Doryanth.	Lupulus,	Lup.
Drosera,	Dros.	Lycopodium,	Lyc.
Dulcamara,	Dulc.	Magnesia carb,	Mgn-c.
Elaps cor,	Elaps.	Magnesia mur,	Mgn-m.
Elaterium,	Elat.	Magnesia sulph,	Mgn-s.
Erigeron,	Erig.	Manganum,	Mang.
Eugenia,	Eugen.	Menyanthes,	Meny.
Eupatorium perf,	Eupator.	Mephites,	Mph.
Euphorbrium,	Euph.	Mercurius,	Merc.
Euphrasia,	Euphr.	Mercurius cor,	Merc-cor.
Evonymus,	Evon.	Mercurius jod,	Merc-jod.
Ferrum,	Ferr.	Mercurius sulph,	Merc sulph.
Ferrum magn.,	Ferr-m.	Mercurial perennis,	Mercurial.
Filix mas.,	Filix.	Mezereum,	Mez.
Fluoric acid,	Fluor-ac.	Millefolium,	M.l.ef.
Formica,	Formica.	Morphium,	Morph.
Fragaria vesca,	Frag.	Moschus,	Mosch.
Gelsimium,	Gels.	Murex,	Murex.
Ginsing	Gins.	Muriatic acid,	Mur-ac.
Glonoine,	Glon.	Natrum carb,	Ntr-c.
Gossypium,	Gossyp.	Natrum mur,	Ntr-m.
Graphites,	Graph.	Natrum nitr,	Ntr-nitr.
Gratiola,	Grat.	Natrum sulph,	Ntr-s.
Gnaphel,	Gnaphel.	Niccolum,	Nicc.
Grajacum,	Guaj	Nigella,	Nig.
Gummi gutti,	Gum-gut.	Nitric acid,	Nitr-ac.
Gymnoclades,	Gymnoc.	Nitrum,	Nitr.
Hamamelis,	Ham.	Nux jugulans.	Nux jug.
Hœmatoxylum,	Hœmatox.	Nux moschata,	Nux-m.
Helleborus,	Hell.	Nux vomica,	Nux.
Helonias,	Helon.	Ocimum canum,	Ocim.
Hepar sulph. calc.	Hep.	Oleander,	O'cand.
Hydrastis,	Hydrast.	Oleum animule,	Ol-an.
Hydrocyanic acid,	Hydroc-ac.	Opium,	Op.
Hydrophobin,	Hydroph.	Osmium,	Osm.
Hyosciamus,	Hyosc.	Oxalic acid,	Ox ac.
Hypericum,	Hyperic.	Palladium,	Pal'ad.
Ignatia amara,	Ig.	Pæonia.	Pœon.
Indigo,	Ind.	Paris quad,	Par.
Ipecacuanha,	Ip.	Petroleum,	Petr.
Iris versicolo,	Iris.	Petroselinum,	Petros.
Jacaranda caroba,	Jac-cor.	Phosphorus,	Phosp.
Jalapa,	Jalap.	Phosphoric acid,	Phosp-ac.
Jatrophn curcas,	Jatr.	Phytolacca dec,	Phyt.
Jodium,	Jod.	Plantago major,	Plant-maj.
Kali bichr,	Kali-b.	Plantago minor,	Plant-min.
Kali carb,	Kali-c.	Platina,	Plat.
Kali-chloric,	Kali-chl.	Plumbum,	Plb.
Kali-ferr-cyn.	Kali ferr-cyc.	Podophyllum,	Pod.
Kali hydr,	Kali-jod.	Pothos foetidus,	Poth.
Kali nitricum,	Kali-nit.	Prunus spinosa,	Prun.
Kalmia,	Kalm.	Psorinum,	Psor.
Kino,	Kino.	Pulsatilla,	Puls.
Kobalt,	**Kobalt.**	**Ranunculus bulb.**	**Ran-b.**

Ranunculus scel,	Ran-sc.	Tanacetum,	Tan.
Raphanus	Raph.	Taraxacum,	Tar.
Rhatania,	Rat.	Tartarus emiticus,	Tart.
Rheum,	Rheum.	Tartaric acid,	Tart-ac.
Rhodendron,	Rhod	Taxus,	Tax.
Rhus radicans,	Rhus-rad.	Tellurium,	Tell.
Rhus tox,	Rhus.	Teplitz.	Teplitz.
Rhus vernix,	Rhus-ver.	Terebinthina,	Tereb.
Rumex crispus,	Rumex.	Thea,	Thea.
Ruta,	Ruta.	Theridion,	Therid.
Sabadilla,	Sabad.	Thlapsi bursa pastoris,	Thlapsi.
Sabina,	Sabin.	Thuja occiden,	Thuj.
Sambucus,	Samb.	Tilia europ,	Tilia.
Sanguinaria,	Sang.	Tongo,	Tong.
Sapo,	Sapo.	Trillium pend,	Trill.
Sassaparilla,	Sass.	Urea,	Urea.
Scilla,	Scill.	Urtica urens,	Urt-ur.
Secale cornutum,	Sec-c.	Uva ursi,	Uva-ursi.
Selenium,	Selen.	Valeriana,	Valer.
Senega,	Seneg.	Veratrum alb.,	Verat.
Senna,	Senna.	Veratrum viridi,	Verat-vir.
Sepia,	Sep.	Verbascum,	Verb.
Silicia,	Sil.	Vinca minor,	Vinc.
Solanum mam,	Sol-m.	Viol oderata,	Viol-od.
Solanum nig,	Sol-nig.	Viol tricolor,	Viol-tr.
Spigilla,	Spig.	Vipra red,	Vipra-red.
Spong a tosta,	Spong.	Vipra torv,	Vipra-torv.
Stannum,	Stann.	Xanthoxyllum,	Xanthox.
Staphysagria,	Staph.	Xiphosara,	Xiph.
Sticta pulmon,	Sticta.	Yuba,	Yuba.
Stramonium,	Stram.	Zanthoxylum,	Zanth-ox.
Strontiana,	Stront.	Zincium,	Zinc.
Sulphur,	Sulph.	Zincum-ox,	Zinc-ox.
Sulphuric acid,	Sulph-ac.	Zingiber,	Zing.
Symphytum,	Symph.	Zizia,	Ziz.
Tabacum,	Tabac.		

ERRATA

P. 15, under Wearisomeness, "Carban." should be "Carb-an."
P. 16, under Weeping, whining, "Br." should be "Bry."
P. 19, under vertigo, when standing, "ycl." should be "Cycl."
P. 39, under Black points, "Gon." should be "Con."
P. 42, Meibomian glands, "ham." should be "Cham."
P. 48, under Looking upwards, "Sabab." should be, "Sabad."
P. 49, under like a leaf or membrane, "Galc." should be "Calc."
P. 51, under Relieved by leaning on head, buzzing, "Kli-c," should be "Kali-c."
P. 57, Ulceration of root visible, should be, Twitching of root visible, "Mez."
P. 60, Eruption in face, "Alum-ambr." should be "Alum." "Ambr."
P. 140, "Agave." "Amsic." should be "Agave americ."
P. 146, under Urine fetid, "Benz-ar." should be "Benz-ac."
P. 156, Boring pain in left ovary, etc., should read, Boring pain in left ovary, worse during menses, "Thuj."
—— —— —— ameliorated during menses, "Zinc."
P. 178, Cough with perspiration, should read "Cimex." instead of "Cinnex."
P. 178, Cough and Sleeplessness, should read, "Ars. Nitr."
P. 230, under Sciatica should read "Plantago-maj."
Sect. 20, in this section glands should be glands.
A few typographical errors in the text are not included in this list.